Handbook of

ANATOMY AND PHYSIOLOGY

for Nurses

(for GNM Students)

Handbook of

ANATOMY AND PHYSIOLOGY

for Nurses
(for GNM Students)

Inderbir Singh

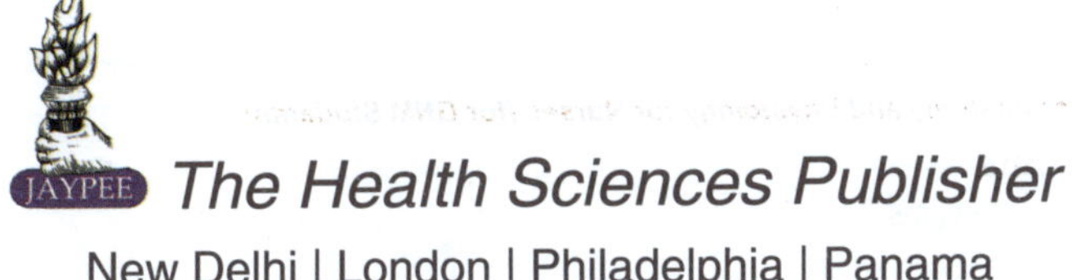

The Health Sciences Publisher

New Delhi | London | Philadelphia | Panama

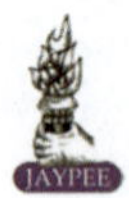

Jaypee Brothers Medical Publishers (P) Ltd

Headquarters
Jaypee Brothers Medical Publishers (P) Ltd
4838/24, Ansari Road, Daryaganj
New Delhi 110 002, India
Phone: +91-11-43574357
Fax: +91-11-43574314
Email: jaypee@jaypeebrothers.com

Overseas Offices

J.P. Medical Ltd
83 Victoria Street, London
SW1H 0HW (UK)
Phone: +44 20 3170 8910
Fax: +44 (0)20 3008 6180
Email: info@jpmedpub.com

Jaypee Medical Inc
The Bourse
111 South Independence Mall East
Suite 835, Philadelphia, PA 19106, USA
Phone: +1 267-519-9789
Email: jpmed.us@gmail.com

Jaypee Brothers Medical Publishers (P) Ltd
Bhotahity, Kathmandu, Nepal
Phone: +977-9741283608
Email: kathmandu@jaypeebrothers.com

Jaypee-Highlights Medical Publishers Inc
City of Knowledge, Bld. 237, Clayton
Panama City, Panama
Phone: +1 507-301-0496
Fax: +1 507-301-0499
Email: cservice@jphmedical.com

Jaypee Brothers Medical Publishers (P) Ltd
17/1-B Babar Road, Block-B, Shaymali
Mohammadpur, Dhaka-1207
Bangladesh
Mobile: +08801912003485
Email: jaypeedhaka@gmail.com

Website: www.jaypeebrothers.com
Website: www.jaypeedigital.com

Inquiries for bulk sales may be solicited at: jaypee@jaypeebrothers.com

Handbook of Anatomy and Physiology for Nurses (for GNM Students)

First Edition: **2015**

ISBN 978-93-5152-590-5

Printed at Sanat Printers, Kundli.

Preface

It is unfortunate that very large number of nursing students are studying the important subjects of Anatomy and Physiology from cheap notes. In this book, all facts about these subjects that a nurse needs to know, are presented in clear, easy-to-understand language.

Further matter that will interest students who want to learn more is presented in the form of color plates illustrating various regions of the body.

This book provides an introduction to common diseases that affect different organs of the body. After studying these descriptions, the nursing student should find it possible to understand most of the terms used by doctors.

Suggestions for improvement of the book will be welcomed.

Inderbir Singh

Text that pertains
MAINLY TO ANATOMY
is printed on
a white background

Text that pertains
MAINLY TO PHYSIOLOGY
is printed on
a light green background

Text that pertains
MAINLY TO CLINICAL ASPECTS
is printed on
a light red background

Contents

PART 1: INTRODUCTION TO THE HUMAN BODY

PART 2: CELLS AND TISSUES OF THE BODY

PART 4: FURTHER LEARNING THROUGH PICTURES

PART ONE

Introduction to the Human Body

CHAPTER
1
Learning the Language of Medicine

THE SUBJECT OF ANATOMY

Anatomy is the science that deals with the structure of the human body. Many features of structure can be seen by naked eye and such a study is called ***gross anatomy*** or ***morphological anatomy***. Many other features can be observed only under a microscope, and a study of these features constitutes the science of ***microscopic anatomy*** or ***histology***. Histology includes the study of details of the structure of cells (***cytology***), and of related chemical considerations (***histochemistry***). Many recent advances in our knowledge of the structure of the body have been made possible by the use of high magnifications available with an electron microscope, and such details are referred to as ***ultrastructure***. The science of anatomy also includes the study of the development of tissues and organs before birth: this is called ***embryology***. Aspects of anatomy that are of particular relevance to understanding of disease and its treatment are referred to as ***applied anatomy*** or ***clinical anatomy***.

MAIN SUBDIVISIONS OF THE HUMAN BODY

For convenience of description the human body is divided into a number of major parts. Many of the parts bear names with which you will be already familiar, but even some of these may require more precise definition.

The uppermost part of the body is the ***head***. The ***face*** is part of the head (and includes the region of the ***forehead***, the ***eyes***, the ***nose***, the ***cheeks*** and the ***chin***). Below the head there is the neck. Below the neck, there is the region that a lay person calls the chest. In anatomical terminology the chest is referred to as the ***thorax***. The thorax is in the form of a bony cage within which the heart and lungs lie. Below the thorax, there is the region commonly referred to as 'stomach' or 'belly'. Its proper name is ***abdomen***. The abdomen contains several organs of vital importance to the body. Traced downwards, the abdomen extends to the hips. A part of the abdomen present in the region of the hips is called the ***pelvis***.

The thorax, the abdomen, the neck and the head together form the ***trunk***. Attached to the trunk there are the upper and lower ***limbs***, or the upper and lower ***extremities***. In relation to the upper limb the terms ***shoulder***, ***elbow***, ***wrist***, ***hand***, ***palm***, ***fingers*** and ***thumb*** will be familiar. A lay person frequently refers to the entire upper limb as the ***arm***, but in anatomy we use this term only for the region between the shoulder and elbow. The region between the elbow and wrist is the ***forearm***. The fingers and thumb are also called ***digits***.

In the lower limbs the terms ***hip***, ***knee***, ***ankle***, ***foot*** and ***toes*** will be familiar. The region between the hip and the knee is the ***thigh***, and that between the knee and the ankle is the ***leg***. Like the fingers, the toes are also called digits. The innermost, and largest toe, is the ***great toe***.

SOME COMMONLY USED DESCRIPTIVE TERMS

A nursing student entering a hospital for the first time is very likely to find that doctors seem to use many strange sounding words. You will become familiar with them over the years. Many of these strange words are really terms used to describe different parts of the body, and they constitute the basis for the study of anatomy and physiology.

The learning of these terms is the basic foundation on which all subsequent studies of the human body depend. In short, the study of anatomy teaches us the language of medicine.

Of all the terms to be learnt the first, and most fundamental, are those used for precise description of the mutual relationships of various structures within the body. In describing such relationships the lay person uses terms like 'in front', 'behind', 'above', 'below' etc. However, in a study of anatomy, such terms are found to be inadequate; and the student's first task is to become familiar with the specialized terms used.

A major problem in describing anatomical relationships is that they keep changing with movement. For example, when a person stands upright the head is the uppermost part of the body and the feet the lowermost. However, on lying down the head and feet are at the same level. The problem is overcome by always describing relationships within the body presuming that the person is standing upright, looking directly forwards, with the arms held by the sides of the body, and with the palms facing forwards. (This posture is referred to as the ***anatomical position***.) We will now consider some descriptive terms one by one.

(1) When structure **A** lies nearer the front of the body as compared to structure **B**, **A** is said to be ***anterior*** to **B** (Fig.1.1).

The opposite of anterior is ***posterior***. In the above example, it follows that **B** is posterior to **A**. Using these terms we can say that the nose is anterior to the ears; and the ears are posterior to the nose.

(2) When structure **C** lies nearer the upper end of the body as compared to structure **D**, **C** is said to be ***superior*** to **D** (Fig. 1.1). The opposite of superior is ***inferior***. In the above example **D** is inferior to **C**. (No difference in the quality of the structures is implied!). Using these terms we can say that the nose is superior to the mouth, but is inferior to the forehead.

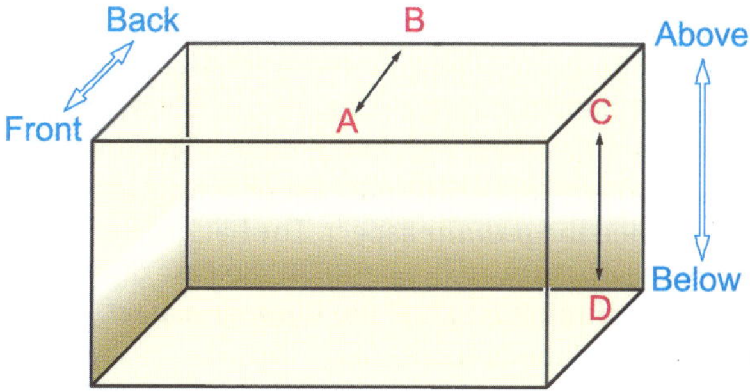

Fig. 1.1 Scheme to explain the terms anterior, posterior, superior, and inferior.

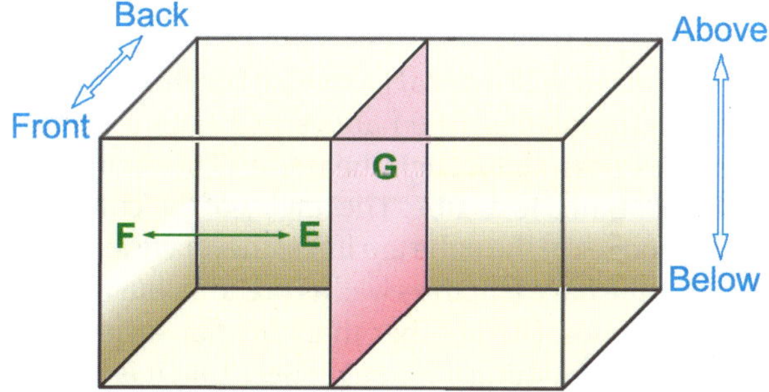

Fig. 1.2 Scheme to explain the terms medial, lateral and median.

(3) The body can be divided into two equal halves, right and left, by a plane passing vertically through it. (A plane is like a sheet of paper. It has length and breadth, but no thickness). The plane separating the right and left halves of the body is called the ***median plane*** (Fig. 1.2). When a structure lies in the median plane it is said to be ***median*** in position (e.g., G in Fig. 1.2). When structure **E** lies nearer the median plane than structure **F**, **E** is said to be ***medial*** to **F**. The opposite of medial is ***lateral***. In the above example **F** is lateral to **E**.

In the anatomical position the palm faces forwards and the thumb lies along the outer side of the hand. Starting from the side of the thumb (or first digit) the fingers are named index finger (second digit), middle finger (third digit), ring finger (fourth digit) and little finger (fifth digit). To describe the medial-lateral relationships of the fingers we can say that the thumb lies lateral to the index finger. The index finger is medial to the thumb, but is lateral to the middle finger.

Various combinations of the descriptive terms mentioned above are frequently used. For example, each eye is anterior to the corresponding ear; and is also medial to it. Therefore, the eye can be said to be ***anteromedial*** to the ear. The tip of the nose is inferior and medial to each eye: we can say the nose is ***inferomedial*** to the eye.

We must now consider terms that are sometimes used as equivalent to some of the terms introduced above. The anterior aspect of the body corresponds to the ventral aspect of the body of four-footed animals. Hence the term ***ventral*** is often used as equivalent to anterior. (However, we shall see later that the two terms are not always equivalent, e.g., in the thigh). The opposite of ventral is ***dorsal***. In the hand the palm is on the anterior or ventral aspect. This aspect of the hand is often called the ***palmar*** aspect. The back of the hand is the dorsal aspect, or simply the ***dorsum***, of the hand. In the case of the foot the surface towards the sole is ventral: it is called the ***plantar aspect***. The upper side of the foot is the ***dorsum*** of the foot.

While referring to structures in the trunk the term ***cranial*** (= towards the head) is sometimes used instead of superior; and ***caudal*** (= towards the tail) in place of inferior. In the limbs the term superior is sometimes replaced by ***proximal*** (= nearer) and inferior by ***distal*** (= more distant). Using this convention the phalanges of the hands are designated proximal, middle and distal. In the case of the forearm (or hand) the medial side is often referred to as the ***ulnar*** side, and the lateral side as the ***radial*** side. Similarly, in the leg (or foot) we can speak of the ***tibial*** (= medial) or ***fibular*** (= lateral) sides.

In addition to the terms described above there are some terms that are used to define planes passing through the body. (The concept of planes can be understood by reference to a cube. The angles of the cube are points: they have no length. The edges of the cube are lines: they have length but no width. The surfaces of the cube have length as well as breadth, but no thickness: these can be regarded as planes. (Remember than any flat surface is also called a plane surface: the essential thing about a plane is that it is absolutely flat).

We have already seen that a plane passing vertically through the midline of the body, so as to divide the body into right and left halves, is called the ***median plane***. It is also called the ***mid-sagittal plane***. Vertical planes to the right or left of the median plane, and parallel to the latter, are called ***paramedian*** or ***sagittal planes*** (Fig. 1.3). A vertical plane placed at right angles to the median plane (dividing the body into anterior and posterior parts) is called a ***coronal plane*** or a ***frontal plane*** (Fig. 1.4). Planes passing horizontally across the body

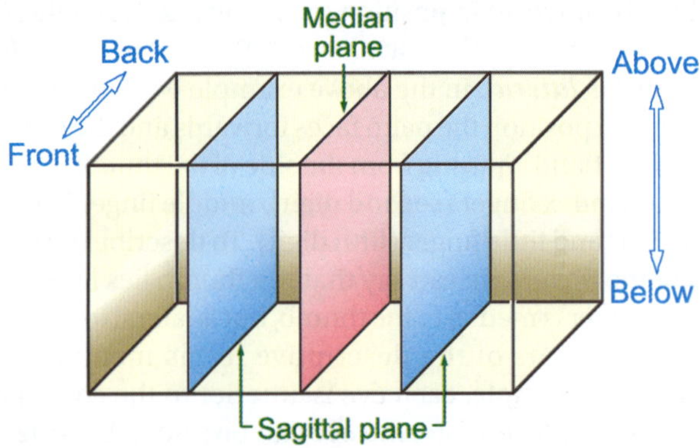

Fig. 1.3 Scheme showing median and sagittal or paramedian planes.

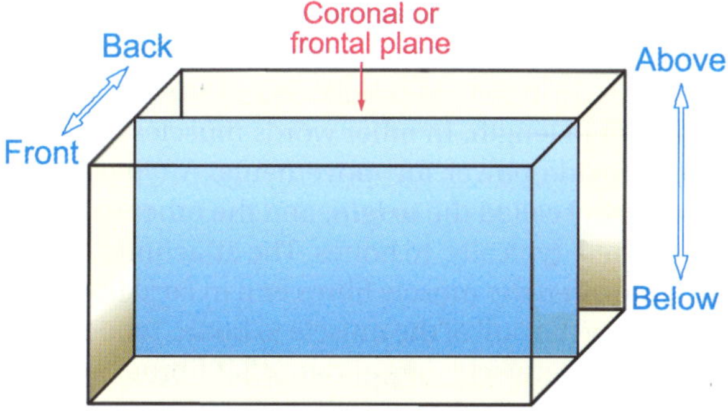

Fig. 1.4 Scheme showing a frontal or coronal plane.

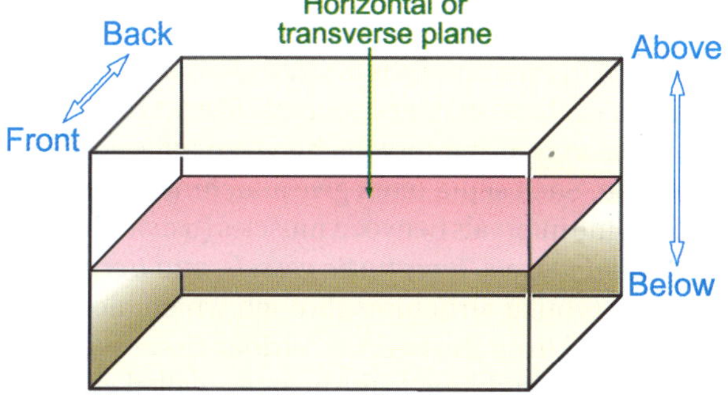

Fig. 1.5 Scheme showing a horizontal or transverse plane.

(i.e., at right angles to both the sagittal and coronal planes) and dividing it into upper and lower parts, are called ***transverse*** or ***horizontal planes*** (Fig. 1.5). In addition there are innumerable oblique planes intermediate between those described above. Sections through any part of the body in any of the planes mentioned above are given corresponding names. Thus we speak of median sections, sagittal sections, coronal or frontal sections, transverse sections and oblique sections.

STRUCTURES CONSTITUTING THE HUMAN BODY

The animal body is made up of various elements. The basic framework of the body is provided by a large number of ***bones*** that collectively form the ***skeleton***. As bones are hard they not only maintain their own shape, but also provide shape to the part of the body within which they lie. In some situations (e.g., the nose or the ear) part of the skeleton is made up, not of bone but of, a firm but flexible tissue called ***cartilage***. Bones meet each other at ***joints***, many of which allow movements to be performed. At joints, bones are united to each other by fibrous bands called ***ligaments***. Overlying (and usually attached to) bones we see ***muscles***. Muscles are what the layman refers to as flesh. In the limbs, muscles form the main bulk. Muscle tissue has the property of being able to shorten in length. In other words muscles can contract, and by contraction they provide power for movements. A typical muscle has two ends one (traditionally) called the ***origin***, and the other called the ***insertion***. Both ends are attached, typically, to bones. The attachment to bone may be a direct one, but quite often the muscle fibres end in cord like structures called ***tendons*** which convey the pull of the muscle to bone. Tendons are very strong structures. Sometimes a muscle may end in a flat fibrous membrane. Such a membrane is called an ***aponeurosis***.

Within a limb we find that the muscles are separated from skin, and from one another, by a tissue in which fibres are prominent. Such tissue is referred to as ***fascia***. Immediately beneath the skin the fibres of the fascia are arranged loosely and this loose tissue is called ***superficial fascia***. Over some parts of the body the superficial fascia may contain considerable amounts of fat. Deep to the superficial fascia the muscles are covered by a much better formed and stronger membrane. This membrane is the ***deep fascia***. In the limbs, and in the neck, the deep fascia encloses deeper structures like a tight sleeve. Membranes similar to deep fascia may also intervene between adjacent muscles forming ***intermuscular septa***. Such septa often give attachment to muscle fibres.

Running through the intervals between muscles (usually in relation to fascial septa) there are ***blood vessels***, ***lymphatic vessels***, and ***nerves***.

Blood vessels are tubular structures through which blood circulates. The vessels that carry blood from the heart to various tissues are called ***arteries***. Those vessels that return this blood to the heart are called ***veins***. Within tissues arteries and veins are connected by plexuses of microscopic vessels called ***capillaries***.

Lymphatic vessels are delicate, thin walled tubes. They are difficult to see. They often run alongside veins. Along the course of these lymphatic vessels small bean shaped structures are present in certain situations. These are ***lymph nodes***. Lymphatic vessels and lymph nodes are part of a system that plays a prominent role in protecting the body in various ways that you will study later.

Running through tissues, often in the company of blood vessels, we have solid cord like structures called ***nerves***. Each nerve is a bundle of a large number of ***nerve fibres***. Each nerve fibre is a process arising from a ***nerve cell*** (or ***neuron***). Most nerve cells are located in the brain and in the spinal cord. Nerves transmit impulses from the brain and spinal cord to various tissues. They also carry information from tissues to the brain. Impulses passing through nerves are responsible for contraction of muscle, and for secretions by glands. Sensations like touch, pain, sight and hearing are all dependent on nerve impulses traveling through nerve fibres.

Bones, muscles, blood vessels, nerves etc., that we have spoken of in the previous paragraphs are to be seen in all parts of the body. In addition to these many parts of the body have specialized ***organs***, also commonly called ***viscera***. Some of the viscera are solid (e.g., the liver, or the kidney), while others are tubular (e.g., the intestines) or sac like (e.g., the stomach). The viscera are grouped together in accordance with function to form various ***organ systems***. Some examples of organ systems are the ***respiratory system*** responsible for providing the body with oxygen; the ***alimentary*** or ***digestive system*** responsible for the digestion and absorption of food; the ***urinary system*** responsible for removal of waste products from the body through urine; and the ***genital system*** which contains organs concerned with reproduction.

CHAPTER

2

A Brief Introduction to Bones, Joints and Muscles of the Body

THE SKELETON

The basic foundation of the body is provided by the skeleton. Any student embarking on a study of anatomy needs to have a general idea of the skeleton as a whole. The purpose of this section is to provide such information.

The human skeleton may be divided into:

a. The ***axial skeleton*** consisting of the bones of the head, neck and trunk; and
b. The ***appendicular skeleton*** consisting of the bones of the limbs.

THE SKULL

The skeleton of the head is called the skull. It is seen from the lateral side in Fig. 2.1 and from above in Fig. 2.2. The skull contains a large ***cranial cavity*** in

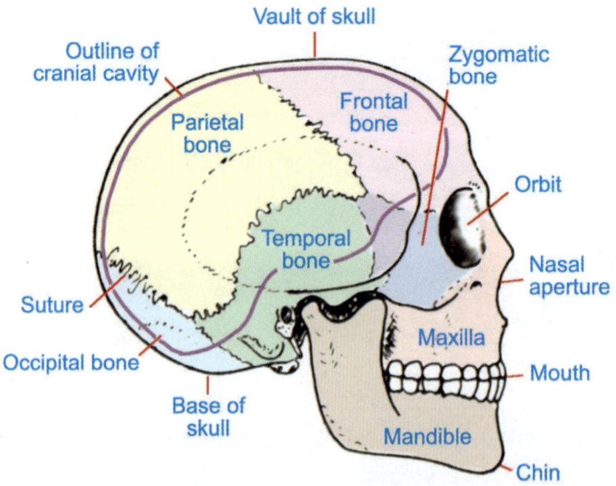

Fig. 2.1 Skull, seen from the right side.

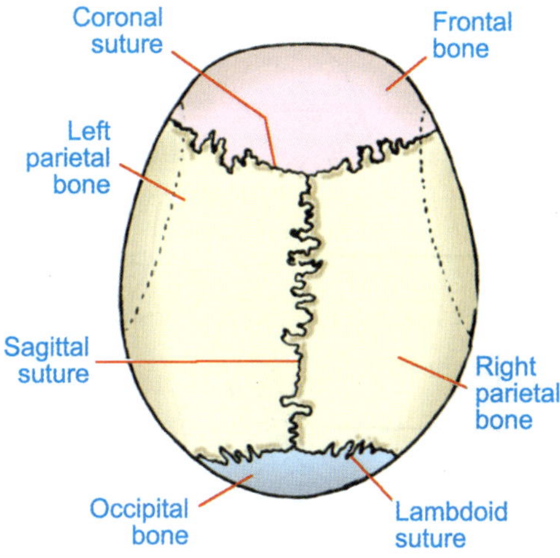

Fig. 2.2 Skull, seen from above.

which the brain is lodged. Just below the forehead the skull shows two large depressions, the right and left ***orbits***, in which the eyes are lodged. In the region of the nose and mouth there are apertures that lead into the interior of the skull.

The skull is made up of a large number of bones that are firmly joined together. Some of these are as follows. In the region of the forehead there is the ***frontal bone***. At the back of the head (also called the ***occiput***) there is the ***occipital bone***. The top of the skull, and parts of its side-walls, are formed mainly by the right and left ***parietal bones***. The region of the head just above the ears is referred to as the ***temple***, and the bone here is the ***temporal bone*** (right or left). The bone that forms the upper jaw, and bears the upper teeth, is the ***maxilla***. The prominence of the cheek is formed by the ***zygomatic bone***. In the floor of the cranial cavity there is an unpaired bone called the ***sphenoid bone***. The bone of the lower jaw is called the ***mandible***. It is separate from the rest of the skull. In addition to these large bones there are several smaller ones.

THE VERTEBRAL COLUMN

Below the skull the central axis of the body is formed by the backbone or ***vertebral column*** (Fig. 2.3). The vertebral column is made up of a large number of bones of irregular shape called ***vertebrae***. There are seven ***cervical vertebrae*** in the neck. Below these there are twelve ***thoracic vertebrae*** that take part in forming the skeleton of the thorax. Still lower down there are five ***lumbar vertebrae*** that lie in the posterior wall of the abdomen. The lowest part of the vertebral column is made up of the ***sacrum***, which consists of five sacral vertebrae that are fused together; and of a small bone called the ***coccyx***. The coccyx is made up of four rudimentary vertebrae fused together. There are thus thirty-three vertebrae in all. Taking the sacrum and coccyx as single bones the vertebral column has twenty-six bones.

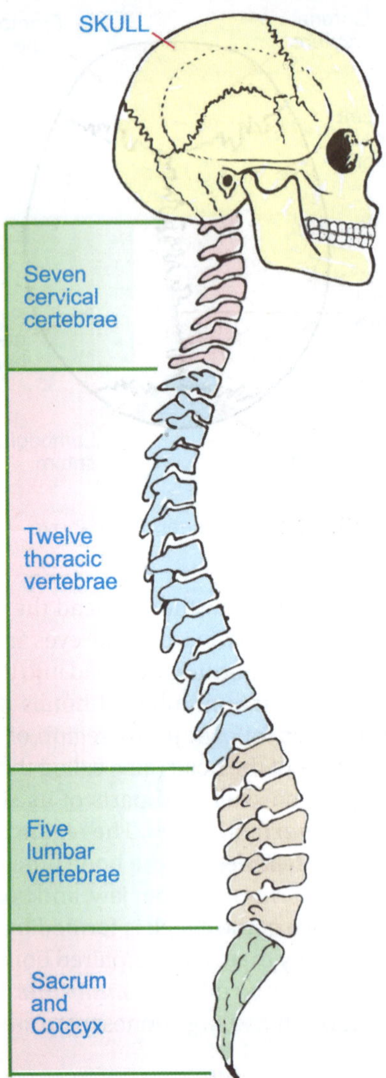

Fig. 2.3 Skull and vertebral column (side view).

Parts of a Typical Vertebra

The parts of a typical vertebra are shown in Fig. 2.4. The anterior part of the vertebra is made up of a solid, cylindrical mass of bone, which is called the ***body***. The bodies of adjoining vertebrae are firmly united to one another, and in this way the vertebral column forms a strong pillar of support to other structures.

Just behind the body of the vertebra we see a rounded ***vertebral foramen***. The foramina of adjoining vertebrae are accurately aligned to one another to form a long ***vertebral canal***. The spinal cord lies in the vertebral canal. At its

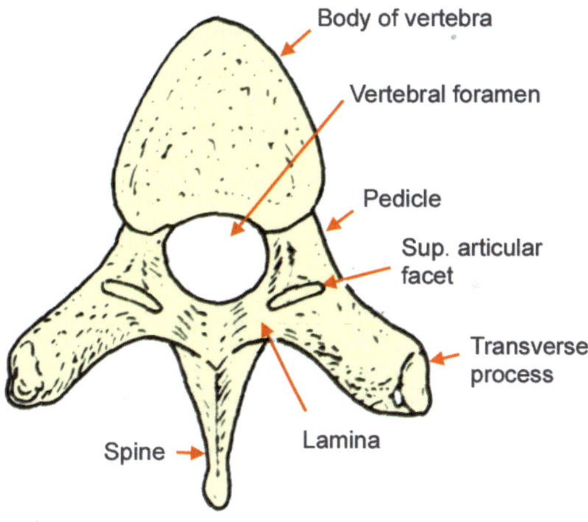

Fig. 2.4 A typical vertebra, seen from above.

upper end the vertebral canal becomes continuous with the cranial cavity, and the spinal cord becomes continuous with the brain.

On either side the vertebral foramen is bounded by right and left ***pedicles***. Posteriorly the foramen closed by the right and left ***laminae***. The laminae meet in the middle line to complete the posterior wall of the vertebral foramen.

Passing backwards and laterally, from the junction of pedicle and lamina, there are right and left ***transverse processes***. Passing backwards from the junction of the right and left laminae there is the ***spine*** (or spinous process) of the vertebra.

The bodies of adjoining vertebrae are joined to each other by a thick plate of fibro-cartilage. This plate is called the ***intervertebral disc***. The central part of the disc is relatively soft and is called the ***nucleus pulposus***. (Also see structure of secondary cartilaginous joint on page 18).

SKELETON OF THE THORAX

The skeleton of the thorax forms a bony cage that protects the heart, the lungs, and some other organs (Fig. 2.5). Behind, it is made up of twelve thoracic vertebrae. In front, it is formed by a bone called the ***sternum***. The sternum consists of an upper part, the ***manubrium***; a middle part, the ***body***; and a lower part, the ***xiphoid process***. The side walls of the thorax are formed by twelve ribs on either side.

Each rib is a long curved bone that is attached posteriorly to the vertebral column. It curves round the sides of the thorax. Its anterior end is attached to a bar of cartilage (the ***costal cartilage***) through which it gains attachment to the sternum. This arrangement is seen typically in the upper seven ribs (***true ribs***). The 8th, 9th and 10th costal cartilages do not reach the sternum, but

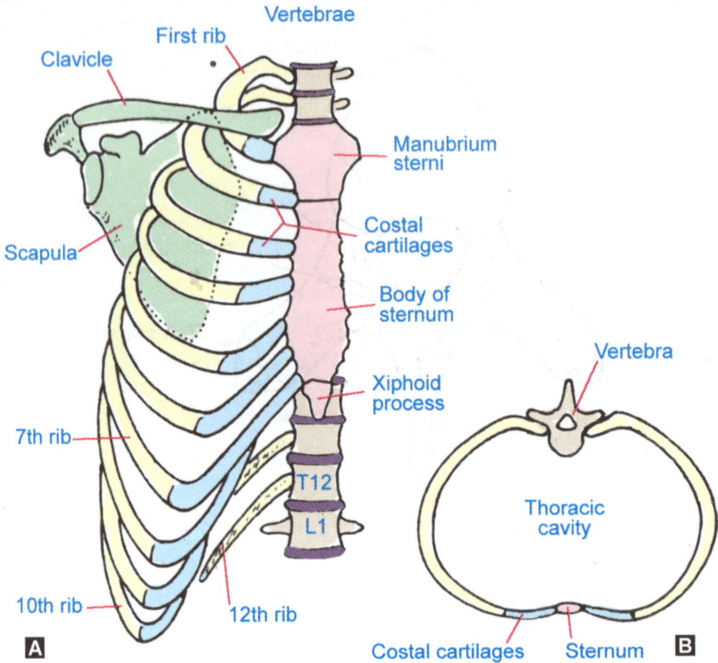

Fig. 2.5 A. Skeleton of the thorax, seen from the front. The bones of the shoulder girdle are also shown. B. Scheme to show how the thorax is formed.

end by getting attached to the next higher cartilage (***false ribs***). The anterior ends of the 11th and 12th ribs are free: they are, therefore, called ***floating ribs***.

SKELETON OF THE UPPER LIMB

The skeleton of each upper limb (Fig. 2.6) consists of the bones of the ***pectoral girdle*** (or ***shoulder girdle***) that lie in close relation to the upper part of the thorax (Fig. 2.5), and those of the ***free limb***.

The pectoral girdle consists of the collar bone or ***clavicle***, and the ***scapula***. The clavicle is a rod like bone placed in front of the upper part of the thorax. Medially, it is attached to the manubrium of the sternum, and laterally to the scapula. The scapula is a triangular plate of bone placed behind the upper part of the thorax.

The bone of the arm is called the ***humerus***. There are two bones in the forearm: the bone that lies laterally (i.e., towards the thumb) is called the ***radius***; and the bone that lies medially (i.e., towards the little finger) is called the ***ulna***. The humerus, radius and ulna are long bones each having a cylindrical middle part called the ***shaft***, and expanded upper and lower ***ends***.

In the wrist there are eight small, roughly cuboidal, ***carpal bones***. The skeleton of the palm is made up of five rod like ***metacarpal bones***, while the skeleton of the fingers (or digits) is made up of the ***phalanges***. There are three phalanges — ***proximal, middle and distal*** — in each digit except the thumb which has only two phalanges (proximal and distal).

The upper end of the humerus is joined to the scapula at the ***shoulder joint***, and its lower end is joined to the upper ends of the radius and ulna to form the ***elbow joint***. The ***wrist joint*** is formed where the lower ends of the radius and ulna meet the carpal bones. The upper and lower ends of the radius and ulna are united to one another at the ***superior*** and ***inferior radioulnar joints***. There are numerous small joints in the hand: the ***intercarpal*** between the carpal bones themselves; the ***carpometacarpal*** between the carpal and metacarpal bones; the ***metacarpo-phalangeal*** between each metacarpal bone and the proximal phalanx; and the ***inter-phalangeal*** joints between the phalanges themselves.

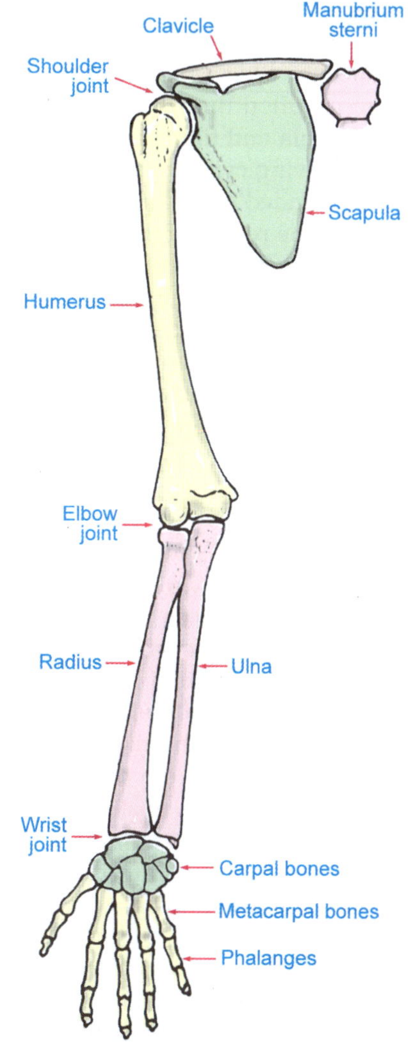

Fig. 2.6 Skeleton of the right upper limb. The manubrium sterni is not a bone of the limb, but is included for orientation.

SKELETON OF THE LOWER LIMB

The skeleton of the lower limb consists of the bones of the ***pelvic girdle***, and those of the ***free limb*** (Fig. 2.7). The pelvic girdle is made up of one ***hip bone*** on either side. Each hip bone is made up of three parts that are fused together. The upper expanded part of the bone is called the ***ilium***. A small part in front (shaded in the figure) is called the ***pubis***. The lower part of the bone is called the ***ischium***. Anteriorly, the two pubic bones meet in the midline to form a joint called the ***pubic symphysis***. Posteriorly, the sacrum is wedged in between the two hip bones. The hip bones and sacrum (along with the coccyx) form the ***bony pelvis***.

The bones of the free part of the limb are arranged in a pattern similar to that in the upper limb. The bone of the thigh is called the ***femur***. There are two bones in the leg. The medial of the two (lying towards the great toe) is called the ***tibia***, while the outer bone is called the ***fibula***. The femur, tibia and fibula are long bones having cylindrical shafts with expanded upper and lower ends. In the region of the ankle, and the posterior part of the foot, there are seven roughly cuboidal ***tarsal bones***. The largest of these is the ***calcaneus,*** which forms the heel. Next in size we have the ***talus***. In the anterior part of the foot there are five ***metatarsal bones***. Each digit (or toe) has three ***phalanges*** — proximal, middle and distal: however, the great toe has only two phalanges — proximal and distal.

The upper end of the femur fits into a deep socket in the hip bone (called the ***acetabulum***) to form the ***hip joint***. The lower end of the femur meets the tibia to form the ***knee joint***. A small bone, the ***patella***, is placed in front of the knee. The tibia and fibula are joined to each other at their upper and lower ends to form the superior and inferior ***tibiofibular joints***. The lower ends of the tibia and fibula join the talus to form the ***ankle joint***. Within the foot there are ***intertarsal, tarsometatarsal, metatarso-phalangeal*** and ***interphalangeal joints*** on a pattern similar to those in the hand.

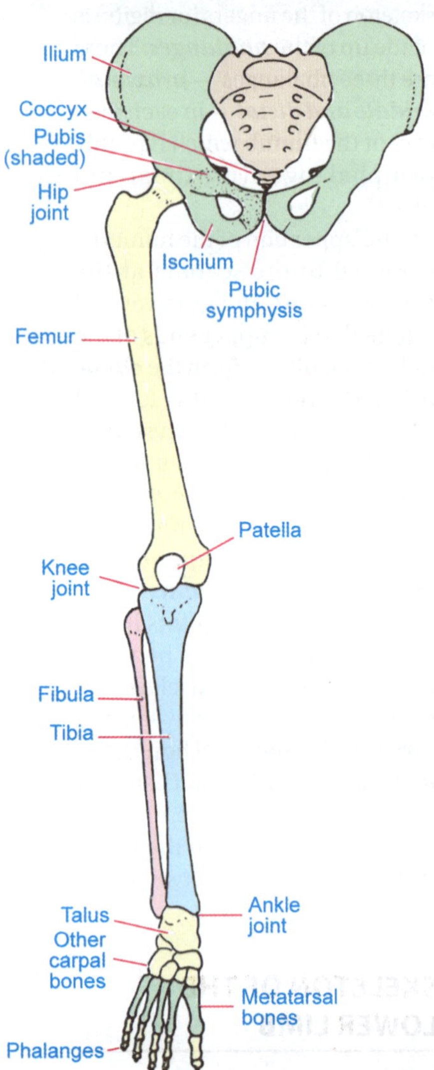

Fig. 2.7 Skeleton of the pelvis and right lower limb.

Variation in Bone Structure

From the brief review of bones of the skeleton, given above, it will be clear that bones come in many sizes and shapes. Some bones are like flat plates (e.g., skull bones). Bones of the carpus and tarsus are solid masses of irregular shape. However, many bones of the body are long bones e.g., humerus or femur, and these share some features in common that are briefly described below.

Some Facts about Long Bones

The greater part of a typical long bone is shaped somewhat like a cylinder. This part is called the ***shaft***. The shaft has a wall of dense bone. Bounded by this wall there is the ***marrow cavity***, containing bone marrow. The two ends of the bone are enlarged. The shape of the enlargement varies from bone to bone. It is adapted for taking part in joints. For example, the upper end of the humerus bears a rounded head that fits into a cavity (glenoid cavity) on the scapula, to form the shoulder joint.

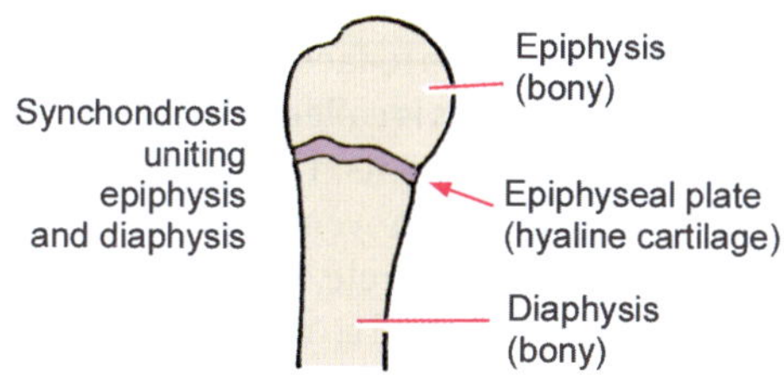

Fig. 2.8 Diagram showing one end of a long bone in a child.

In a growing child, the shaft of the bone (also called the ***diaphysis***) is separated from each bone end by a plate of cartilage (Fig. 2.8). This is the ***epiphyseal plate***. At this stage the bony end is called the ***epiphysis***. The epiphyseal plate unites the epiphysis with the diaphysis. The importance of the epiphyseal plate is that it is the site at which a long bone grows in length. When the bone has attained its full length (generally by the age of eighteen) the epiphyseal plate is replaced by bone. The bone of the epiphysis thus becomes fused with that of the diaphysis.

SOME FEATURES OF JOINTS

We have seen that joints are formed where two (or more) bones meet. Some joints are merely bonds of union between different bones and do not allow movement. Joints of the skull (sutures) belong to this category. Some joints allow slight movement, while some (like the shoulder joint) allow great freedom of movement. In describing movements we use certain terms which the student must understand clearly.

In Chapter 1 we have introduced the concept of planes. Movements at any joint can take place in various planes. Movements taking place in a sagittal plane are referred to as ***flexion*** (= bending), and ***extension*** (= straightening). For example when we bend the upper limb at the elbow joint so that the front of the forearm tends to approach the front of the arm this movement is called flexion. Straightening the limb at the elbow is called extension. Bending the neck forwards is flexion of the neck, and straightening it is extension. Similarly, when we bow, the vertebral column is being flexed, and when the body is made upright the spine is being extended.

Movements in the coronal plane are referred to as ***abduction*** (= taking away) or ***adduction*** (= bringing near). When a limb is moved laterally so that it moves away from the trunk it is said to undergo abduction. For example, such a movement takes place at the shoulder joint when the upper limb is raised sidewards. A similar movement takes place at the hip joint. Adduction and abduction can also take place at the wrist and at metacarpo-phalangeal joints.

Some joints allow ***rotatory movements***. When the forearm is rotated so that the palm comes to face forwards, the movement is called ***supination***. The opposite movement is called ***pronation***. Side to side movements of the neck are also rotatory movements. The movement of the arm performed by a cricketer in bowling is a rotatory movement at the shoulder. Note that during this movement the hand moves in a circle. This movement is, therefore, called ***circumduction***. When the foot is turned so that the sole looks somewhat inwards the movement is called ***inversion***. The opposite movement is called ***eversion***.

CLASSIFICATION OF JOINTS

Joints can be divided into three main types on the basis of structure.

Fibrous Joints

The two bone ends are connected directly by fibrous tissue. Examples of such joints areas follows.

a. Joints between flat bones of the skull (called ***sutures***) (Fig. 2.9).
b. Joints between teeth and jaw (***peg and socket joints***).
c. Joint between lower ends of tibia and fibula (***syndesmosis***) (Fig. 2.10).

Pericranium
-- fibrous layer
-- cellular layer
BONE
BONE
Endocranium
--fibrous layer
--cellular layer
Sutural ligament

Fig. 2.9 Section across a suture between two bones of the skull.

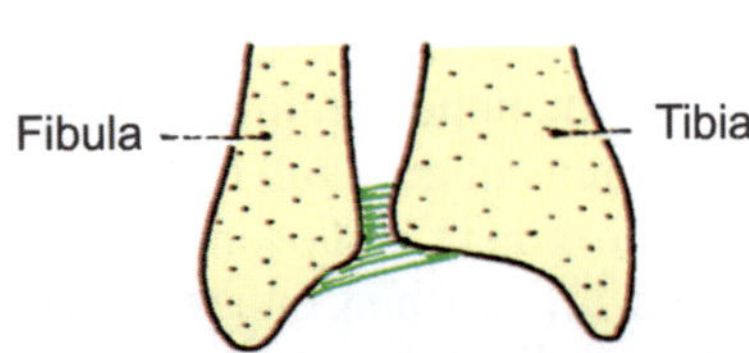

Fig. 2.10 Diagram showing the lower ends of the tibia and fibula united by fibrous tissue. Such a joint is classified as a syndesmosis.

Cartilaginous Joints

The two bones are joined by cartilage. Such joints are of two types.

a. We have seen that in growing individuals the shaft (diaphysis) of a long bone is united to the bone end (epiphysis) by the epiphyseal plate (Fig. 2.8). This plate is made of hyaline cartilage, and this kind of joint is called a ***synchondrosis***. As explained above these joints serve as areas of growth and disappear after growth is completed.
b. Some cartilaginous joints are permanent. These are secondary cartilaginous joints or ***symphyses***. The structure is such a joint is shown in Fig. 2.11. The bone ends forming the joint are covered by a thin layer of hyaline cartilage. The two layers of hyaline cartilage are united by an intervening plate of fibrocartilage.

Examples of this type of joint are the pubic symphysis, and joints between bodies of vertebrae.

Layer of hyaline cartilage covering bone end
Bone end
Bone end
Plate of fibrocartilage

Fig. 2.11 Structure of the pubic symphysis, which is an example of a secondary cartilaginous joint, or symphysis

Synovial Joints

Most of the joints of the body are of this type. The articulating surfaces are not directly connected to each other, by any tissue. They are covered by a layer of hyaline cartilage (called ***articular cartilage***). This makes the surfaces smooth and helps them to glide over each other (Fig. 2.12).

The two bone ends are held together by a ***capsule*** made up of fibrous tissue. The capsule encloses the articular surfaces within a cavity.

The inside of the capsule is lined by a ***synovial membrane*** which secretes synovial fluid. This fluid has a lubricating and nutritive function.

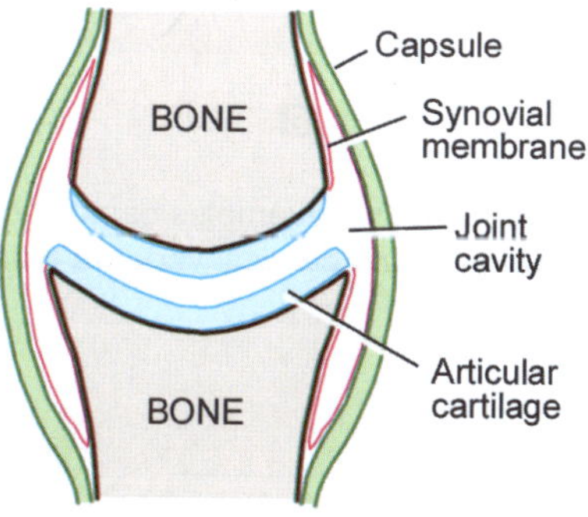

Fig. 2.12 Structure of a typical synovial joint

Synovial joints are of various types as follows.

1. In many small joints the articulating surfaces are flat. These are ***plane joints***.

2. In several joints, a convex articular surface on one bone fits into a concavity on the other (as shown in Fig. 2.12). When the convex surface is rounded (like part of a sphere) and the concave surface is cup-shaped, the joint is said to be of the ***ball and socket*** variety. The shoulder joint and the hip joint are of this type. They allow the maximum movement.

3. In some joints the convex surface is elliptical rather than rounded. These are ***ellipsoid joints***, and the wrist joint is of this type.

4. In some cases one bone end may have two convex surfaces (or condyles) that fit into two cavities on the opposite bone. Such joints are ***condylar joints***. The knee joint is of this type (Fig. 2.13).

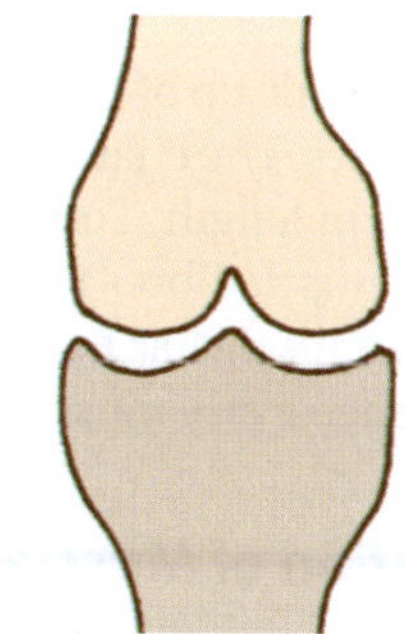

Fig. 2.13 Scheme to show a condylar joint.

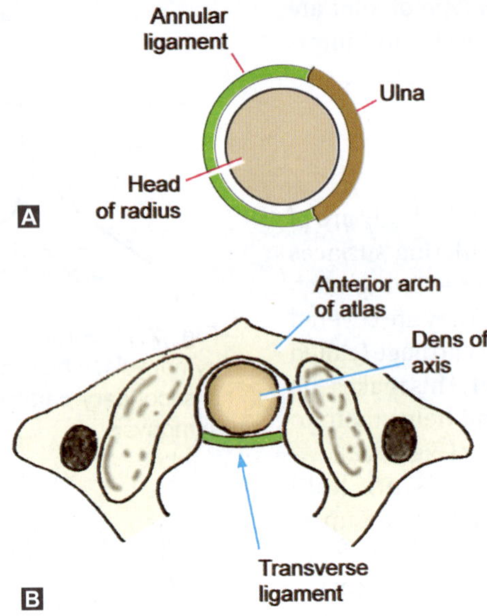

Fig. 2.14 Two examples of pivot joints. A. Superior radioulnar joint. B. Joint between the first cervical vertebra (atlas), and the second cervical vertebra (axis).

5. In a ***pivot joint*** one bone end is rod shaped. It fits into a ring made up partly of bone and partly of a ligament. Two examples are shown in Fig. 2.14.

SOME FACTS ABOUT MUSCLES

Muscles are made up of tissue that a layperson calls flesh. Muscles are made up of muscle fibres. The characteristic feature of a muscle fibre is that can contract and shorten in length. The contraction results in movement. The greater the number of muscle fibres in a muscle the greater its strength. For contraction to begin the muscle has to receive a stimulus. The normal stimulus is through a nerve. Hence every muscle needs a nerve supply.

Organisation of Muscle Fibres in Muscles

Within a muscle, the muscle fibres are arranged in the form of bundles or fasciculi. The number of fasciculi in a muscle, and the number of fibres in each fasciculus, are both highly variable. In small muscles concerned with fine movements (like those of the eyeball, or those of the vocal folds) the fasciculi are delicate and their number small. In large muscles (in which strength of contraction is the main consideration) fasciculi are coarse and numerous.

Muscles differ in the way their fasciculi are arranged. Some muscles (e.g., the sartorius) are strap-like, the fasciculi running the whole length of the muscle. Other muscles are fusiform, the fasciculi being attached at one or both ends to tendons. In still other muscles, the fasciculi are much shorter than the total length of the muscle, and gain attachment to tendinous intersections within the muscle. Some variations in fascicular architecture are illustrated in Figs. 2.15 A to F.

Variations in the fascicular architecture are to be correlated with the kind of movements performed by a muscle. A muscle fibre can shorten to about two-thirds of its full length. The total displacement that a muscle can produce is, therefore, proportional to the length of its fibres. In contrast the strength of contraction of a muscle depends on the number of fibres in a muscle (irrespective of their length). In some muscles a large number of short fasciculi are packed into a relatively small total volume (e.g., in a multipennate muscle like the deltoid: Fig. 2.15F). Such a muscle can exert much greater force than a long strap muscle having the same total volume.

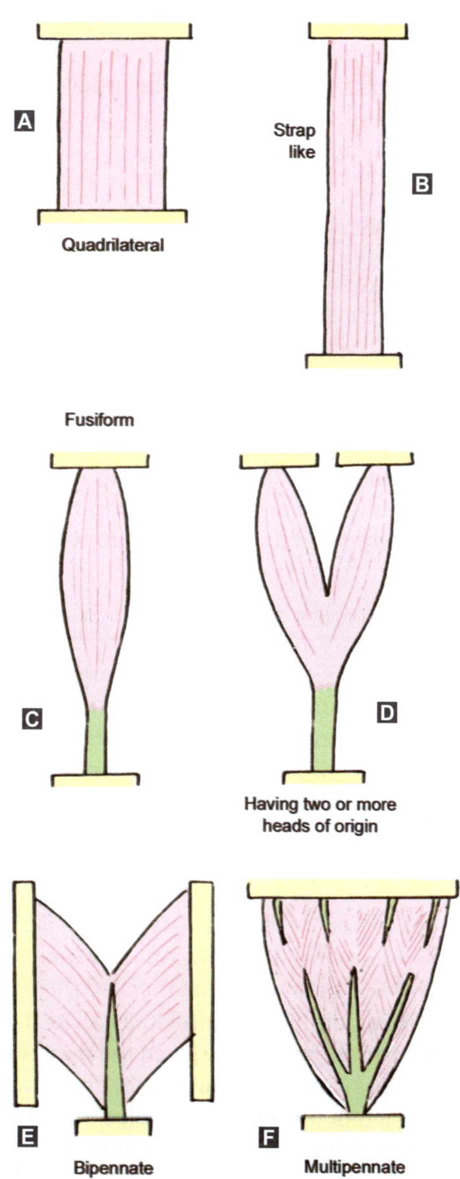

Fig. 2.15 Scheme to show some ways in which the fasciculi of a muscle may be arranged.

Connective Tissue Framework of Muscles

Muscles are pervaded by a network of connective tissue fibres that support muscle fibres and unite them to each other. Individual muscle fibres are surrounded by delicate connective tissue that is called the ***endomysium***. Individual fasciculi are surrounded by a stronger sheath of connective tissue called the ***perimysium***. Connective tissue that surrounds the entire muscle is called the ***epimysium***. At the junction of a muscle with a tendon the fibres of the endomysium, the perimysium and the epimysium become continuous with the fibres of the tendon.

Tendons

Many muscles are attached to bone through very strong cord like structures that are called tendons. Tendons are are shiny white. They are composed of collagen fibres that run parallel to each other. The fibres are arranged in the form of bundles.

Tendons serve to concentrate the pull of a muscle on a relatively small area of bone. By curving around bony pulleys, or under retinacula, they allow alterations in the direction of pull. Tendons also allow the muscle mass to be placed at a convenient distance away from its site of action. (Imagine what would happen if there were no tendons in the fingers!).

How Muscles are Named

The human body contains a very large number of muscles, each of which bears a name. A muscle may be named on the basis of its action, its shape and size, and the region in which it lies. The name of a given muscle usually consists of two or more words based on these characteristics. How muscles are named will be clear from the following examples.

Some Names based on Region

1. The region on the front of the chest is called the ***pectoral region***. There are two muscles in this region. The larger of the two is called the ***pectoralis major***. The smaller one is called the ***pectoralis minor***.
2. The region of the buttock is called the ***gluteal region***. It contains three large muscles that are given the names ***gluteus maximus*** (largest), ***gluteus medius*** (intermediate in size) and ***gluteus minimus*** (smallest).

In each of the above examples note that the first word refers to the region concerned, and the second to relative size.

Some Names based on Shape

1. Muscles that are straight are given the name ***rectus*** (compare with 'erect'). One such muscle present in the wall of the abdomen is called the ***rectus abdominis***. Another in the thigh is called the ***rectus femoris***. (Femoris = thigh: that is why the bone of the thigh is the femur).
2. Over the shoulder there is a strong triangular muscle called the ***deltoid*** (after the Greek letter delta, which is shaped like a triangle).

3. A quadrilateral muscle present in the lumbar region is called the ***quadratus lumborum***.
4. Most muscles have a fusiform shape. The central thicker part is muscular and is called the ***belly***. The ends are usually tendinous. Some muscles have two (or more) bellies each with a distinct origin (or head). A muscle having two heads is given the name ***biceps***. There is one such muscle in the arm and another in the thigh. The one in the arm is the ***biceps brachii*** (brachium = arm); and that in the thigh is the ***biceps femoris***. On the back of the arm there is a muscle that arises by three heads. It is called the ***triceps***. On the front of the thigh there is a muscle that has four heads. It is called the ***quadriceps femoris***.

Some Names based on Action

Muscles that produce flexion may be named ***flexors***; and those that cause extension may be called ***extensors***. Similarly, a muscle may be an ***abductor***, an ***adductor***, a ***supinator*** or a ***pronator***. In each case the word indicating action is followed by another word indicating the part on which the action is produced. For example, on the back of the forearm there is a muscle that is an extensor of the digits: it is called the ***extensor digitorum***. Sometimes we can have more than one muscle that qualifies for such a name. In that case we add a third word indicative of position. On the front of forearm there are two muscles that produce flexion at the wrist (or carpus). One of them, which lies towards the medial (or ulnar) side is called the ***flexor carpi ulnaris*** (= ulnar flexor of the carpus). The second muscle lies towards the lateral (or radial) side and is called the ***flexor carpi radialis***. Sometimes it is necessary to add a fourth word to the name. On the back of the forearm there are two radial extensors of the wrist: we call the longer one the ***extensor carpi radialis longus*** and the shorter one is named the ***extensor carpi radialis brevis***. On the medial side of the thigh there are three muscles that adduct it. Because of variations in size they are called the ***adductor longus***, the ***adductor brevis***, and the ***adductor magnus*** (magnus = largest).

Appreciation of these principles, used in naming muscles, can go a long way in easing the burden of remembering the names of muscles and their actions.

CHAPTER

3

A Brief Introduction to Organ Systems of the Body

We have seen that the body contains a number of organ systems that are essential to its working. We shall take a brief look at each system in the paragraphs that follow. Each of the organs mentioned will be studied in detail later.

INTRODUCTION TO THE RESPIRATORY SYSTEM

The respiratory system is meant, primarily, for the oxygenation of blood. The chief organs of the system are the right and left ***lungs***. Oxygen contained in air reaches the lungs by passing through a series of respiratory passages, which also serve for removal of carbon dioxide released from the blood.

The respiratory passages are shown in Figs. 3.1 and 3.2. Air from the outside enters the body through the right and left ***anterior nares*** (or ***external nares***) which open into the right and left ***nasal cavities.*** Apart from their respiratory function, the nasal cavities have olfactory areas that act as end organs for smell. At their posterior ends the nasal cavities have openings called the ***posterior nares*** (or ***internal nares***) through which they open into the ***pharynx.*** The pharynx is a single cavity not divided into right and left halves. It is divisible, from above downwards, into an upper part the ***nasopharynx*** (into which the nasal cavities open); a middle part the ***oropharynx*** (which is continuous with the posterior end of the oral cavity); and a lower part the ***laryngopharynx***. Air from the nose enters the nasopharynx and passes down through the oropharynx and laryngopharynx. Air can also pass through the mouth directly into the oropharynx and from there to the laryngopharynx. Air from the laryngopharynx enters a box like structure called the ***larynx.*** The larynx is placed on the front of the upper part of the neck. Apart from being a respiratory passage it is the organ where voice is produced. It is, therefore, sometimes called the voice box.

Inferiorly the larynx is continuous with a tube called the ***trachea.*** The trachea passes through the lower part of the neck into the upper part of the thorax. At the level of the lower border of the manubrium sterni the trachea bifurcates into the right and left ***principal bronchi***, which carry air to the

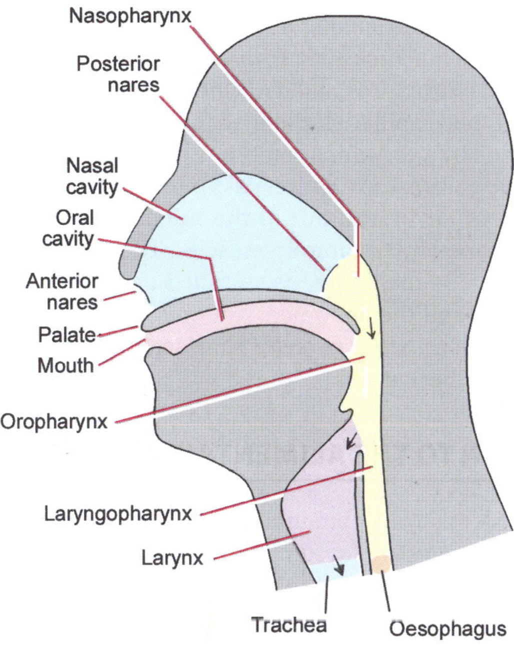

Fig. 3.1 Simplified diagram showing intercommunications between the nasal cavities, the mouth, the pharynx, the larynx and the oesophagus.

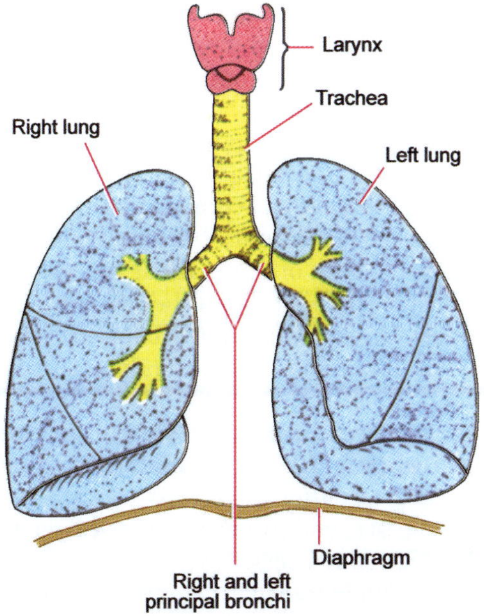

Fig. 3.2 Diagram to show the main parts of the respiratory system.

right and left lungs. Within the lung each principal bronchus divides, like the branches of a tree, into smaller and smaller ***bronchi*** that ultimately end in microscopic tubes that are called ***bronchioles.*** The bronchioles open into microscopic sac-like structures called ***alveoli.*** The walls of the alveoli contain a rich network of blood capillaries. Blood in these capillaries is separated from the air in the alveoli by a very thin membrane through which oxygen can pass into the blood and carbon dioxide can pass into the alveolar air.

The pumping of air in and out of the lungs is a result of respiratory movements performed by respiratory muscles. The most important of these is the ***diaphragm***. The diaphragm is so called because it forms a partition between the thorax and the abdomen. Another important set of respiratory muscles are the ***intercostals muscles*** that occupy the intercostal spaces (intervals between adjacent ribs).

INTRODUCTION TO THE ALIMENTARY SYSTEM

In ordinary English the word 'alimentary' means 'pertaining to nourishment'. The alimentary (or digestive) system includes all those structures that are concerned with eating, and with the digestion and absorption of food. The system consists of an alimentary canal that starts at the ***mouth*** and ends at the ***anus***.

The external opening of the mouth is the ***oral fissure*** bounded by the upper and lower lips. Within the mouth cavity (or ***oral cavity***) there are the ***teeth*** with which food is chewed; and the ***tongue*** which helps the processes of chewing and swallowing in addition to being an organ of taste. The roof of the mouth is formed by the ***palate*** (which separates the mouth from the nasal cavities). Posteriorly, the mouth opens into the ***oral part of the pharynx***. We have already seen that this part of the pharynx is continuous, below, with the ***laryngeal part of the pharynx***. The latter becomes continuous with the ***oesophagus***. The oesophagus is a tube that descends through the lower part of the neck, and then through the entire length of the thorax, to pierce the diaphragm and reach the abdomen (Fig. 3.3). Here the oesophagus ends by joining the ***stomach***. The stomach is a large sac-like organ that acts as a store of swallowed food. After this food is partially digested in the stomach it passes into the ***small intestine***. The small intestine is in the form of a tube about 5 meters long. It is divided, (rather arbitrarily) into three parts. These are the ***duodenum***, the ***jejunum*** and the ***ileum*** (in that order). The small intestine is followed by the ***large intestine***. The large intestine is about one and a half meters long. (It is described as large because it has a wider diameter). Its main subdivisions are the ***caecum***, the ***ascending colon***, the ***transverse colon***, the ***descending colon***, the ***sigmoid*** (or ***pelvic***) ***colon***, the ***rectum*** and the ***anal canal***. These are shown in Fig. 3.3. The anal canal opens to the exterior at the ***anus***.

After food has been digested and absorbed the useless remnants that remain are passed out to the exterior as faeces.

Closely related to the alimentary canal there are several accessory organs. In the region of the mouth there are three pairs of ***salivary glands,*** which produce

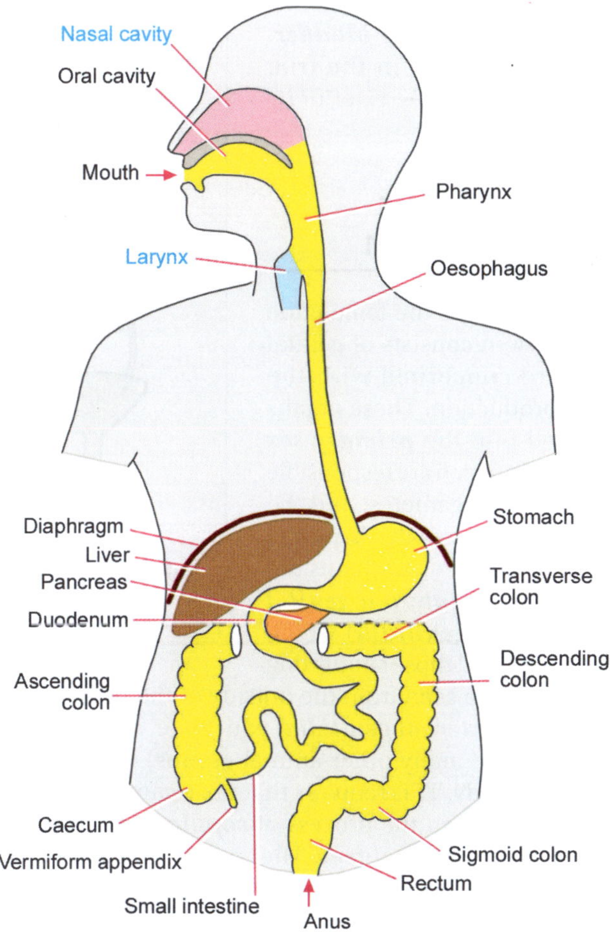

Fig. 3.3 Diagram to show the main parts of the digestive system.

a fluid the ***saliva***, that helps to keep the oral cavity moist. In the abdomen we have two large glands: the ***liver*** and the ***pancreas***. The liver occupies the upper right part of the abdomen. It is a very important organ having numerous functions. The pancreas lies transversely on the posterior wall of the abdomen. It produces digestive juices that are poured into the duodenum and help in digestion. It is also an important endocrine organ.

INTRODUCTION TO THE URINARY SYSTEM

The organs of the body that are concerned with the formation of urine and its elimination from the body are referred to as urinary organs. Urine is produced in the right and left ***kidneys,*** which lie on the posterior wall of the abdomen (Fig. 3.4). This urine passes through narrow tubes, the right and left ***ureters***, to reach a sac like reservoir called the ***urinary bladder***. The urinary bladder lies in the true pelvis. It is connected to the exterior by a tube called the ***urethra***.

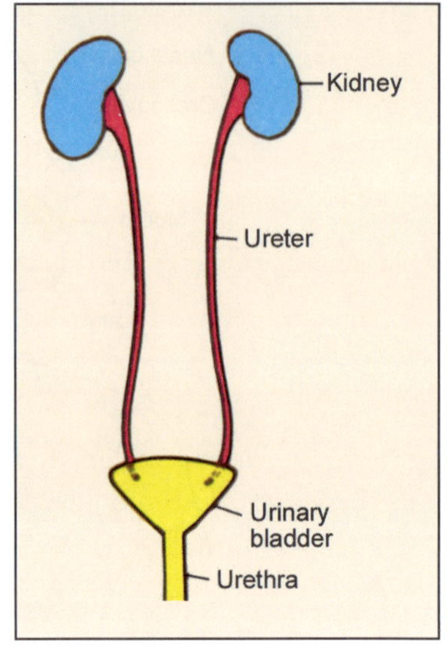

Fig. 3.4 Diagram to show the urinary organs

INTRODUCTION TO THE REPRODUCTIVE SYSTEM

Both in the male and in the female the reproductive system consists of genital organs that are concerned with the function of reproduction. These organs may be divided into the ***primary sex organs,*** or ***gonads,*** which are responsible for the production of gametes; and the ***accessory sex organs,*** which play a supporting role. The genital organs are also divided into the ***internal genital organs*** (or ***internal genitalia***) which include the gonads and those supporting organs that cannot be seen from the outside of the body; and the ***external genital organs*** (or ***external genitalia***) which are visible on the outside. In human beings (as in many other animal groups) fertilization takes place within the female body. This requires that male gametes be introduced into the female body through the process of ***copulation*** or ***coitus*** (commonly referred to as sexual intercourse). The male and female organs that are concerned with copulation are referred to as ***copulatory organs***. The region of the body where the external genitalia (and anus) are located is referred to as the ***perineum***.

Male Reproductive Organs

The male gonads are the right and left ***testes*** (singular = testis) (Fig. 3.5). They produce the male gametes, which are called ***spermatozoa*** (singular = ***spermatozoon***). From each testis the spermatozoa pass through a complicated system of genital ducts. The most obvious of these are the ***epididymis*** and the ***ductus deferens.*** Near its termination, the ductus deferens is joined by the duct of the ***seminal vesicle*** (a sac like structure), to form the ***ejaculatory duct.*** The right and left ejaculatory ducts open into the urethra.

The testis, epididymis and the initial part of the ductus deferens of both sides lie in a sac like structure covered by skin: this sac is called the ***scrotum***. From here the ductus deferens passes upwards and enters the abdomen by passing through an oblique passage in the anterior abdominal wall: this passage is called the ***inguinal canal***. Here the ductus deferens is surrounded by several structures that collectively form the ***spermatic cord***.

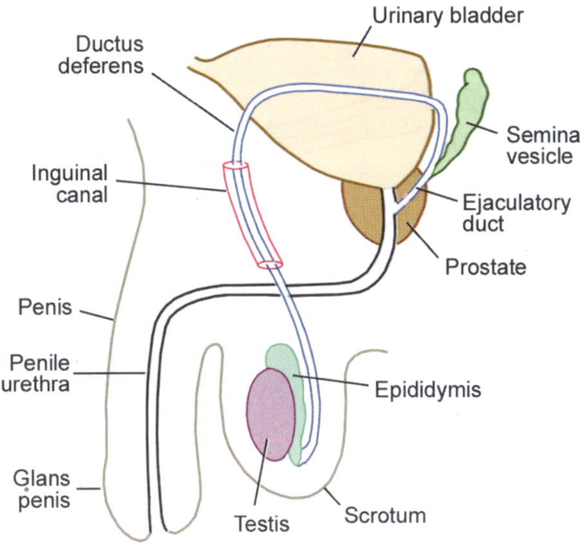

Fig. 3.5 Diagram to show the male reproductive organs

As spermatozoa pass through the genital ducts, named above, they undergo maturation. They get mixed up with secretions produced by the seminal vesicle and the prostate to form the ***seminal fluid*** or ***semen.*** The process of ejection of semen from the body is called ***ejaculation.*** In this process semen is poured into the urethra and passes through it to the exterior. The male urethra is, therefore, both a urinary and a genital passage.

The ***penis*** is the male external genital organ. It is the organ of copulation. Because it is capable of becoming rigid it can be introduced into the vagina of the female, and semen can be injected into the vaginal cavity.

Female Reproductive Organs

The female reproductive organs are shown in Fig. 3.6. The female gonads are the right and left ***ovaries.*** The female internal genital organs are the ***uterus,*** the ***uterine tubes*** and the ***vagina.*** The vagina is the female organ of copulation. It opens to the exterior through a depression in the perineum called the ***vestibule.*** The female external genital organs are present around the vestibule. They are the ***labia majora,*** the ***labia minora*** and the ***clitoris***; and some deeper structures that are associated with them. The ***mammary glands*** are accessory organs of reproduction.

In a mature female one ovum is produced every month (in the right or left ovary). It travels into the uterine tube towards the uterus. Spermatozoa introduced into the vagina can travel from the vagina into the uterus to reach the uterine tube. If a spermatozoon encounters an ovum, fertilization can take place. (Fertilization normally takes place in the uterine tube). The fertilized ovum then travels to the uterus where it gets lodged and starts developing into a fetus (unborn child in the process of development).

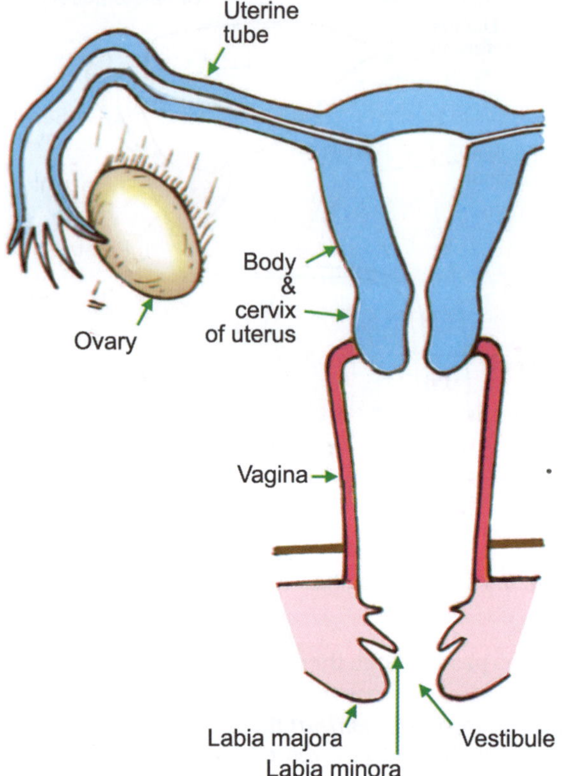

Fig. 3.6 Diagram to show the female reproductive organs.

The uterus provides the fetus with nutrition and with a suitable environment for its growth. The period during which a fetus is growing in the uterus is called ***pregnancy***. During pregnancy a fetus receives nutrition and oxygen from the mothers' blood. Transfer of these from mother to fetus takes place through an organ called the ***placenta***. The uterus enlarges greatly during pregnancy. At the end of pregnancy the fetus is expelled out of the uterus. It passes through the vagina to the exterior as a newborn infant. The process of childbirth is called ***parturition***. The mammary glands provide the newborn baby with nourishment in the form of milk.

INTRODUCTION TO THE ENDOCRINE GLANDS

Some organs of the body produce secretions. Such organs are called ***glands***. In the case of many glands the secretions produced by them pass through one or more ducts to be poured into a cavity. The salivary glands are of this type. Such glands are called ***exocrine glands***. In contrast, there are other glands that have no duct. Their secretions are poured into blood. Such glands are called ***endocrine glands***, and their secretions are called ***hormones***. Hormones can travel through blood to distant organs and can influence their functions. One endocrine gland may produce more than one hormone. Some hormones influence only one organ, while some can have more widespread effects. Some endocrine glands constitute independent anatomical entities. These are the ***hypophysis cerebri*** (or ***pituitary gland)*** and the ***pineal body*** located within the cranial cavity; the ***thyroid*** and ***parathyroid glands*** located in the neck; and the ***suprarenal glands*** that lie in the abdomen just above the kidneys. Other endocrine glands are present in the form of histological elements embedded within organs having other functions. There are aggregations of cells having an endocrine function in the pancreas, the testes, and the ovaries. Some cells with endocrine functions are also present in the thymus, the kidney, the gastrointestinal tract, and the placenta.

THE LYMPHOID ORGANS

We have seen that tissues contain lymph vessels, and that small rounded bodies called ***lymph nodes*** are associated with them. Within lymph nodes we find aggregations of large numbers of cells called ***lymphocytes***. Similar aggregations of lymphocytes are also present in some other organs. All these are referred to as ***lymphoid organs***.

The largest lymphoid organ is the ***spleen***. It is located in the upper and left part of the abdomen, close to the stomach.

Another, very important, lymphoid organ is the ***thymus***. It is located in the thorax just deep to the sternum.

In the lateral walls of the oropharynx we have small lymphoid organs called the ***tonsils*** (one right and one left). These are frequently inflamed (***tonsillitis***) resulting in sore throat.

Many aggregations of lymphocytes are also present in the walls of some organs including the intestines and the respiratory passages.

INTRODUCTION TO THE CARDIOVASCULAR SYSTEM

The cardiovascular system consists of the ***heart*** and ***blood vessels***. The system is responsible for the circulation of blood through the tissues of the body. The heart acts as a pump and provides the force for this circulation. Blood vessels taking blood from the heart to the tissues are called ***arteries***.

The largest artery in the body is called the ***aorta***. Arising from the heart it divides, like the branches of a tree, into smaller and smaller branches. The smallest arteries are called ***arterioles***. The arterioles end in a plexus of thin-walled vessels that permeate the tissues. These thin walled vessels are called ***capillaries***. Oxygen, nutrition, waste products etc., can pass through the walls of capillaries from blood to tissue cells and ***vice versa***. In some organs these vessels are somewhat different in structure from capillaries and are called ***sinusoids***. Blood from capillaries or sinusoids is collected by another set of vessels that carry it back to the heart: these are called ***veins.*** The veins adjoining the capillaries are very small and are called ***venules.*** Smaller veins join together (like tributaries of a river) to form larger and larger veins. Ultimately the blood reaches two large veins, the ***superior vena cava*** and the ***inferior vena cava***, which pour it back into the heart. This blood reaching the heart through the veins has lost its oxygen. A special set of arteries and veins circulates this blood through the lungs where it is again oxygenated. This circulation through the lungs, for the purpose of oxygenation of blood, is called the ***pulmonary circulation,*** to distinguish it from the main or ***systemic circulation.***

For further consideration of the cardiovascular system see Chapter 14.

INTRODUCTION TO THE NERVOUS SYSTEM

The nervous system may be divided into two parts.

a. The ***central nervous system*** (CNS) is made up of the ***brain*** (lying in the cranial cavity) and the ***spinal cord*** (lying in the vertebral canal).
b. The ***peripheral nervous system*** is made up nerves that arise from the brain and spinal cord.

The brain consists of the following parts (Fig. 3.7):

1. The ***cerebrum*** made of two large ***cerebral hemi-spheres***;
2. The ***cerebellum***,
3. The ***midbrain***,

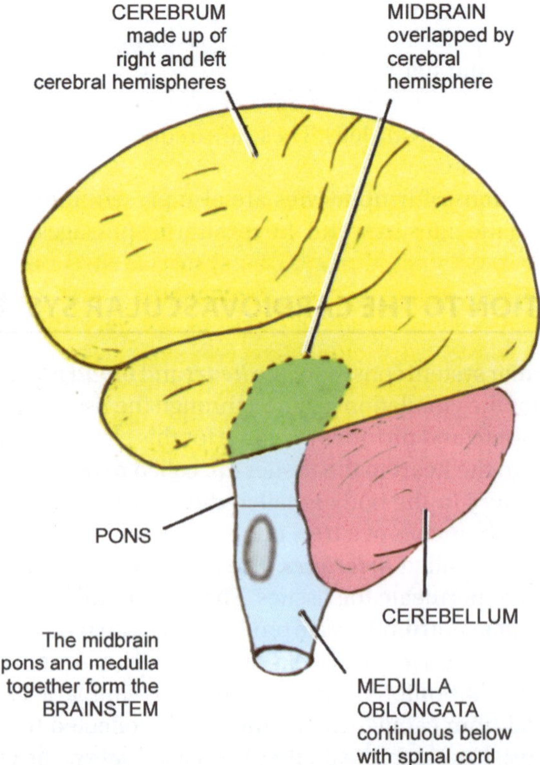

Fig. 3.7 Diagram to show the main parts of the brain.

4. The ***pons***, and
5. The ***medulla oblongata.***

The midbrain, pons and medulla together constitute the ***brainstem***. The medulla is continuous, inferiorly, with the spinal cord.

Peripheral nerves attached to the brain are called ***cranial nerves***; and those attached to the spinal cord are called ***spinal nerves***.

The Cranial Nerves

There are twelve pairs of cranial nerves. They are identified by number and also bear names.

The **first** cranial nerve is called the ***olfactory*** nerve. It is the nerve of smell (olfaction = smell). It passes from the nose to the brain.

The **second** cranial nerve is called the ***optic nerve***. It is the nerve of sight and passes from the eyeball to the brain.

The **third** cranial nerve is called the ***oculomotor*** nerve. It supplies several muscles that move the eyeball.

The **fourth** cranial nerve is called the ***trochlear*** nerve. It is so called because it supplies a muscle (superior oblique, of the eyeball) that passes through a pulley (trochlea = pulley).

The **fifth** cranial nerve is called the ***trigeminal*** nerve because it has three major divisions. These are the ***ophthalmic division*** to the orbit, the ***maxillary division*** to the upper jaw, and the ***mandibular division*** to the lower jaw.

The **sixth** cranial nerve is called the ***abducent*** nerve because it supplies a muscle (lateral rectus) which 'abducts' the eyeball.

The **seventh** cranial nerve is the ***facial*** nerve because it supplies the muscles of the face.

The **eighth** cranial nerve is called the ***vestibulo-cochlear*** nerve because it supplies structures in the vestibular and cochlear parts of the internal ear. It is sometimes called the ***auditory*** nerve (auditory = pertaining to hearing) or the ***stato-acoustic*** nerve (stato = pertaining to equilibrium; acoustic = pertaining to sound).

The **ninth** cranial nerve is called the ***glossopharyngeal*** nerve as it is distributed to the pharynx and to part of the tongue (glossal = pertaining to the tongue).

The **tenth** cranial nerve is called the ***vagus***. It has an extensive course through the neck, the thorax and the abdomen. (The word vagus may be correlated with 'vagrant' = wandering from place to place).

The **eleventh** cranial nerve is called the ***accessory*** nerve because it appears to be a part of the vagus nerve (or 'accessory' to the vagus).

The **twelfth** cranial nerve is called the ***hypoglossal*** nerve (because it runs part of its course below the tongue before supplying the muscles in it (hypo = below; glossal = pertaining to tongue).

Spinal Nerves

We have seen that spinal nerves arise from the spinal cord. In the thoracic, lumbar and sacral regions the number of spinal nerves corresponds to that

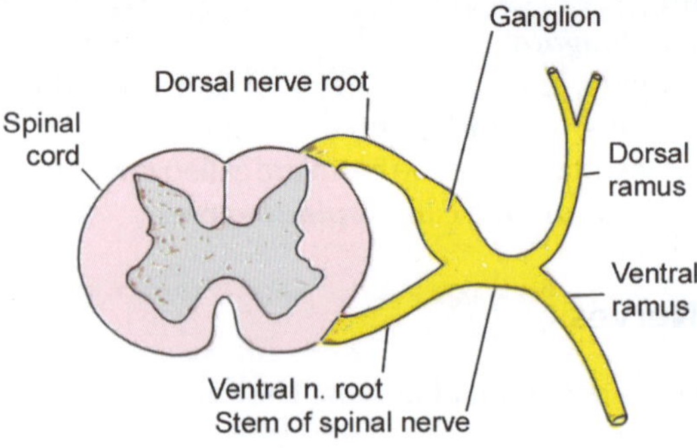

Fig. 3.8 Diagram to show the roots and main divisions of a typical spinal nerve.

of the vertebrae. On each side (right or left) there are twelve thoracic nerves, five lumbar nerves, and five sacral nerves. In the cervical region there are eight cervical nerves (but only seven vertebrae). Below the sacral nerves there is one coccygeal nerve.

Each spinal nerve arises from the spinal cord by two roots, one dorsal and one ventral (Fig. 3.8). After a very short course the spinal nerve divides into a dorsal primary ramus (ramus = branch) and a ventral primary ramus. As a rule the dorsal ramus is smaller than the ventral ramus. It passes backwards and divides into medial and lateral branches which supply the muscles and skin of the back. The ventral primary ramus passes forwards. In the thoracic region each ventral ramus remains distinct and forms an ***intercostal nerve***. In the cervical, lumbar and sacral regions the ventral rami join those of neighbouring spinal nerves to form complicated plexuses.

Branches arising from these plexuses supply muscles and skin. In the upper cervical region we have a ***cervical plexus***. In the lower cervical region there is the ***brachial plexus*** that gives origin to the nerves of the upper limb. In the lumbar region we have a ***lumbar plexus***, and in the sacral region we have a ***sacral plexus***. The lumbar and sacral plexuses send branches into the lower limb.

The cervical plexus gives off several branches to tissues in the head and neck. It also gives off the ***phrenic nerve*** which descends into the thorax to supply the diaphragm.

There are three prominent nerves in the upper limb. These are the ***median***, ***ulnar*** and ***radial*** nerves. They are all branches of the brachial plexus and are so named because of their relative position in the forearm.

There are two main nerves in the lower limb. The ***femoral nerve*** is seen in the front of the thigh. It is a branch of the lumbar plexus. The ***sciatic nerve*** is seen on the back of the thigh. It is derived from the sacral plexus. It descends to the back of the knee where it divides into the ***tibial nerve*** (which supplies the back of the leg) and the ***common peroneal nerve*** (which supplies the front and lateral side of the leg). Branches of both these nerves descend into the foot.

Most of the nerves mentioned above supply tissues like skin and muscle. From the skin they carry impulses of touch, pain, temperature, etc. Such nerves are called ***sensory nerves***. Nerves that supply muscles are called ***motor nerves***. Nerves that contain both sensory and motor nerve fibres are ***mixed nerves***, and the large majority of nerves belong to this category.

The segment of the spinal cord that gives origin to one spinal nerve is called a ***spinal segment***. The number of spinal segments corresponds to the number of spinal nerves.

AUTONOMIC NERVOUS SYSTEM

Most internal organs of the body, (including the blood vessels), are supplied by nerves that belong to the autonomic nervous system. This system is divisible into two large subdivisions, ***sympathetic*** and ***para-sympathetic***. Most autonomic nerves are very thin and difficult to see. They often form plexuses around blood vessels and in relation to viscera. The most prominent components of this system are the right and left ***sympathetic trunks***. Each trunk extends vertically from the base of the skull (above) to the coccyx (below). The trunks lie along the sides of the vertebral column. Each trunk bears a large number of thickenings along its length. These thickenings are ***sympathetic ganglia***.

The vagus nerve provides a parasympathetic supply to many organs of the body.

CHAPTER

4

Introduction to Body Functions

External Environment

A living organism is in constant interaction with the external environment surrounding it. It is from this environment that the organism obtains food. This food provides energy required to perform various functions. Waste products left after utilisation of ingested food are thrown back into the external environment.

In addition to food, the animal body needs oxygen, and this is also obtained from the environment.

The body has to react to changes in the environment, for example changes in temperature. In mammals the body is maintained at a more or less constant temperature. When the environment is cold the body need mechanisms to provide it with heat. Conversely, when the environment is too warm, the body has to be cooled.

Internal Environment

The animal body is made up of very large numbers of cells. The cells are surrounded by intercellular fluid. The composition of this fluid is in constant change, but in a healthy person these changes are maintained within very narrow limits. The maintenance of the environment within these limits is called ***homeostasis***. There are many mechanisms in the body for homeostasis.

Negative Feedback Mechanism

When the temperature of the body rises beyond normal, it triggers mechanisms that lower body temperature, e.g., by perspiration. In this example, the stimulus produces an effect (cooling) opposite to that of the stimulus. Such a mechanism is, therefore, called a negative feedback mechanism. Most central mechanisms of the body are of this variety.

Positive Feedback Mechanism

In such a mechanism the response is similar to the original stimulus and makes it stronger. For example, during childbirth (labour) the onset of uterine contractions acts as a stimulus for further strengthening of the contractions.

SOME ESSENTIAL BODY FUNCTIONS

Every animal body has to perform certain basic functions that are necessary for survival.

Procuring and Ingestion of Food

Every animal needs regular intake of nutrition. Substances that provide nutrition are called ***nutrients***. The most important nutrients are water, carbohydrates, proteins, and fats. Small quantities of vitamins and mineral salts are also required. We obtain carbohydrates from sugar, and from food grains like wheat or rice. The richest sources of protein are the flesh of animals, and milk. Proteins are also available in some vegetarian foods specially in lentils (*daal*) and various kinds of beans (specially soya bean). Fats are present in milk (and milk products), in the flesh of animals, and in vegetable oils like mustard oil, groundnut oil and sunflower oil.

The nutrients taken into the body provide us with energy for various internal and external needs. Food is also necessary for growth in children, and for maintenance of tissues at all ages.

When ingested, food enters the alimentary canal. This is a long canal consisting of many parts. As food passes through the canal it undergoes a process of digestion. Sugar and carbohydrates are broken down into glucose. Proteins are broken down into amino acids; and fats are broken down into fatty acids and glycerol. It is in this form that food is absorbed from the intestine and is transported to various parts of the body for use.

Respiration

In addition to food, the body requires a constant supply of oxygen. This is obtained from the air we breathe. The parts of the body responsible for intake of air and absorption of oxygen into the blood constitute the respiratory system. The main organs of the system are the right and left lungs.

Excretion of Waste Products

1. After useful elements have been extracted from food, waste products are expelled from the body in the form of faeces.
2. When any fuel is burnt, oxygen is used and carbon dioxide is produced. This happens in the animal body too. Oxygen is necessary for "burning" food to create heat and energy. Carbon dioxide produced during this process has to be expelled from the body, and this is done through the lungs.
3. Many chemical reactions take places in various organs of the body and result in formation of chemicals (e.g., urea) that are harmful to the body. Most of these chemicals are excreted through urine. Urine is produced in the kidneys. It passes through a series of passages before being expelled to the exterior. The kidneys and the passages through which urine passes constitute the urinary system.

The Need for Movement

The capacity for movement is a fundamental characteristic of animals. Unicellular organisms (like amoeba) can move away from unpleasant stimuli. They can alter their shape in order to absorb particulate matter from the environment.

In the animal body the capacity for movement serves many functions that are essential to survival of the animal.

Movement in relation to the environment

1. Movement enables an animal to procure food.
2. Movement enables an animal to move away from danger. The same purpose is also served when animals come together to live in groups.
3. Movement is also essential for finding a mate. This is in turn, essential for preservation of the species.

Movement in relation the environment is made possible by:

A. A skeleton made up of many bones. Movements occur at joints between the bones.
B. Movements are produced by action of muscles.

The skeleton, joints and muscles collectively form the anatomical basis for production of movements in relation to the environment.

Movement within the body

1. Movement is necessary for eating food, and for its transport through the alimentary canal. This transport is dependent on muscle present in the walls of the canal.
2. The taking of air into the body (inspiration) and expelling it out of the body (expiration) is dependent on the action of muscles present in the walls of the thorax (chest) and abdomen.
3. Food absorbed from the intestines, and oxygen absorbed through the lungs, reach all parts of the body through blood. Blood is in constant circulation through all parts of the body. The power for the circulation of blood is provided by the heart. The heart is a pump made up mainly of muscle.
   The circulation is also necessary for transporting waste products to excretory organs (e.g., kidneys, sweat glands) and for transporting numerous substances from one part of the body to another.
4. Movement is required for expelling faeces and urine from the body, and for childbirth.
   From what has been said above it will be clear that movement is essential for life. Cessation of heart-beat, or of respiratory movements, results in death.

MODES OF COMMUNICATION WITHIN THE BODY

We have seen that substances can travel from one part of the body to another through circulating blood. This is one mode of communication. Apart from nutrients and oxygen, blood carries chemical messengers (called ***hormones***) through which one organ can have profound effect on the working of another.

The brain exerts a control on all parts of the body through nerves. Nerves can be compared to wires carrying an electric current. Contraction of muscles takes place through orders starting in the brain and travelling through nerves. The brain influences many other functions of the body in a similar manner.

The brain receives information about the external environment through sense organs like the eyes, the ears and the skin. Such information travels through nerves. Information is also received from various organs of the body. It provides the input on the basis of which the working of the organs is controlled.

In the chapters that follow we will consider the structure and functions of organs involved in the various functions very briefly introduced this chapter.

CHAPTER

5

Essential Chemistry

INTRODUCTION

The earliest attempts at understanding the structure of the body, were limited to what could be seen by eye; or at best by use of simple magnifying lenses. Today we refer to structure thus studied as ***gross anatomy***. A great leap forward was made when compound microscopes capable of high magnifications (up to x1500) were developed. Structure as seen through microscopes is referred to as ***histology***. Still further impetus was achieved with the invention of electron microscopes. With these, we could for the first time much greater details of structure (***ultrastructure***). Using the highest magnifications of electron microscopes it was even possible to see individual molecules of some substances. In combination with other techniques it now became possible to correlate physical structure of some substances, present in the body, with their chemical composition. All physical structure is ultimately to be understood in terms of chemistry. At this level, the disciplines of anatomy, physiology and biochemistry all merge into one and enable understanding of structure and function in a way that was unimaginable a few decades ago.

This introduction tells us why knowledge of chemistry is essential for understanding the human body. In this chapter we will consider some very elementary aspects of chemistry only.

ATOMS AND ELEMENTS

All matter, living or non-living is made up of particles called ***atoms***. An atom is the smallest unit in which matter can exist (in a stable form).

Atoms exist in various sizes, but the size is constant for a given type of matter. Matter in which all atoms are similar is called an ***element***. There are 92 elements in nature. Some examples, are hydrogen and oxygen, which exist as gases; mercury which is a liquid; and iron, gold or silver which exist as solids.

Basic Structure of an Atom

The basic structure of an atom is shown in Fig. 5.1. The central part of the atom is called the ***nucleus***. It contains two kinds of particles, namely ***neutrons*** and ***protons***.

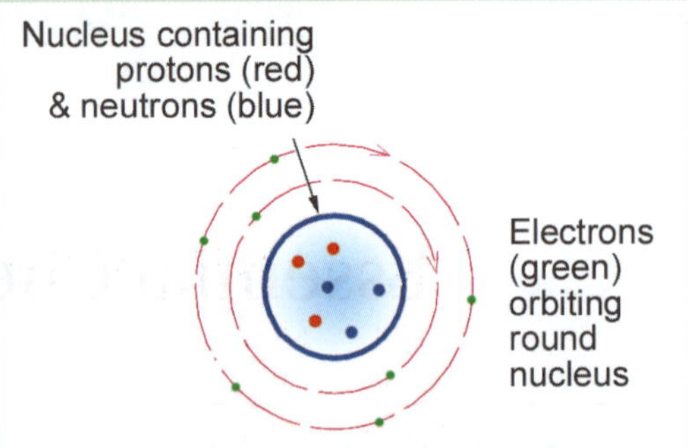

Fig. 5.1 Structure of a typical atom.

The region around the nucleus contains particles called ***electrons***. Electrons are in constant motion along circular paths surrounding the nucleus.

Concept of Electrical Charge

Many particles occurring in nature bear an electrical charge. Some facts about electrical charge are as follows:

1. An electrical charge can be positive (+) or negative (-).
2. Positive and negative charges are attracted to each other. When a positively charged particle lies next to a negatively charged one, the attraction between them makes the combined structure a stable one.
3. Protons, present in the nucleus of an atom, are positively charged. Electrons, revolving around the nucleus, are negatively charged. Neutrons are so called as they are electrically neutral (They do not have any charge, positive or negative).

Variation in Structure of Atom

The number of protons present in the nucleus is different for each element. Hydrogen is the lightest element and an atom of hydrogen bears only one proton (Fig. 5.2). An atom of oxygen has 8 protons (Fig. 5.3), while an atom of sodium has 11 protons. Each element can therefore, be identified by the number of protons in it. This is called the ***atomic number***. The atomic number of hydrogen is 1, and that of oxygen is 8.

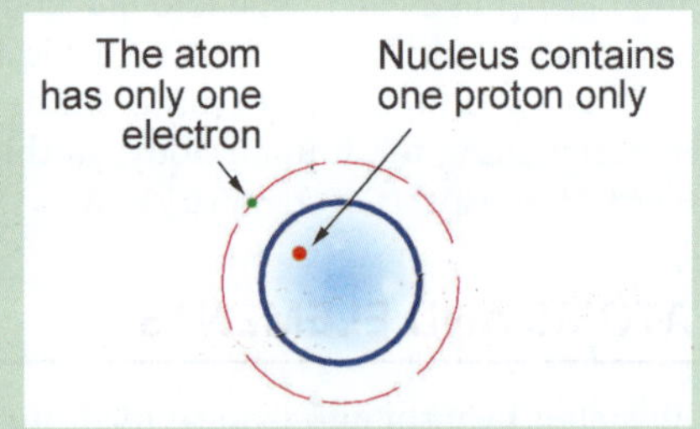

Fig. 5.2 Structure of an atom of hydrogen.

We can presume that each proton has the same weight. We have seen than in addition to protons the nucleus of an atom also contains neutrons. One neutron can be presumed to have the same weight as one proton. An atom of hydrogen has one proton only (there is no neutron). An atom of oxygen has 8 protons and 8 neutrons (the total being 16). Hence, an atom of oxygen is 16 times as heavy as an atom of hydrogen. In addition to its atomic number (explained above) each element has its own ***atomic weight***.

In calculating atomic weight we do not attach any significance to the number of electrons present in an atom. This is because electrons are very light compared to protons or neutrons. One atom of hydrogen has one proton and one electron (no neutron) and its atomic weight is one. One atom of oxygen has 8 protons, and 8 neutrons. It atomic weight is, therefore, (8 + 8) = 16.

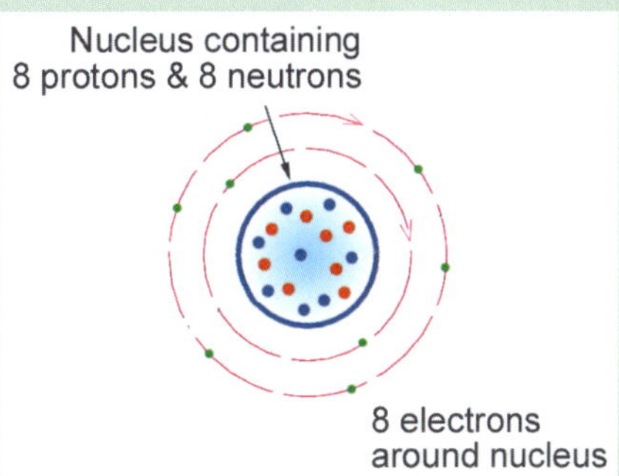

Fig. 5.3 Structure of an atom of oxygen.

Isotopes

Very rarely, an atom of hydrogen may have one neutron (in addition to the normal proton) (Fig. 5.4); and every more rarely it may have two neutrons. Thus, there can be three different forms of hydrogen each with a different atomic weight. When an element exists in more than one form the various forms are referred to as ***isotopes***.

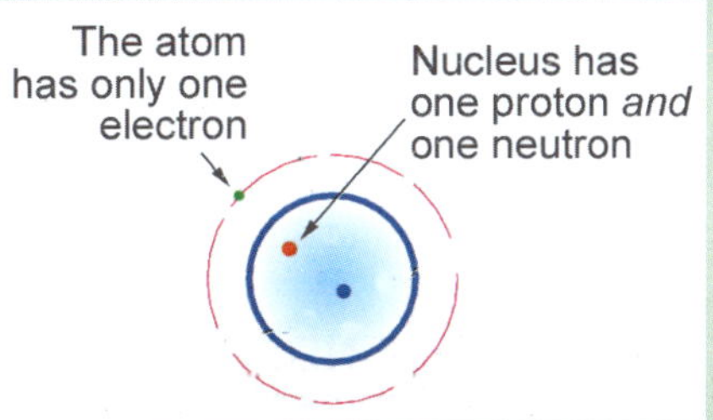

Fig. 5.4 Isotopes of hydrogen having one proton and one neutron in ♥the nucleus.

COMPOUNDS AND MOLECULES

Although some elements can exist in nature in pure form, it is much more common for an element to be bound with one or more other elements. When a substance is made up of two (or more) elements it is called a ***compound***. For example, water is a compound containing hydrogen and oxygen. The smallest unit of a compound is called a ***molecule***. One molecule of water contains two atoms of hydrogen and one atom of oxygen. Hence, the structure of the water is expressed by the formula H_2O.

Examine this formula. The letter H (capital) is the symbol for hydrogen. The letter O is the symbol for oxygen. The number 2 following the H indicates that the molecule contains 2 atoms of hydrogen. There is no number after O as there is only one atom of oxygen.

Each element has a symbol. The symbol for sodium is **Na** (Capital N followed by 'a' which is not capital). The symbol for chlorine is **Cl**. When Na + Cl combine they form the compound sodium chloride. This is common salt used in cooking. Its formula is NaCl.

Molecular Weight

The weight of a molecule is equal to the sum of the atomic weights of the elements in it. Take the example of water.

Atomic weight of hydrogen is 1. As there are two hydrogen atoms their combined weight is 1 + 1 = 2. The atomic weight of oxygen is 16. Hence, the molecular weight of water is 2 + 16 = 18.

Similarly the molecular weight of sodium chloride is:
(Atomic weight of sodium = 23) + (Atomic weight of chlorine = 35) = 58.

Mole

Please note that molecular weight (like atomic weight) is just a number. It is not expressed in terms of any unit of weight (e.g., grams, milligrams).

If we express the molecular weight of a substance in grams, the quantity is called a ***mole***. Thus one mole of sodium chloride is equal to 58 grams (for reasons which we need not go into, it is actually taken as 58.5 g).

Sometimes instead of a mole we speak of smaller units. A millimole is one thousandth of a mole. A micromole is one thousandth of a millimole (= one millionth of a mole).

Molar Solution

If one mole of a substance is dissolved in one litre of water, we get what is called a ***molar solution***. To make a molar solution of sodium chloride we take 58.5 g of the salt and dissolve it in 1 litre of water.

CHEMICAL BONDS

When two (or more) elements join together to form a compound, the stability of the compound depends on bonds between the elements.

We have seen that the nucleus of an atom is surrounded by electrons (moving in orbits round the nucleus). The electrons are kept in place by the "attraction" exerted on them by the nucleus. (Compare this with the gravitational pull exerted on the moon by the earth). When two elements form a compound some electrons behave as it they were "shared" by nuclei of both elements. In other words, these electrons are attracted towards both nuclei. This binds the two nuclei strongly. Such bonds are called ***covalent bonds*** (Fig. 5.5).

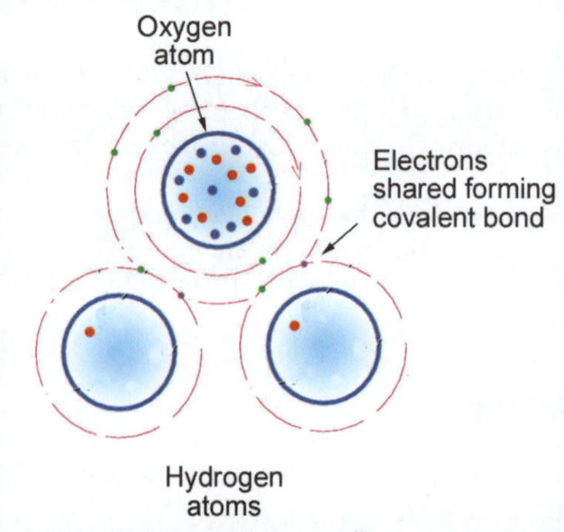

Fig. 5.5 Water molecule. Two hydrogen atoms are united to one oxygen atom through covalent bonds.

We have seen that in an atom the number of electrons is equal to the number of protons. The positive charge of one proton neutralizes the negative charge of one electron. Hence the atom is electrically neutral. One atom of sodium contains 11 protons + 11 electrons. One atom of chloride contain 17 protons + 17 electrons.

When one atom of sodium combines with one atom of chlorine (to form sodium chloride), one electron is transferred from sodium to chlorine. The sodium atom now has 11 protons and only 10 electrons and is, therefore, positively charged. The chloride atom has 17 protons + 18 electrons and is negatively charged. The positively charged sodium atom is attracted to the negatively charged chlorine atom forming an ***ionic bond*** (Fig. 5.6).

Ionic bond are not as strong as covalent bonds. When we dissolve sodium chloride in water, the sodium and chloride atoms separate and are now called ***ions***. (That is why the bond is called an ionic bond). The sodium ion bears a positive charge (expressed as Na^+) and the Cl ion bear a negative charge (expressed as Cl^-).

We have seen that when sodium chloride is dissolved in water the ions formed are electrically charged. Another property of the solution is that an electric current can pass through it. Because of this property a solution of sodium chloride is called an ***electrolyte***. Apart from sodium chloride there are many other electrolytes in the body. In some cases the ion may contain more than one element. When sodium bicarbonate $NaHCO_3$ is dissolved the ions formed are sodium (Na^+) and bicarbonate (HCO_3^-). Note that the bicarbonate ion contains hydrogen (H), carbon (C) and oxygen (O).

There are many chemical compounds in the body that are not ionic (i.e., they do not split into ions when dissolved in water). Such solutions do not conduct electricity.

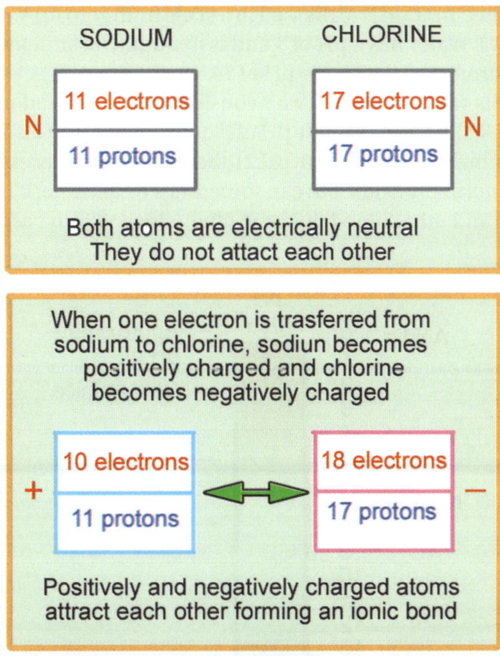

Fig. 5.6 Sodium chloride formed by union of sodium and chlorine through an ionic bond.

Importance of Electrolytes

As we have seen electrolytes can conduct electricity. We shall see later that this fact is of great significance in functioning of muscles and nerves. When two solutions, containing varying concentrations of electrolytes, are separated by a very thin membrane, ions tend to pass (through the membrane) from the more concentrated solution to the less concentrated one. This process is called ***osmosis***. The difference in concentration of the two solutions is called a ***concentration gradient***. The force that causes the ions to pass through the membrane is called ***osmotic pressure***.

Ions are also of importance is determining whether a solution is acid, alkaline or neutral as explained below.

Acids and Alkalies

Some naturally occurring substances have a sour taste, e.g., lemon juice and vinegar. Such substances are said to be acidic and contain acids. In contrast, some other substance are bitter in taste e.g., sodium bicarbonate used in cooking. Sodium bicarbonate is an alkali. Water is neither acidic nor alkaline.

We know that water contains two atoms of hydrogen and one of oxygen. However, these exist as two ions H^+ and OH^-. H^+ ions are responsible for making a solution acidic. The more the number of free H^+ in the solution, the stronger the acid. The OH^- ion is called a hydroxyl ion. It is responsible for alkalinity. Water is neither acid or alkaline as it contains equal number of H^+ and OH^- ions.

We have seen that the acidity of a solution is related to the number of free H^+ ions in it. This is spoken of as ***hydrogen ion concentration***. For sake of convenience hydrogen ion concentration is expressed in a scale from zero to14. This is called the pH scale (Fig. 5.7). Water has a pH of 7 and is neutral. The strongest acid has a pH of zero and the strongest alkali has a pH of 14.

Fluids presents within the body vary considerably in pH and most of them are mildly acidic or alkaline. For example pH of blood is about 7.4. Gastric juice, present in the stomach, is highly acidic, (about pH 2), the acidity being necessary for digestion of food. Urine is normally acidic but can sometimes be alkaline. It is very important that pH of blood and other blood fluids be maintained within narrow limits.

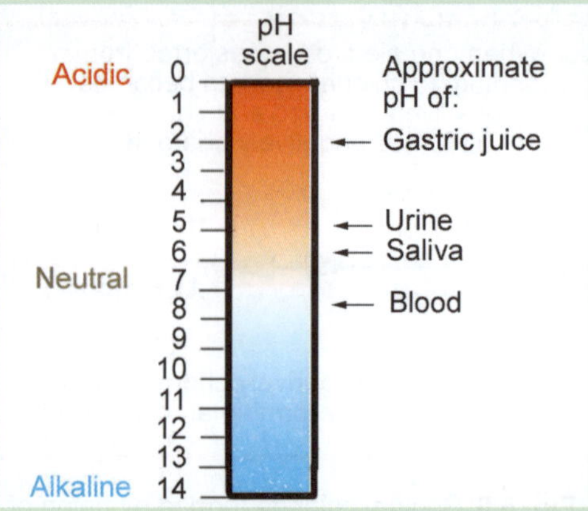

Fig. 5.7 The pH scale.

Buffers

The pH of body fluids is kept within normal limits by buffers. When H^+ ions are in excess, these get attached to some buffers and this prevents the fluid from becoming too acidic. In a similar manner OH^- (hydroxyl) ions get fixed to some buffers preventing the solution from becoming too alkaline.

Some substances that act as buffers are phosphates, bicarbonates and certain proteins. The extent to which buffers can control pH is limited by the availability of buffers. Under certain circumstances all available buffer is used up and the body may then contain too much acid. This condition is called ***acidosis***. The reverse condition in which there is too much alkali is called ***alkalosis***.

INTRODUCTION TO SOME IMPORTANT CHEMICAL CONSTITUENTS OF THE BODY

Most of the chemical molecules to be found in the body belong to one (or more) of the following:

1. Carbohydrates.
2. Proteins
3. Fats.

The same substances constitute the bulk of the food we eat.

Carbohydrates

Food grains such as wheat and rice, are made up predominantly of starch, which is a complex form of carbohydrate. Another form of carbohydrate, which is well known to us, is sugar.

Carbohydrates are so called because they contain carbon, oxygen and hydrogen.

The simplest form in which carbohydrates exist is that of ***glucose***. Carbohydrates in food are ultimately broken down (by the process of digestion) to glucose. Glucose is absorbed into blood and reaches all part of the body. The chemical structure of glucose is shown in Fig. 5.8. The carbon atoms are arranged in the form of a ring. Atoms of hydrogen and oxygen are attached to the carbon atoms.

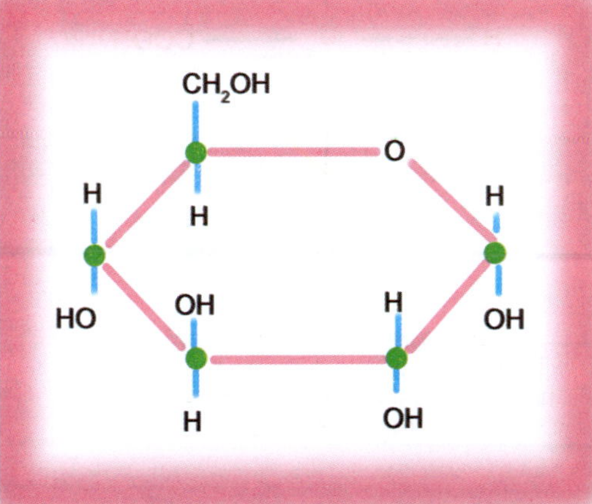

Fig. 5.8 Structure of a molecule of glucose.♥

Sugars, like glucose, which exist as single molecules, are called ***monosaccharides***. Another example of a monosaccharide is fructose (fruit sugar). Sugars made up of two molecules are called ***disaccharides***. The sugar we use in homes is a disaccharide called ***sucrose***. It is made up of one molecule of glucose plus one of fructose.

Carbohydrates, derived from food, constitute the most important source of energy required for various needs. When available in excess, glucose is converted to glycogen, which is stored in the body. Excess carbohydrate is also converted into fat.

Proteins

Animal flesh is made up mainly of proteins. Egg-white (albumin) is also a common form of protein. Proteins are also present in many plant foods specially beans and lentils.

Proteins in food are broken down by digestion, into ***amino acids***. (In other words proteins are formed by joining together of amino acids). Each amino acid contains carbon, hydrogen, oxygen, and nitrogen. Some of them contain sulphur. The simplest amino acid is ***glycine***. Its structure is shown in Fig. 5.9.

Amino acids join together to form proteins. Proteins exist in various forms. Some proteins form the structural basis of cells and tissues, while others serve as enzymes, hormones, antibodies and many other biologically active substances.

Proteins are essential for growth and repair of tissues. When available in excess, proteins can be used to provide energy for storage as fat, but normally carbohydrates are used for this purpose.

Fats or Lipids

Lipids are important constituents of cells and tissues. We obtain fats through milk and milk products (butter, cheese, ghee, cream) and also through vegetable oils

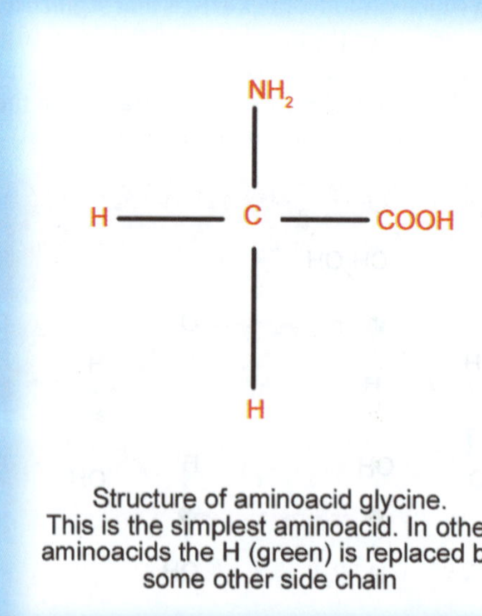

Fig. 5.9 Structure of amino acids.

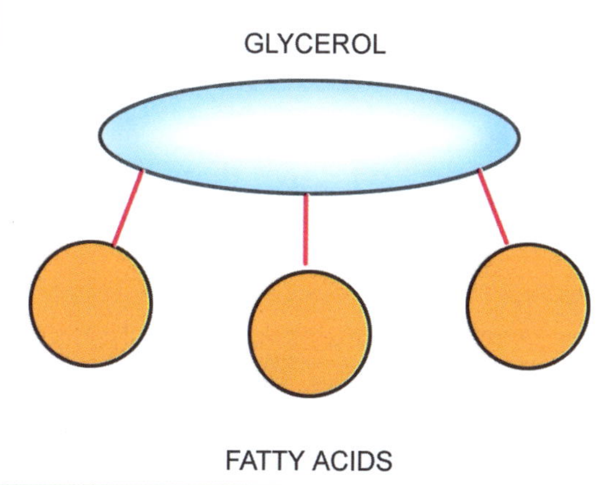

Fig. 5.10 Basic structure of fat.

(groundnut oil, mustard oil, sunflower oil and many others). Considerable fat is also present in many non-vegetarian foods.

Like carbohydrates, fats also contain carbon, hydrogen and oxygen. Some lipids contain phosphorus (phospholipids).

The basic structure of a molecule of fat is shown in Fig. 5.10. It consists of a core of glycerol to which three fatty acids are attached. During digestion, fats are broken down into fatty acids and glycerol. Fats present in food are absorbed in the form of these end products.

Like carbohydrates, lipids are a source of energy for the body. When available in excess, fat is stored in the body. Fats are essential constituents of many tissues e.g., of cell membranes and of myelin sheaths of nerves.

PART TWO

Cells and Tissues of the Body

CHAPTER

6

Cell Structure

CELL STRUCTURE

A cell is bounded by a ***cell membrane*** (or ***plasma membrane***) within which is enclosed a complex material called ***protoplasm***. The protoplasm consists of a central, dense, part called the ***nucleus***; and an outer less dense part called the ***cytoplasm***. The nucleus is separated from the cytoplasm by a nuclear membrane. The cytoplasm has a fluid base (matrix) that is referred to as the ***cytosol*** or ***hyaloplasm***. The cytosol contains a number of ***organelles*** that have distinctive structure and functions. Many of them are in the form of membranes that enclose spaces. These spaces are collectively referred to as the ***vacuoplasm***.

From what has been said above it is evident that membranes play an important part in the constitution of the cell. The various membranes within the cell have a common basic structure that we will consider before going on to study cell structure in detail.

BASIC MEMBRANE STRUCTURE

When suitable preparations are examined by EM the average cell membrane is seen to be about 7.5 nm (nm = nanometer) thick. It consists of two densely stained layers separated by a lighter zone, thus creating a trilaminar appearance (Fig. 6.1A).

Cell membranes are made up predominantly of lipids. Proteins and carbohydrates are also present.

Lipids in cell membranes

It is now known that the trilaminar structure of membranes is produced by the arrangement of lipid molecules (predominantly phospholipids) that constitute the basic framework of the membrane (Fig. 6.1B).

Each phospholipid molecule consists of an enlarged head in which the phosphate portion is located; and of two thin tails (Fig. 6.2). The head end is also called the ***polar end*** while the tail end is the ***non-polar end***. The head end is soluble in water and is said to be ***hydrophilic***. The tail end is insoluble and is said to be ***hydrophobic***.

When such molecules are suspended in an aqueous medium they arrange themselves so that the hydrophilic ends are in contact with the medium; but the hydrophobic ends are not. They do so by forming a bi-layer.

The dark staining parts of the membrane (seen by EM) are formed by the heads of the molecules, while the light staining intermediate zone is occupied by the tails, thus giving the membrane its trilaminar appearance.

Because of the manner of its formation, the membrane is to be regarded as a fluid structure that can readily reform when its continuity is disturbed. For the same reasons proteins present within the membrane (see below) can move freely within the membrane.

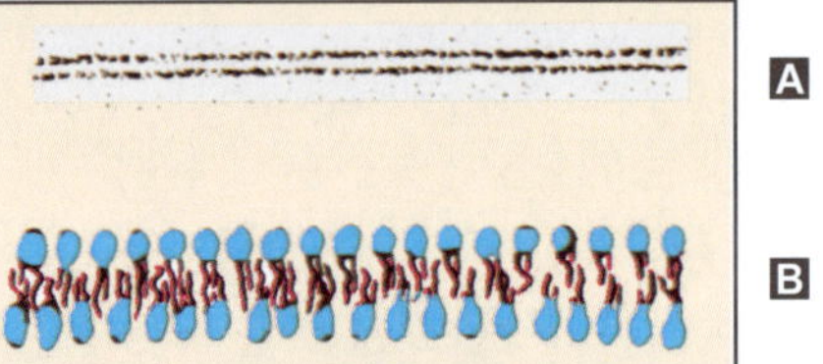

Fig. 6.1 A. Trilaminar structure of a cell membrane as revealed by high magnifications of EM; B. Diagram showing the arrangement of phospholipid molecules forming the membrane.

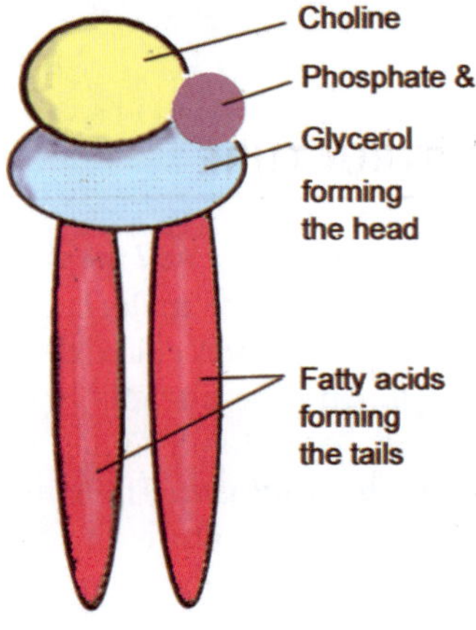

Fig. 6.2 Diagram showing the structure of a phospholipid molecule (phosphatidyl choline) seen in a cell membrane.

Proteins in Cell Membranes

In addition to molecules of lipids the cell membrane contains several proteins. It was initially thought that the proteins formed a layer on each side of the phospholipid molecules (forming a protein-phospholipid sandwich). However, it is now known that this is not so. The proteins are present in the form of irregularly rounded masses. Most of them are embedded within the thickness of the membrane and partly project on one of its surfaces (either outer or inner). However, some proteins occupy the entire thickness of the membrane and may project out of both its surfaces (Fig. 6.3). These are called transmembrane proteins.

The proteins of the membrane are of great significance as follows.

a. They may form an essential part of the structure of the membrane i.e., they may be structural proteins.
b. Some proteins play a vital role in transport across the membrane and act as pumps. Ions get attached to the protein on one surface and move with the protein to the other surface.

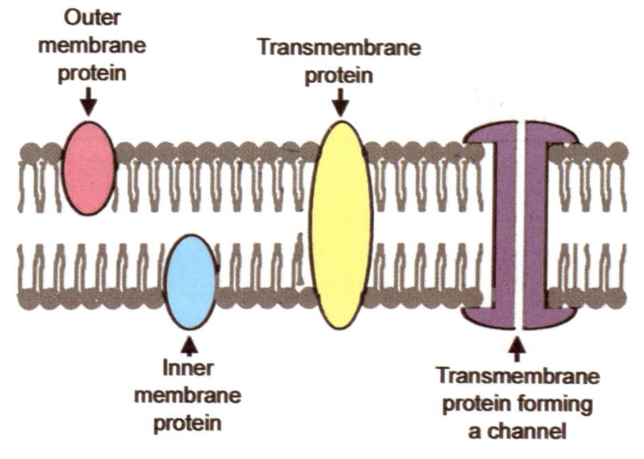

Fig. 6.3 Some varieties of membrane proteins.

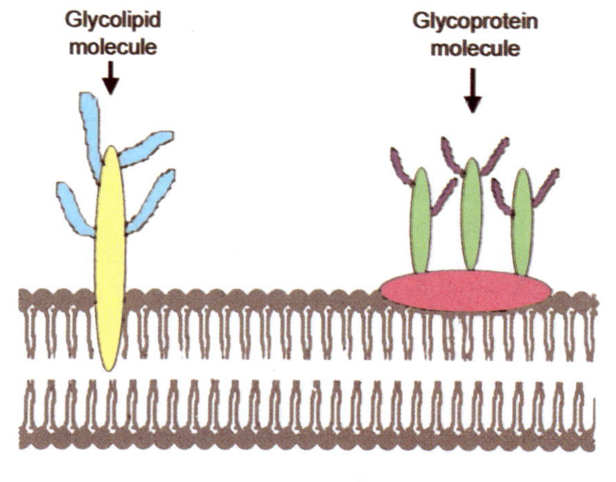

Fig. 6.4 Glycolipid and glycoprotein molecules attached to the outer aspect of cell membrane.

c. Some proteins are so shaped that they form passive channels through which substances can diffuse through the membrane. However, these channels can be closed by a change in the shape of the protein.
d. Other proteins act as receptors for specific hormones or neurotransmitters.
e. Some proteins act as enzymes.

Carbohydrates of Cell Membranes

In addition to the phospholipids and proteins, carbohydrates are present at the surface of the membrane. They are attached either to the proteins (forming glycoproteins) or to the lipids (forming glycolipids) (Fig. 6.4). The carbohydrate layer is specially well developed on the external surface of the plasma membrane forming the cell boundary. This layer is referred to as the cell coat or ***glycocalyx***.

Membranes in cells are highly permeable to water, and to oxygen, but charged ions (Na^+, K^+) do not pass through easily.

THE CELL MEMBRANE

The membrane separating the cytoplasm of the cell from surrounding structures is called the ***cell membrane*** or the ***plasma membrane***. It has the basic structure described above. We have seen that the carbohydrate layer, or ***glycocalyx***, is specially well formed on the external surface of this membrane.

The cell membrane is of great importance in regulating the activities of the cell as follows.

a. The membrane maintains the shape of the cell.
b. It controls the passage of all substances into or out of the cell. Some substances (consisting of small molecules) pass through the passive channels already described: this does not involve deformation of the membrane. Larger molecules enter the cell by the process of endocytosis described below.
c. The cell membrane forms a sensory surface. This function is most developed in nerve and muscle cells. The plasma membranes of such cells are normally polarized: the external surface bears a positive charge and the internal surface bears a negative charge. When suitably stimulated there is a selective passage of sodium and potassium ions across the membrane reversing the charge. This is called ***depolarisation***: it results in contraction in the case of muscle, or in generation of a nerve impulse in the case of neurons.
d. The surface of the cell membrane bears ***receptors*** that may be specific for particular molecules (e.g., hormones or enzymes). Stimulation of such receptors (e.g., by the specific hormone) can produce profound effects on the activity of the cell. Receptors also play an important role in absorption of specific molecules into the cell as described below.

Enzymes present within the membrane may be activated when they come in contact with specific molecules. Activation of the enzymes can influence metabolism within the cell.

Role of Cell Membrane in Transport of Material Into or Out of the Cell

Movement of various substances through cell membranes is an essential feature of cell function. Nutrients enter cells, and waste materials are expelled, in this way. The movement of some ions through cell membranes plays a very important role in functioning of nerve cells, muscle cells and others.

Transport through the cell membrane can take place in two distinct ways:

a. Transport can take place by diffusion or osmosis (from higher concentration to lower). For such transport the force required is provided by the concentration gradient, and no energy is used. It is, therefore, called ***passive transport***.
b. Sometimes substances have to be moved against the concentration gradient (from lower concentration to higher). For this to happen energy is required, and such transport is called ***active transport***. Active transport is used for moving sodium and potassium ions across cell membranes (to neutralise their movement by diffusion).

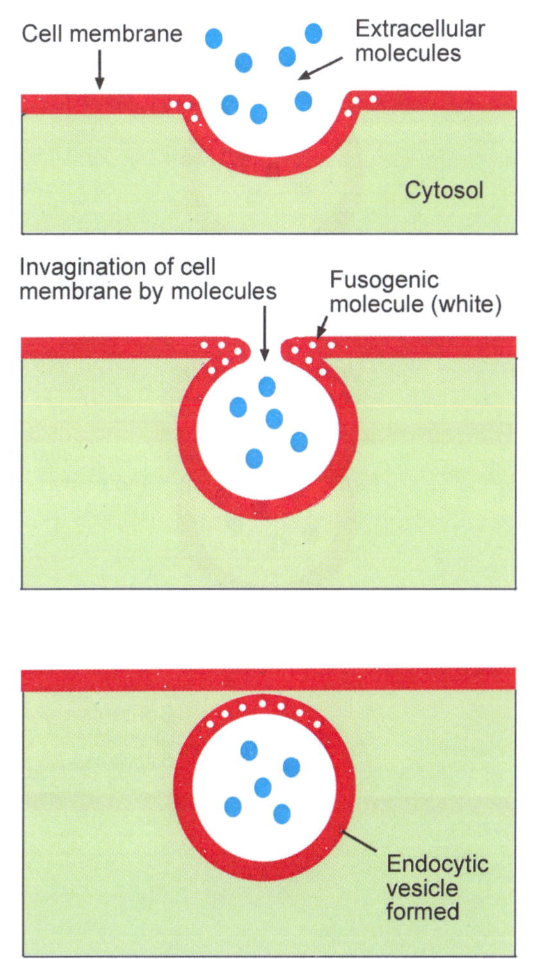

Fig. 6.5 Three stages in the absorption of extra-cellular molecules by endocytosis.

We have seen, above, that some molecules can enter cells by passing through passive channels in the cell membrane. Large molecules enter the cell by the process of ***endocytosis*** (Fig. 6.5). In this process the molecule invaginates a part of the cell membrane, which first surrounds the molecule, and then separates (from the rest of the cell membrane) to form an ***endocytic vesicle***. This vesicle can move through the cytosol to other parts of the cell.

The term ***pinocytosis*** is applied to a process similar to endocytosis when the vesicles (then called ***pinocytotic vesicles***) formed are used for absorption of fluids (or other small molecules) into the cell.

Some cells use the process of endocytosis to engulf foreign matter (e.g., bacteria). The process is then referred to as ***phagocytosis***.

Molecules produced within the cytoplasm (e.g., secretions) may be enclosed in membranes to form vesicles that approach the cell membrane and fuse with its

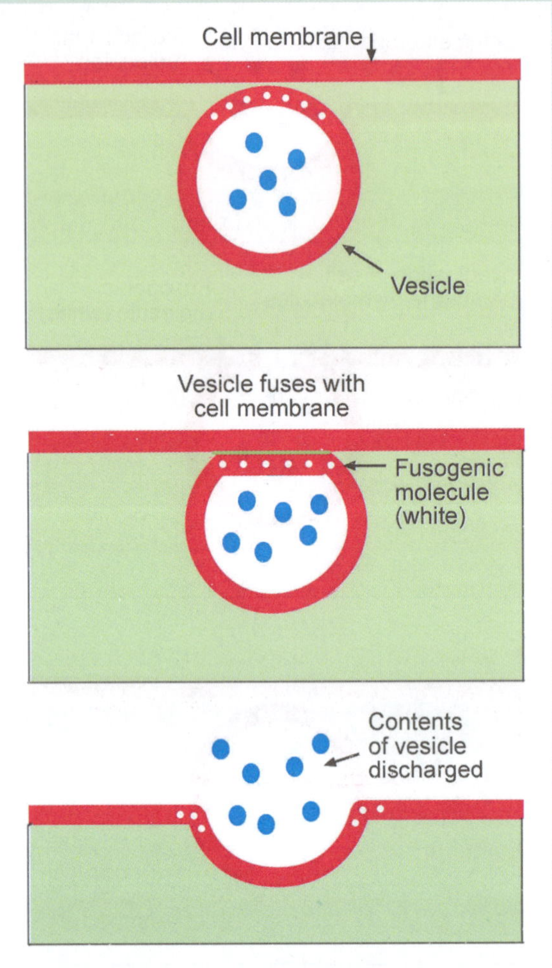

Fig. 6.6 Three stages in exocytosis. The fusogenic proteins facilitate adhesion of the vesicle to the cell membrane.

internal surface. The vesicle then ruptures releasing the molecule to the exterior. The vesicles in question are called ***exocytic vesicles***, and the process is called ***exocytosis*** or ***reverse pinocytosis*** (Fig. 6.6).

CELL ORGANELLES

We have seen that (apart from the nucleus) the cytoplasm of a typical cell contains various structures that are referred to as organelles. They include the endoplasmic reticulum, ribosomes, mitochondria, the Golgi complex, and various types of vesicles (Fig. 6.7). The cytosol also contains a cytoskeleton made up of microtubules, microfilaments, and intermediate filaments.

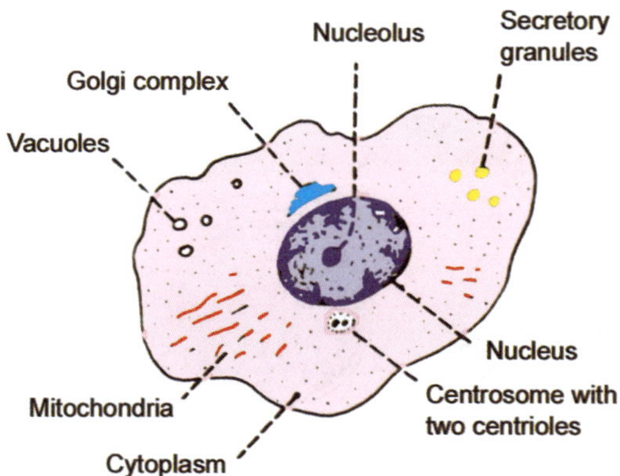

Fig. 6.7 Some features of a cell that can be seen with a light microscope.

Centrioles are closely connected with microtubules. We shall deal with these entities one by one.

Endoplasmic Reticulum

The cytoplasm of most cells contains a system of membranes that constitute the endoplasmic reticulum (ER). The membranes form the boundaries of channels that may be arranged in the form of flattened sacs (or cisternae) or of tubules.

Because of the presence of the ER the cytoplasm is divided into two components, one within the channels and one outside them (Fig. 6.8). The cytoplasm within the channels is called the ***vacuoplasm***, and that outside the channels is the ***hyaloplasm*** or ***cytosol***.

In most places the membranes forming the ER are studded with minute particles of RNA called ***ribosomes***. The presence of these ribosomes gives the membrane a rough appearance. Membranes of this type form what is called the rough (or granular) ER. In contrast some membranes are devoid of ribosomes and constitute the smooth or agranular ER (Fig. 6.8).

Rough ER represents sites at which proteins are synthesized. The attached ribosomes play an important role in this process.

Ribosomes

We have seen above that ribosomes are present in relation to rough ER. They may also lie free in the cytoplasm. They may be present singly in which case they are called ***monosomes***; or in groups which are referred to as ***polyribosomes*** (or ***polysomes***).

Mitochondria

Mitochondria can be seen with the light microscope in specially stained preparations. They are so called because they appear either as granules or as

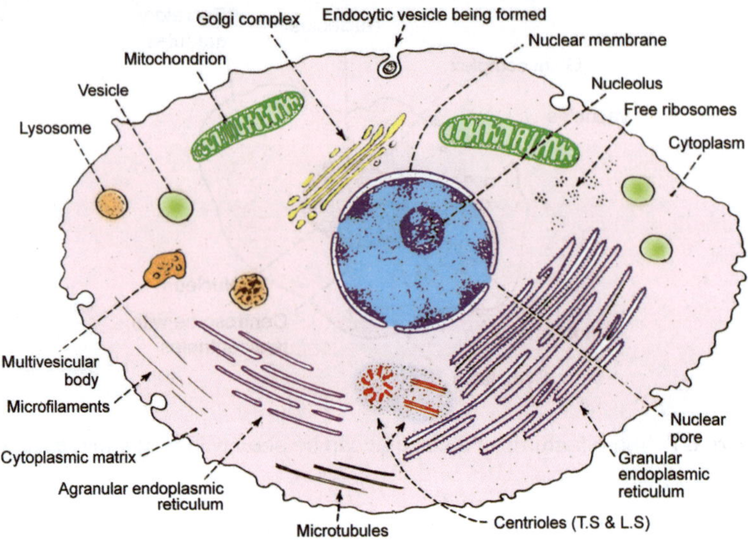

Fig. 6.8 Schematic diagram to show the various organelles to be found in a typical cell. The various structures shown are not drawn to scale.

rods (mitos = granule; chondrium = rod). The number of mitochondria varies from cell to cell being greatest in cells with high metabolic activity (e.g., in secretory cells). Mitochondria vary in size, most of them being 0.5 to 2 μm in length (μm=micrometer). Mitochondria are large in cells with a high oxidative metabolism.

A schematic presentation of some details of the structure of a mitochondrion (as seen by EM) is shown in Fig. 6.9. The mitochondrion is bounded by a smooth ***outer membrane*** within which there is an ***inner membrane***, the two being separated by an ***intermembranous space***. The inner membrane is highly folded on itself forming incomplete partitions called ***cristae***. The space bounded by the inner membrane is filled by a granular material called the ***matrix***. This matrix contains numerous enzymes. It also contains some RNA and DNA: these are believed to carry information that enables mitochondria to duplicate themselves during cell division. An interesting fact, discovered recently, is that all mitochondria are derived from those in the fertilized ovum, and are entirely of maternal origin.

Mitochondria are of great functional importance. They contain many enzymes including some that play an important part in Kreb's cycle (TCA cycle). ATP and GTP are formed in mitochondria from where they pass to other parts of the cell and provide energy for various cellular functions. These facts can be correlated with the observation that within a cell mitochondria tend to concentrate in regions where energy requirements are greatest.

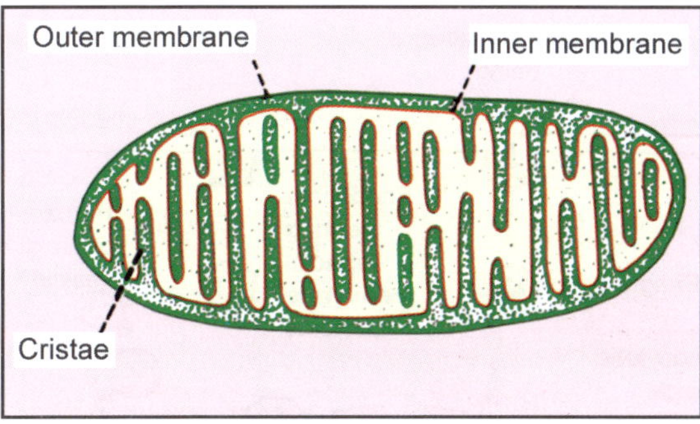

Fig. 6.9 Structure of a mitochondrion.

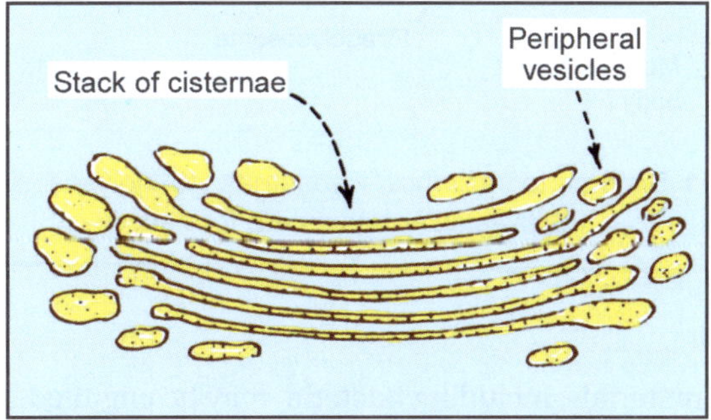

Fig. 6.10 Structure of the Golgi complex.

Golgi Complex

The Golgi complex (Golgi apparatus, or merely Golgi) was known to microscopists long before the advent of electron microscopy. In light microscopic preparations suitably treated with silver salts the Golgi complex can be seen as a small structure of irregular shape, usually present near the nucleus (Fig. 6.7).

When examined with the EM the complex is seen to be made up of membranes similar to those of smooth ER. The membranes form the walls of a number of flattened sacs that are stacked over one another. Towards their margins the sacs are continuous with small rounded vesicles (Fig. 6.10).

Membrane Bound Vesicles

The cytoplasm of a cell may contain several types of vesicles. The contents of any such vesicle are separated from the rest of the cytoplasm by a membrane which forms the wall of the vesicle.

Some vesicles serve to store material. Others transport material into or out of the cell, or from one part of a cell to another. Vesicles also allow exchange of membrane between different parts of the cell.

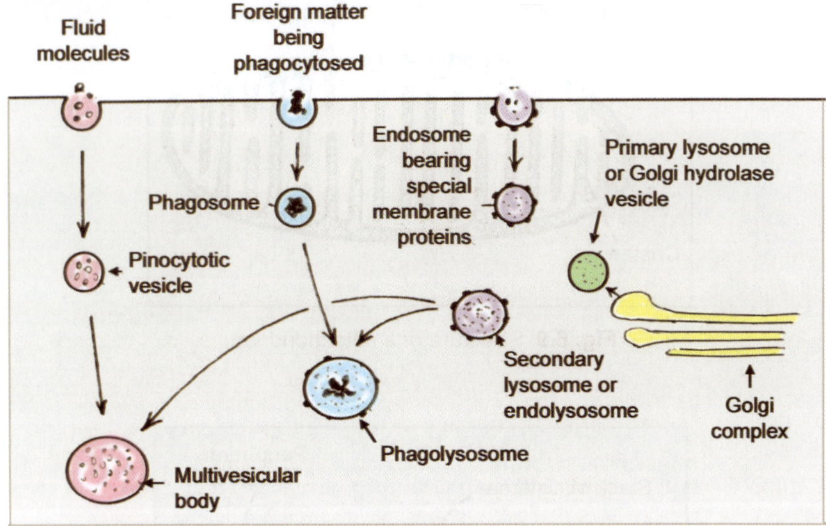

Fig. 6.11 Scheme to show how lysosomes, phagolysosomes and multivesicular bodies are formed.

Phagosomes

Solid 'foreign' materials, including bacteria, may be engulfed by a cell by the process of ***phagocytosis***. In this process the material is surrounded by a part of the cell membrane. This part of the cell membrane then separates from the rest of the plasma membrane and forms a free floating vesicle within the cytoplasm. Such membrane bound vesicles, containing solid ingested material are called ***phagosomes***.

Pinocytotic Vesicles

Some fluid may also be taken into the cytoplasm by a process similar to phagocytosis. In the case of fluids the process is called ***pinocytosis*** and the vesicles formed are called ***pinocytotic vesicles***.

Exocytic Vesicles

Just as material from outside the cell can be brought into the cytoplasm by phagocytosis or pinocytosis, materials from different parts of the cell can be transported to the outside by vesicles. Such vesicles are called ***exocytic vesicles***, and the process of discharge of cell products in this way is referred to as ***exocytosis*** (or ***reverse pinocytosis***).

Secretory Granules

The cytoplasm of secretory cells frequently contains what are called ***secretory granules***. These can be seen with the light microscope. With the EM each

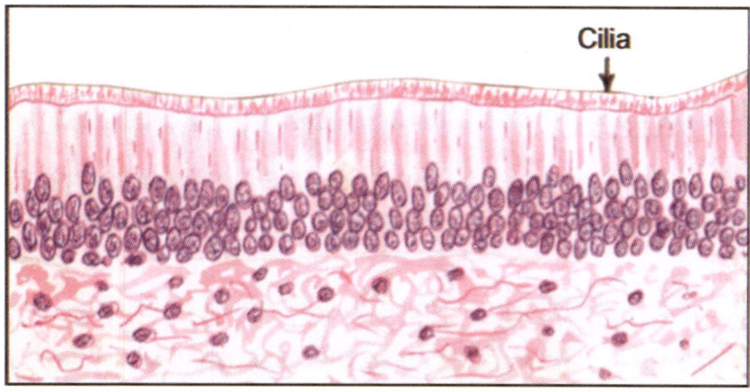

Fig. 6.12 Pseudostratified columnar epithelium showing cilia.

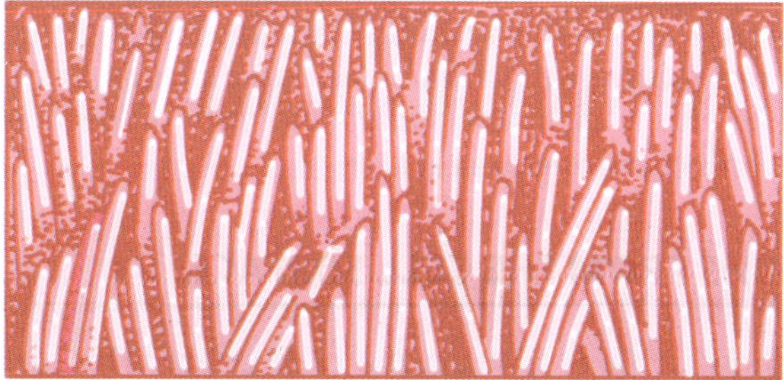

Fig. 6.13 Drawing of cilia as seen by scanning electronmicroscopy.

'granule' is seen to be a membrane bound vesicle containing secretion. The appearance, size and staining reactions of these secretory granules differ depending on the type of secretion. These vesicles are derived from the Golgi complex.

Lysosomes

These vesicles contain enzymes that can destroy unwanted material present within a cell. Such material may have been taken into the cell from outside (e.g., bacteria); or may represent organelles that are no longer of use to the cell (Fig. 6.11).

THE CYTOSKELETON

The cytoplasm is permeated by a number of fibrillar elements that collectively form a supporting network. This network is called the cytoskeleton. Apart from maintaining cellular architecture the cytoskeleton facilitates cell motility (e.g., by forming cilia), and helps to divide the cytosol into functionally discrete areas. It also facilitates transport of some constituents through the cytosol, and plays a role in anchoring cells to each other.

The elements that constitute the cytoskeleton consist of the following.

1. Microfilaments.
2. Microtubules.
3. Intermediate filaments.

Centrioles

All cells capable of division (and even some which do not divide) contain a pair of structures called centrioles. With the light microscope the two centrioles are seen as dots embedded in a region of dense cytoplasm which is called the ***centrosome***. With the EM the centrioles are seen to be short cylinders that lie at right angles to each other. When we examine a transverse section across a centriole (by EM) it is seen to consist essentially of a series of microtubules arranged in a circle. There are nine groups of tubules, each group consisting of three tubules.

Centrioles play an important role in the formation of various cellular structures that are made up of microtubules. These include the mitotic spindles of dividing cells, cilia, flagella, and some projections of specialised cells (e.g., the axial filaments of spermatozoa).

PROJECTIONS FROM THE CELL SURFACE

Many cells show projections from the cell surface. The various types of projections are described below.

Cilia

These can be seen, with the light microscope, as minute hair-like projections from the free surfaces of some epithelial cells (Fig. 6.12 to 6.14). In the living animal cilia can be seen to be motile.

Functional Significance of Cilia

The cilia lining an epithelial surface move in co-ordination with one another the total effect being that like a wave. As a result fluid, mucous, or small solid objects lying on the epithelium can be caused to move in a specific direction. Movements of cilia lining the respiratory epithelium help to move secretions in the trachea and bronchi towards the pharynx. Ciliary action helps in the movement of ova through the uterine tube, and of spermatozoa through the male genital tract.

Flagella

These are somewhat larger processes having the same basic structure as cilia. In the human body the best example of a flagellum is the tail of the spermatozoon.

Microvilli

Microvilli are finger-like projections from the cell surface that can be seen by EM (Fig. 6.15). Each microvillus consists of an outer covering of plasma

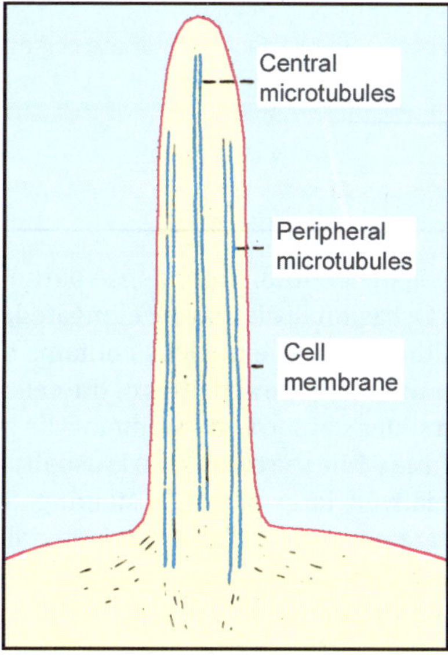

Fig. 6.14 Longitudinal section through a cilium.

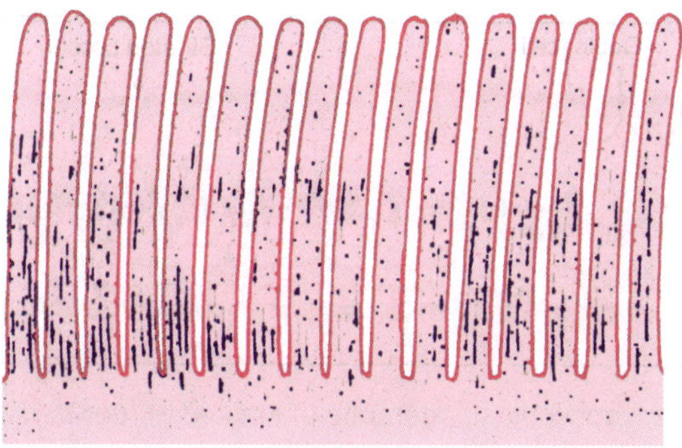

Fig. 6.15 Microvilli as seen in longitudinal section. The regular arrangement of microvilli is characteristic of the striated border of intestinal absorptive cells.

membrane and a cytoplasmic core in which there are numerous microfilaments (actin filaments).

With the light microscope the free borders of cells lining the small intestine appear to be thickened: the thickening has striations perpendicular to the surface. This ***striated border*** of light microscopy (Fig. 6.16) has been shown by EM to be made up of long microvilli arranged parallel to one another.

In some cells the microvilli are not arranged so regularly. With the light microscope the microvilli of such cells give the appearance of a ***brush border***.

Microvilli greatly increase the surface area of the cell and are, therefore, seen most typically at sites of active absorption e.g., the intestine, and the proximal and distal convoluted tubules of the kidneys.

THE NUCLEUS

The nucleus constitutes the central, more dense part of the cell. It is usually rounded or ellipsoid. Occasionally it may be elongated, indented or lobed. It is usually 4-10 μm in diameter. The nucleus contains inherited information which is necessary for directing the activities of the cell as we shall see below.

In usual class room slides stained with haematoxylin and eosin, the nucleus stains dark purple or blue while the cytoplasm is usually stained pink. In some cells the nuclei are relatively large and light staining. Such nuclei appear to be made up of a delicate network of fibres: the material making up the fibres of the network is called ***chromatin*** (because of its affinity for dyes). At some places (in the nucleus) the chromatin is seen in the form of irregular dark masses that are called ***heterochromatin***. At other places the network is loose and stains lightly: the chromatin of such areas is referred to as ***euchromatin***. Nuclei which are large and in which relatively large areas of euchromatin can be seen are referred to as ***open-face nuclei.*** Nuclei which are made up mainly of heterochromatin are referred to as ***closed-face nuclei*** (Fig. 6.17).

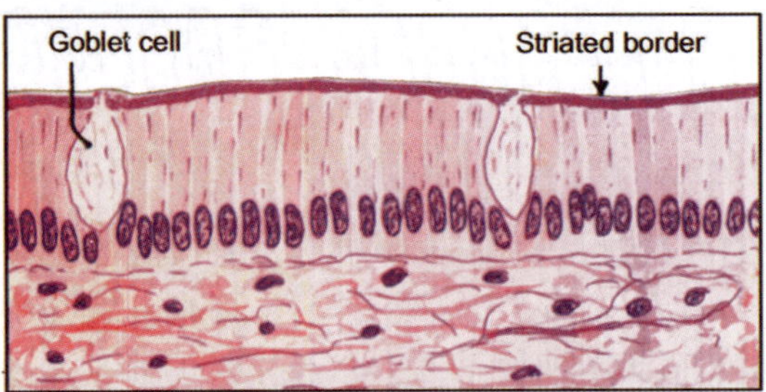

Fig. 6.16 Light microscopic appearance of striated border formed by microvilli.

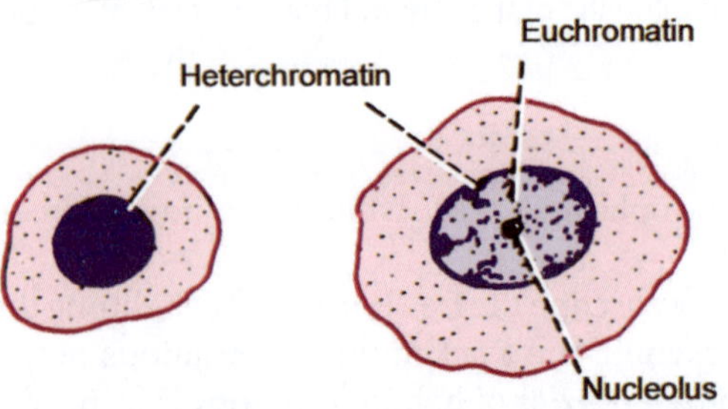

Fig. 6.17 Comparison of a heterochromatic nucleus (left), and a euchromatic nucleus (right).

In addition to the masses of heterochromatin (which are irregular in outline), the nucleus shows one or more rounded, dark staining bodies called ***nucleoli*** (See below). The nucleus also contains various small granules, fibres and vesicles (of obscure function). The spaces between the various constituents of the nucleus described above are filled by a base called the ***nucleoplasm***.

With the EM the nucleus is seen to be surrounded by a double layered ***nuclear membrane*** or ***nuclear envelope***. At several points the inner and outer layers of the nuclear membrane fuse leaving gaps called ***nuclear pores***. Nuclear pores represent sites at which substances can pass from the nucleus to the cytoplasm and vice versa (Fig. 6.8).

Nature and Significance of Chromatin

In recent years there has been a considerable advance in our knowledge of the structure and significance of chromatin. It is made up of a substance called ***deoxyribonucleic acid*** (usually abbreviated to DNA); and of proteins.

Heterochromatin represents areas where chromatin fibres are tightly coiled on themselves forming 'solid' masses. In contrast euchromatin represents areas where coiling is not so marked. During cell division the entire chromatin within the nucleus becomes very tightly coiled and takes on the appearance of a number of short, thick, rod-like structures called ***chromosomes***. Chromosomes are made up of DNA and proteins. Proteins stabilise the structure of chromosomes.

Nucleoli

We have seen that nuclei contain one or more nucleoli. These are spherical and about 1-3 μm in diameter. They stain intensely both with haematoxylin and eosin, the latter giving them a slight reddish tinge. In ordinary preparations they can be distinguished from heterochromatin by their rounded shape. (In contrast masses of heterochromatin are very irregular). Nucleoli are larger and more distinct in cells that are metabolically active.

Using histochemical procedures that distinguish between DNA and RNA it is seen that the nucleoli have a high RNA content.

Nucleoli are sites where ribosomal RNA is synthesized. This RNA leaves the nucleolus, passes through a nuclear pore, and enters the cytoplasm where it takes part in protein synthesis.

CHROMOSOMES

Haploid and Diploid Chromosomes

We have seen that during cell division the chromatin network in the nucleus becomes condensed into a number of thread-like or rod-like structures called chromosomes. The number of chromosomes in each cell is fixed for a given species, and in man it is 46. This is referred to as the ***diploid number*** (diploid = double). However, in spermatozoa and in ova the number is only half the diploid number i.e., 23: this is called the ***haploid number*** (haploid = half).

Autosomes and Sex Chromosomes

The 46 chromosomes in each cell can again be divided into 44 ***autosomes*** and two ***sex chromosomes***. The sex chromosomes may be of two kinds, X or Y. In a man there are 44 autosomes, one X chromosome, and one Y chromosome; while in a woman there are 44 autosomes and two X chromosomes in each cell. When we study the 44 autosomes we find that they really consist of 22 pairs, the two chromosomes forming a pair being exactly alike (***homologous chromosomes***). In a woman the two X chromosomes form another such pair; but in a man this pair is represented by one X and one Y chromosome. We shall see later that one chromosome of each pair is obtained (by each individual) from the mother, and one from the father.

As the two sex chromosomes of a female are similar the female sex is described as ***homogametic***; in contrast the male sex is ***heterogametic***.

Significance of Chromosomes

Each cell of the body contains within itself a store of information that has been inherited from precursor cells. This information (which is necessary for the proper functioning of the cell) is stored in chromatin. Each chromosome bears on itself a very large number of functional segments that are called ***genes***. Genes represent 'units' of stored information which guide the performance of particular cellular functions, which may in turn lead to the development of particular features of an individual or of a species. Recent researches have told us a great deal about the way in which chromosomes and genes store and use information.

The nature and functions of a cell depend on the proteins synthesized by it. Proteins are the most important constituents of our body. They make up the greater part of each cell and of intercellular substances. Enzymes, hormones, and antibodies are also proteins.

It is, therefore, not surprising that one cell differs from another because of the differences in the proteins that constitute it. Individuals and species also owe their distinctive characters to their proteins. We now know that chromosomes control the development and functioning of cells by determining what type of proteins will be synthesized within them.

Chromosomes are made up predominantly of a nucleic acid called ***deoxyribonucleic acid*** (or ***DNA***), and all information is stored in molecules of this substance. When the need arises this information is used to direct the activities of the cell by synthesizing appropriate proteins. To understand how this becomes possible we must consider the structure of DNA in some detail.

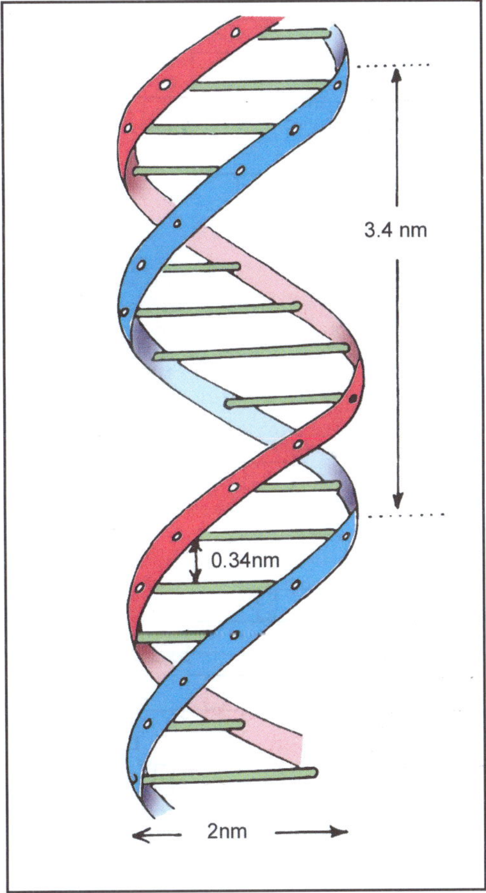

Fig. 6.18 Diagram showing part of a DNA molecule arranged in the form of a double helix.

Basic Structure of DNA

DNA in a chromosome is in the form of very fine fibres. If we look at one such fibre it has the appearance shown in Fig. 6.18. It is seen that each fibre consists of two strands that are twisted spirally to form what is called a ***double helix***. The two strands are linked to each other at regular intervals.

Each strand of the DNA fibre consists of a chain of ***nucleotides***. Each nucleotide consists of a sugar, deoxyribose, a molecule of phosphate and a base (Fig. 6.19). The phosphate of one nucleotide is linked to the sugar of the next nucleotide (Fig. 6.20).

The base which is attached to the sugar molecule may be adenine, guanine, cytosine or thymine. The two strands of a DNA fibre are joined together by the linkage of a base on one strand with a base on the opposite strand (Fig. 6.21).

This linkage is peculiar in that adenine on one strand is always linked to thymine on the other strand, while cytosine is always linked to guanine. Thus the two strands are complementary and the arrangement of bases on one strand can be predicted from the other.

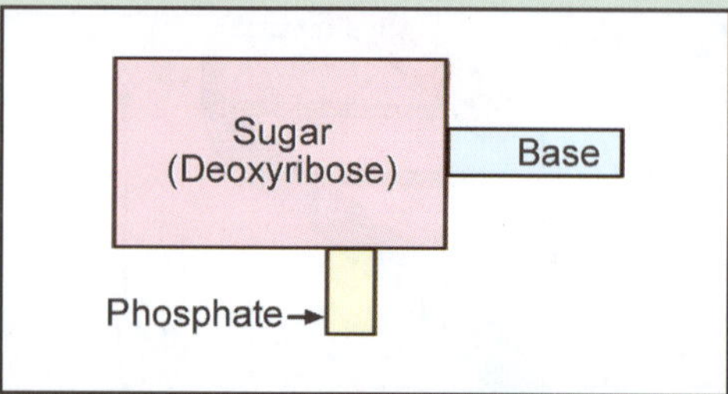

Fig. 6.19 Composition of a nucleotide. The base may be adenine, cytosine, guanine or thymine.

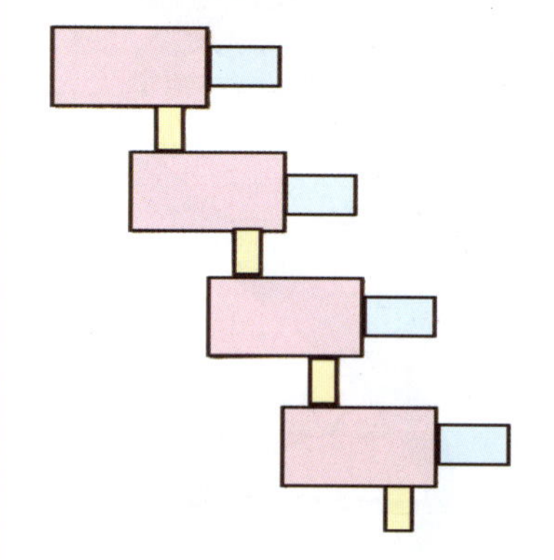

Fig. 6.20 Linkage of nucleotides to form one strand of a DNA molecule.

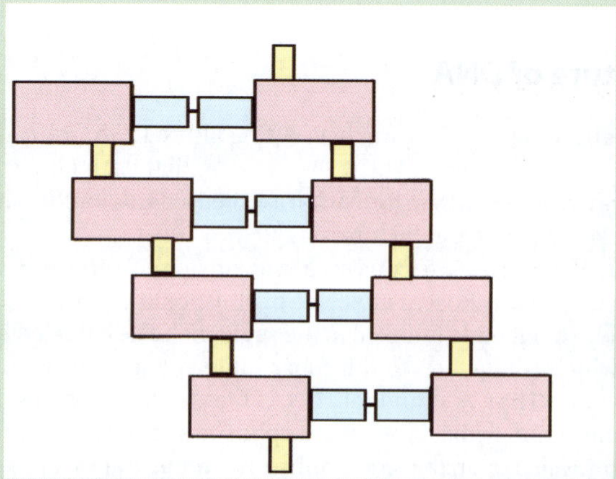

Fig. 6.21 Linkage of two chains of nucleotides to form part of a DNA molecule.

The order in which these four bases are arranged along the length of a strand of DNA determines the nature of the protein that can be synthesized under its influence. Every protein is made up of a series of amino acids; the nature of the protein depending upon the amino acids present, and the sequence in which they are arranged. Amino acids may be obtained from food or may be synthesized within the cell. Under the influence of DNA these amino acids are linked together in a particular sequence to form proteins.

Ribonucleic Acid (RNA)

In addition to DNA, cells contain another important nucleic acid called ***ribonucleic acid*** or ***RNA***. The structure of a molecule of RNA corresponds fairly closely to that of one strand of a DNA molecule, with the following important differences.

a. RNA contains the sugar ribose instead of deoxyribose.
b. Instead of the base thymine it contains uracil.

RNA is present both in the nucleus and in the cytoplasm of a cell. It is present in three main forms namely ***messenger RNA*** (***mRNA***), ***transfer RNA*** (***tRNA***) and ***ribosomal RNA***. Messenger RNA acts as an intermediary between the DNA of the chromosome and the amino acids present in the cytoplasm, and plays a vital role in the synthesis of proteins from amino acids.

Synthesis of Protein

We have seen that a protein is made up of amino acids that are linked together in a definite sequence. This sequence is determined by the order in which the bases are arranged in a strand of DNA. Each amino acid is represented in the DNA molecule by a sequence of three bases (***triplet code***) (Fig. 6.22). It has been mentioned earlier that there are four bases in all in DNA, namely adenine, cytosine, thymine and guanine. These are like letters in a word. They can be arranged in various combinations so that as many as sixty four code 'words' can be formed from these four bases. There are only about twenty amino acids that have to be coded for so that each amino acid has more than one code. The code words for some amino acids are shown in Fig. 6.22. The code for a complete polypeptide chain is formed when the codes for its constituent amino acids are arranged in proper sequence. That part of the DNA molecule that bears the code for a complete polypeptide chain constitutes a ***structural gene*** or ***cistron***.

At this stage it must be emphasised that a chromosome is very long and thread-like. Only short lengths of the fibre are involved in protein synthesis at a particular time.

The main steps in the synthesis of a protein may now be summarised as follows (Fig. 6.23).

1. The two strands of a DNA fibre separate from each other (over the area bearing a particular cistron) so that the ends of the bases that were linked to the opposite strand are now free.
2. A molecule of messenger RNA is synthesized using one DNA strand as a guide (or ***template***), in such a way that one guanine base is formed opposite each cytosine base of the DNA strand, cytosine is formed opposite guanine, adenine is formed opposite thymine, and uracil is formed opposite adenine. In this way the code for the sequence in which amino acids are to be linked is passed on from DNA

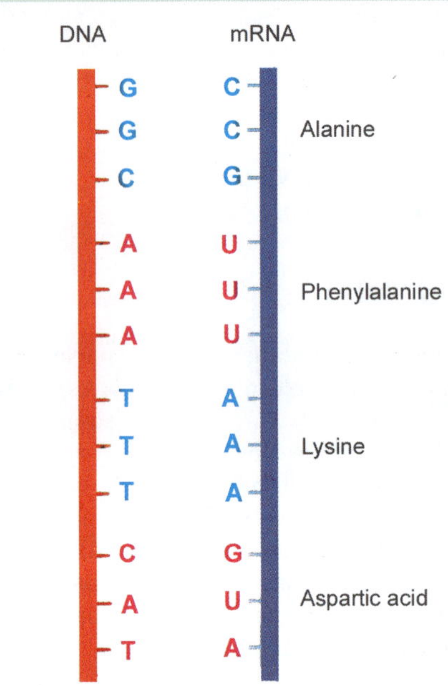

Fig. 6.22 Codes for some amino acids made up of the bases adenine (A), cytosine (C), guanine (G), and thymine (T) on a DNA molecule. When this code is transferred to messenger RNA, cytosine is formed opposite guanine (and vice versa), adenine is formed opposite thymine, while uracil (U)is formed opposite adenine.

of the chromosome to messenger RNA. This process is called ***transcription***. [Transcription takes place under the influence of the enzyme RNA polymerase.] That part of the messenger RNA strand that bears the code for one amino acid is called a ***codon***.

3. This molecule of messenger RNA now separates from the DNA strand and moves from the nucleus to the cytoplasm (passing through a nuclear pore).
4. In the cytoplasm the messenger RNA becomes attached to a ribosome.
5. As mentioned earlier the cytoplasm also contains another form of RNA called transfer RNA. In fact there are about twenty different types of transfer RNA each corresponding to one amino acid. On one side transfer RNA becomes attached to an amino acid. On the other side it bears a code of three bases (***anticodon***) that are complementary to the bases coding for its amino acid on messenger RNA. Under the influence of the ribosome several units of transfer RNA, alongwith their amino acids, become arranged along side the strand of messenger RNA in the sequence determined by the code on messenger RNA. This process is called ***translation***.
6. The amino acids now become linked to each other to form a polypeptide chain. From the above it will be clear that the amino acids are linked up exactly in the order in which their codes are arranged on messenger RNA, which in turn is based on the code on the DNA molecule (but also see below). Chains of amino acids formed in this way constitute polypeptide chains. Proteins are formed by union of polypeptide chains.

The flow of information from DNA to RNA and finally to protein has been described as the "central dogma of molecular biology".

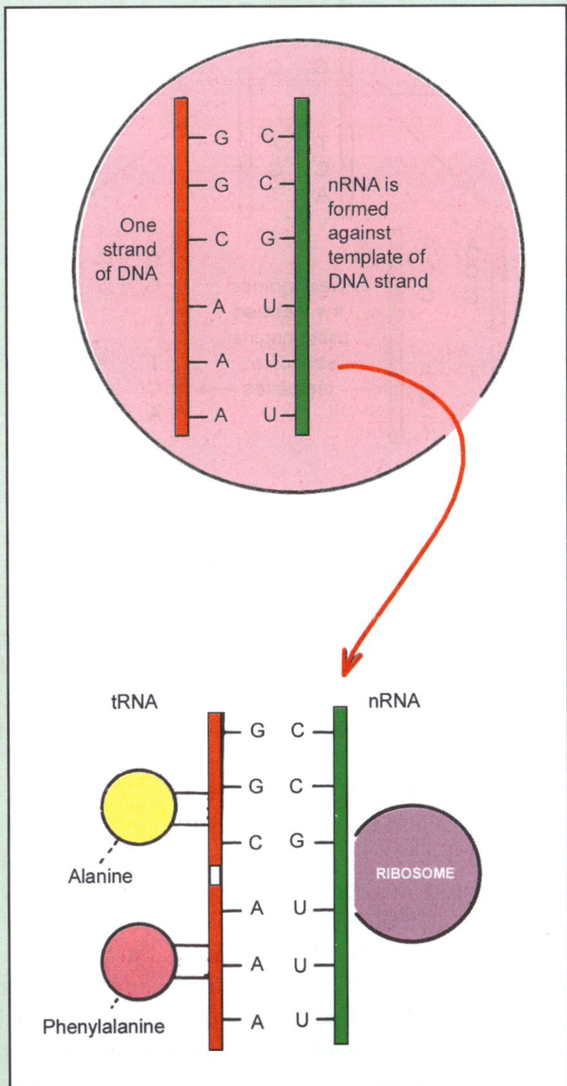

Fig. 6.23 Simplified scheme to show how proteins are synthesized under the influence of DNA. The process is actually more complex as explained in the text.

Role of Ribosomes in Protein Synthesis

Ribosomes play an essential part in protein synthesis. They 'read' the code on mRNA and help to arrange units of tRNA in proper sequence.

Proteins that are to form secretions enter the lumen of rough ER. They pass into the lumen of smooth ER, and then (through vesicles) to the Golgi complex. After being appropriately processed in the Golgi complex they are packaged into vesicles and are discharged from the cell by exocytosis.

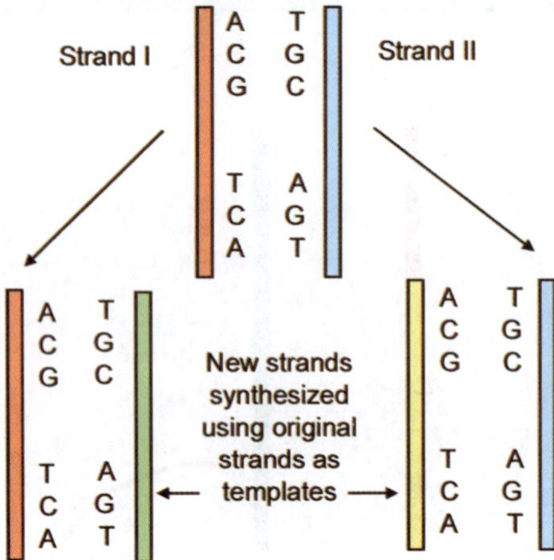

Fig. 6.24 Scheme to show how a DNA molecule is duplicated.

Duplication of Chromosomes

One of the most remarkable properties of chromosomes is that they are able to duplicate themselves. From the foregoing discussion on the structure of chromosomes it is clear that duplication of chromosomes involves the duplication (or replication) of DNA. This takes place as follows (Fig. 6.24).

1. The two strands of the DNA molecule to be duplicated unwind and separate from each other so that their bases are 'free'.
2. A new strand is now synthesized opposite each original strand of DNA in such a way that adenine is formed opposite thymine, guanine is formed opposite cytosine, and *vice versa*. This new strand becomes linked to the original strand of DNA to form a new molecule. As the same process has taken place in relation to each of the two original strands, we now have two complete molecules of DNA. It will be noted that each molecule has one strand that belonged to the original molecule and one strand that is new. It will also be noted that the two molecules formed are identical to the original molecule.

Structure of Fully Formed Chromosomes

Each chromosome consists of two parallel rod-like elements that are called ***chromatids*** (Fig. 6.25). The two chromatids are joined to each other at a narrow area which is light staining and is called the ***centromere*** (or ***kinetochore***). In this region the chromatin of each chromatid is most highly coiled and, therefore, appears to be thinnest. The chromatids appear to be 'constricted' here and this region is called the ***primary constriction***. Typically the centromere is not midway between the two ends of the chromatids, but somewhat towards one end. As a result each chromatid can be said to have a ***long arm*** and a ***short arm***. Such chromosomes are described as being ***submetacentric*** (when the

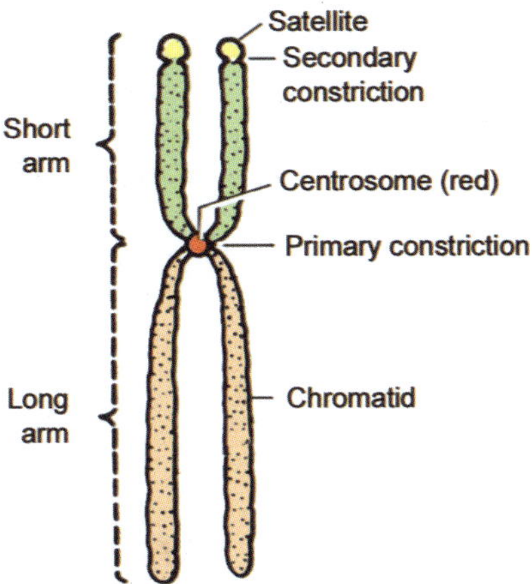

Fig. 6.25 Diagram to show the terms applied to some parts of a typical chromosome. Note that this chromosome is submetacentric.

two arms are only slightly different in length); or as ***acrocentric*** (when the difference is marked) (Fig. 6.26). In some chromosomes the two arms are of equal length: such chromosomes are described as ***metacentric***. Finally, in some chromosomes the centromere may lie at one end: such a chromosome is described as ***telocentric***.

Differences in the total length of chromosomes, and in the position of the centromere are important factors in distinguishing individual chromosomes from each other. Additional help in identification is obtained by the presence in some chromosomes of ***secondary constrictions***. Such constrictions lie near one end of the chromatid. The part of the chromatid 'distal' to the constriction may appear to be a rounded body almost separate from the rest of the chromatid: such regions are called ***satellite bodies***. (Secondary constrictions are concerned with the formation of nucleoli and are, therefore, called ***nucleolar organizing centres***). Considerable help in identification of individual chromosomes is also obtained by the use of special staining procedures by which each chromatid can be seen to consist of a number of dark and light staining transverse bands.

We have noted that chromosomes are distinguishable only during mitosis. In the interphase (between successive mitoses) the chromosomes elongate and assume the form of long threads. These threads are called ***chromonemata*** (Singular = ***chromonema***).

Karyotyping

Using the criteria described above it is now possible to identify each chromosome individually and to map out the chromosomes of an individual. This procedure is called karyotyping. For this purpose a sample of blood from the individual is put into a suitable medium in which lymphocytes can multiply. After a few hours a drug (colchicin, colcemide) that arrests cell division at a stage when chromosomes are most distinct is added to the medium. The dividing cells are then treated with hypotonic saline so that they swell up. This facilitates the proper spreading out of chromosomes. A suspension containing the dividing cells is spread out on a slide and suitably stained. Cells in which the chromosomes are well spread out (without overlap) are photographed. The photographs are cut up and the chromosomes arranged in proper sequence. In this way a map of chromosomes is obtained, and abnormalities in their number or form can be identified. In many cases specific chromosomal abnormalities can be correlated with specific diseases.

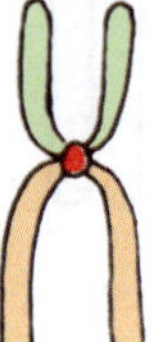

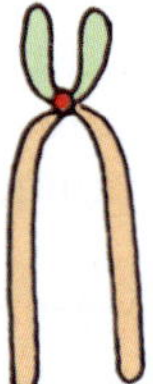

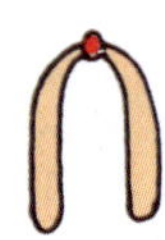

Fig. 6.26 Nomenclature used for different types of chromosomes, based on differences in lengths of the two arms of each chromatid.

CELL DIVISION

Multiplication of cells takes place by division of preexisting cells. Such multiplication constitutes an essential feature of embryonic development. Cell multiplication is equally necessary after birth of the individual for growth and for replacement of dead cells.

We have seen that the chromosomes within the nuclei of cells carry genetic information that controls the development and functioning of various cells and tissues and, therefore, of the body as a whole. When a cell divides it is essential that the whole of the genetic information within it be passed on to both the daughter cells resulting from the division.

In other words the daughter cells must have chromosomes identical in number and in genetic content to those in the mother cell. This type of cell division is called ***mitosis***.

A different kind of cell division called ***meiosis*** occurs during the formation of gametes. This consists of two successive divisions called the first and second meiotic divisions. The cells resulting from these divisions (i.e., the gametes) differ from other cells in the body in that:

a. the number of chromosomes is reduced to half the normal number, and
b. the genetic information in the various gametes produced is not identical.

MITOSIS

Many cells of the body have a limited span of functional activity at the end of which they undergo division into two daughter cells. The daughter cells in turn have their own span of activity followed by another division. The period during which the cell is actively dividing is the phase of mitosis. The period between two successive divisions is called the ***interphase***.

Mitosis is conventionally divided into a number of stages called ***prophase, metaphase, anaphase*** and ***telophase***. The later part of prophase is also called ***prometaphase***. The sequence of events of the mitotic cycle is best understood by starting with a cell in telophase. At this stage each chromosome consists of a single chromatid (Fig. 6.27G). With the progress of telophase the chromatin of the chromosome uncoils and elongates and the chromosome can no longer be identified as such. However, it is believed to retain its identity during the interphase (which follows telophase). This is shown diagrammatically in Fig. 6.27A. During the interphase the DNA content of the chromosome is duplicated so that another chromatid identical to the original one is formed: the chromosome is now made up of two chromatids (Fig. 6.27B). When mitosis begins (i.e., during the prophase) the chromatin of the chromosome becomes gradually more and more coiled so that the chromosome become recognizable as a thread-like structure that gradually acquires a rod-like appearance (Fig. 6.27C). Towards the end of prophase the two chromatids constituting the chromosome become distinct (Fig. 6.27D) and the chromosome now has the typical structure described above.

While the changes described above are occurring in the chromosomes a number of other events are taking place. The two centrioles separate and move to opposite poles of the cell. They produce a number of microtubules that pass from one centriole to the other and form a ***spindle***. Tubules radiating from each centriole create a star-like appearance or ***aster***. The spindle and the two asters collectively form the ***diaster*** (also called ***amphiaster*** or ***achromatic spindle***). Meanwhile the nuclear membrane breaks down and the nucleoli disappear (Fig. 6.27D). With the formation of the spindle the chromosomes move to a position midway between the two centrioles (i.e., at the equator of the cell) where each chromosome becomes attached to microtubules of the spindle by its centromere. This stage is referred to as ***metaphase*** (Fig. 6.27E). The plane along which the chromosomes lie during metaphase is the ***equatorial plate***.

In the ***anaphase*** the centromere of each chromosome splits longitudinally into two so that the chromatids now become independent chromosomes. At this stage the cell can be said to contain 46 pairs of chromosomes. One chromosome of each such pair now moves along the spindle to either pole of the cell (Fig. 6.27F). This is followed by telophase in which two daughter nuclei are formed by appearance of nuclear membranes around them. The chromosomes gradually elongate and become indistinct. Nucleoli reappear. The centriole is duplicated at this stage or in early interphase (Fig. 6.27G).

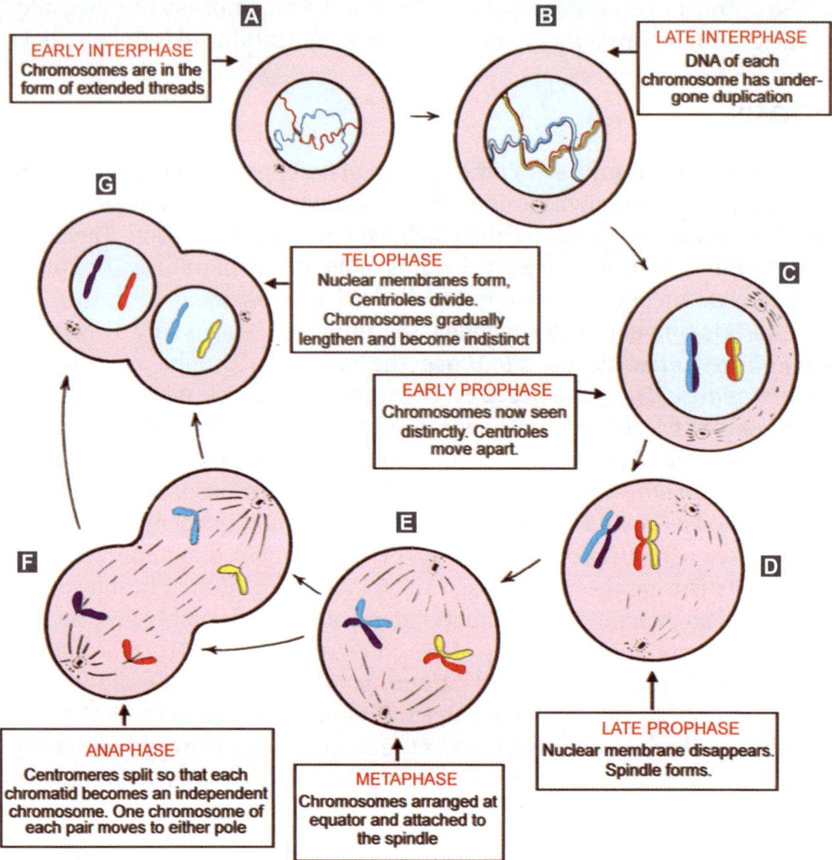

Fig. 6.27 Scheme to show the main steps in mitosis.

The division of the nucleus is accompanied by the division of the cytoplasm. In this process the organelles are presumably duplicated and each daughter cell comes to have a full complement of them. The cleavage into two separate cells is referred to as ***cytokinesis***.

The rate of cell division varies from tissue to tissue, being greatest in those epithelia which lose cells because of friction (e.g., the epidermis and the lining cells of the intestine). The rate varies with demand becoming much greater during repair after injury. The rate is precisely controlled to correlate with demand. Failure of such control results in uncontrolled growth leading to formation of tumours. Abnormalities in mitosis may be produced by exposure to various radiations, the most important being nuclear radiation. Mitosis can be arrested by chemicals. One of them is colchicin (or colcemide). It stops mitosis at metaphase and allows us to study chromosomes at this stage.

Some cells do not undergo mitosis (neurons, cardiac muscle cells). Some cells (e.g., those of the liver) do not normally divide. This may divide to replace cell damage by disease.

MEIOSIS

As already stated meiosis consists of two successive divisions called the first and second meiotic divisions. During the interphase preceding the first division duplication of the DNA content of the chromosomes takes place as in mitosis.

First Meiotic Division

The prophase of the first meiotic division is prolonged and is usually divided into a number of stages as follows.

a. ***Leptotene***: The chromosomes become visible (as in mitosis). Although each chromosome consists of two chromatids these cannot be distinguished at this stage (Fig. 6.28A). During leptotene the chromosomes gradually become thicker and shorter.

b. ***Zygotene***: We have seen that the 46 chromosomes in each cell consist of 23 pairs (the X and Y chromosomes of the male being taken as a pair). The two chromosomes of each pair come to lie parallel to each other, and are closely apposed. This pairing of chromosomes is also referred to as ***synapsis*** or ***conjugation***. The two chromosomes together constitute a ***bivalent*** (Fig. 6.28B).

c. ***Pachytene***: The two chromatids of each chromosome become distinct. The bivalent now has four chromatids in it and is called a ***tetrad***. There are two central and two peripheral chromatids, one from each chromosome (Fig. 6.28C). An important event now takes place. The two central chromatids (one belonging to each chromosome of the bivalent) become coiled over each other so that they cross at a number of points. This is called ***crossing over***. For sake of simplicity only one such crossing is shown in Fig. 6.28D. At the site where the chromatids cross they become adherent: the points of adhesion are called ***chiasmata***.

d. ***Diplotene***: The two chromosomes of a bivalent now try to move apart. As they do so the chromatids 'break' at the points of crossing and the 'loose' pieces become attached to the opposite chromatid. This results in exchange of genetic material between these chromatids. A study of Fig. 6.28E will show that as a result of this ***crossing over*** of genetic material each of the four chromatids of the tetrad now has a distinctive genetic content.

The metaphase follows. As in mitosis the 46 chromosomes become attached to the spindle at the equator, the two chromosomes of a pair being close to each other (Fig. 6.29A).

The anaphase differs from that in mitosis in that there is no splitting of the centromeres. One entire chromosome of each pair moves to each pole of the spindle (Fig. 6.29B). The resulting daughter cells, therefore, have 23 chromosomes, each made up of two chromatids (Fig. 6.29C).

The telophase is similar to that in mitosis.

The first meiotic division is followed by a short interphase. This differs from the usual interphase in that there is no duplication of DNA. Such duplication is unnecessary as the chromosomes of the cells resulting from the first meiotic division already possess two chromatids each (Fig. 6.29C).

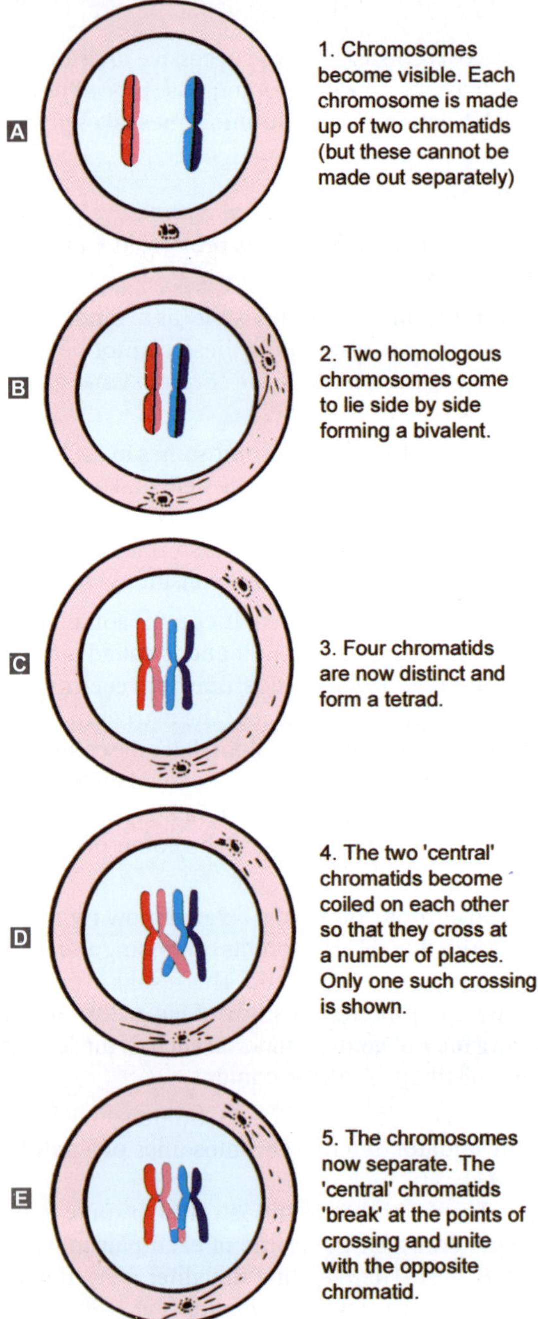

Fig. 6.28 Stages in the prophase of the first meiotic division.

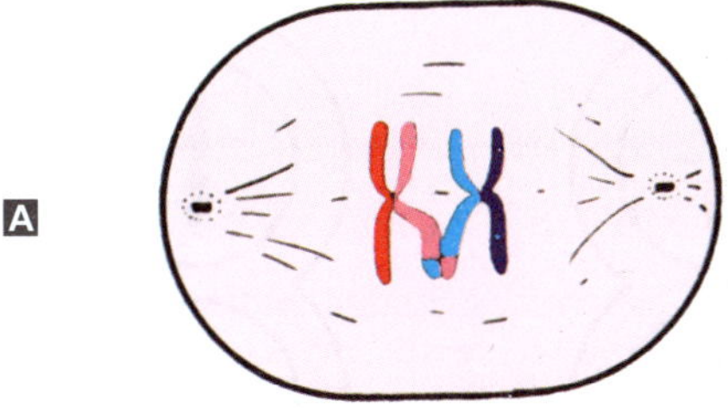

METAPHASE

The nuclear membrane disappears. Spindle forms and chromosomes are attached to it by their centromeres.

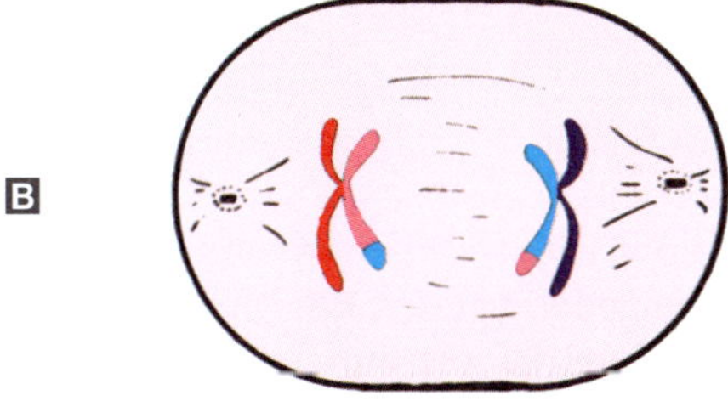

ANAPHASE

One entire chromosome of the pair moves to either pole. Note that the centromeres do not divide.

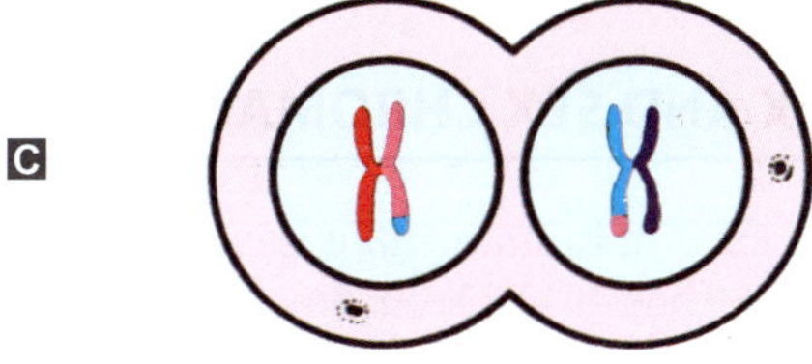

TELOPHASE

Note that the chromosomes in each cell have been reduced to the haploid number

Fig. 6.29 Metaphase (A), anaphase (B), and telophase (C) of the first meiotic division.

Second Meiotic Division

The second meiotic division is usually said to be similar to mitosis, as there is no reduction in chromosome number. However, the DNA content of the daughter cells is reduced to half. Because of the crossing over that has occurred during the first division, the daughter cells are not identical in genetic content (Fig. 6.30). These reasons make the second meiotic division different from a typical mitosis.

At this stage it may be repeated that the 46 chromosomes of a cell consist of 23 pairs, one chromosome of each pair being derived from the mother and one from the father.

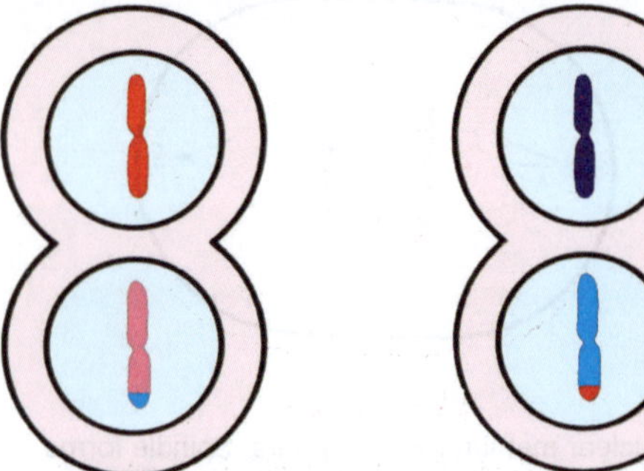

Fig. 6.30 Daughter cells resulting from the second meiotic division. The daughter cells are not alike because of the crossing over during the first division.

During the first meiotic division the chromosomes derived from the father and those derived from the mother are distributed between the daughter cells entirely at random. This, along with the phenomenon of crossing over, results in thorough shuffling of the genetic material so that the cells produced as a result of various meiotic divisions (i.e., ova and spermatozoa) all have a distinct genetic content. A third step in this process of genetic shuffling takes place at fertilization when there is a combination of randomly selected spermatozoa and ova. It is, therefore, not surprising that no two persons (except identical twins) are alike.

CHROMOSOMAL SEX AND SEX CHROMATIN

We have seen that each cell of a human male has 44+X+Y chromosomes; and that each cell of a female has 44+X+X chromosomes. We have also seen that during the formation of gametes by meiosis the chromosome number is reduced to half. As a result all ova contain 22+X chromosomes. Spermatozoa are of two types. Some have the chromosomal constitution 22+X and the others have the constitution 22+Y. If an ovum is fertilised by a sperm bearing an X-chromosome the resulting child has (22+X)+(22+X) = 44+X+X chromosomes and is a girl. On the other hand if an ovum is fertilised by a sperm bearing a Y-chromosome the child has (22+X)+(22+Y) = 44+X +Y chromosomes and is a boy.

Of the two X-chromosomes in a female only one is functionally active. The other (inactive) X-chromosome forms a mass of hetero-chromatin that lies just under the nuclear membrane (Fig. 6.31). This mass of heterochromatin can be identified in suitable preparations and can be useful in determining whether a particular tissue belongs to a male or a female. Because of this association with sex this mass of heterochromatin is called the ***sex chromatin***. It is also called a ***Barr-body*** after the name of the scientist who discovered it. In some cells the sex chromatin occupies a different position from that described above. In neurons it forms a rounded mass lying very close to the nucleolus and is, therefore, called a ***nucleolar satellite***. In neutrophil leucocytes it may appear as an isolated round mass attached to the rest of the nucleus by a narrow band, thus resembling the appearance of a ***drumstick***.

In some cases the sex of an individual may not be clear (at birth) because of abnormalities in the genital organs. In such cases the true sex of the individual may be determined by looking for the sex chromatin. Methods are also available for identifying the Y-chromosome in cells. However, the best thing to do is to make a karyotype.

ABNORMAL CELL GROWTH AND TUMOURS

Normally, cell multiplication is a controlled process and is just sufficient for replacing dead cells, for growth in children, or for repair of wounds and injuries.

Sometimes cell multiplication goes out of control and cells in an organ keep multiplying when more cells are not needed. These cells form an abnormal mass that is called a ***tumour*** or ***neoplasm***.

In some tumours, growth is slow. The cells formed resemble normal cells of the tissue from which they originate (i.e., they are well differentiated). Surrounding connective tissue forms a capsule around the tumour. The tumour remains confined to one organ. Such tumours are said to be ***benign***. They can cause problems by pressure on surrounding structures.

In other tumours the cells grow rapidly, and do not acquire characteristics of normal cells (i.e., they remain undifferentiated). Such tumours can invade adjoining structures. These are called ***malignant*** tumours. A malignant tumour arising from an epithelial cell is called a ***carcinoma*** (cancer). A malignant tumour arising from connective tissue cells is called a ***sarcoma***. Some cells of the tumour can get detached and can travel to lymph nodes through lymphatic vessels. They can also spread to other organs, through blood, and can start growing there forming secondary growths or metastases.

In many cases there is no obvious cause for formation of a carcinoma. Some chemical substances can stimulate cancer formation and are called carcinogens. Other causes are exposure to some radiations (e.g., X-rays, and radiations from radioactive substances). Some viruses can also cause cancer.

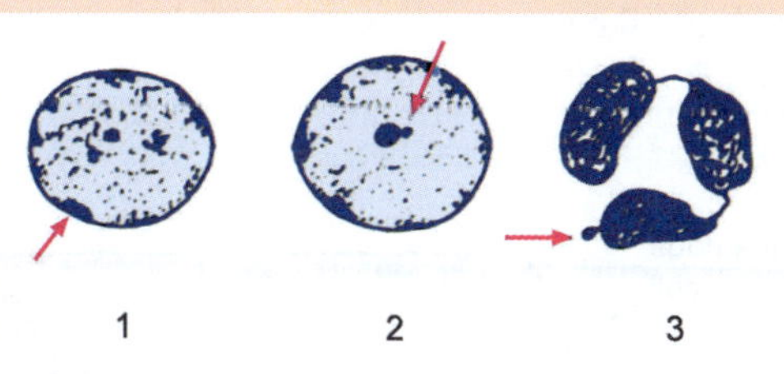

Fig. 6.31 Sex chromatin. 1. Typical position deep to the nuclear membrane. 2. As a nucleolar satellite in neurons. 3. As an appendage shaped like a drum-stick in neutrophil leucocytes. Only the nuclei are drawn.

CHAPTER 7

Epithelia and Glands

The outer surface of the body and the luminal surfaces of cavities within the body are lined by one or more layers of cells that completely cover them. Such layers of cells are called ***epithelia*** (singular=epithelium). Epithelia also line the ducts and secretory elements of glands (which develop as outgrowths from epithelium lined surfaces).

CLASSIFICATION OF EPITHELIA

An epithelium may consist of only one layer of cells when it is called a ***unilayered*** or ***simple*** epithelium. Alternatively, it may be ***multi-layered*** or ***stratified***.

Simple epithelia may be further classified according to the shape of the cells constituting them.

1. In some epithelia the cells are flattened, their height being very little as compared to their width. Such an epithelium is called a ***squamous epithelium*** (Figs. 7.1, 7.2).
2. When the height and width of the cells of the epithelium are more or less equal (i.e., they look like squares in section) it is described as a ***cuboidal epithelium*** (Figs. 7.9, 7.10).

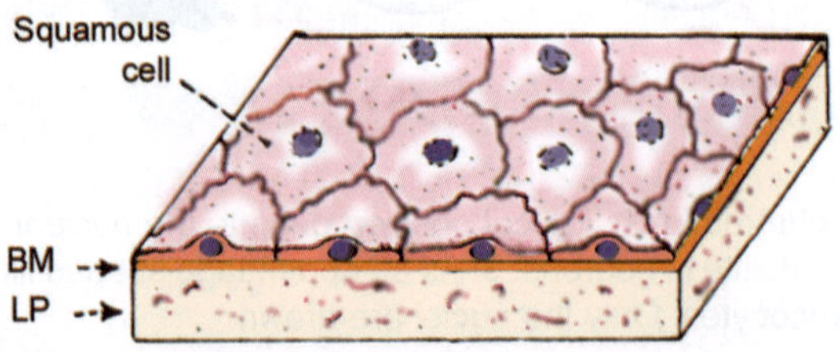

Fig. 7.1 Simple squamous epithelium (diagrammatic). BM= Basement membrane; LP= Lamina propria.

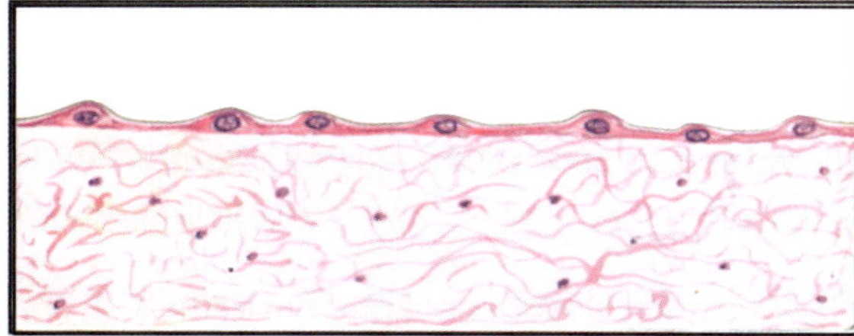

Fig. 7.2 Simple squamous epithelium as seen in a section.

3. When the height of the cells of the epithelium is distinctly greater than their width, it is described as a ***columnar epithelium*** (Figs. 7.3, 7.4).

Multi-layered epithelia are of two main types. In the most common type the deeper layers are columnar, but in proceeding towards the surface of the epithelium the cells become increasingly flattened (or squamous). Such an epithelium is described as ***stratified squamous*** (Fig. 7.15). It may be noted that all cells in this kind of epithelium are not squamous. In the other type of multilayered epithelium all layers are made up of cuboidal, polygonal or rounded cells. The cells towards the surface of the epithelium are not flattened. This type of epithelium is called ***transitional epithelium*** (being transitional

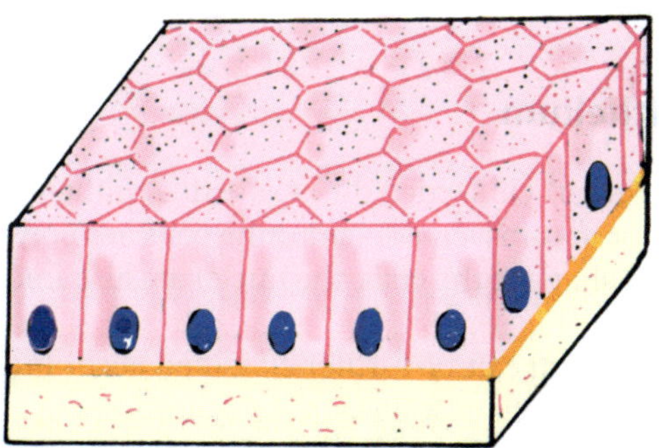

Fig. 7.3 Simple columnar epithelium (diagrammatic). Note the basally placed oval nuclei. The cells appear hexagonal in surface view.

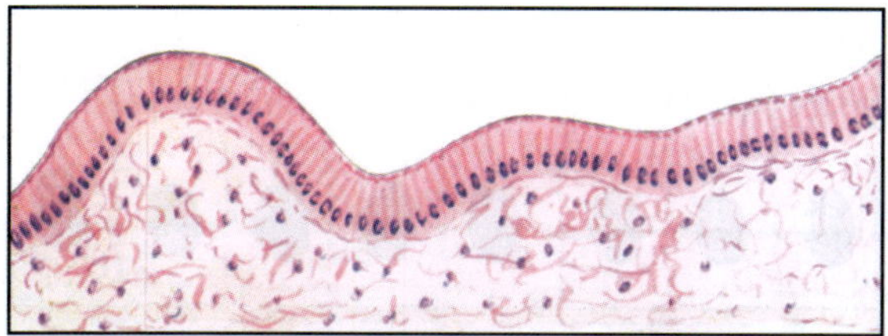

Fig. 7.4 Simple columnar epithelium as seen in a section.

between unilayered epithelia and stratified squamous epithelium) (Fig. 7.17). As transitional epithelium is confined to the urinary tract it is also called ***urothelium***.

A third, rather rare type of multilayered epithelium is made up of two or more layers of cuboidal or columnar cells (***stratified cuboidal*** or ***stratified columnar*** epithelium). Lastly, in some situations a columnar epithelium which is really single layered may give the appearance of a stratified epithelium: such an epithelium is referred to as ***pseudostratified columnar epithelium*** (Figs. 7.13, 7.14).

The various types of epithelia named above are considered further below. All epithelia rest on a very thin ***basement membrane***.

Squamous Epithelium

The cytoplasm of cells in this kind of epithelium forms only a thin layer. The nuclei produce bulgings of the cell surface (Figs. 7.1, 7.2). In surface view the cells have polygonal outlines that interlock with those of adjoining cells.

Squamous epithelium lines the alveoli of the lungs. It lines the free surface of the serous pericardium, of the pleura, and of the peritoneum: here it is called ***mesothelium***. It lines the inside of the heart, where it is called ***endocardium***; and of blood vessels and lymphatics, where it is called ***endothelium***. Squamous epithelium is also found lining some parts of the renal tubules, and in some parts of the internal ear.

Columnar Epithelium

We have seen that in vertical section the cells of this epithelium are rectangular. On surface view (or in transverse section) the cells are polygonal. In keeping with the elongated shape of the cells, the nuclei are also frequently elongated (Figs. 7.3, 7.4).

Columnar epithelium can be further classified according to the nature of the free surfaces of the cells as follows.

a. In some situations the cell surface has no particular specialization: this is ***simple columnar epithelium***.
b. In some situations the cell surface bears cilia. This is ***ciliated columnar epithelium*** (Fig. 7.5).

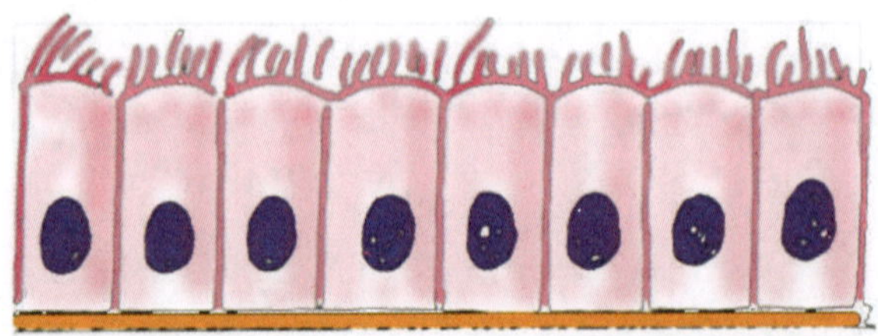

Fig. 7.5 Columnar epithelium showing cilia (diagrammatic).

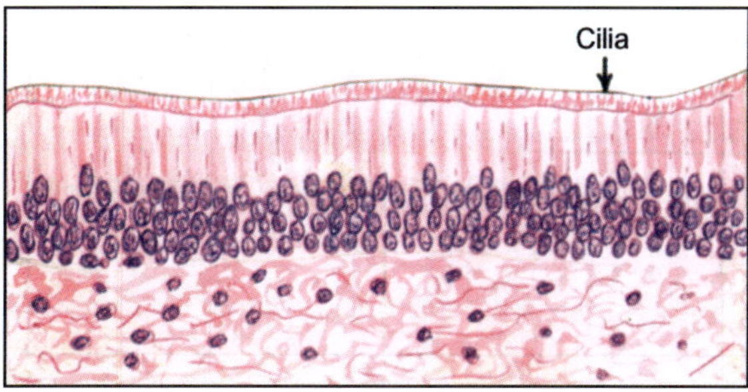

Fig. 7.6 Ciliated epithelium (pseudostratified columnar) as seen in a section.

c. In other situations the surface is covered with microvilli. Although the microvilli are visible only with the EM, with the light microscope the region of the microvilli is seen as a ***striated border*** (when the microvilli are arranged regularly)(Fig. 7.7) or as a ***brush border*** (when the microvilli are irregularly placed).

Some columnar cells have a secretory function. The apical parts of their cytoplasm contain secretory vacuoles.

Simple columnar epithelium (without cilia or microvilli) is present over the mucous membrane of the stomach and the large intestine.

Columnar epithelium with a striated border is seen most typically in the small intestine, and with a brush border in the gall bladder.

Ciliated columnar epithelium lines most of the respiratory tract, the uterus, and the uterine tubes. It is also seen in the efferent ductules of the testis, parts of the middle ear and auditory tube; and in the ependyma lining the central canal of the spinal cord and the ventricles of the brain. In the respiratory tract the cilia move mucous accumulating in the bronchi (and containing trapped dust particles) towards the larynx and pharynx. When excessive this mucous is brought out as sputum during coughing. In the uterine tubes the movements of the cilia help in the passage of ova towards the uterus.

Secretory columnar cells are scattered in the mucosa of the stomach and intestines. In the intestines many of them secrete mucous which accumulates in the apical part of the cell making it very light staining. These cells acquire a characteristic shape (Fig. 7.8) and are called ***goblet cells***. Some columnar cells secrete enzymes.

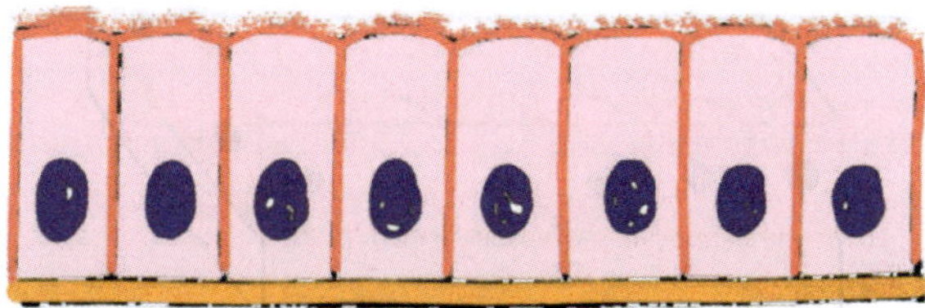

Fig. 7.7 Columnar epithelium showing a striated border made up of microvilli (diagrammatic).

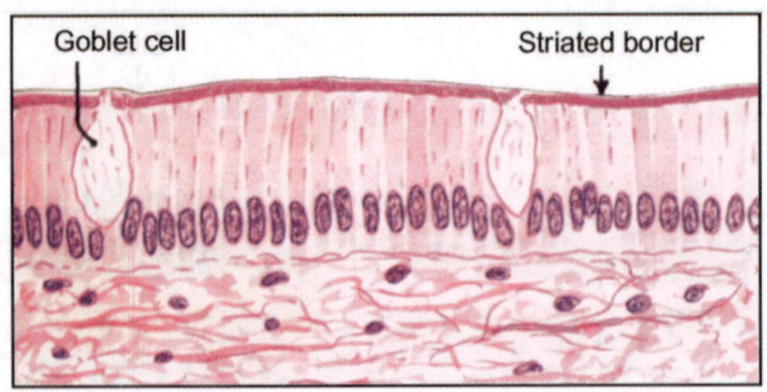

Fig. 7.8 Columnar epithelium with striated border as seen in a section.

Cuboidal Epithelium

Cuboidal epithelium is similar to columnar epithelium, but for the fact that the height of the cells is about the same as their width. The nuclei are usually rounded (Figs. 7.9, 7.10).

A typical cuboidal epithelium may be seen in the follicles of the thyroid gland, in the ducts of many glands, and on the surface of the ovary (where it is called ***germinal epithelium***). Other sites are the choroid plexuses, the inner surface of the lens, and the pigment cell layer of the retina.

An epithelium that is basically cuboidal (or columnar) lines the secretory elements of many glands. In this situation, however, the parts of the cells nearest the lumen are more compressed (against neighbouring cells) than at their bases, giving them a triangular shape (Figs. 7.11, 7.12).

A cuboidal epithelium with a prominent brush border is seen in the proximal convoluted tubules of the kidneys.

Pseudostratified Columnar Epithelium

In usual class-room slides the boundaries between epithelial cells are often not clearly seen. In spite of this we can make out what type of epithelium it is. This is because the shape and spacing of the nuclei gives a good idea of where the cell boundaries must lie.

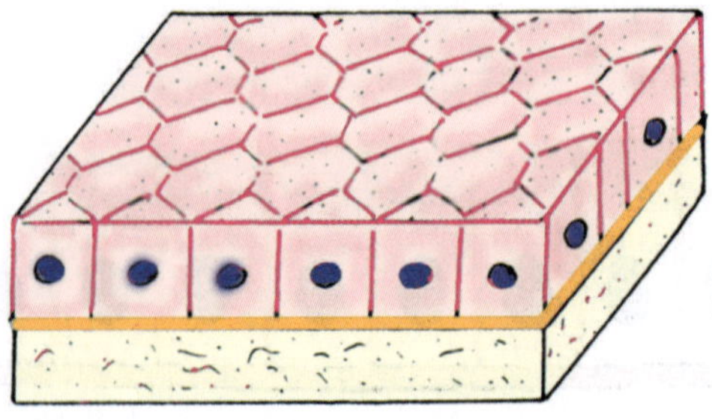

Fig. 7.9 Simple cuboidal epithelium (diagrammatic). Note that the cells appear cuboidal in section and hexagonal in surface view.

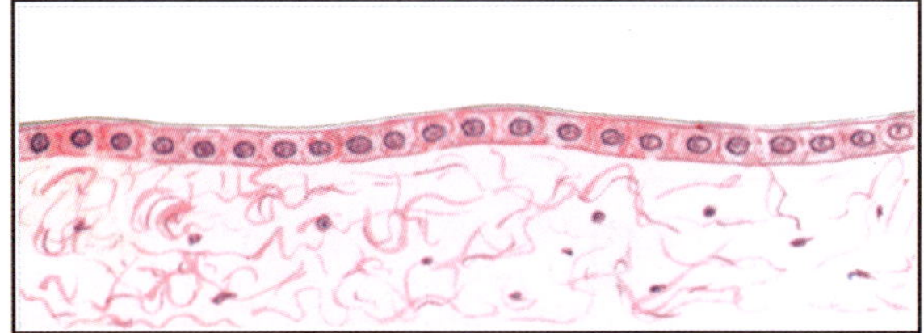

Fig. 7.10 Simple cuboidal epithelium as seen in a section.

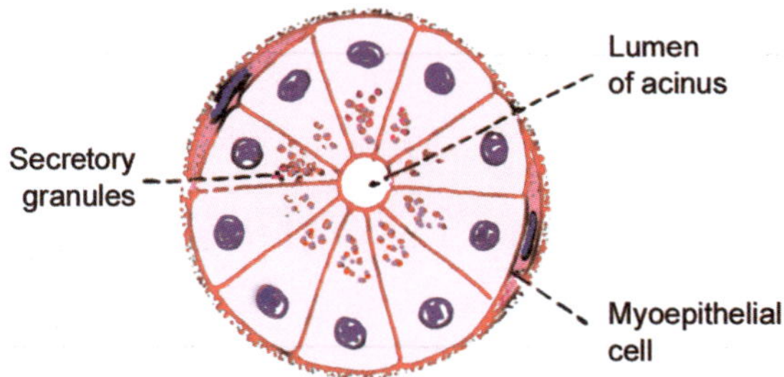

Fig. 7.11 Modified columnar cells in the wall of an acinus (of a gland) (diagrammatic). Note the triangular shape of the cells, the presence of secretory granules, and the myoepithelial cells lying between the gland cells and the basement membrane.

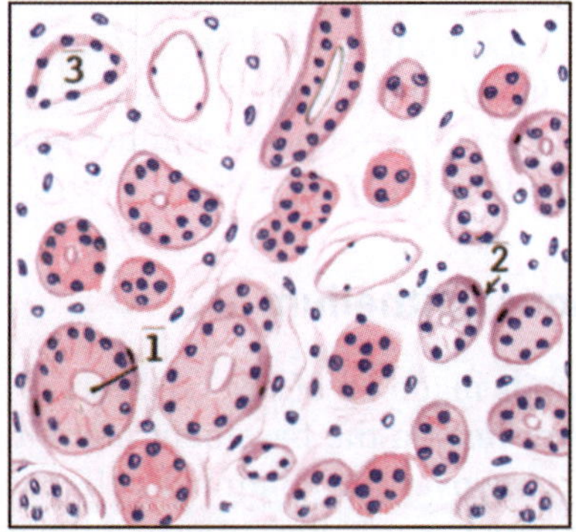

Fig. 7.12 Section through lacrimal gland showing acini of the kind described in Fig. 7.11.

Normally, in columnar epithelium the nuclei lie in a row, towards the bases of the cells. Sometimes, however, the nuclei appear to be arranged in two or more layers giving the impression that the epithelium is more than one cell thick (Fig. 7.14). The reason for this will be understood easily from Fig. 7.13. It is seen that there is actually only one layer of cells, but some cells are broader near the base, and others near the apex. The nuclei lie in the broader part of each cell and are, therefore, not in one layer. To distinguish this kind of

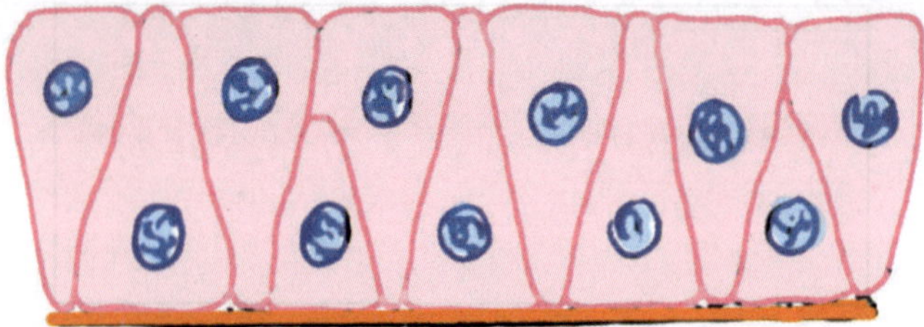

Fig. 7.13 Pseudostratified columnar epithelium (diagrammatic). This figure explains why the nuclei lie at various levels.

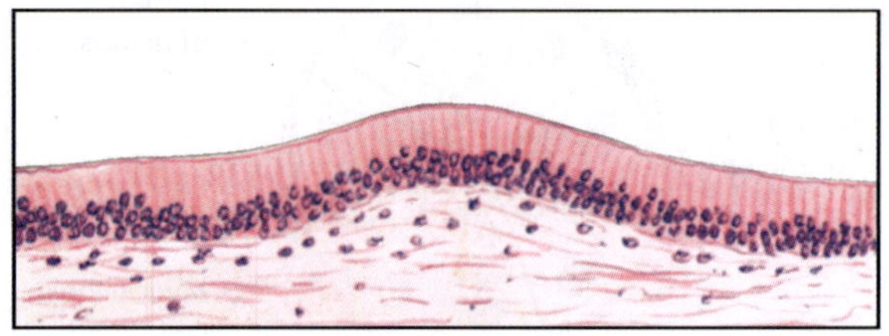

Fig. 7.14 Realistic appearance of pseudostratified columnar epithelium as seen in a section.

epithelium from a true stratified epithelium, it is referred to as ***pseudostratified columnar epithelium***.

A pseudostratified columnar epithelium is found in some parts of the auditory tube, the ductus deferens, and the male urethra (membranous and penile parts). A ciliated pseudostratified columnar epithelium is seen in the trachea and in large bronchi (Fig. 7.6).

Stratified Squamous Epithelium

This type of epithelium is made up of several layers of cells. The cells of the deepest (or basal) layer rest on the basement membrane: they are usually columnar in shape. Lying over the columnar cells there are polyhedral or cuboidal cells. As we pass towards the surface of the epithelium these cells become progressively more flat, so that the most superficial cells consist of flattened squamous cells (Figs. 7.15, 7.16).

Stratified squamous epithelium can be divided into two types: ***non-keratinized*** and ***keratinized***. In situations where the surface of the epithelium remains moist, the most superficial cells are living and nuclei can be seen in them. This kind of epithelium is described as non-keratinized. In contrast, at places where the epithelial surface is dry (as in the skin) the most superficial cells die and lose their nuclei. These cells contain a substance called ***keratin***, which forms a non-living covering over the epithelium. This kind of epithelium constitutes keratinized stratified squamous epithelium.

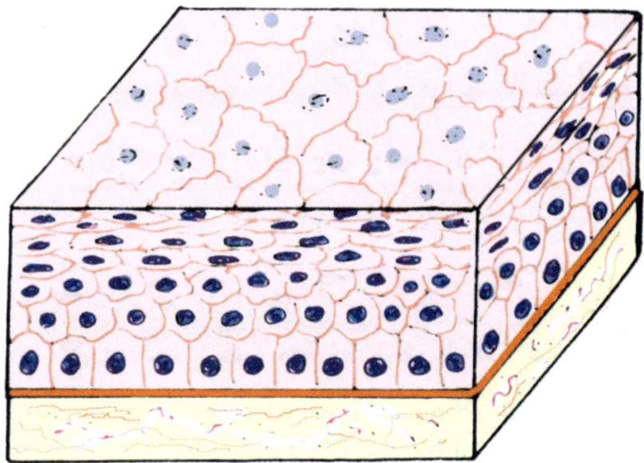

Fig. 7.15 Stratified squamous epithelium. There is a basal layer of columnar cells that rests on the basement membrane. Overlying the columnar cells of this layer there are a few layers of polygonal cells or rounded cells. Still more superficially, the cells undergo progressive flattening, becoming squamous.

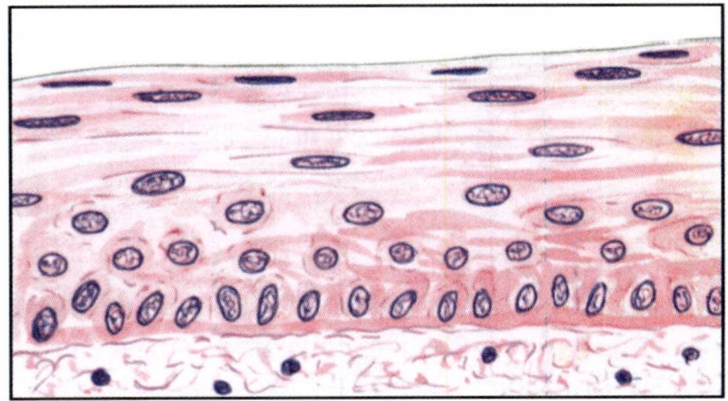

Fig. 7.16 Stratified squamous epithelium (non-keratinized) as seen in a section.

Stratified squamous epithelium (both keratinized and non-keratinized) is found over those surfaces of the body that are subject to friction. As a result of friction the most superficial layers are constantly being removed and are replaced by proliferation of cells from the basal (or germinal) layer. This layer, therefore, shows frequent mitoses.

Keratinized stratified squamous epithelium covers the skin of the whole of the body and forms the epidermis. Non-keratinized stratified squamous epithelium is seen lining the mouth, the tongue, the pharynx, the oesophagus, the vagina and the cornea. Under pathological conditions the epithelium in any of these situations may become keratinized.

Transitional Epithelium

This is a multi-layered epithelium and is 4 to 6 cells thick. It differs from stratified squamous epithelium in that the cells at the surface are not squamous.

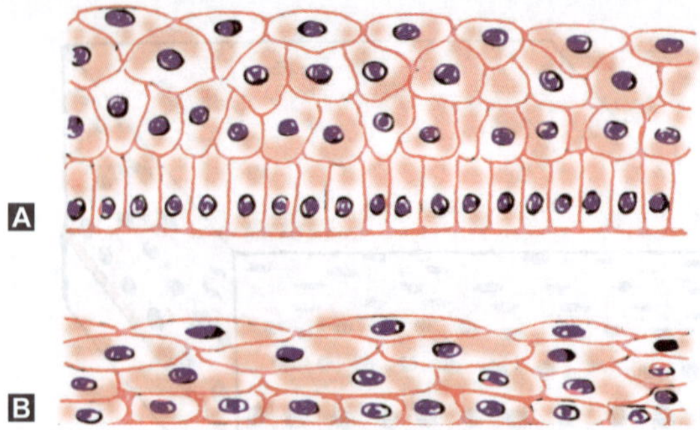

Fig. 7.17 Transitional epithelium (diagrammatic) in unstretched (A), and in stretched (B) conditions.

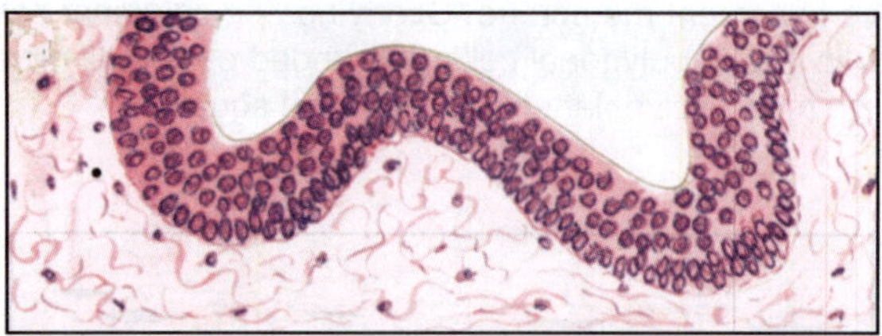

Fig. 7.18 Realistic appearance of transitional epithelium as seen in a section.

The deepest cells are columnar or cuboidal. The middle layers are made up of polyhedral or pear-shaped cells. The cells of the surface layer are large and often shaped like an umbrella (Fig. 7.17).

Transitional epithelium is found in the renal pelvis and calyces, the ureter, the urinary bladder, and part of the urethra. Because of this distribution it is also called ***urothelium***. In the urinary bladder it is seen that transitional epithelium can be stretched considerably without being damaged. When stretched it appears to be thinner and the cells become flattened or rounded.

Mucous Membranes

We have seen that epithelia line many tubular structures within the body. In such structures the epithelium rests on a layer of connective tissue called the ***lamina propria*** (or ***corium***). The layer of epithelium along with its lamina propria is referred to as the ***mucous membrane*** or ***mucosa*** (as its surface is kept moist by secretions of mucous glands).

In the intestines the mucous membrane has a third layer formed by a thin stratum of smooth muscle. This smooth muscle is called the ***muscularis mucosae*** (= muscle of the mucous membrane).

GLANDS

We have seen that some epithelial cells may be specialized to perform a secretory function. Such cells, present singly or in groups, constitute glands.

From this it is obvious that some glands are ***unicellular***. Unicellular glands are interspersed amongst other (non-secretory) epithelial cells. They can be found, for example, in the epithelium lining the intestines.

Most glands are, however, ***multicellular***. Such glands develop as diverticula from epithelial surfaces. The 'distal' parts of the diverticula develop into secretory elements, while the 'proximal' parts form ducts through which secretions reach the epithelial surface.

Those glands that pour their secretions on to an epithelial surface, directly or through ducts are called ***exocrine glands*** (or ***externally secreting glands***). Some glands lose all contact with the epithelial surface from which they develop: they pour their secretions into blood. Such glands are called ***endocrine glands***, ***internally secreting glands***, or ***duct-less glands***.

When all the secretory cells of an exocrine gland discharge into one duct the gland is said to be a ***simple gland***. Sometimes there are a number of groups

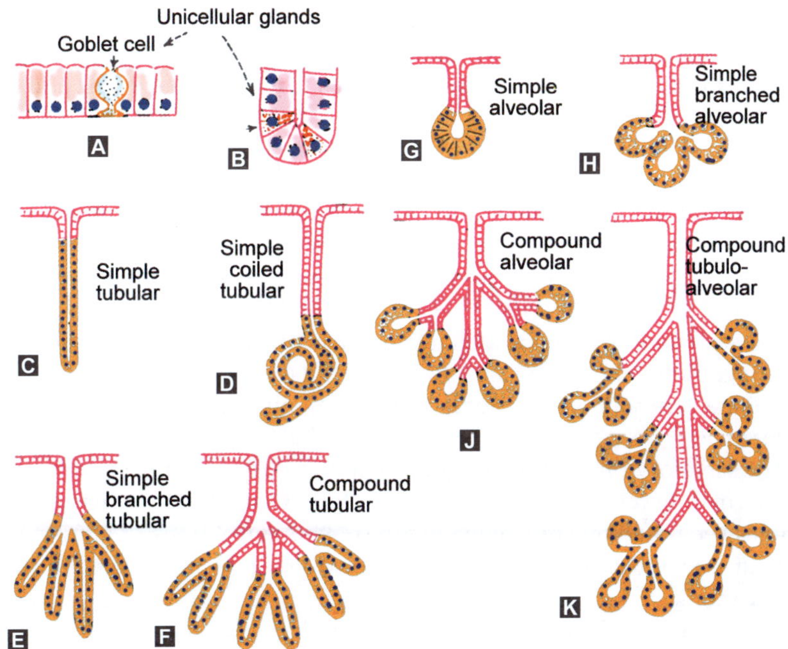

Fig. 7.19 Scheme to show various ways in which the secretory elements of a gland may be organized. A and B are examples of unicellular glands. All others are multicellular. Glands with a single duct are simple glands, while those with a branching duct system are compound glands.

of secretory cells, each group discharging into its own duct. These ducts unite to form larger ducts that ultimately drain on to an epithelial surface. Such a gland is said to be a ***compound gland***.

Both in simple and in compound glands the secretory cells may be arranged in various ways.

a. The secretory element may be ***tubular***. The tube may be straight, coiled, or branched.
b. The cells may form rounded sacs or ***acini***.
c. They may form flask-shaped structures called ***alveoli***. However, it may be noted that the terms acini and alveoli are often used as if they were synonymous. Glands in which the secretory elements are greatly distended are called ***saccular glands***.
d. Combinations of the above may be present in a single gland. From what has been said above it will be seen that an exocrine gland may be:
   1. Unicellular.
   2. Simple tubular.
   3. Simple alveolar (or acinar).
   4. Compound tubular.
   5. Compound alveolar.
   6. Compound tubulo-alveolar (or racemose).

   Some further subdivisions of these are shown in Fig. 7.19.

Exocrine glands may also be classified on the basis of the nature of their secretions into ***mucous glands*** and ***serous glands***. In mucous glands the secretion contains mucopolysaccharides. The secretion collects in the apical parts of the cells. As a result nuclei are pushed to the base of the cell, and may be flattened.

In classroom slides stained with haematoxylin and eosin the secretion within mucous cells remains unstained so that they have an 'empty' look.

However, the stored secretion can be brightly stained using a special procedure called the periodic acid Schiff (PAS) method. Unicellular cells secreting mucous are numerous in the intestines: they are called ***goblet cells*** because of their peculiar shape (See Figs. 7.8 and Fig. 7.19A).

The secretions of serous glands are protein in nature. The cytoplasm of these cells is granular and often stains bluish with haematoxylin and eosin. Their nuclei are centrally placed. Some glands contain both serous and mucous elements.

The secretory elements of exocrine glands are held together by connective tissue (mainly reticular fibres). The glandular tissue is often divisible into lobules separated by connective tissue septa. Aggregations of lobules may form distinct lobes. The connective tissue covering the entire gland forms a ***capsule*** for it.

When a gland is divided into lobes the ducts draining it may be ***intralobular*** (lying within a lobule), ***interlobular*** (lying in the intervals between lobules), or ***interlobar*** (lying between adjacent lobes), in increasing order of size.

Blood vessels and nerves pass along connective tissue septa to reach the secretory elements. As a rule exocrine glands have a rich blood supply. Their activity is under nervous or hormonal control.

The secretory cells of a gland constitute its ***parenchyma***, while the connective tissue in which the former lie is called the ***stroma***.

Endocrine glands are usually arranged in cords or in clumps that are intimately related to a rich network of blood capillaries or of sinusoids. In some cases (for example the thyroid gland) the cells may form rounded follicles.

Endocrine cells and their blood vessels are supported by delicate connective tissue, and are usually surrounded by a capsule.

Neoplasms can arise from the epithelium lining a gland. A benign growth arising in a gland is an ***adenoma***; and a malignant growth is an ***adenocarcinoma***.

In this chapter we have considered the general features of glands. Further details of the structure of exocrine and endocrine glands will be considered while studying individual glands.

CHAPTER

8

General Connective Tissue

INTRODUCTORY REMARKS

What is Connective Tissue?

The term ***connective tissue*** is applied to a tissue that fills the interstices between more specialized elements; and serves to hold them together and support them. Connective tissue serves to hold together, and to support, different elements within an organ. Such connective tissue is to be found in almost every part of the body. It is conspicuous in some regions and scanty in others. This kind of connective tissue is referred to as ***general connective tissue*** to distinguish it from more specialized connective tissues that we will consider separately. It is also called ***fibro-collagenous tissue***.

Basic Components of General Connective Tissue

Many tissues and organs of the body are made up mainly of aggregations of closely packed cells e.g., epithelia, and solid organs like the liver. In contrast, cells are relatively few in connective tissue, and are widely separated by a prominent ***intercellular substance***. The intercellular substance is in the form of a ***ground substance*** within which there are numerous ***fibres*** (Fig. 8.1). Connective tissue can assume various forms depending upon the nature of the ground substance, and of the type of fibres and cells present.

Fibres in Connective Tissue

The most conspicuous components of connective tissue are the fibres within it. These are of three main types.

a. ***Collagen fibres*** are most numerous.
b. ***Reticular fibres*** were once described as a distinct variety of fibres, but they are now regarded as one variety of collagen fibre.
c. ***Elastic fibres***.

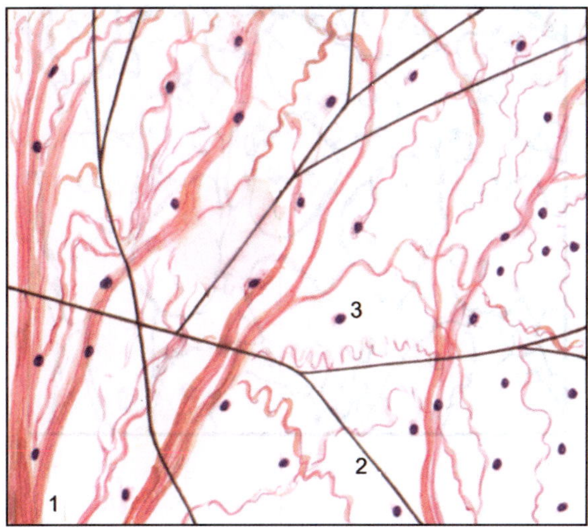

Fig. 8.1 Stretch preparation of omentum showing loose areolar tissue.

The three types of fibres mentioned above are embedded in an amorphous ground substance or ***matrix***.

Cells in General Connective Tissue

Various types of cells are present in connective tissue. These can be classed into two distinct categories.

a. Cells that are intrinsic components of connective tissue:

   In typical connective tissue the most important cells are ***fibroblasts***. Others present are ***undifferentiated mesenchymal cells, pigment cells***, and ***fat cells***. Other varieties of cells are present in more specialized forms of connective tissues.

b. Cells that belong to the immune system and are identical or closely related with certain cells present in blood and in lymphoid tissues:

   These include ***macrophage cells*** (or ***histiocytes***), ***mast cells***, ***lymphocytes, plasma cells***, ***monocytes*** and ***eosinophils***.

Different forms of Connective Tissue

Loose Connective Tissue

If we examine a small quantity of superficial fascia under a microscope, at low magnification, it is seen to be made up mainly of bundles of loosely arranged fibres that appear to enclose large spaces. This is ***loose connective tissue***. Spaces are also called ***areolae***, and such tissue is also referred to as ***areolar tissue*** (Fig. 8.1).

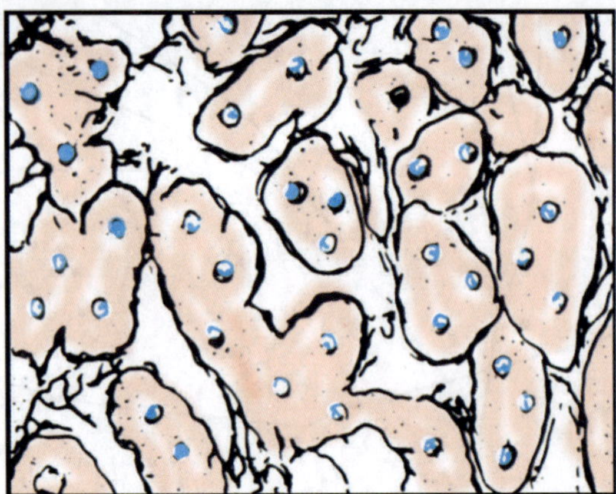

Fig. 8.2 Reticular fibres (black) forming a network in the liver. The white spaces represent sinusoids.

Fibrous Tissue

We have seen that in loose areolar tissue the fibre bundles are loosely arranged with wide spaces in between them. In many situations the fibre bundles are much more conspicuous, and form a dense mass. This kind of tissue is referred to as ***fibrous tissue***. It appears white in colour and is sometimes called ***white fibrous tissue***.

Elastic Tissue

We have seen that some elastic fibres can be seen in loose areolar tissue (Fig. 8.1). Some elastic fibres may also be present in any other variety of connective tissue. However, in some situations, most of the connective tissue is formed by elastic fibres: this is called ***elastic tissue***. In contrast to white fibrous tissue, elastic tissue is yellow in colour. Some ligaments are made up of elastic tissue. These include the ligamentum nuchae (on the back of the neck). The vocal ligaments (of the larynx) are also made up of elastic fibres. Elastic fibres are numerous in membranes that are required to stretch periodically. For example the deeper layer of superficial fascia covering the anterior abdominal wall has a high proportion of elastic fibres to allow for distension of the abdomen.

Elastic fibres may fuse with each other to form sheets. Such sheets form the main support for the walls of large arteries (e.g., the aorta). In smaller arteries they form the internal elastic lamina.

Reticular Tissue

This is made up of reticular fibres. In many situations (e.g., lymph nodes, glands) these fibres form supporting networks for the cells (Fig. 8.2). In some situations (bone marrow, spleen, lymph nodes) the reticular network is closely associated with ***reticular cells***. Most of these cells are fibroblasts, but some may be macrophages.

Other ConnectiveTissues

Bone and cartilage are regarded as forms of connective tissue as the cells in them are widely separated by intercellular substance. The firmness of cartilage, and the hardness of bone, are because of the nature of the ground substance in them. Cartilage and bone will be considered in Chapter 9. Blood is also included amongst connective tissues as the cells are widely dispersed in a fluid intercellular substance, the plasma. Blood is considered in Chapter 11.

Adipose tissue will be considered later in this chapter.

FIBRES OF CONNECTIVE TISSUE

Collagen Fibres

With the light microscope collagen fibres are seen in bundles (Fig. 8.1). The bundles may be straight or wavy depending upon how much they are stretched. The bundles are made up of collections of individual collagen fibres which are 1-12 μm in diameter. The bundles often branch, or anastomose with adjacent bundles, but the individual fibres do not branch.

Staining Characters

Bundles of collagen fibres appear white with the naked eye. In sections stained with haematoxylin and eosin collagen fibres are stained light pink. With special methods they assume different colours depending upon the dye used.

Physical Properties

Collagen fibres can resist considerable tensile forces (i.e., stretching) without significant increase in their length. At the same time they are pliable and can bend easily.

Collagen fibres swell and become soft when treated with a weak acid or alkali. They are destroyed by strong acids. On boiling, collagen is converted into gelatine.

Chemical Nature

Collagen fibres are so called because they are made up mainly of a protein called *collagen*. Collagen is made up of molecules of *tropocollagen*. Carbohydrates are also present.

Reticular Fibres

These fibres are a variety of collagen fibre. They differ from typical collagen fibres as follows.

1. They are much finer.
2. They are uneven in thickness.
3. They form a network (or reticulum) by branching, and by anastomosing with each other. They do not run in bundles.
4. They can be stained specifically by silver impregnation, which renders them black. They can thus be easily distinguished from typical collagen fibres which are stained brown. Because of their affinity for silver salts reticular fibres are sometimes called ***argentophil fibres***.

Reticular fibres provide a supporting network in many situations. These include the spleen, lymph nodes and bone marrow; most glands, including the liver; and the kidneys. Reticular fibres form an essential component of all basement membranes. They are also found in relation to smooth muscle and nerve fibres.

Elastic Fibres

In areolar tissue, elastic fibres are much fewer than those of collagen. They run singly (not in bundles), branch and anastomose with other fibres. Elastic fibres are thinner than those of collagen.

In some situations elastic fibres are thick (e.g., in the ligamenta flava). In other situations (as in walls of large arteries) they form fenestrated membranes.

Physical Properties

As their name implies elastic fibres can be stretched (like a rubber band) and return to their original length when tension is released. Unlike collagen, elastic fibres are not affected by weak acids or alkalies, or by boiling. However, they are digested by the enzyme *elastase.*

Chemical Nature

Elastic fibres are composed mainly of a protein called ***elastin*** which forms their central amorphous core. Elastin is made up of smaller units called ***tropoelastin***. Elastic fibres of connective tissue are produced by fibroblasts.

CELLS OF CONNECTIVE TISSUE

As mentioned earlier, the cells of connective tissue can be divided into those that are intrinsic components of the tissue, and those that belong to the immune system but are commonly seen in connective tissues. In the first group we include fibroblasts, undifferentiated mesenchymal cells, and pigment cells. Fat cells are commonly seen.

Cells of the immune system to be seen are some varieties of leucocytes and their derivatives. They include the following.

1. Lymphocytes, and plasma cells which are derived from lymphocytes.
2. Monocytes, and macrophages that are derived from monocytes.
3. Mast cells that are related to basophils.
4. Neutrophils and eosinophils are occasionally seen.

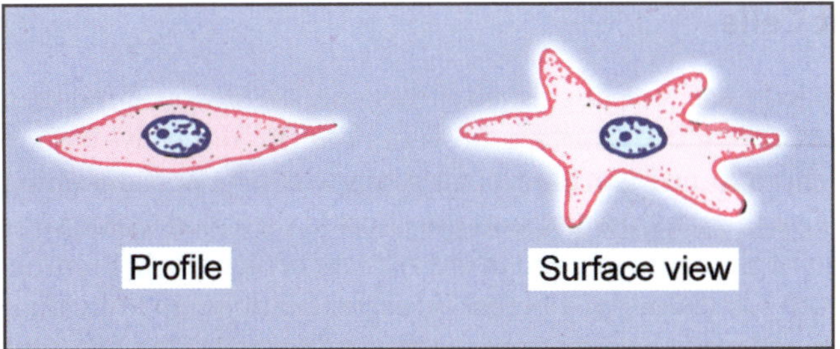

Fig. 8.3 Structure of a fibroblast.

Fibroblasts

These are the most numerous cells of connective tissue. They are called fibroblasts because they are concerned with the production of collagen fibres. They also produce reticular and elastic fibres. Where associated with reticular fibres they are usually called ***reticular cells***.

Fibroblasts are present in close relationship to collagen fibres. They are 'fixed' cells i.e., they are not mobile. In tissue sections these cells appear to be spindle shaped, and the nucleus appears to be flattened. When seen from the surface the cells show branching processes (Fig. 8.3).

Fibroblasts become very active when there is need to lay down collagen fibres. This occurs, for example, in wound repair. When the need arises fibroblasts can give rise, by division, to more fibroblasts.

Undifferentiated Mesenchymal Cells

Embryonic connective tissue is called ***mesenchyme***. It is made up of small cells with slender branching processes that join to form a fine network (Fig. 8.4).

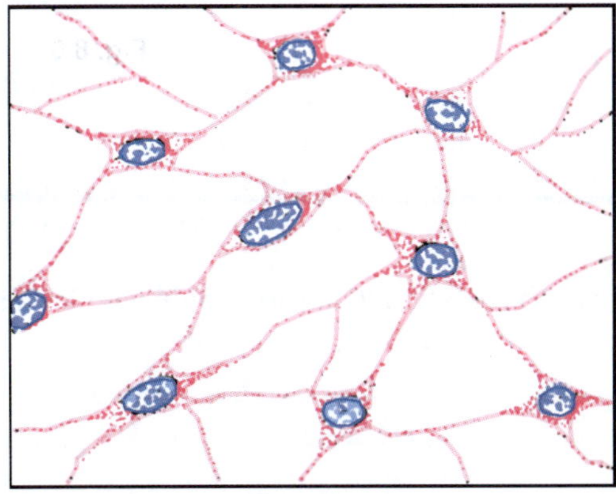

Fig. 8.4 Mesenchymal cells.

Pigment Cells

Pigment cells are easily distinguished as they contain brown pigment (melanin) in their cytoplasm (Fig. 8.5). They are most abundant in connective tissue of the skin, and in the choroid and iris of the eyeball. Along with pigment containing epithelial cells they give the skin, the iris, and the choroid their dark colour. Variations in the number of pigment cells, and in the amount of pigment in them accounts for differences in skin colour of different races, and in different individuals.

Pigment cells prevent light from reaching other cells. The importance of this function in relation to the eyeball is obvious. Pigment cells in the skin protect deeper tissues from the effects of light (specially ultraviolet light). The darker skin of races living in tropical climates is an obvious adaptation for this purpose.

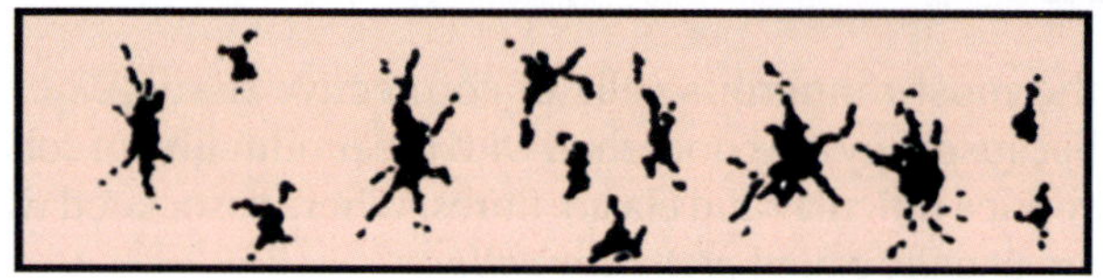

Fig. 8.5 Pigment cells.

Fat Cells (Adipocytes)

Although some amount of fat (lipids) may be present in the cytoplasm of many cells, including fibroblasts, some cells store fat in large amounts and become distended with it (Fig. 8.9). These are called ***fat cells***, ***adipocytes***, or ***lipocytes***. Aggregations of fat cells constitute ***adipose tissue*** (Figs. 8.10, 8.11).

Macrophage Cells

Macrophage cells of connective tissue are part of a large series of cells present in the body that have similar functions. These collectively form the ***mononuclear phagocyte system***.

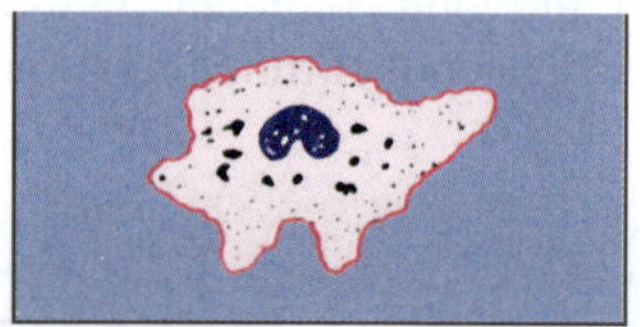

Fig. 8.6 Macrophage cell (histiocyte)

Macrophage cells of connective tissue are also called ***histiocytes*** or ***clasmatocytes*** (Fig. 8.6). They have the ability to phagocytose (eat up) unwanted material. Such material is usually organic: it includes bacteria invading the tissue, and damaged tissues. Macrophages also phagocytose inorganic particles injected into the body (e.g., India ink).

Apart from direct phagocytic activity, macrophages play an important role in immunological mechanisms.

Mast Cells

These are small round or oval cells. They are also called ***mastocytes***, or ***histaminocytes*** (Fig. 8.7). The nucleus is small and centrally placed.

The distinguishing feature of these cells is the presence of numerous granules in the cytoplasm. The granules can be demonstrated by special stains.

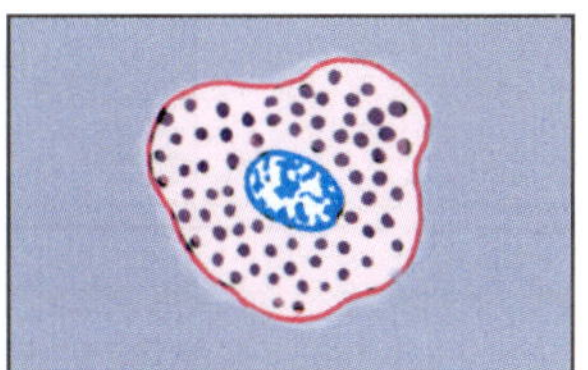

Fig. 8.7 Mast cell.

Mast cells are believed to release various substances when appropriately stimulated. The most important of these is histamine. Release of histamine is associated with the production of allergic reactions when a tissue is exposed to an antigen to which it is sensitive (because of previous exposure). In this context it is believed that the cell membranes of mast cells contain antibodies which react with the antigen. This leads to rupture of the cells with discharge of histamine. The discharge in turn leads to local reactions like urticaria, or to severe general reactions like anaphylactic shock.

Lymphocytes

Lymphocytes represent one variety of leucocytes (white blood cells) present in blood. Large aggregations of lymphocytes are present in lymphoid tissues. They reach connective tissue from these sources, and are specially numerous when the tissue undergoes inflammation. Lymphocytes play an important role in defence of the body against invasion by bacteria and other organisms. They have the ability to recognize substances that are foreign to the host body; and to destroy these invaders by producing antibodies against them. Lymphocytes will be considered in detail in Chapter 11. Here it will suffice to note that lymphocytes are derived from stem cells present in bone marrow. They are of two types. ***B-lymphocytes*** pass through blood to reach other tissues directly. Some B-lymphocytes mature into ***plasma cells*** described below. The second type of lymphocytes, called ***T-lymphocytes***, travel (through blood) from bone marrow to the thymus. After undergoing a process of maturation in this organ they again enter the blood stream to reach other tissues. Both B-lymphocytes and T-lymphocytes can be seen in connective tissue.

Other Leucocytes

Apart from lymphocytes two other types of leucocytes may be seen in connective tissue. ***Monocytes*** are closely related in function to macrophages. ***Eosinophils*** (so called because of the presence of eosinophilic granules in the cytoplasm) are found in the connective tissue of many organs. They increase in number in allergic disorders.

Plasma Cells or Plasmatocytes

Very few plasma cells can be seen in normal connective tissue. Their number increases in the presence of certain types of inflammation. It is believed that plasma cells represent B-lymphocytes that have matured and have lost their power of further division.

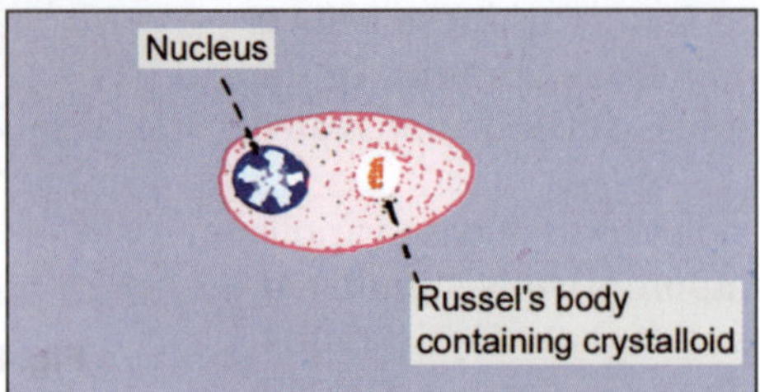

Fig. 8.8 Plasma cell.

With the light microscope a plasma cell is seen to be small and rounded (Fig. 8.8). It can be recognized by the fact that the chromatin in its nucleus forms four or five clumps near the periphery (of the nucleus) thus giving the nucleus a resemblance to a cart-wheel.

Plasma cells produce antibodies which may be discharged locally; may enter the circulation; or may be stored within the cell itself in the form of inclusions called ***Russell's bodies***.

ADIPOSE TISSUE

Structure of Adipose Tissue

Adipose tissue is basically an aggregation of fat cells, also called adipocytes. Each fat cell contains a large droplet of fat that almost fills it (Fig. 8.9). As a result the cell becomes rounded. (When several fat cells are closely packed, they become polygonal because of mutual pressure). The cytoplasm of the cell forms a thin layer just deep to the plasma membrane. The nucleus is pushed against the plasma membrane and is flattened.

Distribution of Adipose Tissue

Adipose tissue is distributed as follows.

1. It is present in the superficial fascia over most of the body. This subcutaneous layer of fat is called the ***panniculus adiposus***. It is responsible for giving a smooth contour to the skin. However, fat is not present in the superficial fascia of the eyelids, the scrotum and the penis. The distribution of subcutaneous fat in different parts of the body is also different in the male and female and is responsible (to a great extent) for the differences in body contours in the two sexes. In women it forms a thicker and more even layer: this is responsible for the soft contours of the female body. Subcutaneous fat is not present in animals which have a thick coat of fur.
2. Adipose tissue fills several hollow spaces in the body. These include the orbits, the axillae and the ischiorectal fossae. In the adult much of the space in marrow cavities of long bones is filled by fat in the form of yellow bone marrow. Much fat is also present in synovial folds of many joints filling spaces that would otherwise have been empty during certain phases of movement.

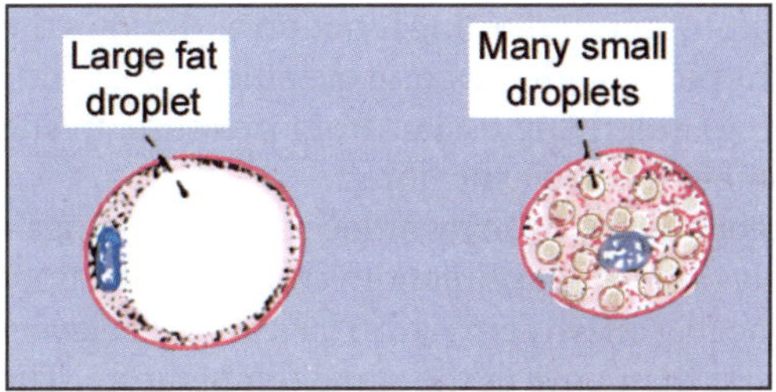

Fig. 8.9 Comparison of a normal fat cell with one in brown fat.

3. Fat is present around many abdominal organs, specially the kidneys (***perinephric fat***).
4. Considerable amounts of fat may be stored in the greater omentum, and in other peritoneal folds.

Functions of Adipose Tissue

Various functions have been attributed to adipose tissue.

a. It acts as a store-house of nutrition, fat being deposited when available in excess; and being removed when deficient in the diet.
b. In many situations fat performs a mechanical function. The fat around the kidneys keeps them in position. If there is a sudden depletion of this fat the kidneys may become mobile (***floating kidney***). The fat around the eyeball

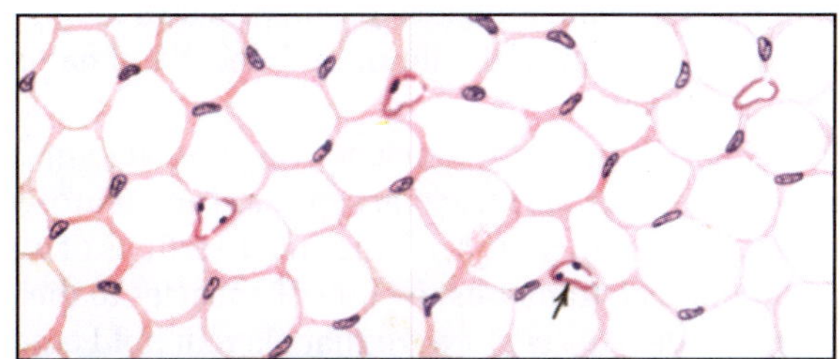

Fig. 8.10 Adipose tissue as seen in a routine paraffin section. The cells look empty as the fat dissolves during processing of tissue.

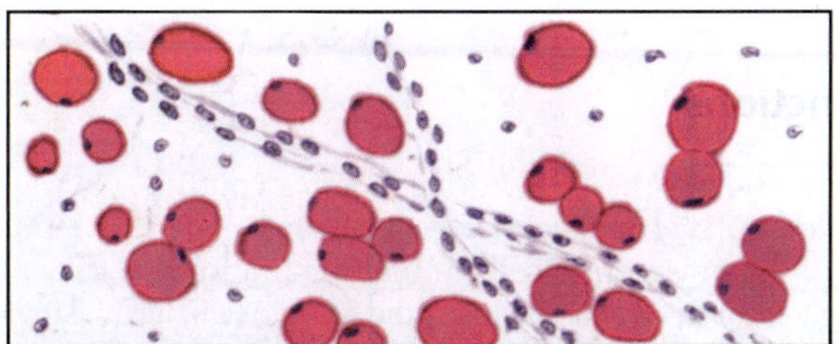

Fig. 8.11 Fat cells in a stretch preparation of omentum stained with a specific stain for fat (Sudan IV).

performs an important supporting function and allows the eyeball to move smoothly. In the palms and soles, and over the buttocks fat has a cushioning effect protecting underlying tissues from pressure. In such areas adipose tissue may contain many elastic fibres.

c. The subcutaneous fat has been regarded as insulation against heat loss, and would certainly perform this function if the layer of adipose tissue is thick. This may be one reason why girls (who have a thicker layer of subcutaneous fat) feel less cold than boys at the same temperature. The whale (a warm blooded mammal) can survive in very cold water because it has a very thick layer of subcutaneous fat.

SUMMARY OF THE FUNCTIONS OF CONNECTIVE TISSUES

Mechanical Functions

1. In the form of loose connective tissue, it holds together structures like skin, muscles, blood vessels, etc. It binds together various layers of hollow viscera. In the form of areolar tissue and reticular tissue it forms a framework that supports the cellular elements of various organs like the spleen, lymph nodes, and glands, and provides capsules for them.
2. The looseness of areolar tissue facilitates movement between structures connected by it. The looseness of superficial fascia enables the movement of skin over deep fascia. In hollow organs this allows for mobility and stretching.
3. In the form of deep fascia connective tissue provides a tight covering for deeper structures (specially in the limbs and neck) and helps to maintain the shape of these regions.
4. In the form of ligaments it holds bone ends together at joints.
5. In the form of deep fascia, intermuscular septa and aponeuroses, connective tissue provides attachment for the origins and insertions of many muscles.
6. In the form of tendons it transmits the pull of muscles to their insertion.
7. Thickened areas of deep fascia form retinacula that hold tendons in place at the wrist and ankle.
8. Both areolar tissue and fascial membranes provide planes along which blood vessels, lymphatics, and nerves travel. The superficial fascia provides passage to vessels and nerves going to the skin, and supports them.
9. In the form of dura mater it provides support to the brain and spinal cord.

Other Functions

a. In the form of adipose tissue it provides a store of nutrition. In cold weather the fat provides insulation and helps to generate heat.
b. Because of the presence of cells of the immune system (macrophages and plasma cells), connective tissue helps the body to fight against invading foreign substances (including bacteria) by destroying them, or by producing antibodies against them.

c. Because of the presence of fibroblasts connective tissue helps in laying down collagen fibres necessary for wound repair.
d. By virtue of the presence of undifferentiated mesenchymal cells connective tissue can help in regeneration of tissues (e.g., cartilage and bone) by providing cells from which specialized cells can be formed.
e. Deep fascia plays a very important role in facilitating venous return from the limbs (specially the lower limbs). When muscles of the limb contract, their outward expansion is limited by the deep fascia. As a result, veins deep to the fascia are pressed upon. Because of the presence of valves in the veins, this pressure causes blood to flow towards the heart. In this way deep fascia enables muscles to act as pumps that push venous blood towards the heart.

CHAPTER

9

Cartilage and Bone

CARTILAGE

Cartilage is a tissue that forms the 'skeletal' basis of some parts of the body e.g., the auricle of the ear, or the lower part of the nose. Feeling these parts readily demonstrates that while cartilage is sufficiently firm to maintain its form, it is not rigid like bone. It can be bent, returning to its original form when the bending force is removed.

Cartilage is considered to be a modified connective tissue. It resembles ordinary connective tissue in that the cells in it are widely separated by a considerable amount of intercellular material or ***matrix***. The latter consists of a homogeneous ***ground substance*** within which fibres are embedded. Cartilage differs from typical connective tissue mainly in the nature of the ground substance: this is firm and gives cartilage its characteristic consistency. Three main types of cartilage can be recognised depending on the number and variety of fibres in the matrix. These are ***hyaline cartilage***, ***fibrocartilage***, and ***elastic cartilage***.

As a rule, the free surfaces of hyaline cartilage are covered by a fibrous membrane called the ***perichondrium***, but fibrocartilage is not.

Cartilage Cells

The cells of cartilage are called ***chondrocytes***. They lie in spaces (or ***lacunae***) present in the matrix. At first the cells are small. As the cartilage cells mature they enlarge considerably, often reaching a diameter of 40 μm or more.

Ground Substance

The ground substance of cartilage is made up of complex molecules containing proteins and carbohydrates (proteoglycans). These molecules form a meshwork that is filled by water and dissolved salts.

HYALINE CARTILAGE

Hyaline cartilage is so called because it is transparent (hyalos = glass). Its intercellular substance appears to be homogeneous, but using special techniques it can be shown that many collagen fibres are present in the matrix.

Towards the centre of a mass of hyaline cartilage the chondrocytes are large and are usually present in groups (of two or more) (Fig. 9.1). The groups are formed by division of a single parent cell. The cells tend to remain together as the dense matrix prevents their separation. Groups of cartilage cells are called ***cell-nests*** (or ***isogenous cell groups***). Immediately around lacunae housing individual chondrocytes, and around cell nests the matrix stains deeper than elsewhere giving the appearance of a capsule. Towards the periphery of the cartilage the cells are small, and elongated in a direction parallel to the surface. Just under the perichondrium the cells become indistinguishable from fibroblasts.

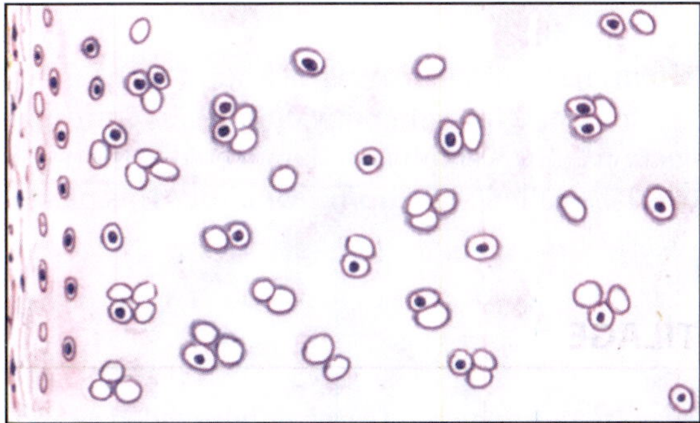

Fig. 9.1 Hyaline cartilage. Note groups of chondrocytes surrounded by homogenous matrix. Perichondrium is seen at the left end of the figure.

Embedded in the ground substance of hyaline cartilage, there are numerous collagen fibres. The fibres are arranged so that they resist tensional forces. Hyaline cartilage has been compared to a tyre. The ground substance (corresponding to the rubber of the tyre) resists compressive forces, while the fibres (corresponding to the treads of the tyre) resist tensional forces.

Distribution of Hyaline Cartilage

Hyaline cartilage is widely distributed in the body as follows.

1. *Costal Cartilages*

These are bars of hyaline cartilage that connect the ventral ends of the ribs to the sternum, or to adjoining costal cartilages. They show the typical structure of hyaline cartilage described above.

2. *Articular Cartilage*

The articular surfaces of most synovial joints are lined by hyaline cartilage. These articular cartilages provide the bone ends with smooth surfaces between which there is very little friction. They also act as shock absorbers. Articular cartilages are not covered by perichondrium. Their surface is kept moist by synovial fluid that also provides nutrition to them.

3. *Other Sites where Hyaline Cartilage is Found*

a. The skeletal framework of the larynx is formed by a number of cartilages. Of these the thyroid cartilage, the cricoid cartilage and the arytenoid cartilage are composed of hyaline cartilage.
b. The walls of the trachea and large bronchi contain incomplete rings of cartilage. Smaller bronchi have pieces of cartilage of irregular shape in their walls.
c. Parts of the nasal septum, and of the lateral wall of the nose are made up of pieces of hyaline cartilage.
d. In growing children long bones consist of a bony ***diaphysis*** (corresponding to the shaft) and of one or more bony ***epiphyses*** (corresponding to bone ends or projections). Each epiphysis is connected to the diaphysis by a plate of hyaline cartilage called the ***epiphyseal plate***. This plate is essential for bone growth.

FIBROCARTILAGE

On superficial examination this type of cartilage (also called ***white fibrocartilage***) looks very much like dense fibrous tissue (Fig. 9.2). However, in sections it is seen to be cartilage because it contains typical cartilage cells surrounded by capsules. The matrix is pervaded by numerous collagen bundles amongst which there are some fibroblasts. The fibres merge with those of surrounding connective tissue, there being no perichondrium over the cartilage. This kind of cartilage has great tensile strength combined with considerable elasticity.

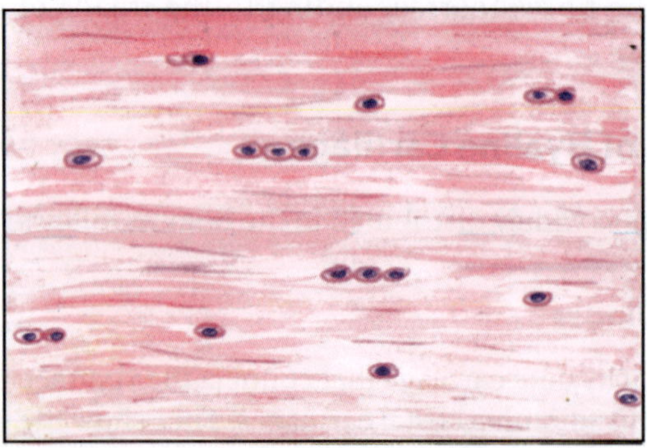

Fig. 9.2 Fibrocartilage. Cartilage cells are embedded amongst thick bundles of collagen fibres.

White fibrocartilage is found at the following sites.

1. Fibrocartilage is most conspicuous in secondary cartilaginous joints or ***symphyses***. These include the joints between bodies of vertebrae (where the cartilage forms intervertebral discs); the pubic symphysis; and the manubriosternal joint.
2. In some synovial joints the joint cavity is partially or completely subdivided by an articular disc. These discs are made up of fibrocartilage. (Examples are discs of the temporo-mandibular and sternoclavicular joints, and menisci of the knee joint).
3. The glenoidal labrum of the shoulder joint and the acetabular labrum of the hip joint are made of fibrocartilage.
4. In some situations where tendons run in deep grooves on bone, the grooves are lined by fibrocartilage. Fibrocartilage is often present where tendons are inserted into bone.

ELASTIC CARTILAGE

Elastic cartilage (or yellow fibrocartilage) is similar in many ways to hyaline cartilage. The main difference is that instead of collagen fibres, the matrix contains numerous elastic fibres which form a network (Fig. 9.3). The fibres are difficult to see in haematoxylin and eosin stained sections, but they can be clearly visualised if special methods for staining elastic fibres are used. The surface of elastic cartilage is covered by perichondrium.

Elastic cartilage possesses greater flexibility than hyaline cartilage, and readily recovers its shape after being deformed.

The sites where elastic cartilage is found are as follows.

1. It forms the 'skeletal' basis of the auricle (or pinna), and of the lateral part of the external acoustic meatus.
2. The wall of the medial part of the auditory tube is made of elastic cartilage.
3. The epiglottis and two small laryngeal cartilages (corniculate and cuneiform) consist of elastic cartilage. The apical part of the arytenoid cartilage contains elastic fibres but the major portion of it is hyaline.

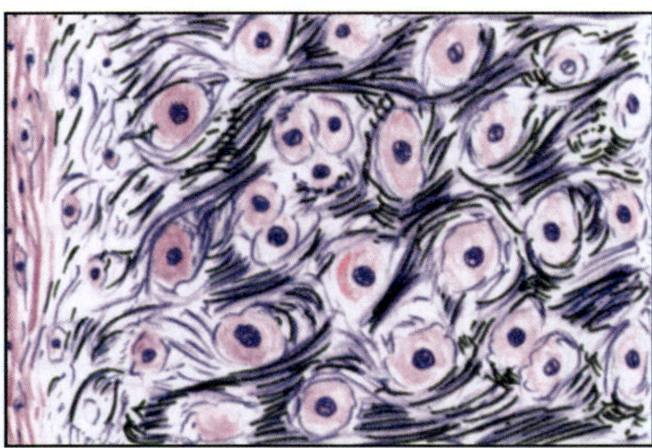

Fig. 9.3 Elastic cartilage. Note chondrocytes surrounded by bundles of elastic fibres. The section has been stained by Verheoff's method in which elastic fibres are stained bluish black.

Note that all the sites mentioned above are concerned either with the production or reception of sound.

Cartilage is derived (embryologically) from mesenchyme. Some mesenchymal cells differentiate into cartilage forming cells or ***chondroblasts***. Chondroblasts produce the intercellular matrix as well as the collagen fibres that form the intercellular substance of cartilage. Chondroblasts that become imprisoned within this matrix become chondrocytes. Some mesenchymal cells that surround the developing cartilage form the ***perichondrium***. Apart from collagen fibres and fibroblasts, the perichondrium contains cells that are capable of transforming themselves into cartilage cells when required.

During fetal life cartilage is much more widely distributed than in the adult. The greater part of the skeleton is cartilaginous in early fetal life. The ends of most long bones are cartilaginous at the time of birth, and are gradually replaced by bone. The replacement is completed only after full growth of the individual (i.e., by about 18 years of age).

Replacement of cartilage by bone is called ***ossification***. Ossification of cartilage has to be carefully distinguished from ***calcification*** in which the matrix hardens because of the deposition in it of calcium salts, but true bone is not formed.

Calcification of hyaline cartilage is often seen in old people. The costal cartilages or the large cartilages of the larynx are commonly affected. In contrast to hyaline cartilage, elastic cartilage and fibrocartilage do not undergo calcification. Although articular cartilage is a variety of hyaline cartilage it does not undergo calcification or ossification.

BONE

Some Features of Gross Structure

If we examine a longitudinal section across a bone (such as the humerus) we see that the wall of the shaft is tubular and encloses a large ***marrow cavity*** (Fig. 9.4). The wall of the tube is made up of a hard dense material that appears, on naked eye examination, to have a uniform smooth texture with no obvious spaces in it. This kind of bone is called ***compact bone***. It is seen further, that compact bone is thickest midway between the two ends of the bone and gradually tapers towards the ends.

When we examine the bone ends we find that the marrow cavity does not extend into them. They are filled by a meshwork of tiny rods or plates of bone and contain numerous spaces, the whole appearance resembling that of a sponge. This kind of bone is called ***spongy*** or ***cancellous bone*** (cancel= cavity).

Where the bone ends take part in forming joints they are covered by a layer of articular cartilage. With the exception of the areas covered by articular cartilage, the entire outer surface of bone is covered by a membrane called the ***periosteum***. The wall of the marrow cavity is lined by a membrane called the ***endosteum***.

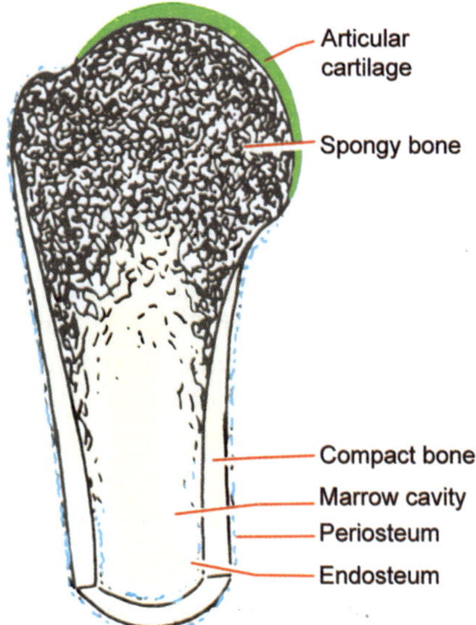

Fig. 9.4 Some features of bone structure as seen in a longitudinal section through one end of a long bone.

The marrow cavity and the spaces of spongy bone (present at the bone ends) are filled by a highly vascular tissue called ***bone marrow***. At the bone ends the marrow is red in colour. Apart from blood vessels this ***red marrow*** contains numerous masses of blood forming cells (***haemopoietic tissue***). In the shaft of the bone of an adult, the marrow is yellow. This ***yellow marrow*** is made up predominantly of fat cells. Some islands of haemopoietic tissue may be seen here also. In bones of a fetus, or of a young child, the entire bone marrow is red. The marrow in the shaft is gradually replaced by yellow marrow with increasing age.

BASIC FACTS ABOUT BONE STRUCTURE

Elements Comprising Bone Tissue

Like cartilage, bone is a modified connective tissue. It consists of bone cells or ***osteocytes*** that are widely separated from one another by a considerable amount of intercellular substance. The latter consists of a homogeneous ground substance or matrix in which collagen fibres and mineral salts (mainly calcium and phosphorus) are deposited.

In addition to mature bone cells (osteocytes) two additional types of cells are seen in developing bone. These are bone producing cells or ***osteoblasts***, and bone removing cells or ***osteoclasts*** (Fig. 9.11). Other cells present include ***osteoprogenitor cells*** from which osteoblasts and osteocytes are derived.

Lamellar Bone

When we examine the structure of any bone of an adult, we find that it is made up of layers or ***lamellae*** (Fig. 9.5). This kind of bone is called ***lamellar bone***. Each lamellus is a thin plate of bone consisting of collagen fibres and mineral salts that are deposited in a gelatinous ground substance. Even the smallest piece of bone is made up of several lamellae placed over one another.

Between adjoining lamellae we see small, flattened spaces or ***lacunae***.

Each lacuna contains one osteocyte (Fig. 9.6). Spreading out from each lacuna there are fine canals or ***canaliculi*** that communicate with those from other lacunae. The canaliculi are occupied by delicate cytoplasmic processes of osteocytes.

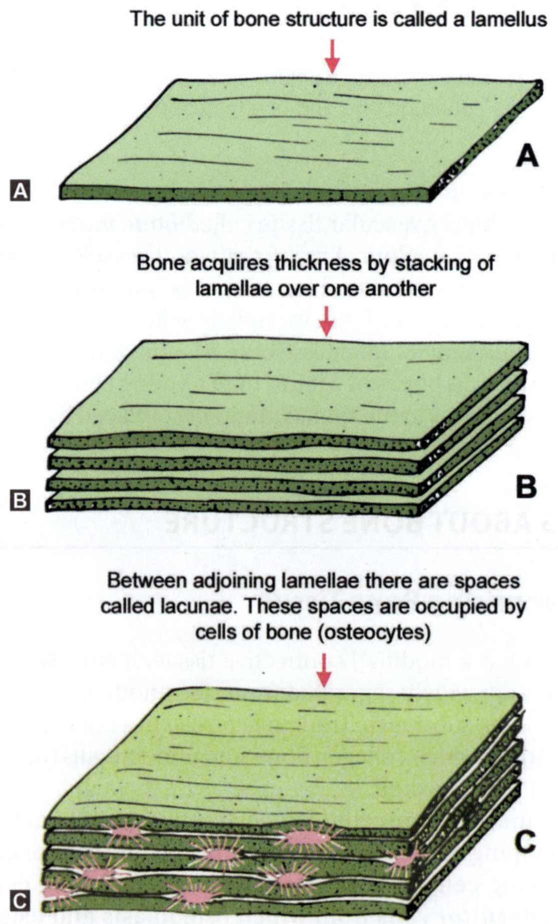

Fig. 9.5 Scheme to show how lamellae constitute bone.

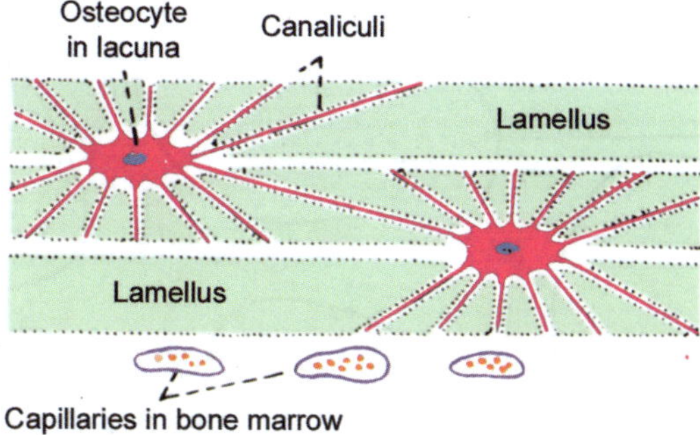

Fig. 9.6 Diagram to show the relationship of osteocytes to bone lamellae.

Woven Bone

In contrast to mature bone, newly formed bone does not have a lamellar structure. The collagen fibres are present in bundles that appear to run randomly in different directions, interlacing with each other. Because of the interlacing of fibre bundles, this kind of bone is called ***woven bone***. All newly formed bone is woven bone. It is later replaced by lamellar bone.

We have seen that bone may be classified as compact or cancellous, and as lamellar or woven. On the basis of the manner of its development, bone can also be classified as ***cartilage bone*** or as ***membrane bone.***

Structure of Cancellous Bone

The bony plates or rods that form the meshwork of cancellous bone are called ***trabeculae***. Each trabeculus is made up of a number of lamellae (described above) between which there are lacunae containing osteocytes. Canaliculi, containing the processes of osteocytes, radiate from the lacunae.

The trabeculae enclose wide spaces which are filled in by bone marrow. They receive nutrition from blood vessels in the bone marrow (Figs. 9.7, 9.8)

Structure of Compact Bone

When we examine a section of compact bone we find that this type of bone is also made up of lamellae, and is pervaded by lacunae (containing osteocytes), and by canaliculi (Figs. 9.9, 9.10). Most of the lamellae are arranged in the form of concentric rings that surround a narrow ***Haversian canal*** present at the centre of each ring. The Haversian canal is occupied by blood vessels, nerve fibres, and some cells. One Haversian canal and the lamellae around it constitute a ***Haversian system*** or ***osteon.***

Compact bone consists of several such osteons. Between adjoining osteons there are angular intervals that are occupied by ***interstitial lamellae***. Near

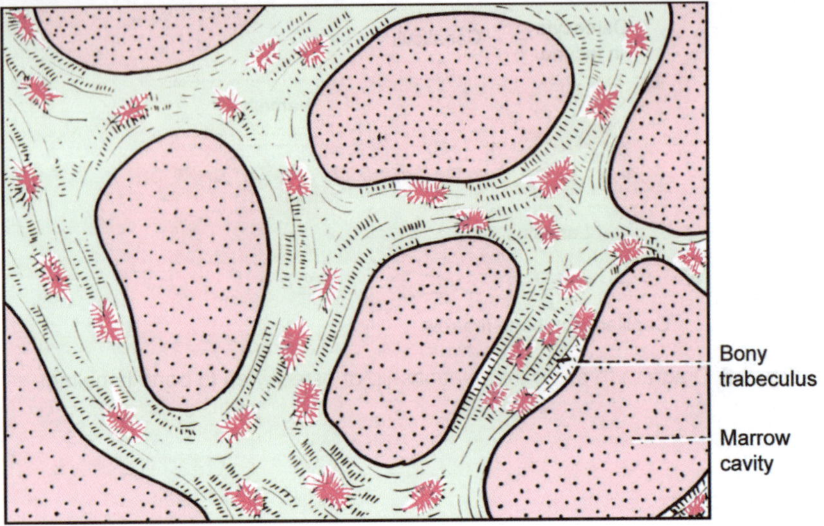

Fig. 9.7 Structure of cancellous bone (diagrammatic).

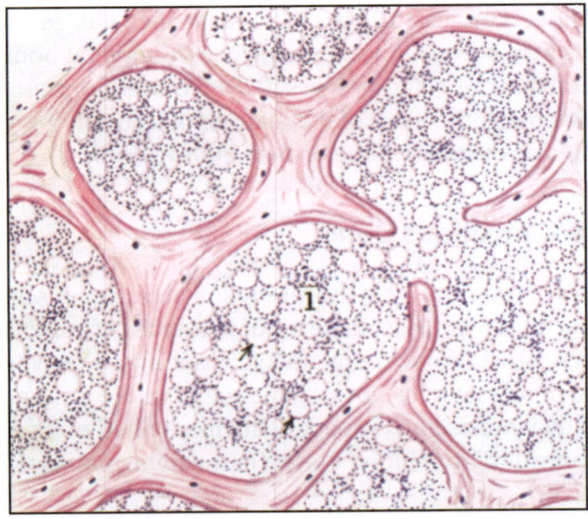

Fig. 9.8 Structure of cancellous bone as seen in a section. 1-Bone marrow.

the surface of compact bone the lamellae are arranged parallel to the surface: these are called ***circumferential lamellae***.

From what has been said above it will be appreciated that there is an essential similarity in the structure of cancellous and compact bone. Both are made up of lamellae. The difference lies in the relative volume occupied by bony lamellae and by the spaces. In compact bone the spaces are small and the solid bone is abundant; whereas in cancellous bone the spaces are large and actual bone tissue is sparse.

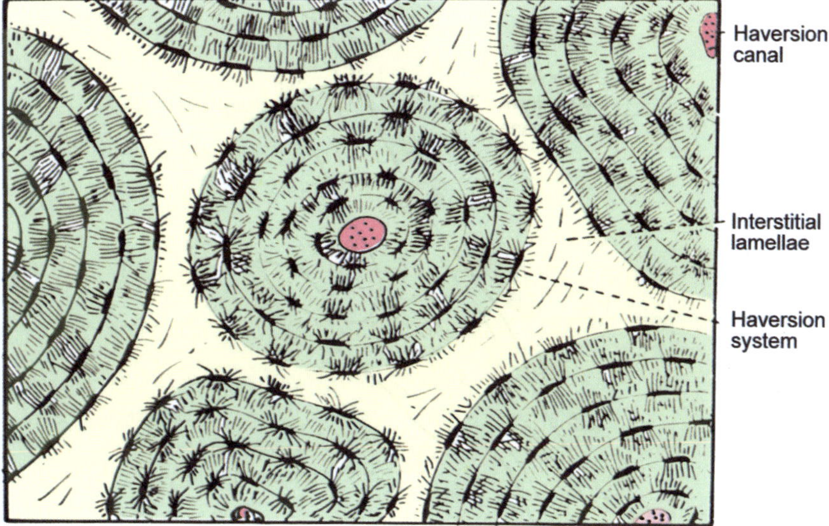

Fig. 9.9 Structure of compact bone (diagrammatic).

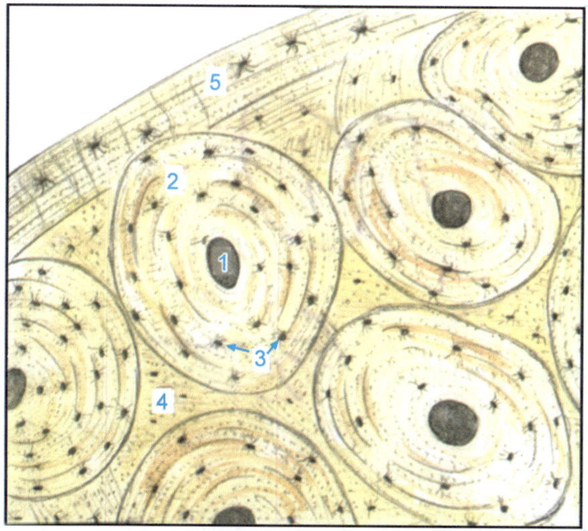

Fig. 9.10 Structure of compact bone as seen in a ground section. 1. Haversian canal. 2.Concentric lamellae forming Haversian system. 3. Lacunae. 4. Interstitial lamellae. 5. Circumferential lamellae.

The Periosteum

We have seen that the external surface of any bone is, as a rule, covered by a membrane called periosteum. (The only parts of the bone surface devoid of periosteum are those that are covered with articular cartilage). The periosteum consists of two layers, outer and inner. The outer layer is a fibrous membrane.

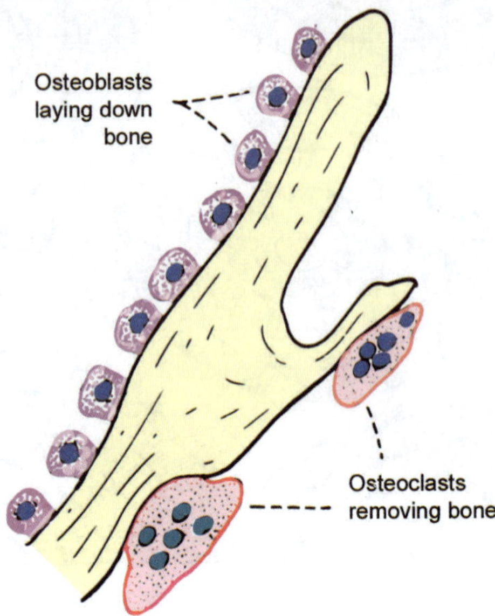

Fig. 9.11 Relationship of osteoblasts and osteoclasts to developing bone.

The inner layer is cellular. In young bones the inner layer contains numerous osteoblasts, and is called the ***osteogenetic layer***. In the periosteum covering the bones of an adult osteoblasts are not conspicuous, but osteoprogenitor cells present here can form osteoblasts when need arises e.g., in the event of a fracture. Periosteum is richly supplied with blood. Many vessels from the periosteum enter the bone and help to supply it.

Functions of Periosteum

1. The periosteum provides a medium through which muscles, tendons and ligaments are attached to bone.
2. Because of the blood vessels passing from periosteum into bone, the periosteum performs a nutritive function.
3. Because of the presence of osteo-progenitor cells in its deeper layer the periosteum can form bone when required. This role is very important during development. It is also important in later life for repair of bone after fracture.

FORMATION OF BONE

The process of bone formation is called ***ossification***. Formation of most bones is preceded by the formation of a cartilaginous model, which is subsequently replaced by bone. This kind of ossification is called ***endochondral ossification***; and bones formed in this way are called ***cartilage bones***. In some situations (e.g., the vault of the skull) formation of bone is not preceded by formation of a cartilaginous model. Instead bone is laid down directly in a fibrous membrane.

This process is called ***intramembranous ossification***; and bones formed in this way are called ***membrane bones***. The bones of the vault of the skull, the mandible, and the clavicle are membrane bones.

Development of a Typical Long Bone

In the region where a long bone is to be formed mesenchymal cells get converted to cartilage producing chondroblasts. These cells produce a cartilaginous model of the bone. This cartilage is covered by perichondrium. Endochondral ossification starts in the central part of the cartilaginous model (i.e., at the centre of the future shaft).

This area is called the ***primary centre of ossification***. Gradually, bone formation extends from the primary centre towards the ends of shaft. This is accompanied by progressive enlargement of the cartilaginous model.

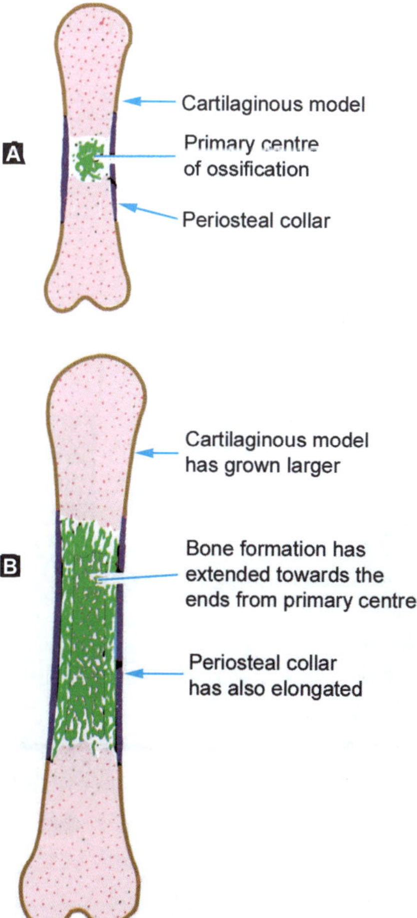

Fig. 9.12 Formation of a typical long bone: primary centre of ossification and periosteal collar.

Soon after the appearance of the primary centre, and the onset of endochondral ossification in it, the perichondrium (which may now be called periosteum) becomes active. The osteoprogenitor cells in its deeper layer lay down bone on the surface of the cartilaginous model by ***intramembranous ossification***. This periosteal bone completely surrounds the cartilaginous shaft and is, therefore, called the ***periosteal collar*** (Fig. 9.12).

At about the time of birth the developing bone consists of (a) a part called the ***diaphysis*** (or shaft), that is bony, and has been formed by extension of the primary centre of ossification, and (b) ends that are cartilaginous (Fig. 9.13). At varying times after birth ***secondary centres*** of endochondral ossification appear in the cartilages forming the ends of the bone (Fig. 9.13B). These centres enlarge until the ends become bony (Fig. 9.14). More than one secondary centre of ossification may appear at either end. The portion of bone formed from one secondary centre is called an ***epiphysis***.

For a considerable time after birth the bone of the diaphysis and the bone of any epiphysis are separated by a plate of cartilage called the ***epiphyseal cartilage***, or ***epiphyseal plate***. This is formed by cartilage into which ossification has not extended either from the diaphysis or from the epiphysis. This plate plays a vital role in growth of the bone (Fig. 9.16).

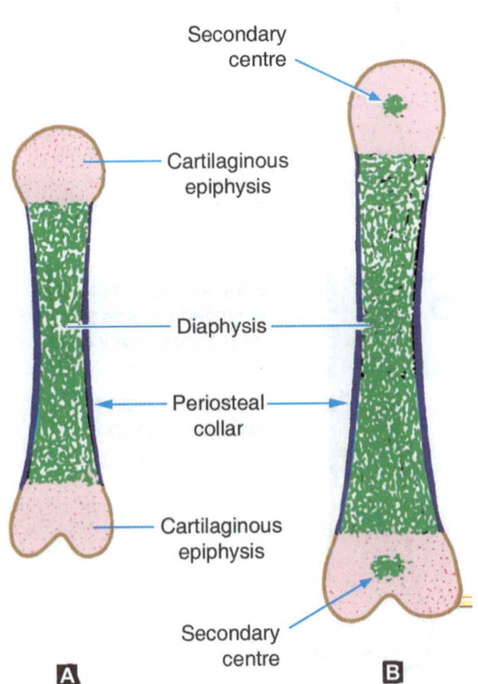

Fig. 9.13 Formation of a typical long bone: secondary centres of ossification.

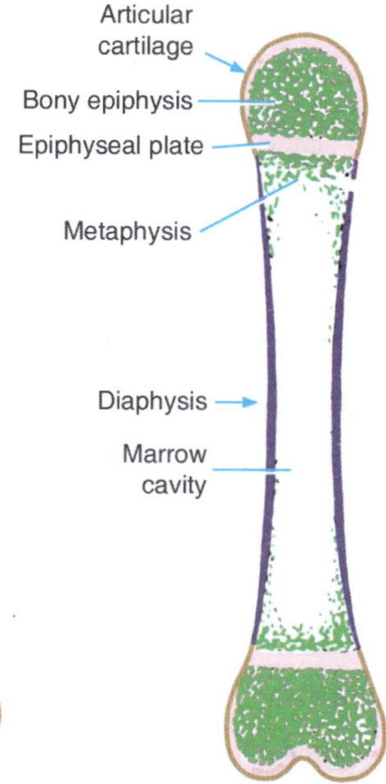

Fig. 9.14 Formation of a typical long bone: bony epiphyses and epiphyseal plates.

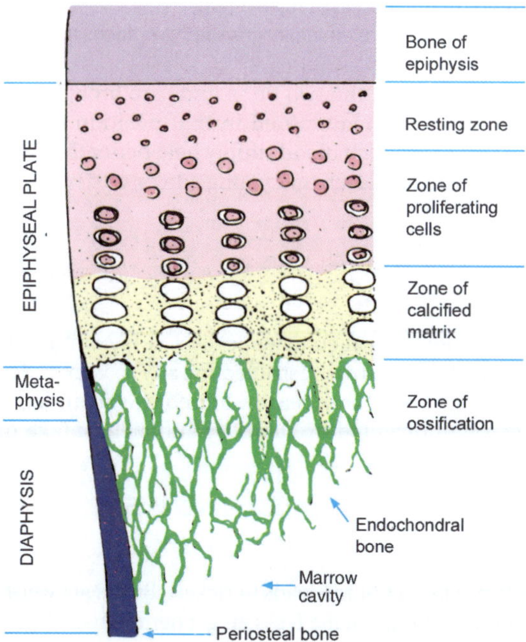

Fig. 9.15 Structure of an epiphyseal plate.

Metaphysis

The portion of the diaphysis adjoining the epiphyseal plate is called the metaphysis (Fig. 9.14). It is a region of active bone formation and, for this reason, it is highly vascular. The metaphysis does not have a marrow cavity. Numerous muscles and ligaments are usually attached to the bone in this region. The metaphysis acts as a store house of calcium from which calcium is released into blood when required. The metaphysis is frequently the site of infection.

SOME DISORDERS OF BONE

Fractures

The most common condition affecting a bone is fracture. Nature tries to rejoin the broken ends. The process of fracture healing is described below.

Fracture Healing

1. When a bone fractures, there is bleeding at the site, and a haematoma forms between the two bone ends.
2. An inflammatory reaction sets in. Macrophages collect in the region and gradually remove clotted blood and bone fragments. Granulation tissue consisting of new capillaries and fibroblasts is formed.
3. Osteoblasts (present in periosteum) multiply and lay down new bone, that joins the bone ends. This new bone is temporary and is called ***callus***. The union is at first weak but gradually increases in strength.
4. Activity of osteoblasts and osteoclasts gradually replaces the callus with normal bone.

Fracture healing is best if the two bone ends are brought close together (= reduction of fracture); and maintained in that position (= immobilisation). Regions of bone that have a rich blood supply heal better than areas with scanty supply. Healing is best in children and young adults, and is often delayed in the elderly.

Osteoporosis

Reduced density of bone is called osteoporosis. It is common in old persons, and in those in whom mobility is restricted for any reason. Calcium content of bone decreases so that bones break easily. Vertebrae can undergo compression. Osteoporosis can be prevented or cured by sufficient intake of calcium and vitamin D.

Rickets

Deficiency of vitamin D in children leads to rickets. Bones are weak, and growth of the body is not normal. Bones of the legs can get bent (bowed legs).

Osteomalacia

Deficiency of vitamin D in adults leads to osteomalacia. The bones become soft and can be deformed. Such deformity of the pelvis, in women, causes difficulty during childbirth.

Osteomyelitis

Infection in bone is called osteomyelitis. It is difficult to treat and easily becomes chronic. Sinuses discharging pus may form, and spicules of bone may come out through the sinus.

Tumours

Both benign and malignant tumours can arise in bone. A benign tumour arising from osteoblasts is called an ***osteoma***. A malignant tumour arising from the same cells is called an ***osteosarcoma***. Osteosarcomas are most commonly seen in bones adjoining the knee joint. They can spread to distant sites in the body through the blood stream.

Paget's Disease

This is caused by abnormal persistence of woven bone. Bones are weak and there may be deformities.

CHAPTER
10

Muscle and Nerve Tissue

MUSCLE

Introductory Remarks

Muscle tissue is composed predominantly of cells that are specialized to shorten in length by contraction. This contraction results in movement. It is in this way that virtually all movements within the body, or of the body in relation to the environment, are ultimately produced.

Muscle tissue is made up basically of cells that are called ***myocytes***. Myocytes are elongated in one direction and are, therefore, often referred to as ***muscle fibres***. We shall see, however, that in some cases muscle fibres are made up of several myocytes joined to each other; or of greatly elongated myocytes containing multiple nuclei.

The force generated by contraction of a muscle fibre is transmitted to other structures through connective tissue. Each muscle fibre is closely invested by connective tissue which is continuous with that around other muscle fibres. Because of this fact the force generated by various muscle fibres gets added together. In some cases a movement may be the result of simultaneous contraction of thousands of muscle fibres.

The connective tissue framework of muscle also provides pathways along which blood vessels and nerves reach muscle fibres.

From the point of view of its histological structure muscle is of three types.

1. The first variety of muscle tissue is present mainly in the limbs and in relation to the body wall. Because of its close relationship to the bony skeleton, this variety is called ***skeletal muscle***. When examined under a microscope fibres of skeletal muscle show prominent transverse striations. Skeletal muscle is, therefore, also called ***striated muscle***. Skeletal muscle can normally be made to contract under our will (to perform movements we desire). It is, therefore, also called ***voluntary muscle***. Skeletal muscle is supplied by somatic motor nerves.

2. The second variety of muscle is present mainly in relation to viscera. It is seen most typically in the walls of hollow viscera. As fibres of this variety do not show transverse striations it is called ***smooth muscle***, or ***nonstriated muscle***. As a rule, contraction of smooth muscle is not under our control; and smooth muscle is, therefore, also called ***involuntary muscle***. It is supplied by autonomic nerves.
3. The third variety of muscle is present exclusively in the heart and is called ***cardiac muscle***. It resembles smooth muscle in being involuntary; but it resembles striated muscle in that the fibres of cardiac muscle also show transverse striations. Cardiac muscle has an inherent rhythmic contractility the rate of which can be modified by autonomic nerves that supply it.

SKELETAL MUSCLE

Elementary Facts about Skeletal Muscle

Skeletal muscle is made up essentially of long, cylindrical 'fibres'. The length of the fibres is highly variable, the longest being as much as 30 cm in length. The diameter of the fibres also varies considerably (10 to 60 µm: usually 50-60 µm). Each 'fibre' is really a syncytium with hundreds of nuclei along its length. (The 'fibre' is formed, during development, by fusion of numerous myoblasts). The nuclei are elongated and lie along the periphery of the fibre, just under the cell membrane (which is called the ***sarcolemma***) (Figs. 10.1 to 10.3). The cytoplasm (or ***sarcoplasm***) is filled with numerous longitudinal fibrils that are called ***myofibrils***.

The most striking feature of skeletal muscle fibres is the presence of transverse striations in them. After staining with haematoxylin the striations are seen as alternate dark and light bands that stretch across the muscle fibre (Fig. 10.4). The dark bands are called ***A-bands***, while the light bands are called ***I-bands***. (As an aid to memory note that 'A' and 'I' correspond to the second letters in the words d**a**rk and l**i**ght.

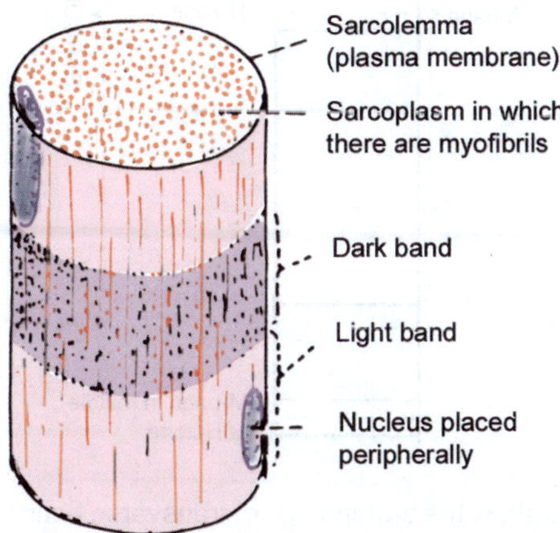

Fig. 10.1 Scheme to show the structure of a muscle fibre.

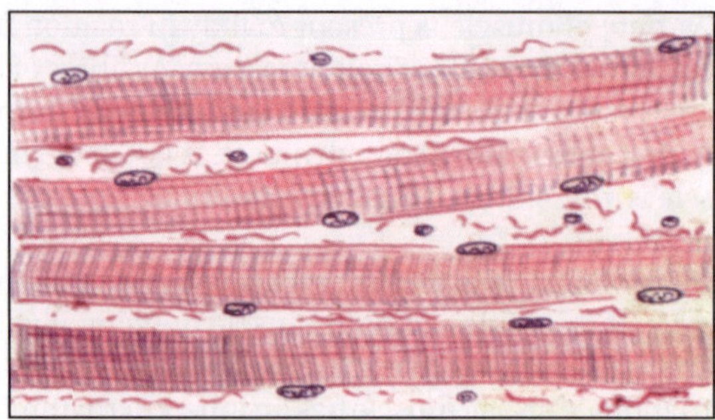

Fig. 10.2 Skeletal muscle seen in longitudinal section.

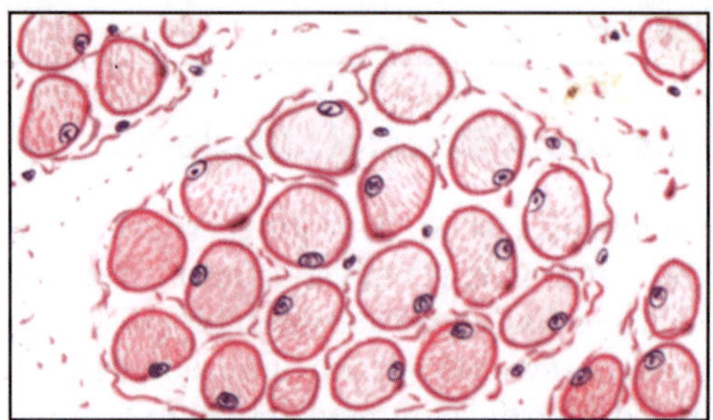

Fig. 10.3 Skeletal muscle seen in transverse section.

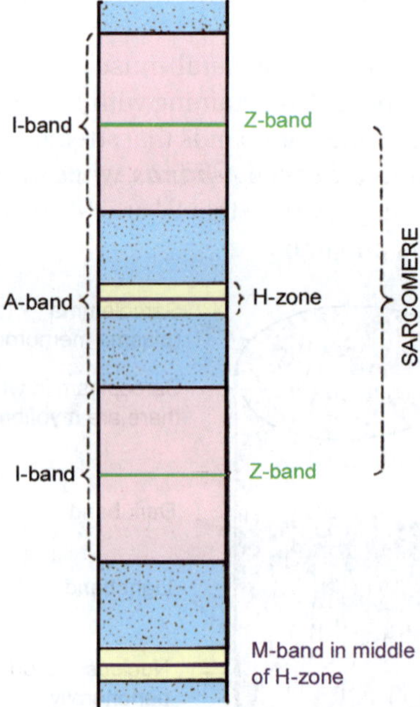

Fig. 10.4 Scheme to show the terminology of transverse bands in a myofibril. Note that the A-band is confined to one sarcomere, but the I-band is made up of parts of two sarcomeres that meet at the Z-band.

Running across the middle of each I-band there is a thin dark line called the ***Z-band***. The centre of the A-band is traversed by a lighter band called the ***H-band*** (or ***H-zone***). Running through the centre of the H-band a thin dark line can be made out. This is the ***M-band***. The various bands described are really present in myofibrils. They appear to run transversely across the whole muscle fibre because corresponding bands in adjoining myofibrils lie exactly opposite one another.

The part of a myofibril situated between two consecutive Z-bands is called a ***sarcomere***. The significance of the striations of myofibrils has to be understood in terms of their ultrastructure which is described later in this chapter.

In addition to myofibrils the sarcoplasm of a muscle fibre contains the usual cell organelles which tend to aggregate near the nuclei. Mitochondria are numerous. Substantial amounts of glycogen are also present. Glycogen provides energy for contraction of muscle.

Innervation of Skeletal Muscle

The nerve supplying a muscle enters it (along with the main blood vessels) at an area called the ***neurovascular hilus.*** This hilus is usually situated nearer the origin of the muscle than the insertion. After entering the muscle the nerve breaks up into many branches that run through the connective tissue of the perimysium and endomysium to reach each muscle fibre. The nerve fibres supplying skeletal muscle are axons arising from large neurons in the anterior (or ventral) grey columns of the spinal cord (or of corresponding nuclei in the brain stem). These ***alpha-efferents*** have a large diameter and are myelinated. Because of repeated branching of its axon, one anterior grey column neuron may supply many muscle fibres all of which contract when this neuron 'fires.' One anterior grey column neuron and the muscle fibres supplied by it constitute one ***motor unit*** (Fig. 10.5). The number of muscle

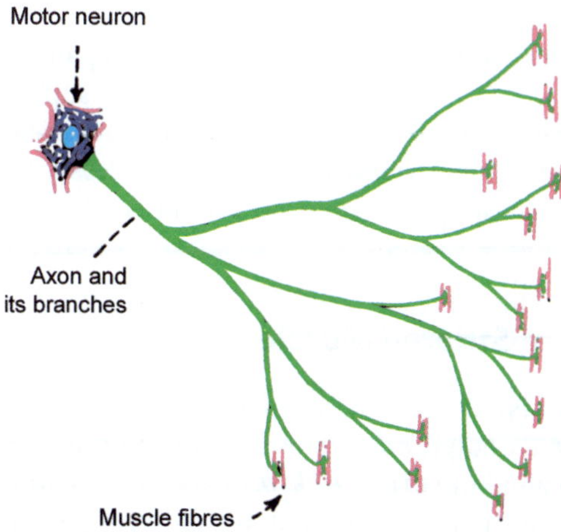

Fig. 10.5 Scheme to illustrate the concept of a motor unit.

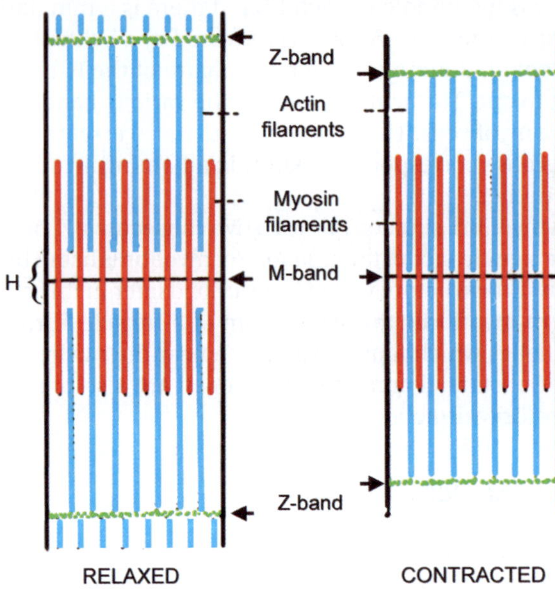

Fig. 10.6 Scheme to show how a myofibril shortens by sliding of actin filaments into the intervals between the myosin filaments. Note that the width of the I-band becomes less, and that the H-zone disappears when the myofibril contracts.

fibres in one motor unit is variable. The units are smaller where precise control of muscular action is required (as in ocular muscles), and much larger in limb muscles where force of contraction is more important. The strength with which a muscle contracts at a particular moment depends on the number of motor units that are activated.

The junction between a muscle fibre and the nerve terminal that supplies it is highly specialized and is called a ***motor end plate***. The structure of a motor end plate is described later in this chapter.

Apart from the alpha efferents described above every muscle receives smaller myelinated ***gamma-efferents*** that arise from gamma neurons in the ventral grey column of the spinal cord. These fibres supply special muscle fibres that are present within sensory receptors called ***muscle spindles***. These special muscle fibres are called ***intrafusal fibres***. Nerves to muscles also carry autonomic fibres that supply smooth muscle present in the walls of blood vessels.

Ultrastructure of Striated Muscle

Each muscle fibre is covered by a plasma membrane that is called the ***sarcolemma***. The sarcolemma is covered on the outside by a ***basement membrane*** (also called the ***external lamina***) which establishes an intimate connection between the muscle fibre and the fibres (collagen, reticular) of the endomysium.

The cytoplasm (***sarcoplasm***) is permeated with myofibrils which push the elongated nuclei to a peripheral position. Between the myofibrils there is an elaborate system of membrane lined tubes called the ***sarcoplasmic reticulum***. Elongated mitochondria (***sarcosomes***) and clusters of glycogen are also scattered amongst the myofibrils. Perinuclear Golgi bodies, ribosomes, lysosomes, and lipid vacuoles are also present.

Structure of Myofibrils

When examined by EM each myofibril is seen to be made of fine myofilaments. These are of two types: ***actin*** and ***myosin***, made up of molecules of corresponding proteins. (Each myosin filament is about 12 nm in diameter, while an actin filament is about 8 nm in diameter. They are therefore referred to as thick and thin filaments respectively). The arrangement of actin and myosin filaments within a sarcomere is shown in Fig. 10.6. It will be seen that myosin filaments are confined to the A-band, the width of the band being equal to the length of the myosin filaments. The actin filaments are attached at one end to the Z-band. From here they pass through the I-band and extend into the 'outer' parts of the A-band, where they interdigitate with the myosin filaments. Note that the I-band is made up of actin filaments alone. The H-band represents the part of the A-band into which actin filaments do not extend. The Z-band is really a complicated network at which the actin filaments of adjoining sarcomeres meet. The M-band is produced by fine interconnections between adjacent myosin filaments.

In an uncontracted myofibril, overlap between actin and myosin filaments is minimal. During contraction the fibril shortens by sliding in of actin filaments more and more into the intervals between the myosin filaments. As a result the width of the I-band decreases, but that of the A-band is unchanged. The H-bands are obliterated in a contracted fibril.

Sarcoplasmic Reticulum

In the intervals between myofibrils, the sarcoplasm contains an elaborate system of tubules called the sarcoplasmic reticulum (Fig. 10.7). The larger elements of this reticulum run in planes at right angles to the long axes of the myofibrils, and form rings around each myofibril. At the level of every junction between an A and I band the myofibril is encircled by a set of three closely connected tubules which constitute a ***muscle triad***. For purposes of description each such triad can be said to be composed of an upper, a middle, and a lower tubule (Fig. 10.7). The upper and lower tubules of the triad are connected to the tubules of adjoining triads through a network of smaller tubules. There is one such network opposite each A-band, and another opposite each I-band. These networks, along with the upper and lower tubules of the triad, constitute the sarcoplasmic reticulum. This reticulum is a closed system of tubes.

The middle tube of the triad is an entity independent of the sarcoplasmic reticulum. It is called a ***centrotubule*** and belongs to what is called the ***T-system*** of membranes. The centrotubules are really formed by invagination

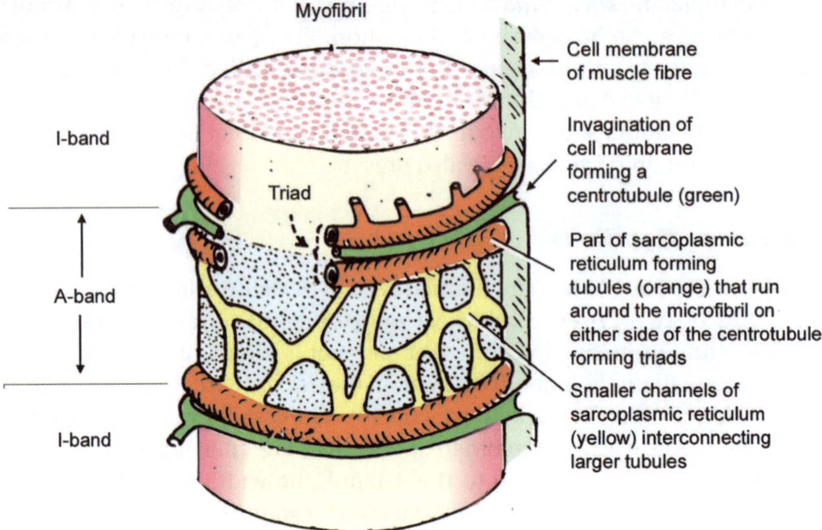

Fig. 10.7 Diagram to show relationship of the sarcoplasmic reticulum, and of the T-tubes to a myofibril.

of the sarcolemma into the sarcoplasm. Their lumina are, therefore, in communication with the exterior of the muscle fibre. As already noted the centrotubules permeate the entire muscle fibre as they form networks around myofibrils as part of the muscle triads.

Contraction of muscle is dependent on release of calcium ions into myofibrils. In a relaxed muscle these ions are strongly bound to the membranes of the sarcoplasmic reticulum. When a nerve stimulus reaches a motor end plate the sarcolemma is depolarized. The wave of depolarization is transmitted to the interior of the muscle fibre through the centrotubules. As a result of this wave calcium ions are released from the sarcoplasmic reticulum into the myofibrils causing their contraction.

Blood Vessels and Lymphatics of Skeletal Muscle

Skeletal muscle is richly supplied with blood vessels. The arteries form a plexus in the epimysium and in the perimysium, and end in a network of capillaries that surrounds each muscle fibre. Veins leaving the muscle accompany the arteries. A lymphatic plexus extends into the epimysium and the perimysium, but not into the endomysium.

PHYSIOLOGY OF SKELETAL MUSCLE

Muscle is an excitable tissue. The exciting stimulus can be chemical, mechanical or electrical. The muscle responds to the stimulus by contraction. Within the body, a muscle contracts on receiving a nerve impulse.

Electrical Phenomena in Muscle

A muscle fibre is covered by a cell membrane, the sarcolemma. In the resting fibre the membrane is polarised. Its internal surface (towards sarcoplasm) has a negative charge, while its outer surface (towards extracellular fluid) as a positive charge. The difference in potential on the two sides of the membrane is the resting membrane potential. By convention, it is expressed in terms of the voltage inside the muscle cell, and is about -90 millivolts.

When a stimulus is applied to the muscle, the membrane undergoes depolarisation. This means that voltage on the two sides of the membrane becomes equal. This is the action potential. The action potential lasts only for 2-4 ms (milliseconds) at a given site. Depolarisation begins at the motor end plate. It spreads through the sarcolemma like a wave, succeeding segments being depolarised followed by repolarisation. In this way the entire muscle fibre is stimulated to contract.

Ionic Basis of Resting Membrane Potential

Positively charged sodium and potassium ions and negatively charged chloride ions are present on both sides of the membrane. However, there are more positively charged ions on the external surface than inside the cell. This is the reason for the resting membrane potential. This potential is kept constant by movement of ions as described below.

Ions can move across a cell membrane, by passive transport, in two ways. When the concentration of ions is greater on one side of the membrane than on the other, this concentration gradient tends to move ions from region of higher concentration to lower. Similarly an electric gradient can move positive ions towards the side having a lower potential, and negative ions towards the side of higher potential.

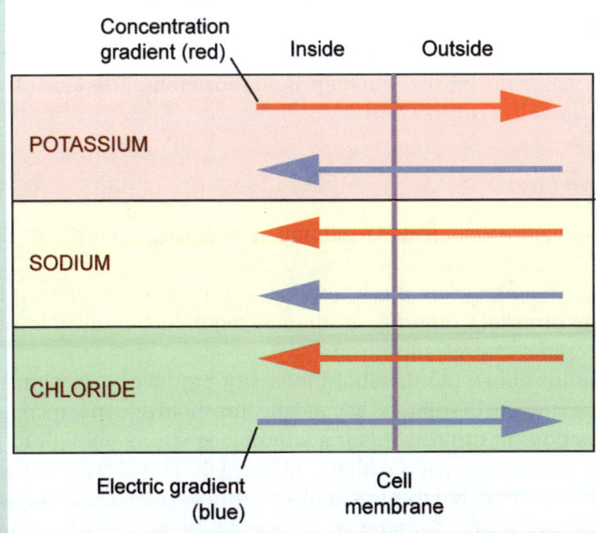

Fig. 10.8 Movement of ions across cell membrane.

These two forces may act in the same direction or in opposing directions. In the first instance the two reinforce one another, and in the second instance the two forces oppose one another.

Chloride ions (Cl^-)are present in higher concentration outside the cell, than inside it. Hence the concentration gradient tends to move chloride ions into the cell (Fig. 10.8). On the other hand the electric gradient tends to move negatively charged Cl^- ions out of the cell and equilibrium is reached when the two forces are equal. In the case of potassium (K^+) ions, the concentration gradient pushes the ions out of the cell, but the electric gradient tends to move K^+ ions into the cell. In the case of sodium (Na^+) both the concentration gradient and the electric gradient tend to move ions inwards. Such passive movement of ions would have the effect of changing the resting membrane potential. However, this is not allowed to happen. Sodium ions are moved out of the cell by active transport (using Na^+-K^+ATPase).

Contraction of Muscle

1. When the nerve supplying a muscle is stimulated the muscle contracts once and then relaxes. This is called a muscle twitch.
2. If a second stimulus is given before relaxation sets in, a second contraction gets added to the first one, resulting in a higher curve. The adding together of two or more contractions is called ***summation of contractions***.
3. If repeated stimuli are given, the muscle shows a prolonged response. This is called a ***tetanic contraction*** (or ***tetanus***).
4. There is a limit to the number of times a muscle can keep contracting in response to stimuli. After the first few contractions, the force of each contraction gradually decreases. Finally the muscle stops responding. This is called ***fatigue***. Fatigue is caused by exhaustion of acetyl choline in the motor end plate, lack of oxygen and nutrients, and accumulation of lactic acid.
5. If one end of a muscle is fixed, and the other end is free to move, contraction leads to shortening. Because of shortening, tension on the muscle fibres remains more or less constant. This kind of contraction is called ***isotonic contraction***.
6. If both ends of a muscle are fixed, and such a muscle is made to contract, tension develops within the muscle, but there is no shortening. This kind of contraction is called ***isometric contraction***.

All or None Law

When a muscle fibre is subjected to stimuli of increasing intensity we observe the following.

1. A specific strength of stimulus is necessary for contraction of the muscle fibre. This is the ***threshold intensity*** of stimulus required. Stimuli of lesser intensity cannot produce any response.
2. Any stimulus above the threshold intensity produces a maximal response. Increasing strength of stimulus beyond the threshold does not increase strength of contraction. In other words if a stimulus is strong enough to produce a response the fibre contracts with its full strength. This is called the ***all or none law***. However, note that this law applies only a single muscle fibre, and not to the muscle as a whole. The strength of contraction of a muscle depends on the total number of fibres that contract at a given time.

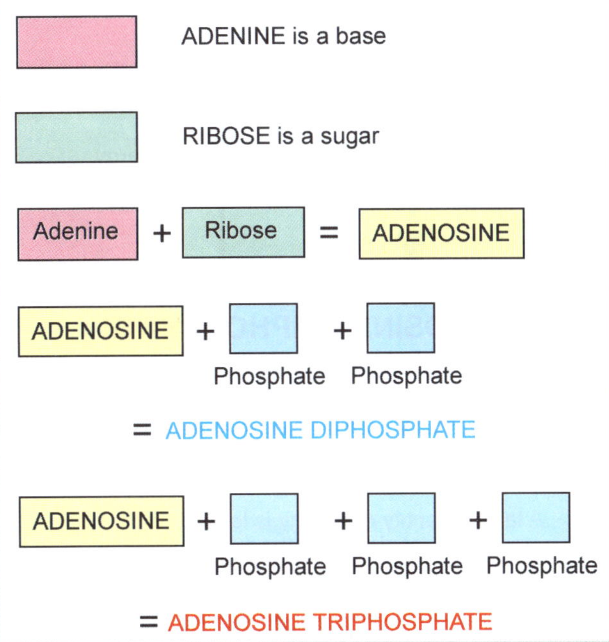

Fig. 10.9 Structure of ATP.

Effect of Temperature

The strength of muscle contraction is increased by moderate increase in temperature (to about 40ºC). The increase is due to increased excitability of muscle, to accleration of chemical processes, and reduced viscosity of muscle. Cooling the muscle (to about 10ºC) has the opposite effect.

CHEMICAL PROCESSES INVOLVED IN MUSCLE CONTRACTION

Muscle contraction requires a large amount of energy, in the form of ATP (adenosine triphosphate). The structure of ATP is explained in Fig. 10.9. The storage and release of energy from ATP is shown in Fig. 10.10. Muscle fibres store large quantities of glygogen. Glycogen is readily converted to glucose. ATP is obtained by metabolism of glucose as shown in Fig. 10.11. The process is efficient when oxygen is available in adequate quantity. Utilization of glucose in the presence of oxygen is called aerobic catabolism. Some utilization of glucose can also take place in the absence of oxygen (anaerobic catabolism) but this process is not efficient. The steps involved in utilization of glucose are summarised below. Remember that energy released is stored in the form of ATP.

Glucolysis

Step 1. Glucose (from the circulation) enters the cytoplasm of a cell. Each molecule of glucose forms two molecules of pyruvic acid. Energy is released in the form of two molecules of ATP. Glucolysis is an anaerobic process (Fig. 10.11).

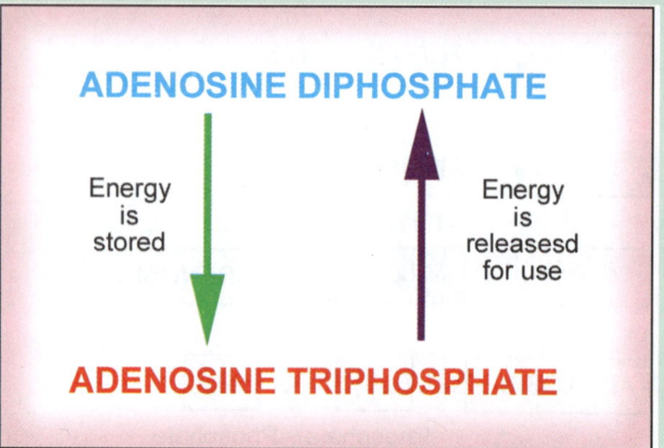

Fig. 10.10 Role of ATP in metabolism.

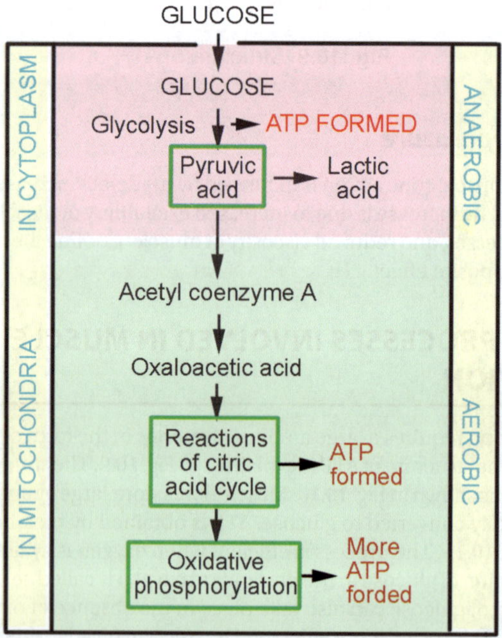

Fig. 10.11 Deriving energy from glucose.

Step 2. The two molecules of pyruvic acid enter mitochondria and undergo a series of reactions that are known as the citric acid cycle or Krebs' cycle. In this process two more molecules of ATP are generated. Oxygen is required for this reaction.

Step 3. Some substances produced in the citric acid cycle undergo oxidative phosphorylation to produce several more molecules of ATP. This takes place within mitochrondria and requires adequate supply of oxygen.

Step 4. When adequate supply of oxygen is not available (e.g., during heavy exercise) the two molecules of pyruvic acid formed by glucolysis (see step 1 above) remain in the cytoplasm and are converted to lactic acid. Accumulation of lactic acid in muscles, leads to pain and cramps (that athletes often complain of). Later when adequate blood supply (oxygen supply) is restored accumulated lactic acid is removed as follows.

Some of it is reconverted into pyruvic acid. Pyruvic acid is oxidized to form CO_2 and water. CO_2 enters blood and is removed through the lungs. Water (if in excess) is removed from the body through urine.

Muscle contains the compound phosphorylcreatine. This compound can be hydrolyzed to creatine and phosphate. This reaction releases considerable energy which can be stored as ATP. This is an alternative source of energy available in muscle. A third source of energy are free fatty acids present in blood. They are oxidised to CO_2 and H_2O releasing energy in the form of ATP.

Oxygen Debt

When a muscle is at rest the oxygen used by it is the ***basal consumption***.

During exertion the oxygen consumption becomes much higher, as oxygen is needed for aerobic metabolism of glucose using the pathway shown in Fig. 10.11. As intensity of exercise increases, oxygen supply falls short of demand. When this happens the muscle uses anaerobic pathways for production of ATP. These are

1. Anaerobic conversion of glucose to pyruvate, and of pyruvate to lactic acid.
2. Hydrolysis of phosphorylcreatine.

The availability of these anaerobic pathways enables muscle contraction to continue for a longer period. When activity of muscle has ceased, for some time the muscle continues to use a higher quantity of oxygen than in the resting state. This oxygen is needed for:

a. Replenishing exhausted stores of ATP.
b. Replenishing exhausted stores of phosphorylcreatine.
c. Reconverting some accumulated lactate to pyruvate.
d. Removal of excessive lactate.

The extra oxygen used to bring the muscle back to the state that existed before beginning of exercise is called the ***oxygen debt***.

Strength, Power and Endurance of Muscle

The term ***strength*** is applied to the maximum force that can be generated by a muscle. It is about 3 to 4 kg per square centimeter of cross sectional area of the muscle. Hence the thicker the muscle, the more its strength. The force generated by shortening of the muscle is called ***contractile strength***. The force required to stretch a contracted muscle is called ***holding strength***.

Power is a measure of work done by a muscle (expressed in Kg per minute). Power depends on strength, its force of contraction and frequency of contraction.

The capacity of a muscle to maintain activity over a period of time is called ***endurance***. This depends mainly on availability of glycogen in the muscle. It is increased by training in athletes, and by a high carbohydrate diet.

General and Cardiorespiratory Endurance

Endurance of muscular activity is only possible by adequate supply of blood and oxygen.

The factors that increase blood supply are as follows.

1. ***Increase in heart rate***: This is produced by increased sympathetic tone and reduced vagal tone. Factors affecting these include proprioceptive impulses from muscle, increased carbon oxide tension, raised body temperature, and increased secretion of catecholamines.
2. ***Increase in cardiac output***: This is produced by increased heart rate and increased stroke volume.
3. ***Increased venous return***: This is a result of the pumping action of muscle, greater activity of respiratory pump and reduced blood supply to viscera.
4. ***Increased blood pressure***: In isotonic exercise systolic blood pressure rises, but the diastolic pressure remains normal, or less than normal. Diastolic pressure increases in isometric exercise.

The factors that increase oxygen supply to muscle are as follows.

1. ***Increased pulmonary ventilation***: This is a result of increase in rate and depth of respiration. These are produced through stimulation of the respiratory centre, by stimulation of chemoreceptors by hypoxia, by increase of body temperature, and by acidosis.
2. ***Increased blood flow*** through pulmonary capillaries increases diffusion capacity for oxygen.
3. ***Increased consumption of oxygen***. The oxygen consumed by tissues, specially by muscle, greatly increases during exercise. This is possible because of increased availability of oxygen through blood.
4. See oxygen debt (page 84) and respiratory quotient (Chapter 15).

Effects of Ageing on Activity

Muscle mass and strength increase as a child grows, reaching a maximum at about the age of 20 years. A person's physical efficiency is at its peak between 20-30 years of age. In most persons physical and muscle strength gradually declines after the age of 50. Endurance is reduced and fatigue sets in faster.

Decrease in activity with age is to be correlated with reduced efficiency of the cardiovascular and respiratory systems. Narrowing of arteries, due to atherosclerosis begins as early as the age of 20 and progressively increases thereafter. This progressively reduces blood and oxygen supply to all parts of the body. Narrowing of arteries leads to increased peripheral resistance, with reduced arterial compliance. Increased resistance leads to elevation of systolic blood pressure and ultimately to some degree of left ventricular hypertrophy. The cardiac output falls and the body is less able to adjust to a rise in heart rate, to dehydration, or to postural changes.

The respiratory system becomes less efficient as lung elasticity decreases, and chest wall stiffness increases.

Changes also take place in the nervous system. Atrophy of brain tissue has been observed. Reflexes become slower. The gait becomes stiff. Orientation of time and space many be impaired. Impairment of vision and hearing are contributory causes. However, many old persons remain mentally sharp till a late age.

CARDIAC MUSCLE

The structure of cardiac muscle has many similarities to that of skeletal muscle; but there are important differences as well (Figs. 10.12, 10.13).

Similarities between Cardiac and Skeletal Muscle

These are as follows. Like skeletal muscle, cardiac muscle is made up of elongated 'fibres' within which there are numerous myofibrils. The myofibrils (and, therefore, the fibres) show transverse striations similar to those of skeletal muscle. A, I, Z and H bands can be made out in the striations. The connective tissue framework, and the capillary network around cardiac muscle fibres are similar to those in skeletal muscle.

With the EM it is seen that myofibrils of cardiac muscle have the same structure as those of skeletal muscle and are made up of actin and myosin

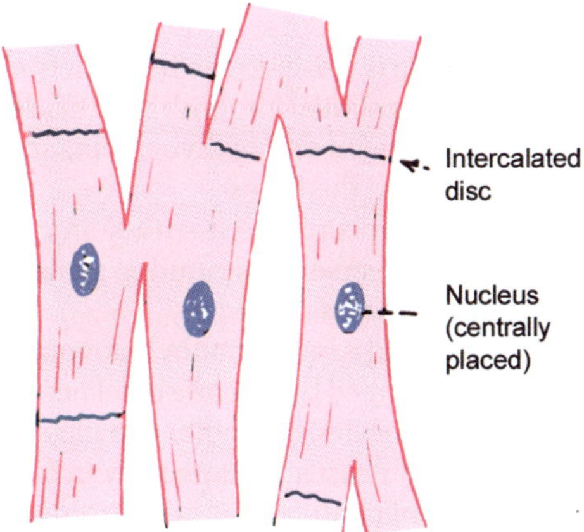

Fig. 10.12 Cardiac muscle (diagrammatic).

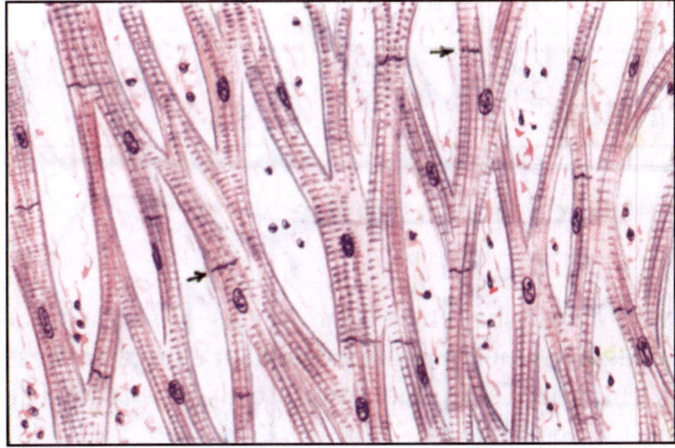

Fig. 10.13 Cardiac muscle as seen in a section.

filaments. A sarcoplasmic reticulum, T-system of centrotubules, numerous mitochondria and other organelles are present.

Differences between Cardiac and Skeletal Muscle

These are as follows.

1. The fibres of cardiac muscle do not run in strict parallel formation, but branch and anastomose with other fibres to form a network.
2. Each fibre of cardiac muscle is not a multinucleated syncytium as in skeletal muscle, but is a chain of cardiac muscle cells (or ***cardiac myocytes***) each having its own nucleus. Each myocyte is about 80 μm long and about 15 μm broad.
3. The nucleus of each myocyte is located centrally (and not peripherally as in skeletal muscle).
4. The sarcoplasm of cardiac myocytes is abundant and contains numerous large mitochondria. The myofibrils are relatively few. At places, the myofibrils merge with each other. As a result of these factors, the myofibrils and striations of cardiac muscle are not as distinct as those of skeletal muscle. In this respect cardiac muscle is closer to the red variety of skeletal muscle than to the white variety. Other similarities with red muscle are the presence of significant amounts of glycogen and of myoglobin, and the rich density of the capillary network around the fibres.
5. With the light microscope the junctions between adjoining cardiac myocytes are seen as dark staining transverse lines running across the muscle fibre. These lines are called ***intercalated discs***.
6. Cardiac muscle is involuntary and is innervated by autonomic fibres (in contrast to skeletal muscle that is innervated by cerebrospinal nerves). Nerve endings terminate near the cardiac myocytes, but motor end plates are not seen.

Isolated cardiac myocytes contract spontaneously in a rhythmic manner. In the intact heart the rhythm of contraction is determined by a pace maker located in the sinuatrial node. From here the impulse spreads to the entire heart through a conducting system made up of a special kind of cardiac muscle. From the above it will be appreciated that a nerve supply is not necessary for contraction of cardiac muscle. Nervous influences do, however, influence the strength and rate of contraction of the heart.

SMOOTH MUSCLE

Basic Facts About Smooth Muscle

Smooth muscle (also called ***non-striated, involuntary*** or ***plain muscle***) is made up of long spindle shaped cells (myocytes) having a broad central part and tapering ends. The nucleus, which is oval or elongated, lies in the central part of the cell. The length of smooth muscle cells (often called fibres) is highly variable (15 μm to 500 μm) (Figs. 10.14, 10.15).

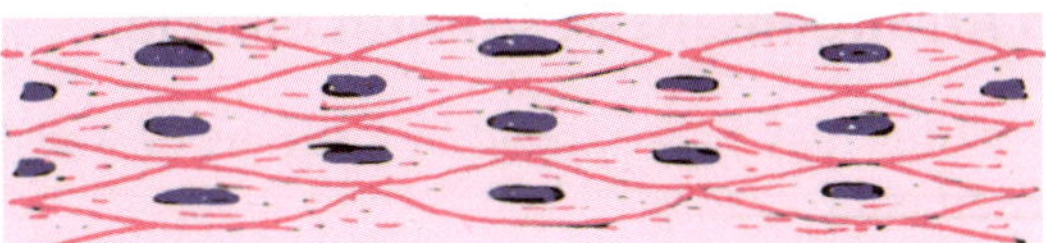

Fig. 10.14 Smooth muscle cells (diagrammatic).

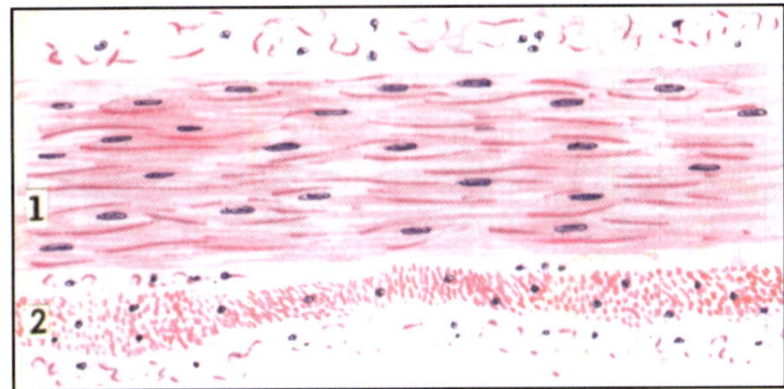

Fig. 10.15 Smooth muscle as seen in section. 1 – L.S. 2 – T.S.

With the light microscope the sarcoplasm appears to have indistinct longitudinal striations, but there are no transverse striations.

Smooth muscle cells are usually aggregated to form bundles, or fasciculi, that are further aggregated to form layers of variable thickness. In such a layer the cells are so arranged that the thick central part of one cell is opposite the thin tapering ends of adjoining cells. Aggregations of smooth muscle cells into fasciculi and layers is facilitated by the fact that each myocyte is surrounded by a network of delicate fibres (collagen, reticular, elastic) that holds the myocytes together. The fibres between individual myocytes become continuous with the more abundant connective tissue that separates fasciculi or layers of smooth muscle.

Distribution of Smooth Muscle

a. Smooth muscle is seen most typically in the walls of hollow viscera including the stomach, the intestines, the urinary bladder and the uterus.
b. It is present in the walls of several structures that are in the form of narrow tubes e.g., arteries, veins, bronchi, ureters, deferent ducts, uterine tubes, and the ducts of several glands.
c. The muscles that constrict and dilate the pupil are made up of smooth muscle.
d. Some smooth muscle is present in the orbit (orbitalis); in the upper eyelid (Muller's muscle); in the prostate; in the skin of the scrotum (Dartos muscle). In the skin delicate bundles of smooth muscle are present in relation to hair follicles. These bundles are called the ***arrector pili*** muscles.

Variations in Arrangement of Smooth Muscle

Smooth muscle fibres may be arranged in a variety of ways depending on functional requirements.

a. In some organs (e.g., the gut) smooth muscle is arranged in the form of two distinct layers: an inner circular and an outer longitudinal. Within each layer the fasciculi lie parallel to each other. Such an arrangement allows peristaltic movements to take place for propulsion of contents along the tube.

   In some organs (e.g., the ureter) the arrangement of layers may be reversed, the longitudinal layer being internal to the circular one. In yet other situations there may be three layers: inner and outer longitudinal with a circular layer in between.
b. In some regions (e.g., urinary bladder, uterus) the smooth muscle is arranged in layers, but the layers are not distinctly demarcated from each other. Even within layers the fasciculi tend to run in various directions and may form a network. In these organs contraction of muscle makes the lumen of the organ smaller and expels its contents.
c. In some tubes (e.g., the bile duct) a thick layer of circular muscle may surround a segment of the tube forming a ***sphincter***. Contraction of the sphincter occludes the tube.
d. In the skin, and in some other situations, smooth muscle occurs in the form of narrow bands.

Innervation of Smooth Muscle

Smooth muscle is innervated by autonomic nerves, both sympathetic and parasympathetic. The two have opposite effects. For example, in the iris, parasympathetic stimulation causes constriction of the pupil, and sympathetic stimulation causes dilatation. It may be noted that sympathetic or parasympathetic nerves may cause contraction of muscle at some sites, and relaxation at other sites.

SOME CLINICAL CORRELATIONS OF MUSCLE

1. Contraction of skeletal muscle can take place only if the nerve supply is intact. When nerve supply is interrupted (by injury or disease) and the muscle cannot contract, the condition is called ***paralysis***. Partial paralysis leads to weakness or ***paresis***. Paralysis of one half of the body is called ***hemiplegia***. Paralysis of both lower limbs is called ***paraplegia***. Paralysis of respiratory muscles leads to death. When muscles are paralysed because of injury to a peripheral nerve, they gradually undergo atrophy.
2. All varieties of muscle can hypertrophy when exposed to greater stress. Hypertrophy takes place by enlargement of existing fibres, and not by formation of new fibres. Skeletal muscle hypertrophies with exercise. Cardiac muscle hypertrophies if the load on a chamber of the heart is increased for any reason. An example is the hypertrophy of muscle in the wall of the left ventricle in hypertension. Hypertrophy of smooth muscle is seen most typically in the uterus

where myocytes may increase from a length of about 15 to 20 μm at the beginning of pregnancy to as much as 500 μm towards the end of pregnancy.

3. Smooth muscle and cardiac muscle have very little capacity for regeneration. Any defects produced by injury or disease are usually repaired by formation of fibrous tissue.

Skeletal muscle fibres can undergo some degree of regeneration. When large segments of a muscle are destroyed the gap is filled in by fibrous tissue.

4. Overactivity of smooth muscle is responsible for many symptoms. Constriction of bronchi leads to asthma. Spasm of smooth muscle can give rise to severe pain (***colic***) which may originate in the intestines (***intestinal colic***), ureter (***renal colic***), or bile duct (***biliary colic***). These symptoms can be relieved by drugs which cause relaxation of smooth muscle.
5. Progressive degeneration of muscle takes place in a group of inherited disorders called ***myopatheis***. Several types of myopathy are known.
6. ***Myasthenia gravis*** is a condition in which muscles become very weak. It is believed to be an autoimmune disease.
7. If a large volume of muscle is damaged by extreme pressure (as in accidents) the fibres undergo necrosis. Myoglobin is released into blood. The kidneys try to excrete this myoglobin, but they can themselves get damaged in the process.

NERVOUS TISSUE

The nervous system is made up, predominantly, of tissue that has the special property of being able to conduct impulses rapidly from one part of the body to another. The specialized cells that constitute the functional units of the nervous system are called ***neurons***. Within the brain and spinal cord neurons are supported by a special kind of connective tissue that is called ***neuroglia.*** Nervous tissue, composed of neurons and neuroglia, is richly supplied with blood.

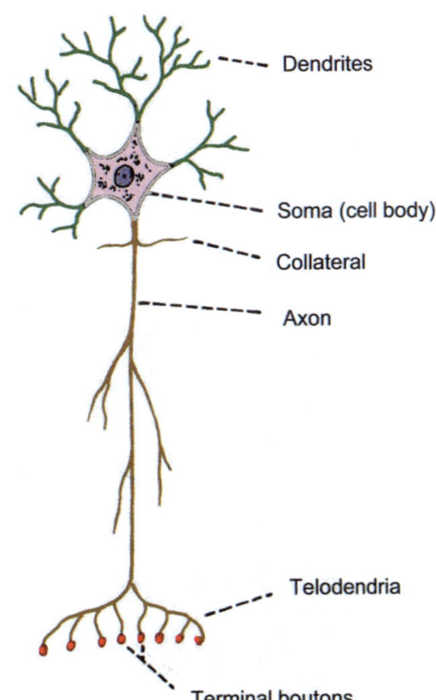

Fig. 10.16 Scheme to show some parts of a neuron.

The nervous system of man is made up of innumerable neurons. The neurons are linked together in a highly intricate manner. It is through these connections that the body is made aware of changes in the environment, or of those within itself; and appropriate responses to such changes are produced e.g., in the form of movement or in the modified working of some organ of the body. There is no doubt that higher functions of the brain, like those of memory and intelligence, are also to be explained on the basis of connections between neurons, but as yet little is known about the mechanisms involved. Neurons are, therefore, to be regarded not merely as simple conductors, but as cells that are specialized for the reception, integration, interpretation and transmission of information.

NEURON STRUCTURE

Elementary Structure of a Typical Neuron

Neurons vary considerably in size, shape and other features. However, most of them have some major features in common and these are described below (Figs. 10.16 to 10.20).

A neuron consists of a ***cell body*** which gives off a variable number of ***processes*** (Fig. 10.16). Like a typical cell it consists of a mass of cytoplasm surrounded by a cell membrane. The cytoplasm contains a large central

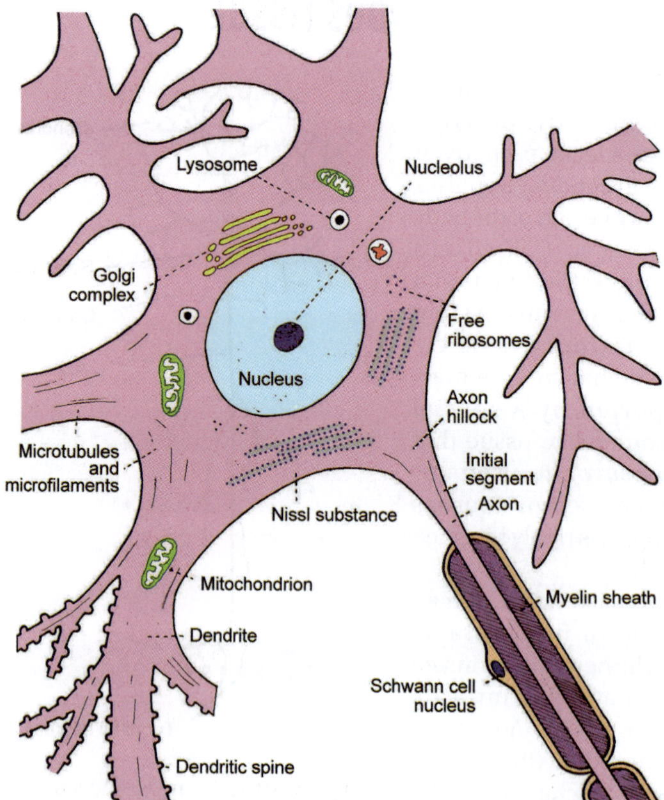

Fig. 10.17 Schematic presentation of some features of the structure of a neuron as seen by EM.

nucleus (usually with a prominent nucleolus), numerous mitochondria, lysosomes and a Golgi complex (Fig. 10.17). In addition to these features, the cytoplasm of a neuron has some distinctive characteristics not seen in other cells. The cytoplasm shows the presence of a granular material that stains intensely with basic dyes; this material is the ***Nissl substance*** (Fig. 10.18). When examined by EM, this substance is seen to be composed of rough surfaced endoplasmic reticulum (Fig. 10.17). The presence of abundant granular endoplasmic reticulum is an indication of the high level of protein synthesis in neurons. The proteins are needed for maintenance and repair, and for production of neurotransmitters and enzymes.

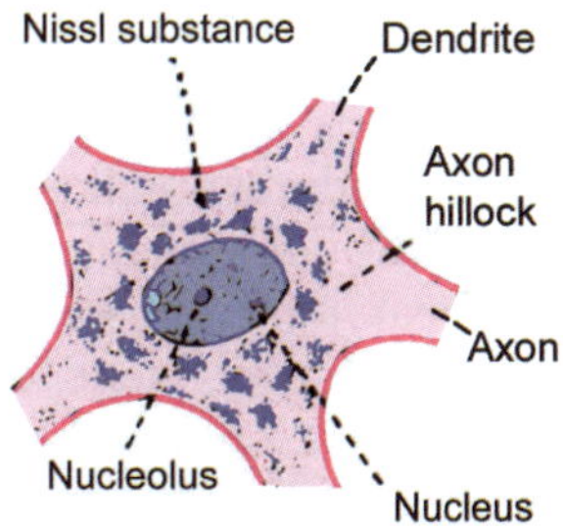

Fig. 10.18 Neuron stained to show Nissl substance. Note that the Nissl substance extends into the dendrites but not into the axon.

Another distinctive feature of neurons is the presence of a network of fibrils permeating the cytoplasm (Fig. 10.20). These ***neurofibrils*** are seen, with the EM, to consist of microfilaments and microtubules. Some neurons contain pigment granules.

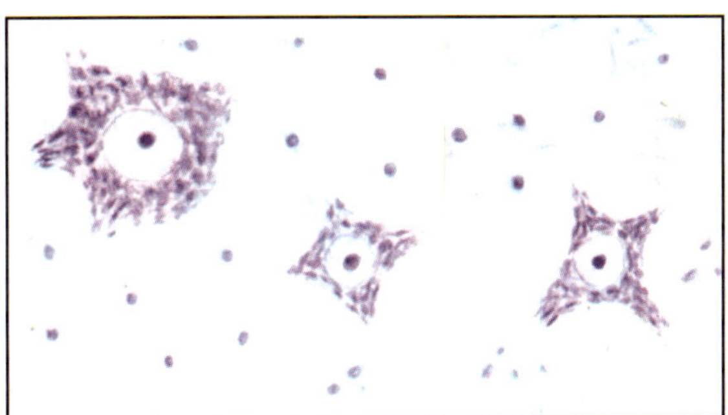

Fig. 10.19 Section of spinal cord showing large neurons in the ventral grey column.

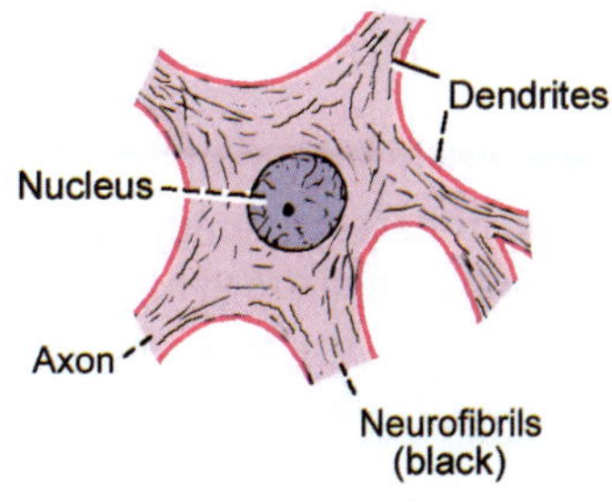

Fig. 10.20 Neuron stained to show neurofibrils. Note that the fibrils extend into both axons and dendrites.

The processes arising from the cell body of a neuron are called ***neurites.*** These are of two kinds. Most neurons give off a number of short branching processes called ***dendrites*** and one longer process called an ***axon.***

The dendrites are characterized by the fact that they terminate near the cell body. They are irregular in thickness, and Nissl granules extend into them. They bear numerous small spines which are of variable shape.

The axon may extend for a considerable distance away from the cell body. The longest axons may be as much as a metre long. Each axon has a uniform diameter, and is devoid of Nissl substance.

In addition to these differences in structure, there is a fundamental functional difference between dendrites and axons. In a dendrite, the nerve impulse travels ***towards the cell body*** whereas in an axon the impulse travels ***away from the cell body.***

We have seen above that the axon is free of Nissl granules. The Nissl-free zone extends for a short distance into the cell body: this part of the cell body is called the ***axon hillock.*** The part of the axon just beyond the axon hillock is called the ***initial segment*** (Fig. 10.17).

Some axons are surrounded by a ***myelin sheath***. In peripheral nerves, the myelin sheath is formed by ***Schwann cells***. Outside the myelin sheath a thin layer of Schwann cell cytoplasm persists to form an additional sheath which is called the ***neurilemma*** (also called the neurilemmal sheath or Schwann cell sheath). Axons lying within the central nervous system are provided a myelin sheath by a kind of neuroglial cell called an ***oligodendrocyte***

Axons having a myelin sheath are called ***myelinated axons***. The presence of a myelin sheath increases the velocity of conduction (for a nerve fibre of the same diameter). It also reduces the energy expended in the process of conduction.

An axon is related to a large number of Schwann cells over its length. Each Schwann cell provides the myelin sheath for a short segment of the axon. At the junction of any two such segments there is a short gap in the myelin sheath. These gaps are called the ***nodes of Ranvier*** (Fig. 10.21).

There are some axons that are devoid of myelin sheaths. These are ***unmyelinated axons***.

An axon may give off a variable number of branches (Fig. 10.16). Some branches, that arise near the cell body and lie at right angles to the axon are called ***collaterals***. At its termination the axon breaks up into a number of fine branches called ***telodendria*** which may end in small swellings (***terminal boutons*** or ***bouton terminaux***).

An axon (or its branches) can terminate in two ways. Within the central nervous system, it always terminates by coming in intimate relationship with another neuron, the junction between the two neurons being called a ***synapse***. Outside the central nervous system, the axon may end in relation to an effector organ (e.g., muscle or gland), or may end by synapsing with neurons in a peripheral ganglion.

Axons (and some dendrites that resemble axons in structure: see below) constitute what are commonly called ***nerve fibres.***

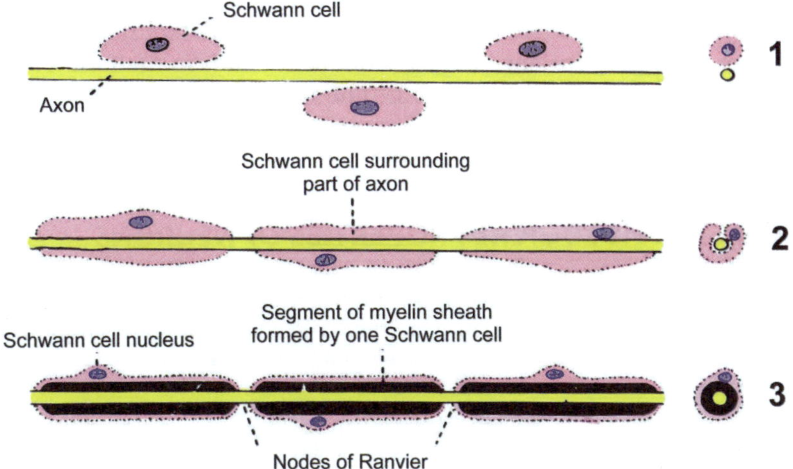

Fig. 10.21 Scheme to show that one Schwann cell forms a short segment of the myelin sheath of a nerve fibre.

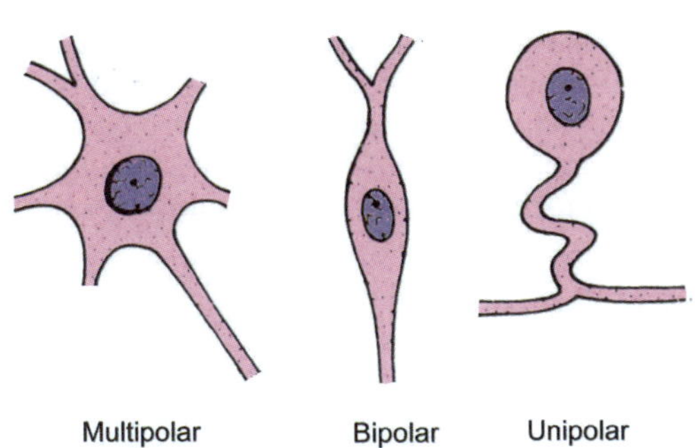

Fig. 10.22 Diagram showing three types of neurons.

Variability in Neuron Structure

Neurons vary considerably in the size and shape of their cell bodies (somata) and in the length and manner of branching of their processes. The shape of the cell body is dependent on the number of processes arising from it. The most common type of neuron gives off several processes and the cell body is, therefore, ***multipolar*** (Fig. 10.22). Some neurons have only one axon and one dendrite and are ***bipolar.***

Another type of neuron has a single process. This process divides into two. One of the divisions represents the axon; the other is functionally a dendrite, but its structure is indistinguishable from that of an axon. This neuron is described as ***unipolar***, but from a functional point of view it is to be regarded as bipolar. Depending on the shapes of their cell bodies some neurons are referred to as ***stellate*** (star shaped) or ***pyramidal.***

In addition to the variations in size and shape, the cell bodies of neurons may show striking variations in the appearance of the Nissl substance. In some neurons, the Nissl substance is very prominent and is in the form of large clumps. In some others, the granules are fine and uniformly distributed in the cytoplasm, while yet other neurons show gradations between these extremes. These differences can be correlated with function.

SOME PHYSIOLOGICAL PROPERTIES OF NEURONS

Earlier in this chapter we have discussed the concepts of membrane potential, depolarisation and repolarisation. The chemical and electrical aspects of these phenomena have been studied. These should be reviewed as they are equally applicable in neurons also. Some differences are given below.

1. The resting membrane potential in a neuron is -70mV.
2. Neurons have a lower threshold for excitation. The neuron 'fires' when depolarisation reaches -55mV.
3. When a neuron is stimulated an action potential is produced. This happens if the strength of the stimulus is adequate (i.e., it is above threshold value). The action potential obeys the all or none law. If the stimulus is adequate to produce a response, a maximal response is obtained, and further increase in strength of stimulation does not increase the response. The action potential is transmitted along the axon as a nerve impulse. As in muscle, the basis for a nerve impulse is the spread of a wave of depolarisation. In unmyelinated axons the impulse travels along the cell membrane, and such conduction is relatively slow. However, in myelinated axons conduction is much faster because depolarisation jumps from one node of Ranvier to the next. This is called ***saltatory conduction***.

The Synapse

We have seen that synapses are sites of junction between neurons. Synapses may be of various types depending upon the parts of the neurons that come in contact. In the most common type of synapse, an axon terminal establishes contact with the dendrite of a receiving neuron to form an ***axodendritic synapse.*** The axon terminal may synapse with the cell body (***axosomatic synapse***) or, less commonly, with the axon of the receiving neuron (***axoaxonal synapse***).

A synapse transmits an impulse only in one direction. The two elements taking part in a synapse can, therefore, be spoken of as ***presynaptic*** and ***postsynaptic***. In a typical synapse the terminal part of the axon is enlarged. It is called the ***presynaptic bouton*** (= button). Numerous vesicles are present in the presynaptic bouton. The dendrite terminal taking part in the synapse is called the ***postsynaptic process***. The presynaptic bouton and the postsynaptic process are separated by a synaptic cleft (Fig. 10.23).

The transmission of impulses through synapses involves the release of chemical substances called ***neurotransmitters*** that are present within synaptic vesicles. When a nerve impulse reaches a terminal bouton neurotransmitter is released into the synaptic cleft. Under the influence of the neurotransmitter the postsynaptic surface becomes depolarized resulting in a nerve impulse in the postsynaptic neuron. The neurotransmitter released into the synaptic cleft acts only for a very short duration. It is either destroyed (by enzymes) or is withdrawn into the terminal bouton.

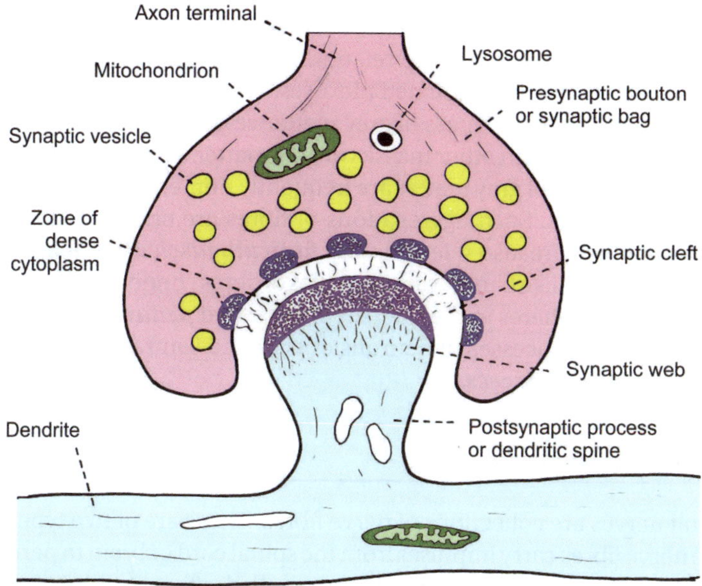

Fig. 10.23 Scheme showing the structure of a typical synapse as seen by EM.

The best known neurotransmitters are acetylcholine, noradrenaline and adrenaline. Many other neurotransmitters are known.

Grey and White Matter

Sections through the spinal cord or through any part of the brain show certain regions that appear whitish, and others that have a darker greyish colour. These constitute the ***white*** and ***grey matter*** respectively. Microscopic examination shows that the cell bodies of neurons are located only in grey matter which also contains dendrites and axons starting from or ending on the cell bodies. Most of the fibres within the grey matter are unmyelinated. On the other hand the white matter consists predominantly of myelinated fibres. It is the reflection of light by myelin that gives this region its whitish appearance. Neuroglia and blood vessels are present in both grey and white matter.

The arrangement of the grey and white matter differs at different situations in the brain and spinal cord. In the spinal cord and brainstem the white matter is on the outside whereas the grey matter forms one or more masses embedded within the white matter. In the cerebrum and cerebellum there is an extensive, but thin, layer of grey matter on the surface. This layer is called the ***cortex.*** Deep to the cortex there is white matter, but within the latter several isolated masses of grey matter are present. Such isolated masses of grey matter present anywhere in the central nervous system are referred to as ***nuclei.*** As grey matter is made of cell bodies of neurons (and the processes arising from or terminating on them) nuclei can be defined as groups of cell bodies of neurons. Aggregations of the cell bodies of neurons may also be found outside the central nervous system. Such aggregations are referred to as ***ganglia.*** Some neurons are located in ***nerve plexuses*** present in close relationship to some viscera. These are, therefore, referred to as ganglionated plexuses.

The axons arising in one mass of grey matter very frequently terminate by synapsing with neurons in other masses of grey matter. The axons connecting two (or more) masses of grey matter are frequently numerous enough to form recognisable bundles. Such aggregations of fibres are called ***tracts***. Larger collections of fibres are also referred to as ***funiculi, fasciculi*** or ***lemnisci***. (A lemniscus is a ribbon like band). Large bundles of fibres connecting the cerebral or cerebellar hemispheres to the brainstem are called ***peduncles.***

Aggregations of processes of neurons outside the central nervous system constitute ***peripheral nerves.***

PERIPHERAL NERVES

Peripheral nerves are collections of nerve fibres. These are of two types.

a. Some nerve fibres carry impulses from the spinal cord or brain to peripheral structures like muscle or gland: they are called ***efferent*** or ***motor*** fibres. Efferent fibres are axons of neurons (the cell bodies of which are) located in the grey matter of the spinal cord or of the brainstem (Fig. 10.24).
b. Other nerve fibres carry impulses from peripheral organs to the brain or spinal cord: these are called ***afferent*** fibres (Fig. 10.25). Many (but not all) afferent fibres are concerned in the transmission of sensations like touch or pain. They are, therefore, also called ***sensory*** fibres.

Afferent nerve fibres are processes of neurons that are located (as a rule) in sensory ganglia. In the case of spinal nerves these ganglia are located on the dorsal nerve roots. In the case of cranial nerves they are located on ganglia situated on the nerve concerned (usually near its attachment to the brain). The neurons in these ganglia are usually of the unipolar type. Each unipolar

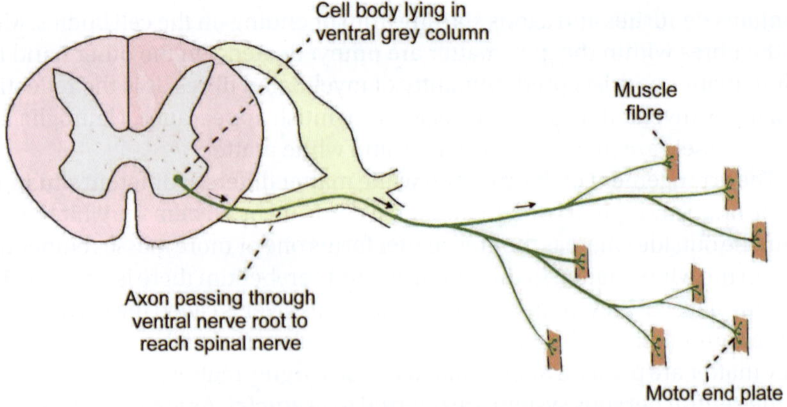

Fig. 10.24 Scheme to show the origin and course of a typical efferent nerve fibre.

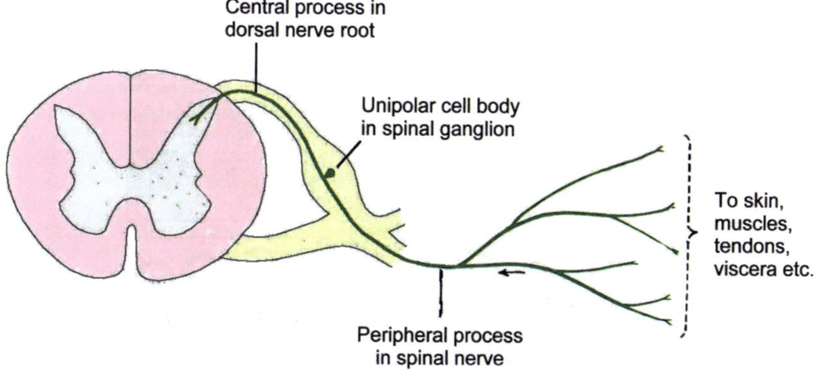

Fig. 10.25 Scheme to show the origin and course of a typical afferent nerve fibre.

neuron gives off a peripheral process which passes into the peripheral nerve forming an afferent nerve fibre. It also gives off a central process that enters the brain or spinal cord.

From what has been said above it will be clear that the afferent nerve fibres in peripheral nerves are functionally dendrites. However, their histological structure is the same as that of axons.

Basic Structure of Peripheral Nerve Fibres

Each nerve fibre has a central core formed by the axon. This core is called the ***axis cylinder***. The plasma membrane surrounding the axis cylinder is the ***axolemma***. The axis cylinder is surrounded by a myelin sheath (Fig. 10.26). This sheath is in the form of short segments that are separated at short intervals called the ***nodes of Ranvier*** (Fig. 10.21). The part of the nerve fibre between two consecutive nodes is the ***internode.*** Each segment of the myelin sheath is formed by one Schwann cell. Outside the myelin sheath there is a thin layer of Schwann cell cytoplasm. This layer of cytoplasm is called the ***neurilemma.***

Each nerve fibre is surrounded by a layer of connective tissue, called the ***endoneurium*** (Fig.10.27). The endoneurium holds adjoining nerve fibres together and facilitates their aggregation to form bundles or ***fasciculi.***

Each fasciculus is surrounded by a thicker layer of connective tissue called the ***perineurium.***

A very thin nerve may consist of a single fasciculus, but usually a nerve is made up of several fasciculi. The fasciculi are held together by a fairly dense layer of connective tissue that surrounds the entire nerve and is called the ***epineurium.***

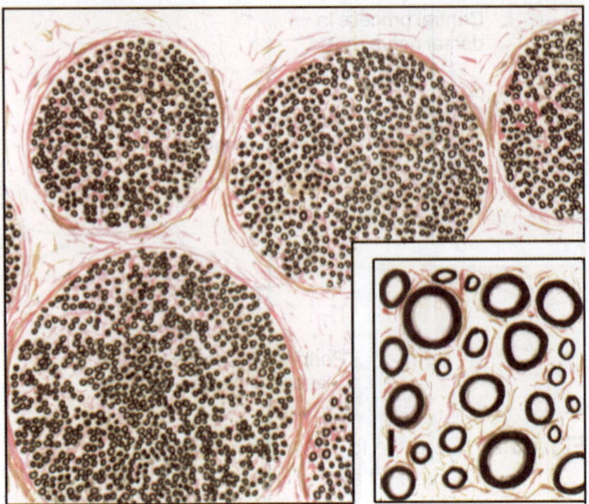

Fig. 10.26 Section through peripheral nerve stained by a method in which the myelin sheaths become black. The inset shows fibres at high magnification.

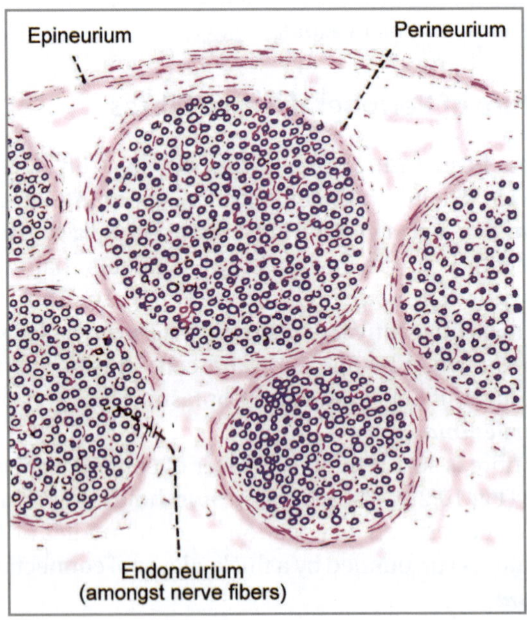

Fig. 10.27 Diagram to show the connective tissue supporting nerve fibres in a peripheral nerve.

DEGENERATION AND REGENERATION OF NEURONS

When the axon of a neuron is cut across a series of degenerative changes are seen in the axon distal to the injury, in the axon proximal to the injury, and in the cell body.

The changes in the part of the axon distal to the injury are referred to as ***anterograde degeneration*** or ***Wallerian degeneration***. They take place in the entire length of this part of the axon. A few hours after injury the axon becomes swollen and irregular in shape, and in a few days it breaks up into small fragments (Fig. 10.28). The neurofibrils within it break down into granules. The myelin sheath breaks up into small segments. It also undergoes chemical changes that enable degenerating myelin to be stained selectively. The region is invaded by numerous macrophages that remove degenerating axons, myelin and cellular debris. These macrophages probably secrete substances that cause proliferation of Schwann cells. The Schwann cells increase in size and produce a large series of membranes that help to form numerous tubes. We shall see later that these tubes play a vital role in regeneration of nerve fibres.

Degenerative changes in the neuron proximal to the injury are referred to as ***retrograde degeneration***. These changes take place in the cell body and in the axon proximal to injury.

The cell body of the injured neuron undergoes a series of changes that constitute the phenomenon of ***chromatolysis***. The cell body enlarges tending to become spherical. The nucleus moves from the centre to the periphery. The Nissl substance becomes much less prominent and appears to dissolve away: hence the term chromatolysis.

Changes in the proximal part of the axon are confined to a short segment near the site of injury (Fig. 10.28). If the injury is sharp and clean the effects extend only up to one or two nodes of Ranvier proximal to the injury. If the injury is severe a longer segment of the axon may be affected. The changes in the affected part are exactly the same as described for the distal part of the axon. They are soon followed by active growth at the tip of the surviving part of the axon. This causes the terminal part of the axon to swell up (Fig. 10.28 F). It then gives off a number of fine branches. These branches grow into the connective tissue at the site of injury in an effort to reach the distal cut end of the nerve (Fig. 10.28 G.H). We have seen that the Schwann cells of the distal part of the nerve proliferate to form a series of tubes. When one of the regenerating axonal branches succeeds in reaching such a tube, it enters it and then grows rapidly within it. The tube serves as a guide to the growing fibre. The axon terminal growing through the Schwann cell tube ultimately reaches, and establishes contact with, an appropriate peripheral end organ. The new axon formed in this way is at first very thin and devoid of a myelin sheath (Fig. 10.28 I). However, there is progressive increase in its thickness and a myelin sheath is formed around it. (Fig. 10.28 J).

From the above account it will be clear that chances of regeneration of a cut nerve are considerably increased if the two cut ends are near each other, and if scar tissue does not intervene between them.

PERIPHERAL NERVE ENDINGS

We have seen that peripheral nerves contain afferent (or sensory) fibres, and efferent (or motor fibres). In relation to the peripheral endings of afferent nerve fibres there are ***receptors*** that respond to various kinds of stimuli. Most efferent

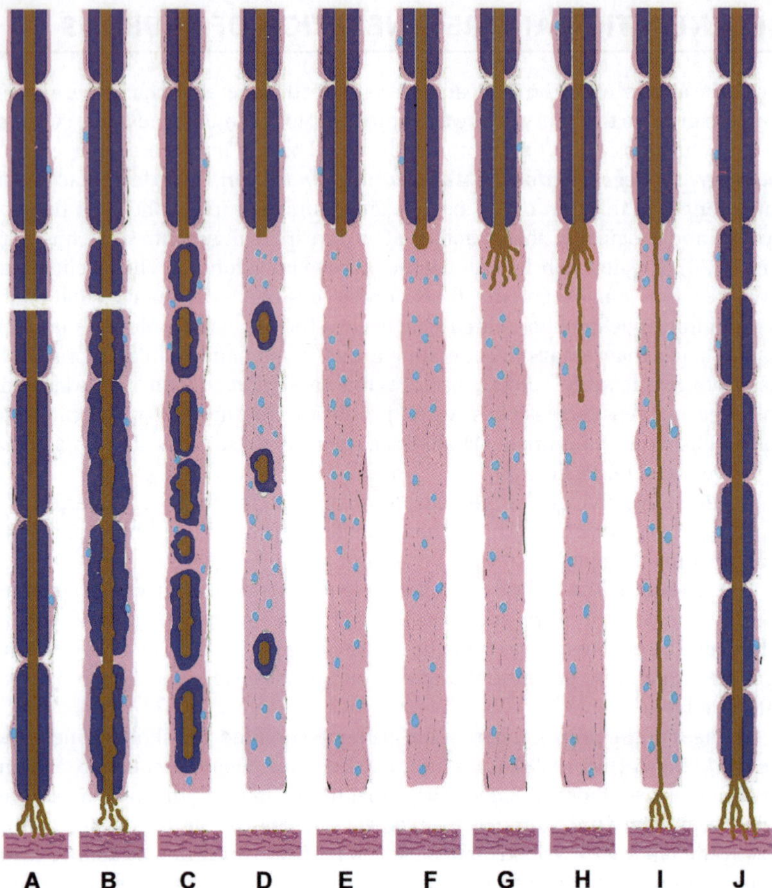

Fig. 10.28 Stages in the degeneration of a nerve fibre after injury (A to E) and its subsequent regeneration (F to J). For explanation see text.

nerve fibres supply muscle, and at the junction of a nerve fibre with muscle we see neuromuscular junctions. In paragraphs that follow we will study the structure of various kinds of sensory receptors, and of neuromuscular junctions

SENSORY RECEPTORS

Preliminary remarks about receptors and their classification

The peripheral terminations of afferent fibres are responsible for receiving stimuli and are, therefore, referred to as ***receptors.*** Receptors can be classified in various ways.

1. From a functional point of view receptors can be classified on the basis of the kind of information they provide. They may be of the following types.

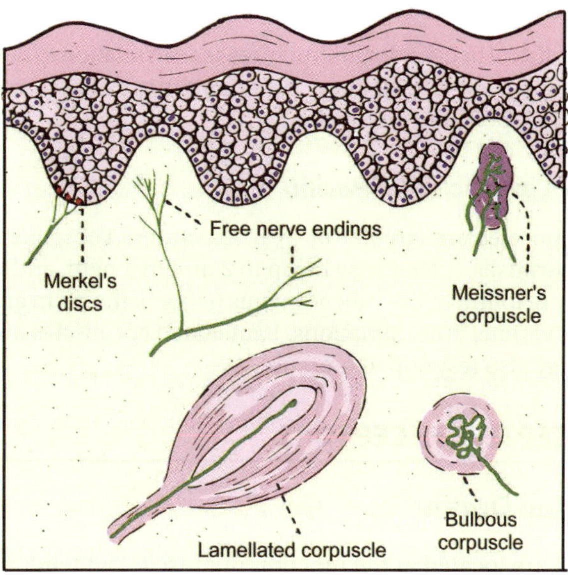

Fig. 10.29 Some sensory receptors present in relation to skin.

a. ***Cutaneous receptors*** are concerned with touch, pain, temperature and pressure. These are also called ***exteroceptive receptors*** or ***exteroceptors*** (Fig. 10.29).
b. ***Proprioceptive receptors*** (or ***proprioceptors***) provide information about the state of contraction of muscles, and of joint movement and position (Fig. 10.30). This information is necessary for precise control of movement and for maintenance of body posture. By and large these activities occur as a result of reflex action and the information from these receptors may or may not be consciously perceived.
c. ***Interoceptive receptors*** (or ***interoceptors***) are located in thoracic and abdominal viscera and in blood vessels. These include specialized structures like the carotid sinus and the carotid body.
d. The above three categories also include receptors that are stimulated by damaging influences which are perceived as pain, discomfort or irritation. Such receptors are referred to as ***nociceptors.***
e. ***Special sense receptors*** of vision, hearing, smell and taste are present in the appropriate organs.

EXTEROCEPTIVE RECEPTORS

Free Nerve Endings

When the terminals of sensory nerves do not show any particular specialization of structure they are called free nerve endings. Such endings are widely distributed in the body. They are found in connective tissue. They are also seen in relation to the epithelial lining of the skin, cornea, alimentary canal, and respiratory system.

Tactile Corpuscles (of Meissner)

These are small oval or cylindrical structures seen in relation to dermal papillae in the hand and foot, and in some other situations. These corpuscles are believed to be responsible for touch.

Lamellated Corpuscles (of Pacini)

Pacinian corpuscles are circular or oval structures. These are much larger than tactile corpuscles. They may be up to 2 mm in length, and up to 0.5 mm across. They are found in the subcutaneous tissue of the palm and sole, in the digits, and in various other situations. Lamellated corpuscles are sensitive to vibration. They also respond to pressure.

PROPRIOCEPTIVE RECEPTORS

Golgi Tendon Organs

These organs are located at the junction of muscle and tendon. Each organ is about 500 μm long and about 100 μm in diameter. It consists of a capsule made up of concentric sheets of cytoplasm (Fig. 10.30). Inside the capsule there are small bundles of tendon fibres. The organ is innervated by one or more myelinated nerve fibres. These receptors are stimulated by pull upon the tendon during active contraction of the muscle, and to a lesser degree by passive stretching.

Muscle Spindles

These are spindle-shaped sensory end organs located within striated muscle (Fig. 10.30). The spindle is bounded by a fusiform connective tissue covering (forming an external capsule) within which there are a few muscle fibres of a special kind. These are called ***intrafusal fibres*** in contrast to ***extrafusal fibres*** that constitute the main bulk of the muscle.

Each muscle spindle is innervated by sensory as well as motor nerves. Spindles provide information to the CNS about the extent and rate of changes in length of muscle.

NEUROMUSCULAR JUNCTIONS

We have seen that skeletal muscle fibres are supplied by ramifications of efferent neurons. We have also seen that axonal branches arising from one neuron may innervate a variable number of muscle fibres (that constitute a motor unit).

Each skeletal muscle fibre receives its own direct innervation. The site where the nerve ending comes into intimate contact with the muscle fibre is a ***neuromuscular (or myoneural) junction***.

The nerve terminal comes in contact with a specialized area near the middle of the muscle fibre. This area is roughly oval or circular, and is referred to as the ***sole plate***. The sole plate plus the axon terminal constitute the ***motor end plate*** (Fig. 10.31).

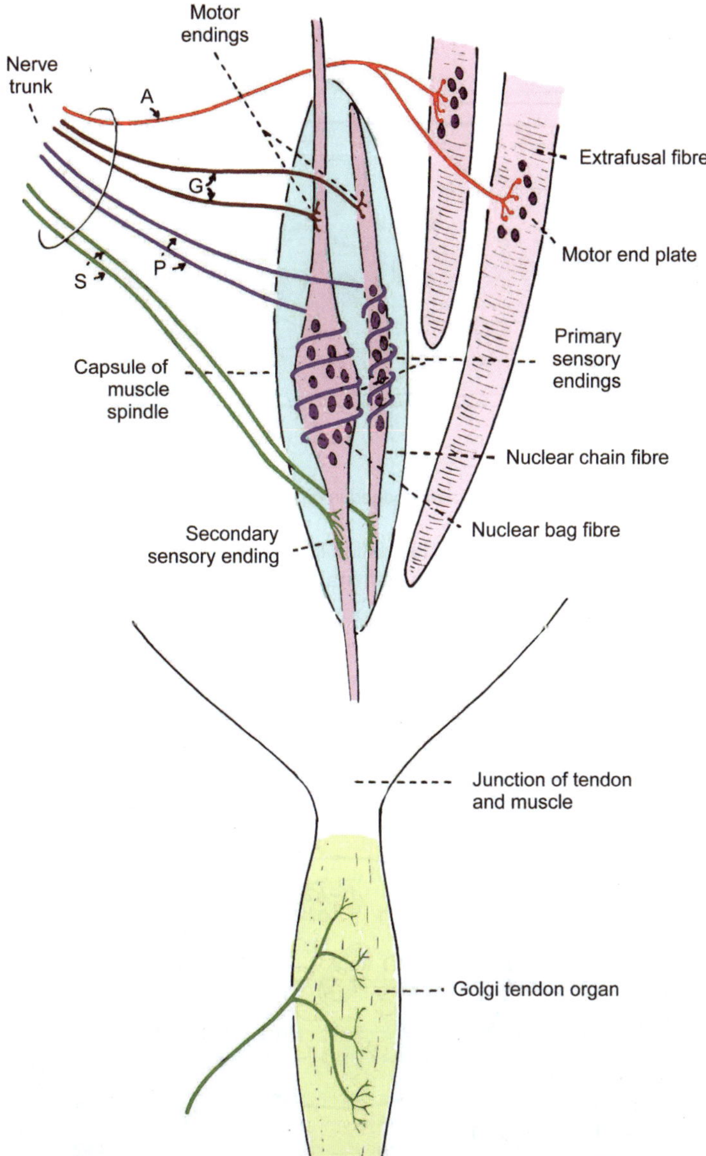

Fig. 10.30 Scheme to show the structure of a muscle spindle and of a Golgi tendon organ.

Structure of a Typical Motor End Plate

In the region of the motor end plate axon terminals are lodged in grooves in the sarcolemma covering the sole plate. Between the axolemma (over the axon) and the sarcolemma (over the muscle fibre) there is a narrow gap. It follows that there is no continuity between axoplasm and sarcoplasm.

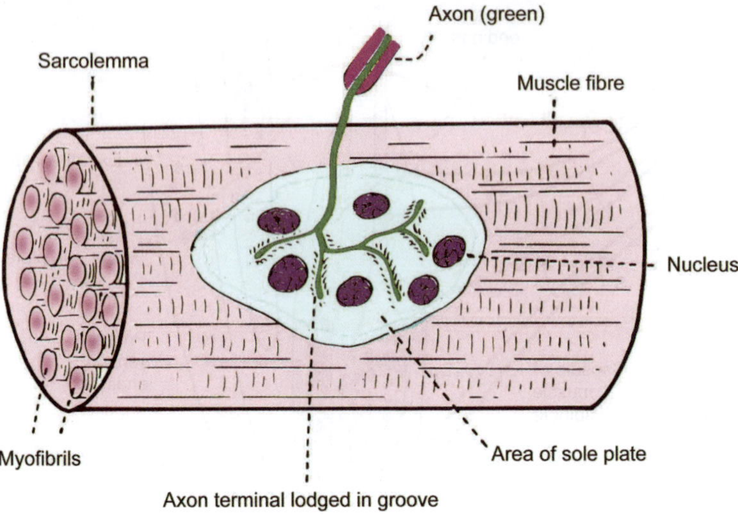

Fig. 10.31 Motor end plate seen in relation to a muscle fibre (surface view). Schwann cell cytoplasm covering the nerve terminal has not been shown for sake of clarity.

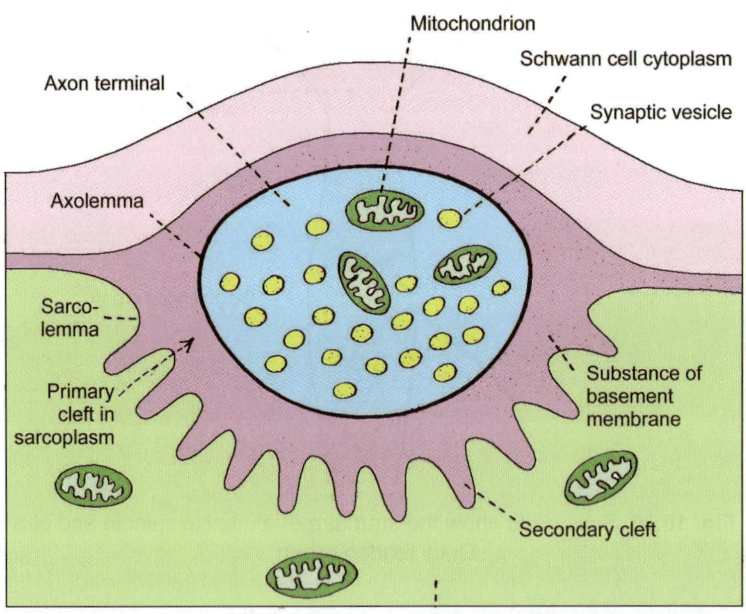

Fig. 10.32 Neuromuscular junction. This figure is a section across one of the axon terminals (and related structures) shown in Fig. 9.25. These details are seen only by EM.

Axon terminals are lodged in grooves in the sarcolemma covering the sole plate. In section (Fig. 10.32) this groove is seen as a semicircular depression. This depression is the ***primary cleft.*** The sarcolemma in the floor of the primary cleft is thrown into numerous small folds resulting in the formation of ***secondary (or subneural) clefts.***

Axon terminals contain vesicles similar to those seen in presynaptic boutons. The vesicles contain the neurotransmitter acetyl choline. Acetyl choline is released when nerve impulses reach the neuromuscular junction. It initiates a wave of depolarisation in the sarcolemma resulting in contraction of the entire muscle fibre. Thereafter the acetyl choline is quickly destroyed by the enzyme acetyl choline esterase.

GANGLIA

Introductory Remarks

Aggregations of cell bodies of neurons, present outside the brain and spinal cord are known as ganglia. Ganglia are of two main types: sensory, and autonomic.

Sensory ganglia are present on the dorsal nerve roots of spinal nerves, where they are called dorsal nerve root ganglia or spinal ganglia (Fig. 10.33). They are also present on the 5th, 7th, 8th, 9th and 10th cranial nerves. We have seen that the neurons in these ganglia are of the unipolar type (except in the case of ganglia associated with the vestibulo-cochlear nerve in which they are bipolar). The peripheral process of each neuron forms an afferent (or sensory) fibre of a peripheral nerve. The central process enters the spinal cord or brain stem.

Autonomic ganglia are concerned with the nerve supply of smooth muscle or of glands. The pathway for this supply always consists of two neurons: preganglionic and postganglionic. The cell bodies of preganglionic neurons are always located within the spinal cord or brainstem. Their axons leave the spinal cord or brainstem and terminate by synapsing with postganglionic neurons, the cell bodies of which are located in autonomic ganglia. Autonomic ganglia are, therefore, aggregations of the cell bodies of postganglionic neurons. These neurons are multipolar (Fig. 10.34). Their axons leave the ganglia as postganglionic fibres to reach and supply smooth muscle or gland. Autonomic ganglia are subdivisible into two major types: sympathetic and parasympathetic. Sympathetic ganglia are located on the right and left sympathetic trunks. Parasympathetic ganglia usually lie close to the viscera supplied through them.

NEUROGLIA

In addition to neurons, the nervous system contains several types of supporting cells. These are:

a. ***Neuroglial cells***, found in the parenchyma of the brain and spinal cord.
b. ***Ependymal cells***, lining the ventricular system.
c. ***Schwann cells***, forming sheaths for axons of peripheral nerves. They are also called ***lemnocytes*** or ***peripheral glia.***

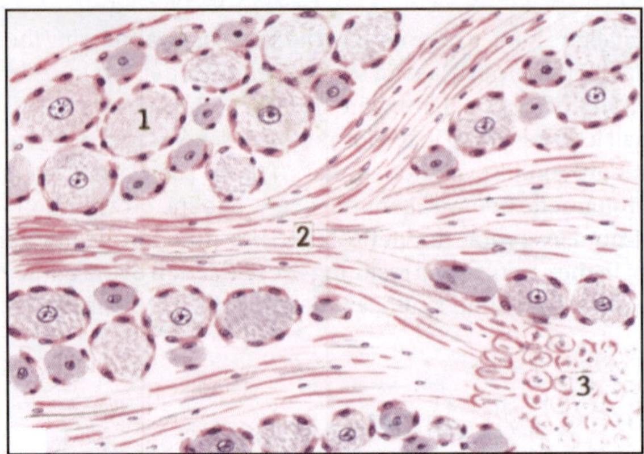

Fig. 10.33 Section through a sensory ganglion. Note large neurons arranged in groups separated by bundles of nerve fibres.

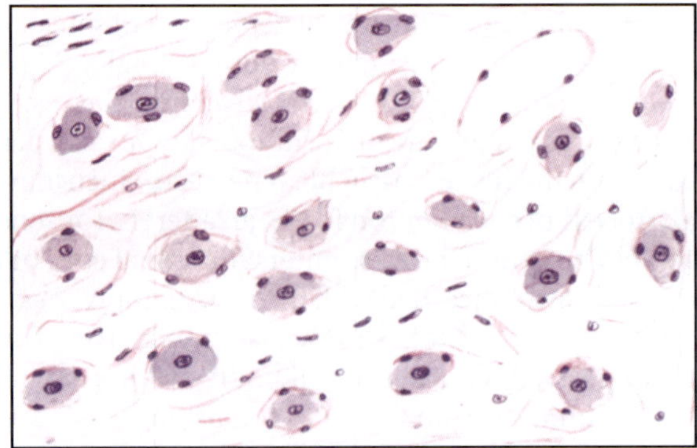

Fig. 10.34 Section through an autonomic ganglion. The neurons are not arranged in groups but are scattered amongst nerve fibres.

d. ***Capsular cells*** (also called ***satellite cells*** or ***capsular gliocytes***) that surround neurons in peripheral ganglia.
e. Various types of supporting cells found in relation to motor and sensory terminals of nerve fibres.

Neuroglial cells may be divided into two major categories (Fig. 10.36).

1. *MACROGLIA (or large glial cells)*

These are of two types.

i. ***Astrocytes,*** which may be subdivided into ***fibrous*** and ***protoplasmic*** astrocytes.
ii. Oligodendrocytes.

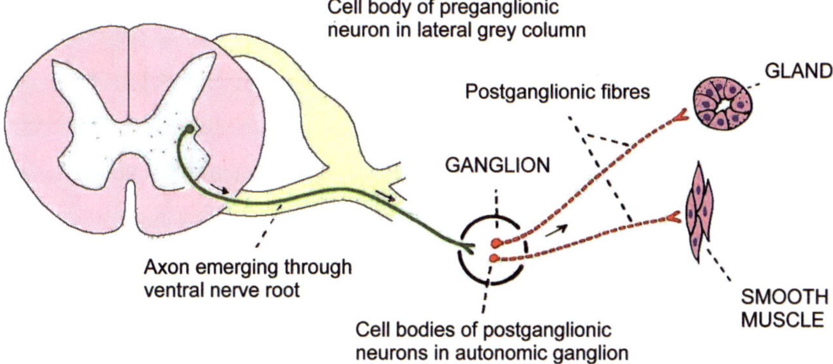

Fig. 10.35 Scheme to show the arrangement of visceral nerve fibres supplying glands and smooth muscle.

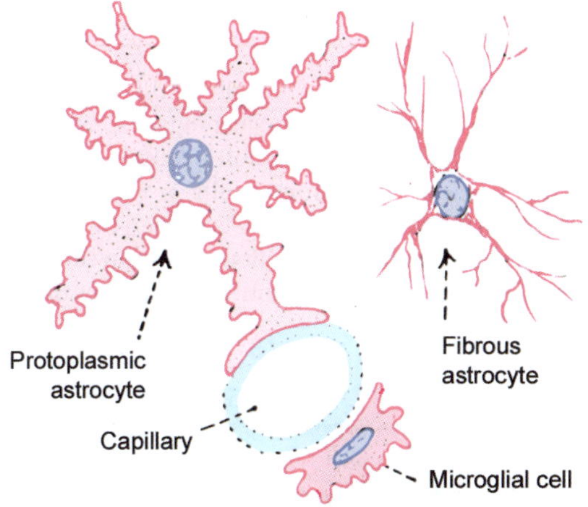

Fig. 10.36 Astrocytes and microglial cells.

2. *MICROGLIA (or small glial cells)*

Macroglial cells are derived from ectoderm of the neural tube. Microglial cells are, on the other hand, of mesodermal origin.

All neuroglial cells are much smaller in size than neurons. However, they are far more numerous. It is interesting to note that the number of glial cells in the brain and spinal cord is ten to fifty times as much as that of neurons. Neurons and neuroglia are separated by a very narrow extracellular space.

In ordinary histological preparations only the nuclei of neuroglial cells are seen. Their processes can be demonstrated by special techniques.

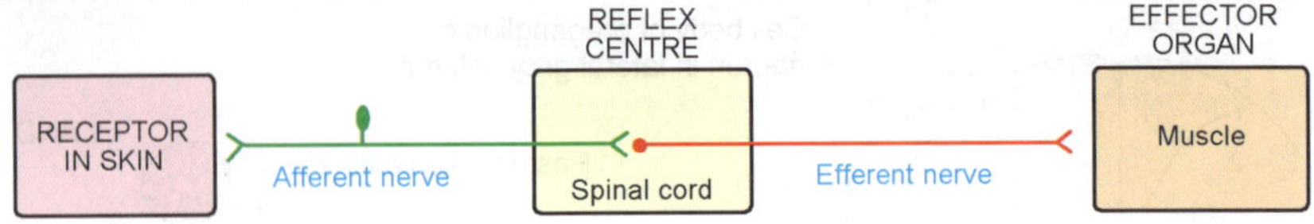

Fig. 10.37 Diagram to show the pathway for a simple reflex action.

Functions of Neuroglia

1. They provide mechanical support to neurons.
2. They serve as insulators.
3. Some neuroglial cells are concerned in providing myelin sheaths to nerve fibres.
4. Neuroglial cells help in regeneration of injured neurons. They also help in controlling the environment of neurons.

REFLEX ACTION

A reflex action is one that takes place automatically, without any conscious effort on our part. For example if you touch the sole of a sleeping person the leg is immediately drawn up. The nervous pathway for such an action is called a ***reflex arc***. The pathway for a simple reflex arc is shown diagrammatically in Fig. 10.37. The stimulus is received by a receptor in skin. A nerve impulse is carried by an afferent nerve to a ***reflex centre*** (in spinal cord). From here an efferent neuron carries an impulse to a muscle (effector organ) causing its contraction. In most cases the actual pathways are more complex.

Reflexes can be classified in various ways.

1. In the reflex arc shown in Fig. 10.37 only one synapse (located in the reflex centre) is involved. Such a reflex is ***monosynaptic***. When the pathway involves more than one synapse it is said to be ***polysynaptic***.
2. ***Location of reflex centre***: Depending on the location of the reflex centre a reflex may be spinal, bulbar (medulla), cerebellar, cortical etc.
3. Reflexes produced by stimulation of skin (or mucous membrane) are ***superficial reflexes***. Those arising from deeper structures (e.g., tendons) are ***deep reflexes***.
4. Reflexes are also named on the structures involved. Those elicited by stimulating skin are ***cutaneous reflexes***, those from tendons are ***tendon reflexes***. Similarly, we have ***pupillary reflexes***, ***visceral reflexes*** etc.
5. Some reflexes are present at birth. These are ***inborn reflexes***. Others develop as a result of experience. These are ***acquired*** (or ***conditioned***) ***reflexes***.
6. Some reflexes are protective e.g., withdrawal of the hand when a hot object is touched. In the movement of withdrawing joints of the extremity are flexed. Such reflexes are, therefore, also called ***flexor reflexes***. When a person is standing a series of reflexes are active to prevent him from falling. As these keep the body straight (with hip and knee joints extended) these are called ***extensor reflexes***, or ***antigravity reflexes***.

Reciprocal innervation

In movements produced by reflexes, some muscles relax while others contract. In a flexor response, the flexors contract and extensors relax. It has been shown that afferent neurons of the reflex arc establish connections with motor neurons supplying both flexors and extensors, inhibiting one group while stimulating the other. This is the law of reciprocal innervation.

CHAPTER

11

Blood

INTRODUCTION

You all know that blood is a red viscous fluid. It is made up of:

a. a liquid base called ***plasma***, and of
b. ***blood cells*** that float in the plasma.

Blood remains liquid only as long as it is within the heart and blood vessels. If we take some blood out of a vein and put it into a tube, it soon loses its fluid nature and becomes gelatinous. This process is called ***coagulation*** or ***clotting*** of blood. Formation of clots blocks any gap in a blood vessel caused by injury. This is nature's way of stopping bleeding, and consequent loss of blood from the body. Some chemicals can prevent coagulation. They are called anticoagulants.

Some important facts about blood are as follows:

1. A normal adult has about 5 litres of blood.
2. Blood is mildly alkaline. Its normal pH is 7.4.
3. Its specific gravity is 1.05 to 1.06.
4. The viscosity of blood is five times that of water.
5. We have seen that blood consists of plasma and blood cells. If we draw some blood from a vein and put it into a bottle containing an anticoagulant it does not clot. This blood is put into a special haematocrit tube and is centrifuged. Blood cells settle at the bottom of the tube leaving a clear layer of plasma in the upper part. We can now see that 55% of the volume of blood is made up of plasma, and 45% is made up of cells. We express this by saying that ***packed cell volume*** (or ***PCV***) is 45%. This is also called the ***haematocrit*** value.

Functions of Blood

As blood circulates through all parts of the body it serves as a very important transport system as follows.

1. Nutrients absorbed from food (including glucose, amino acids lipids and minerals) reach all tissues of the body. Blood also acts as a store of these nutrients.
2. Oxygen absorbed in the lungs is carried to tissues. Carbon dioxide produced in tissues is carried to the lungs.
3. Waste products (e.g., urea) produced in tissues are carried to the kidneys for excretion.

4. Hormones produced in endocrine organs reach their target organs through blood.

White blood cells play an important role in protecting the body from infections by bacteria, and from immune reactions caused by proteins foreign to the body.

Other functions in which blood plays an important role are regulation of water balance, regulation of acid-base balance and regulation of body temperature.

Plasma

Plasma is made up of water (91-92%) and of solids. Solids are organic and inorganic. Dissolved gases are also present.

The main organic substances present in plasma are proteins, carbohydrates and lipids. Other organic substances are amino acids, hormones, enzymes, antibodies and waste products like ammonia, creatinine, urea and uric acid.

The main inorganic substances present in plasma are ions of sodium, potassium, calcium, magnesium, chloride, iodide, phosphate, iron, and copper.

The gases present are oxygen and carbon dioxide.

PLASMA PROTEINS

Proteins present in plasma play an important role in various functions of blood. Hence it is necessary to study some details about them. The proteins present are (a) albumin, (b) globulin and (c) fibrinogen. When blood clots fibrinogen is converted into fibrin which forms part of the clot. Albumin and globulin remain in serum. Plasma proteins can be separated from one another by various methods.

The average amount of total protein in blood (expressed as grams per 100 ml) is 7.3g/100 ml. Of this 4.7 g is present as albumin, 2.3 g as globulin and 0.3 g as fibrinogen. Globulin can be separated into three fractions, alpha globulin, beta globulin and gamma globulin. In terms of percentage albumin is 55%, alpha globulin is 13%, beta globulin is 14%, gamma globulin is 11% and fibrinogen is 7%.

The molecular weight of albumin is 6900; of globulin is 156000, and of fibrinogen is 400000.

Decrease in quantity of protein is called hypoproteinaemia. It can be caused by haemorrhage, by extensive burns, by inadequate nutrition, in cirrhosis of the liver and in chronic infections. An increase in plasma proteins (hyperproteinaemia) is seen in dehydration and in some acute infections.

Functions of Plasma Proteins

1. Fibrinogen is essential for coagulation of blood.
2. Plasma proteins help to maintain the oncotic pressure of blood. Oncotic pressure plays a role in exchange of substances between blood and cells.
3. Gamma globulins play a role in defense mechanisms. They act as antibodies and are therefore called immunoglobulins. The antibodies destroy many disease-causing organisms.
4. Plasma proteins help in transport of substances through blood. The substances include hormones, enzymes, respiratory gases specially carbon dioxide, and some metals.
5. Other functions in which plasma proteins play a role are providing viscosity to blood, erythrocyte sedimentation rate, stability of suspended erythrocytes, and regulation of acid base balance. Plasma proteins serve as reserve proteins when food intake is insufficient.

CELLULAR ELEMENTS OF BLOOD

The cellular or formed elements of blood are of three main types. These are ***red blood corpuscles*** or ***erythrocytes***, ***white blood corpuscles*** or ***leucocytes***, and ***blood platelets***. We refer to them as 'cellular' or 'formed' elements rather than as cells because of the fact that red blood corpuscles are not strictly cells (see below). However, in practice, the terms red blood cells and white blood cells are commonly used.

We have seen that about 55 per cent of the total volume of blood is accounted for by plasma. Most of the remaining 45 per cent is made up of red blood corpuscles, the leucocytes and platelets constituting less than 1 per cent of the volume. If we take one cubic millimetre (mm3 = microlitre or ml) of blood we find that it contains about five million erythrocytes. In comparison there are only about 7000 leucocytes in the same volume of blood.

ERYTHROCYTES (RED BLOOD CORPUSCLES) AND RELATED TOPICS

When seen in surface view each erythrocyte is a circular disc having a diameter of about 7 µm (6.5-8.5 µm). When viewed from the side it is seen to be biconcave, the maximum thickness being about 2 µm (Fig. 11.1). Erythrocytes are cells that have lost their nuclei (and other organelles). They are bounded by a plasma membrane. They contain a red coloured protein called ***haemoglobin***. It is because of the presence of haemoglobin that erythrocytes (and blood as a whole) are red in colour. In a healthy person there are about 15 g of haemoglobin in every 100 ml of blood. Haemoglobin plays an important role in carrying oxygen from the lungs to all tissues of the body. It combines with oxygen to form ***oxyhaemoglobin***. In tissues oxygen is released. Now haemoglobin combines with carbon dioxide to form ***carbaminohaemoglobin***, that is transported to the lungs. Haemoglobin also acts as a buffer.

When erythrocytes are seen in a film of blood spread out on a slide, they appear yellow (or pale red) in colour. Their rims (being thicker) appear darker than the central parts.

Erythrocytes maintain their normal shape only if suspended in an isotonic solution. This is referred to as ***suspension stability***. If the surrounding medium becomes hypotonic the cells absorb water, swell up, and ultimately burst: this is called ***haemolysis***. Alternatively, if erythrocytes are placed in a hypertonic solution, they shrink and their surfaces develop irregularities (***crenation***). Such cells are sometimes called ***echinocytes***.

If blood is placed in a tube the red blood cells pile up over one another. This is called ***rouleaux formation*** (Fig. 11.2).

Erythrocytes are formed in bone marrow from where they enter the blood stream. Each erythrocyte has a life of about 100 to 120 days at the end of which it is removed from blood by cells of the mononuclear phagocyte system (specially in the spleen and bone marrow). The constituents of erythrocytes are broken down and reused to form new erythrocytes.

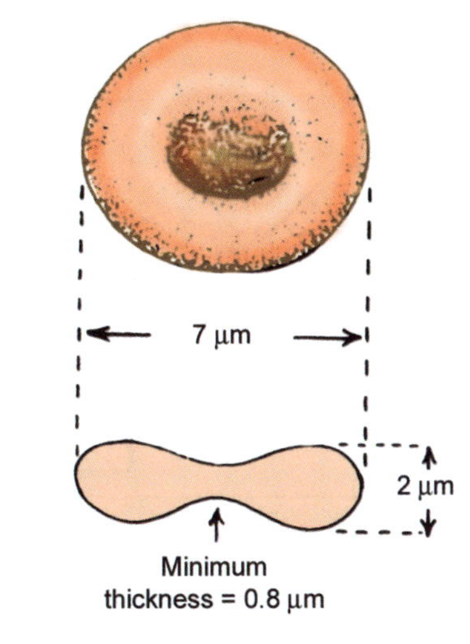

Fig. 11.1 Average dimensions of an erythrocyte. The erythrocyte is seen in surface view (A), and in profile (B).

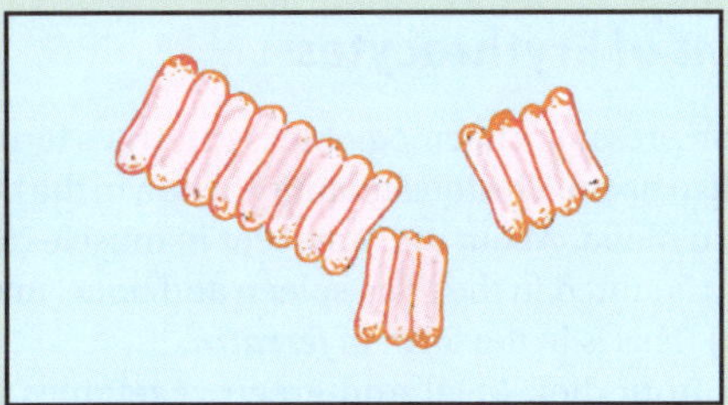

Fig. 11.2 Rouleaux formation.

Like cell membranes of other cells, the plasma membranes of erythrocytes are composed of lipids and proteins. Several types of proteins are present, including ***ABO antigens*** and ***Rh factor*** responsible for a person's blood group.

HAEMOGLOBIN

Haemoglobin is the most important constituent of red blood cells as it is responsible for transport of oxygen from lungs to tissues and of carbon dioxide from tissues to lungs. Some facts about haemoglobin are given below.

1. In a normal male adult, average haemoglobin is 15 g%. In a female adult it is 14.5 g%. At birth it is 25 g%, and at one year of age it is 17g%.
2. Molecules of haemoglobin are large (molecular weight 6800) and complex. They are made up of ***haem*** and ***globin*** (Fig. 11.3). Haem is made up of iron (in ferrous form) and porphyrin. Globin is a protein that has four polypeptide chains (2 alpha and 2 beta). Each molecule of haemoglobin contains four units of haem that are

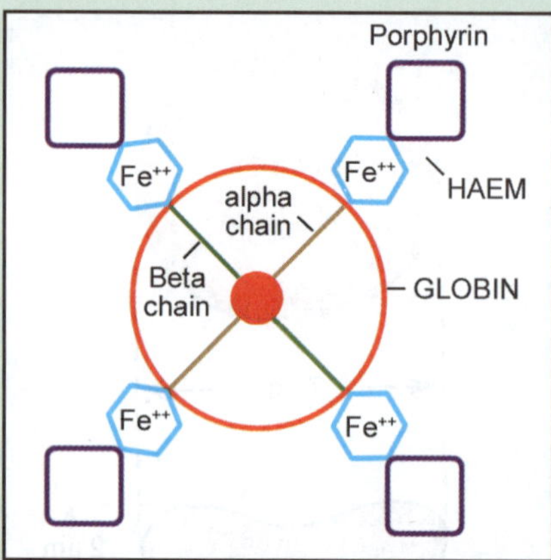

Fig. 11.3 Structure of haemoglobin.

united together by the alpha and beta chains of globin. Each unit of haem can combine with one molecule of oxygen. Hence one molecule of haemoglobin can carry four molecules of oxygen. Carbon dioxide does not combine with haem. It is attached to globin.

Iron Component of Erythrocytes

We have seen that iron present in haemoglobin is in ferrous form. Therefore, oxygen readily attaches itself to haem. The total quantity of iron in the body is about 4 g. Out of this about 65% is in blood. About 4% is present in muscle (as myoglobin). Most of the remaining iron is stored in the liver, spleen and bone marrow (in cells of the macrophage system). This is in the form of ***ferratin***.

Iron is obtained from diet. Meat and green vegetables are rich in it. After absorption in the intestine, iron is transported through plasma in the form of ***transferrin*** (iron plus protein).

About 1 mg of iron is lost from the body daily in feces. A greater quantity is lost in women through menstruation.

Iron absorbed from food is used for formation of haemoglobin. After an erythrocyte has completed its useful life, it is broken down by cells of the macrophage system. Haemoglobin splits into haem and globin. Haem further splits into iron and porphyrin. Iron that is released goes back into circulation as transferrin. It is reused for production of new erythrocytes or is stored in liver, spleen and bone marrow.

Porphyrin released from haem is converted into a yellow pigment called ***bilirubin***. It is in insoluble form. It is taken up by liver cells, changed to soluble form, and excreted into bile. In the large intestine it is converted into ***stercobilinogen*** and then into ***stercobilin***, which is responsible for brown colour of feces. Some stercobilinogen is absorbed into blood and excreted into urine. It is now called ***urobilinogen***. Exposure to air converts into ***urobilin***.

Physiological Factors Influencing RBC number

1. RBC count is very high at birth (8-10 million/mm^3). It remains at this level for about ten days. Even thereafter, the count is higher in children than in adults.

2. RBC count is raised at high altitude, after exercise, after meals, in warm temperature, and during excitement.
3. In women RBC count is relatively low during the reproductive period, and specially during pregnancy.
4. A fall in RBC count is seen when barometric pressure is high (deep sea), and immediately after sleep.

Haemolysis

Destruction of erythrocytes (by bursting) is called haemolysis. Normal RBCs can undergo haemolysis when exposed to hypotonic saline. Water enters the cells and causes them to burst. Haemolysis occurs more readily in aged RBCs because their walls become more fragile i.e., their fragility increases. Fragility is tested by exposing drops of blood to different concentrations of saline.

Haemolysis also takes place when RBCs are exposed to some substances that are, therefore, called haemolysins. A haemolysin may be:

a. A chemical like alcohol or ether, an acid or alkali, or a chemical poison like arsenic.
b. A toxin released by some bacteria.
c. Venom of poisonous snakes.

Destruction of erythrocytes can also be caused by some drugs, by transfusion of incompatible blood, by malarial infection, and by disturbances in the immune system (presence of anti-Rh agglutinin).

Haemolysis is more likely to occur when red blood cells are abnormal. In one such inherited abnormality red blood cells become spherical (***spherocytosis***). Excessive cell destruction also occurs in ***sickle cell disease*** (in which haemoglobin is abnormal).

ANAEMIA

Anaemia is a condition in which the quantity of haemoglobin in blood is less than normal. RBC count and PCV are low. The concentration of haemoglobin in each RBC is also decreased. Depending on how low haemoglobin levels are, anaemia can be described as mild, moderate or severe.

Reduction in RBC count can be a result of less production or of excessive loss.

Reduced Production of RBCs

Several factors are needed for normal production of RBCs.

1. Iron is an important constituent of haemoglobin. A deficiency of iron in diet in a common cause of anaemia in India. In anaemia caused by iron deficiency erythrocytes are smaller than normal (microcytic) and contain less haemoglobin (hypochromic).
2. Anaemia can also be caused by deficiency of vitamin B12 or of folic acid. Such deficiency interferes with maturation of erythrocytes. The erythrocytes become too large (macrocytic). Immature large nucleated precursors of erythrocytes (megaloblasts), normally present only in bone marrow, may appear in blood.
3. Bone marrow is the site of erythrocyte production (and that of leucocytes and platelets). Sometimes activity of bone marrow gets reduced and fewer cells are produced (hypoplastic anaemia). Production can also stop completely (aplastic anaemia).

Excessive Loss of Erythrocytes

Anaemia can be caused by any condition in which there is excessive loss of erythrocytes. This can be caused by:

a. Bleeding as a result of injury, during childbirth, by excessive menstrual flow, or by repeated bleeding from a gastric ulcer or colonic ulcer can cause anaemia.
b. Excessive destruction of erythrocytes. This is called ***haemolytic anaemia***.

Anaemia can also be classified on the basis of the appearance of RBCs in a blood film.

1. When RBC count is below normal, but the size and haemoglobin content of RBCs is normal anaemia is described as ***normocytic normochromic***. This type of anaemia is seen after haemorrhage. This picture is also seen in aplastic anaemia (which is caused by abnormality of bone marrow).
2. When RBCs are larger than normal, but haemoglobin content of cells is normal the anaemia is ***macrocytic normochromic***. This picture is seen in perniceous anaemia. There is deficiency of intrinsic factor and of vitamin B_{12}.
3. When RBCs are smaller than normal, and mean corpuscular haemoglobin is low, the anaemia is ***microcytic hypochromic***. This picture is seen when there is chronic blood loss, and in iron deficiency.

Effects of Anaemia

In patients of anaemia the skin is pale. Heart rate and cardiac output increase. Rate and force of respiration is increased. Breathlessness and dyspnoea (difficulty in breathing) may be seen. Weakness, headache, drowsiness and increased sensitivity to cold are seen. Renal function may be disturbed. Menstrual abnormalities may occur.

ERYTHROCYTE SEDIMENTATION RATE (ESR)

When blood is mixed with anticoagulant, put into a tube, and left undisturbed for some time the RBCs gradually settle to the bottom of the tube leaving a clear layer of plasma in the upper part of the tube. ESR is the distance (in mm) by which the cells settle in one hour. ESR is influenced by number and size of RBCs, viscosity of blood and rouleaux formation.

Two methods of estimation are used. In the ***Westergren*** method we use a graduated tube 300mm long, open at both ends. We take 1.6 ml of blood and mix it with 0.4 ml of 3.8% sodium citrate solution. It is put into the tube up to the zero mark, and the tube fixed in a stand which keeps it upright. Reading of ESR is taken after one hour. With this method normal ESR is 3-7 mm in males and 5-9 mm in females.

In the ***Wintrobe*** method we take 1 ml of blood. The anticoagulant is EDTA. The Wintrobe tube is shorter and broader than the Westergren tube and is closed at one end. It is filled up to the zero mark and reading taken after one hour. With this method the normal value is 0-9 mm for men, and 0-20 mm for women. (Values vary to some extent from laboratory to laboratory).

Variation in ESR

1. As compared to normal male adults ESR is less in children, and more in women (specially during menstruation and pregnancy).

2. ESR is increased in many chronic infections including tuberculosis, in malignancy, and in rheumatoid arthritis and rheumatic fever. It is also increased in anaemia. It is decreased in sickle cell anaemia, polycythemia and in allergic conditions.

PACKED CELL VOLUME (PCV)

To find out packed cell volume blood mixed with EDTA or heparin is taken in a Wintrobe tube which is filled up to the 100 mark. The tube is centrifuged for 30 minutes. RBCs settle down and the volume of the cells can be read. Normal PCV is 40-45% in males and 38-42% in females. Estimation of PCV is useful in treatment of anaemias and some other conditions.

BLOOD INDICES

A number of indices are used to describe the status of anaemia. These are as follows.

Mean Corpuscular Volume (MCV)

$$\text{MCV} = \frac{[\text{PCV}(\%) \times 10]}{\text{RBC count (millions/cu mm)}}$$

Normal value is 78 to 90. Value is raised in macrocytic anaemia, and less in microcytic anaemia.

Mean Corpuscular Haemoglobin (MCH)

This index is expressed in picograms. [One thousandth of a gram is equal to one milligram (mg). One thousandth of a milligram is a microgram (mg). One thousandth of a microgram is a picogram (pg)].

$$\text{MCH} = \frac{\text{Haemoglobin (g) in 1000 ml of blood}}{\text{RBC count (millions/cu. mm)}}$$

Normal value is about 30 pg.

Mean Corpuscular Haemoglobin Concentration (MCHC)

Concentration of haemoglobin in one RBC expressed as a percentage.

$$\text{MCHC} = \frac{\text{Haemoglobin (g/100 ml)}}{\text{PCV (\%)}}$$

Normal value is 30%.

Colour Index

To calculate this index first calculate haemoglobin as percentage as follows.

Haemoglobin % = Haemoglobin of patient / Normal haemoglobin

Next calculate RBC % = RBC count of patient / Normal RBC count

Colour Index = (Haemoglobin %) / (RBC %)

In a person with normal haemoglobin and normal RBC count (both 100%) the colour index is 1 (0.8 to 1.2 is normal). The value is high in macrocytic anaemia and low in microcytic anaemia.

BLOOD GROUPS

When blood of one person is transfused into the blood circulation of another person this is called blood transfusion. It is a life saving measure.

In early attempts at blood transfusion it was observed that some patients developed serious symptoms, and even died, after transfusion. Subsequently, it became known that an individual could safely receive blood from some persons, but not from others. The reason for this is as follows. On the surface of red blood cells there are proteins that act as antigens. These are of different types in different individuals. The serum contains antibodies that are again of different types. When the antigens present in the red cells of one individual are mixed with antibodies present in the serum of a different individual they can behave in two ways. In some cases there may be no reaction, and blood may remain normal. This means that blood of the two persons is compatible. In other cases the red cells collect together (agglutinate) and form clumps, followed by destruction of the red cells. When this happens the blood of the two persons is not compatible. Individuals can be classified into groups depending on the antigens present in their blood. There are many systems of blood groups but the ones that are clinically important are the ABO system and the Rh system.

ABO System

Under this system of classification a person may belong to group A, B, AB or O.

1. Persons of blood group A have antigens of type A on their red blood cells. Their serum contains antibodies of type B.
2. Persons of blood group B have antigens of type B on the red cells. Their serum contains antibodies of type A.
3. Persons of blood group AB have antigens of both type A and type B. They do not have type A or B antibodies.
4. Persons of blood group O have neither antigen A or B. Antibodies of both type A and type B are present.

Group A is further divisible into subgroups A_1 and A_2. Group AB may be A_1B or A_2B.

Determination of Blood Group

You need the following

1. Antiserum A (containing alpha antibody).
2. Antiserum B (containing beta antibody).
3. Suspension of the persons blood in isotonic saline.

BLOOD GROUP	ANTIGENS PRESENT	ANTIBODIES PRESENT	Can receive blood from	Can give blood to
A	A	B	A, O	A, AB
B	B	A	B, O	B, AB
AB	A, B	None	A, B, AB, O Universal recipient	AB only
O	None	A, B	O only	A, B, AB, O Universal donor

Fig. 11.4 ABO blood group.

Place one drop of antiserum A at one end of a glass slide. Put a drop of antiserum B at the other end. Add a drop of blood suspension to each antiserum. Gently rock the slide for two minutes. Occurrence of agglutination is indicated by appearance of clumps. In its absence the drop remains clear.

1. If agglutination occurs with antiserum A, but not with B, the blood group is A.
2. If agglutination occurs with antiserum B, but not with A, the blood group is B.
3. If agglutination occurs with both antisera A and B the blood group is AB.
4. If agglutination occurs neither with antisera A or B the blood group is O.

Compatibilty of Blood Groups

From a practical point of view the most important fact to know about blood groups lies in the answer to the question "What group of blood can safely be given to a patient of a particular blood group?"

Note thc following (Figs. 11.4, 11.5):

1. Persons of group A can receive blood only from other persons of group A, or from persons of group O.
2. Persons of group B can receive blood only from persons of group B, or from persons of group O.
3. Persons of group AB can receive blood only from persons of group A, B or AB.
4. Persons of group O can receive blood only from another person of group O.

The safest thing to do is to give a patient blood from a donor having the same blood as the patient. If a patient (recipient) of group A is given blood from a donor of group O two factors are to be considered.

a. The red cells of the donor blood have neither A or B antigen. So there can be no reaction with antibodies in the patients serum.

PATIENTS BLOOD GROUP	BLOOD GROUP REQUIRED
A	A OR O
B	B or O
AB	AB, A, B, O
O	O only

Fig. 11.5 Which blood does your patient need?

b. The serum of the donor's blood contains antibodies A and B. The A antibody can react with the A antigen on red cells of the recipient. However, as donor serum becomes greatly diluted by the recipients serum, this reaction is not of clinical importance. Therefore, the rule is that in deciding compatibility we consider antigens of the donor's blood, and antibodies of the recipients blood.

However, from the above we can understand why it is better to give a patient of blood group A blood of the same group instead of blood of O group. To be absolutely sure that no adverse reaction takes place we do cross matching.

Cross Matching

For this we mix serum of the recipient and RBCs of the donor. If there is agglutination blood of that donor is not used.

Reactions Due to Transfusion of Mismatched Blood

These are jaundice, cardiac shock and fall of blood pressure, and stoppage of urine production by kidneys. Death can occur.

RH System

In addition to A and B antigens red blood cells bear Rh antigens. (They are termed Rh as they were first discovered in the Rhesus monkey). There are several Rh antigens but the one of clinical importance is the D-antigen. Persons having this antigen are said to be Rh positive, and those without it are Rh negative. About 85% of Indians are Rh positive.

An anti-D antibody does not occur naturally in human blood. However, this antibody is formed if Rh positive blood enters the body of an Rh negative person. The clinical importance of the Rh factor is as follows.

1. An Rh + person can receive Rh- blood without any harmful effect.
2. If Rh+ blood is given to a Rh- person there is no immediate effect (as there are no antibodies against it). However, antibodies develop in about one month or so and destroy the Rh+ cells still in circulation. This reaction is mild. However, if a second transfusion of Rh+ blood is given there is a severe reaction as antibodies are now present.
3. Rh factor is of importance in pregnancy if the mother is Rh- and the fetus is Rh+. Although the Rh antigen of the fetus does not normally pass through the placental barrier, it can do so in some cases. When this happens anti-Rh antibodies form in the mother. These can cross the placenta barrier and enter the fetus. Here they cause haemolysis of fetal red cells. Fetal bone marrow tries to replace the lost red cells and becomes overactive. Immature precursors of red cells appear in blood. The condition is called ***erythroblastosis fetalis***. Destruction of RBCs results in jaundice. If jaundice is severe the increased levels of bilirubin cause damage to the brain of the developing fetus (***kernicterus***).

LEUCOCYTES (WHITE BLOOD CORPUSCLES)

Differences between Erythrocytes and Leucocytes

Leucocytes are different from erythrocytes in several ways.

a. They are true cells, each leucocyte having a nucleus, mitochondria, Golgi complex, and other organelles.
b. They do not contain haemoglobin and, therefore, appear colourless in unstained preparations.
c. Unlike erythrocytes which do not have any mobility of their own, leucocytes can move actively.
d. As a corollary of 'c' erythrocytes do not normally leave the vascular system, but leucocytes can move out of it to enter surrounding tissues. In fact, blood is merely a route by which leucocytes travel from bone marrow to other destinations.
e. Most leucocytes have a relatively short life span.

Features of Different Types of Leucocytes

Leucocytes are of various types. Some of them have granules in their cytoplasm and are, therefore, called ***granulocytes***. Depending on the staining characters of their granules granulocytes are further divided into ***neutrophil leucocytes*** (or ***neutrophils***), ***eosinophil leucocytes*** (or ***eosinophils***), and ***basophil leucocytes*** (or ***basophils***).

Apart from these granulocytes there are two types of agranular leucocytes. These are ***lymphocytes*** and ***monocytes*** (Fig. 11.11).

Apart from the presence or absence of granules, and their nature, the different types of leucocytes show various other differences. In describing

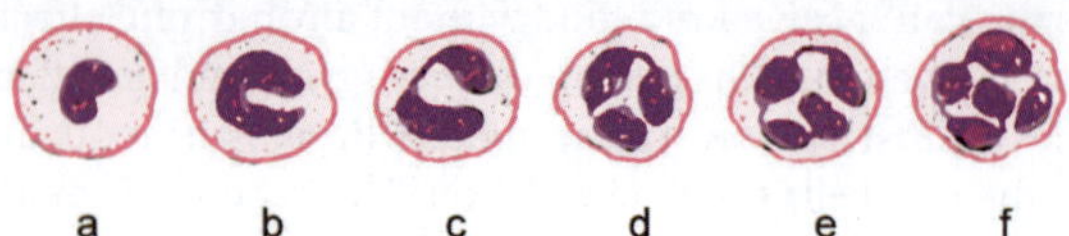

Fig. 11.6 Neutrophil leucocytes (*b* to *f*) showing varying numbers of lobes in their nuclei. A metamyelocyte is shown at '*a*' for comparison.

the differences it is usual for text books to consider all features of one type of leucocyte together. However, in practice, it is more useful to take the features one by one and to compare each feature in the different types of leucocytes as given below.

Relative Number

We have seen that there are about 7000 leucocytes (range 5000-10000) in every cubic millimetre (=mm^3=μl) of blood. Of these about two thirds (60-70%) are neutrophils, and about one fourth (20-30%) are lymphocytes. The remaining types are present in very small numbers. The eosinophils are about 3 per cent, the basophils about 1 per cent, and the monocytes about 5 per cent. The relative and absolute numbers of the different types of leucocytes vary considerably in health; and to a more marked degree in disease. Estimations of their numbers provide valuable information for diagnosis of many diseases. In this connection it is to be stressed that absolute numbers are more significant than percentages. In a healthy individual neutrophils are 3000-6000/μl; lymphocytes 1500-2700/μl; monocytes 100-700/μl; eosinophils 100-400/μl; and basophils 25-200/μl.

Relative Size

Leucocytes are generally examined in thin films of blood that are spread out on glass slides. In the process of making such films the cells are flattened and, therefore, appear somewhat larger than they are when suspended in a fluid medium. In a dry film all types of granulocytes, and monocytes are about 10 μm in diameter. Most lymphocytes are distinctly smaller (6-8 μm) and are called small lymphocytes, but some (called large lymphocytes) measure 12-15 μm.

Nuclei

In lymphocytes the nucleus is spherical, but may show an indentation on one side (Fig. 11.11). It stains densely in small lymphocytes, but tends to be partly euchromatic in large lymphocytes. In monocytes the nucleus is ovoid and may be indented: it is placed eccentrically. In basophils the nucleus is S-shaped. The nucleus of the eosinophil leucocyte is generally made of two lobes that are joined by delicate strands. In neutrophil leucocytes the nucleus is very variable in shape and consists of several lobes (up to 6): that is why these cells are also called ***polymorphonuclear leucocytes***, or simply ***polymorphs***. The number of lobes increases with the life of the cell. (Fig. 11.6)

Cytoplasm

The cytoplasm of a small lymphocyte is scanty and forms a thin rim around the nucleus. It is clear blue in stained preparations. In monocytes the cytoplasm is abundant. It stains blue, but in contrast to the 'transparent' appearance in lymphocytes the cytoplasm of monocytes is like frosted glass. Granules are not present in the cytoplasm of lymphocytes or of monocytes. The cytoplasm of granulocytes is marked by the presence of numerous granules. In neutrophils the granules are very fine and stain lightly with both acidic and basic dyes. The granules of neutrophils are really lysosomes: they are of various types depending upon the particular enzymes present in them. The granules of eosinophil leucocytes are large and stain brightly with acid dyes (like eosin). These are also lysosomes. In basophil leucocytes the cytoplasm contains large spherical granules that stain with basic dyes.

Motility and Phagocytosis

All leucocytes are capable of amoeboid movement. Neutrophils and monocytes are the most active. The eosinophil and basophil leucocytes move rather slowly. Lymphocytes in blood show the least power of movement. However, when they settle on solid surfaces they become freely motile and can pass through various tissues.

Because of their motility leucocytes easily pass through capillaries into surrounding tissues, and can migrate through the latter. Neutrophils collect in large numbers at sites of infection. Here they phagocytose bacteria and use the enzymes in their lysosomes to destroy the bacteria. Eosinophils are phagocytic, but their ability to destroy bacteria is less than that of neutrophils. The number of eosinophils is greatly increased in some allergic conditions. Monocytes are also actively phagocytic.

Life Span

We have seen that erythrocytes have a life span of about 100-120 days. The life of a neutrophil leucocyte is only about 15 hours. Eosinophils live for a few days, while basophils can live for 9 to 18 months. The life span of lymphocytes is variable. Some live only a few days (***short-lived lymphocytes***) while others may live several years (***long-lived lymphocytes***).

FURTHER FACTS ABOUT LYMPHOCYTES

We have seen that lymphocytes are numerous and constitute about 20-30 per cent of all leucocytes in blood. Large numbers of lymphocytes are also present in bone marrow, and as aggregations in various lymphatic tissues.

Formation and Circulation of Lymphocytes

In the embryo lymphocytes are derived from mesenchymal cells present in the wall of the yolk sac, in the liver and in the spleen. These stem cells later migrate to bone marrow. Lymphocytes formed from these stem cells (in bone marrow) enter the blood. Depending on their subsequent behaviour they are classified into two types.

1. Some of them travel in the blood stream to reach the thymus. Here they divide repeatedly and undergo certain changes. They are now called ***T-lymphocytes*** ('T' from thymus). These T-lymphocytes, that have been 'processed' in the thymus re-enter the circulation to reach lymphoid tissue in lymph nodes, spleen, tonsils and intestines.

   In lymph nodes T-lymphocytes are found in the diffuse tissue around lymphatic nodules. In the spleen they are found in white pulp (Chapter 11). From these masses of lymphoid tissue many lymphocytes pass into lymph vessels, and through them they go back into the circulation. In this way lymphocytes keep passing out of blood into lymphoid tissue (and bone marrow), and back from these into the blood. About 85 per cent of lymphocytes seen in blood are T-lymphocytes (Fig. 11.7).

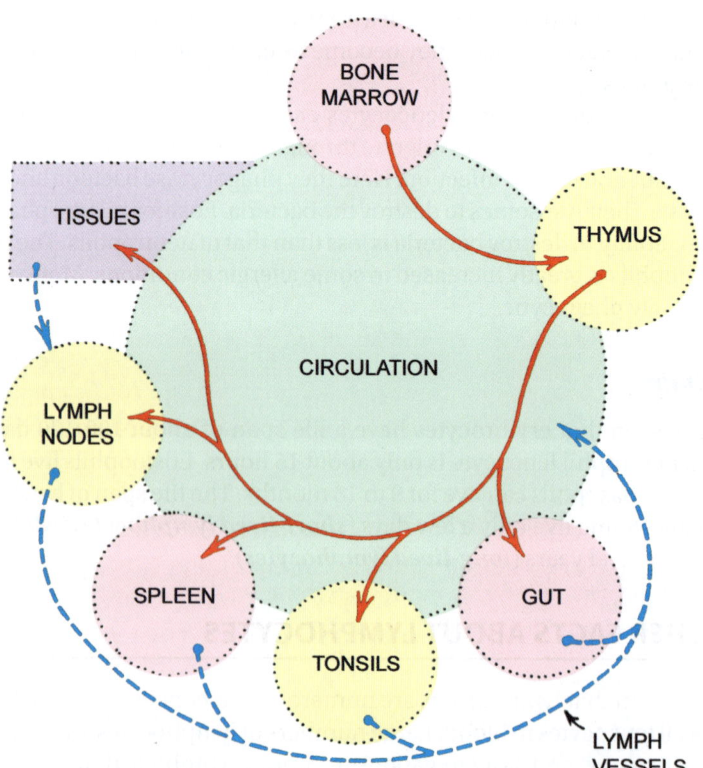

Fig. 11.7 Scheme to show the circulation of T-lymphocytes.

2. Lymphocytes of a second group arising from stem cells in bone marrow enter the blood stream, but do not go to the thymus. They go directly to lymphoid tissues (other than the thymus). Such lymphocytes are called ***B-lymphocytes***. In contrast to T-lymphocytes which lie in the diffuse lymphoid tissue of the lymph nodes and spleen, B-lymphocytes are seen in lymphatic nodules. The germinal centres are formed by actively dividing B-lymphocytes, while the dark rims of lymphatic nodules are formed by dense aggregations of B-lymphocytes. Like T-lymphocytes, B-lymphocytes also circulate between lymphoid tissues and the blood stream (Fig. 11.8).

Lymphocytes play a very important role in the immune system which is considered in Chapter 12.

LUKAEMIAS

Lukaemia is a condition in which there is uncontrolled production of leucocytes by bone marrow. It is a malignant, life threatening, condition. Leucocyte precursors, normally confined to bone marrow, are seen in large numbers in peripheral blood.

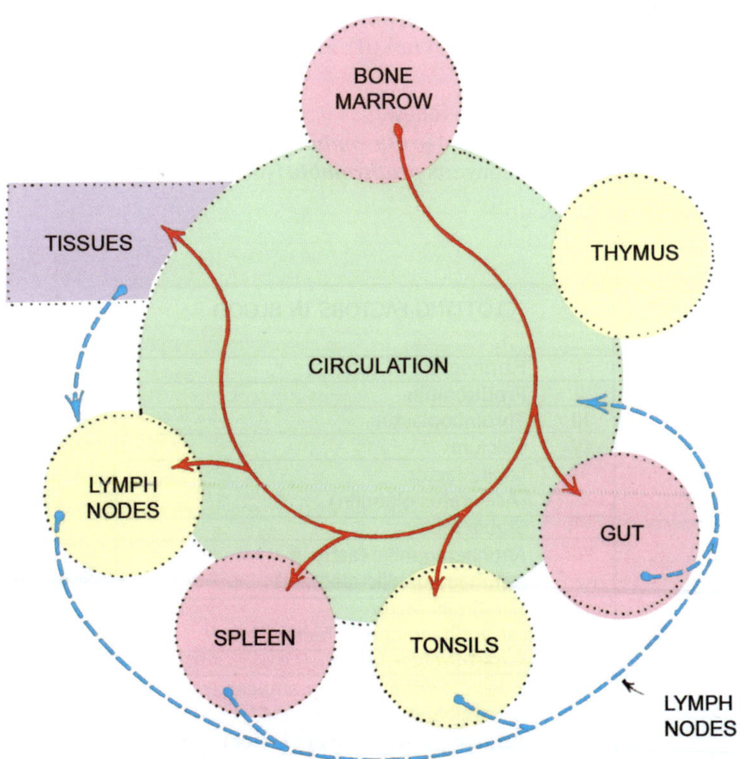

Fig. 11.8 Scheme to show the circulation of B-lymphocytes.

Lukaemias are of different types depending on the type of leucocytes, or leucocyte precursors, that are proliferating. When progress of the disease is slow (chronic lukaemia) the proliferating cells get time to differentiate, and they can be recognized. However, in acute lukaemias the peripheral blood is flooded with undifferentiated precursors of leucocytes.

BLOOD PLATELETS

Blood platelets are round, oval, or irregular discs about 3 µm in diameter. They are also known as ***thrombocytes***. The discs are biconvex. Each disc is bounded by a plasma membrane within which there are mitochondria and membrane bound vesicles. There is no nucleus. In ordinary blood films the platelets appear to have a clear outer zone (***hyalomere***) and a granular central part (***granulomere***). There are about 250,000 to 500,000 platelets per µl of blood. The life of a platelet is about 10 days.

Platelets are concerned with the clotting of blood as described below.

COAGULATION OF BLOOD

We have seen that coagulation of blood is very important for stoppage of bleeding from an injured blood vessel. The process of coagulation is complex and involves many steps, and many factors (most of which are proteins). The factors are identified by roman numerals (I to V and VII to XIII), and are also given names as shown in Fig. 11. 9.

The most important steps are as follows.

1. When a blood vessel is injured ***prothrombin activator*** is produced.
2. Prothrombin activator converts ***prothrombin*** (present in plasma) to ***thrombin*** (an enzyme).

CLOTTING FACTORS IN BLOOD	
I	Fibrinogen
II	Prothrombin
III	Thromboplastin
IV	Calcium
V	Labile factor (Acclerator globulin)
VII	Stable factor
VIII	Antihaemophilic factor A (antihaemophilic globulin)
IX	Christmas factor (or antihaemophilic factor B)
X	Stuart-Prower factor
XI	Plasma thromboplastin antecedent (PTA) (or antihaemophilic factor C)
XII	Hegman factor (Contact factor)
XIII	Fibre stabilizing factor

Fig. 11.9 Coagulation factors.

3. Thrombin acts on the plasma protein ***fibrinogen*** and converts it into insoluble fibres of ***fibrin***. These fibres form a meshwork in which blood cells get entangled to form a solid clot.

Prothrombin Activator

Prothrombin is formed only after injury to a blood vessel. There are two pathways for prothrombin formation. There is an intrinsic pathway (in blood), and one extrinsic pathway (in tissue). Each pathway consists of a number of steps that are shown in Fig. 11.10 Both pathways end in the production of prothrombin activator. As stated above this activator converts prothrombin to thrombin.

Lack of factors VIII or IX leads to an inherited disease in which the blood does not clot. It is called ***haemophilia.*** Lack of factor VII can also interfere with clotting. The presence of Calcium ions is very important for clotting of blood. The presence of vitamin K is important for synthesis of clotting factors.

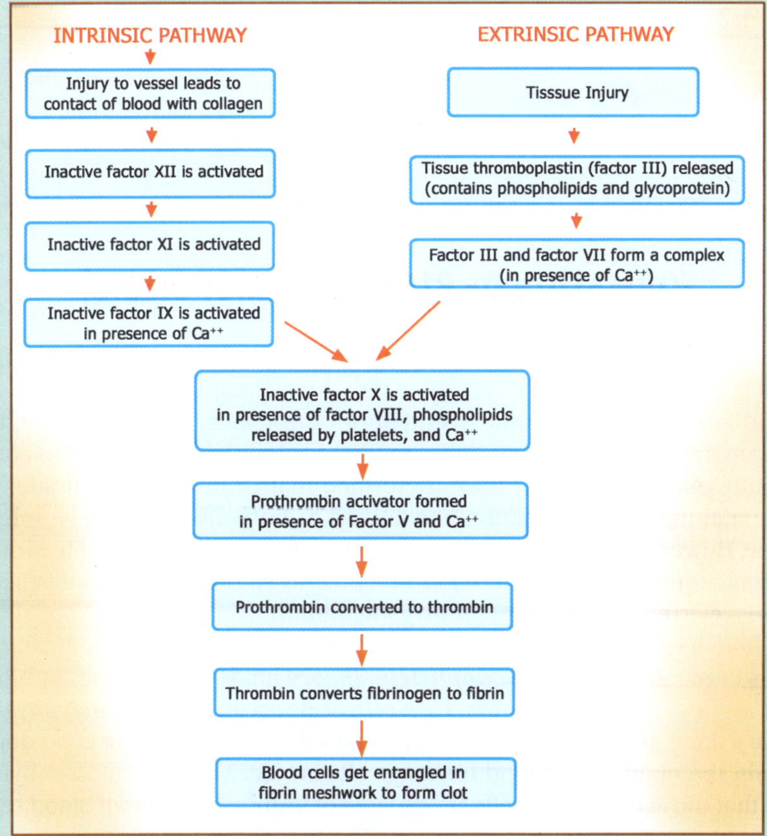

Fig. 11.10 Pathways for generation of prothrombin factor.

ANTICOAGULANTS

Chemicals that prevent clotting of blood are called anticoagulants. Some of them act within the body (in vivo), some outside the body (in vitro), and some in both situations.

Heparin

This is produced by mast cells and by basophil leucocytes. It suppresses activity of thrombin, removes thrombin from blood and inactivates several clotting factors.

Heparin injected intravenously prevents coagulation for a few hours. It is useful in conditions in which avoidance of intravenous clotting is desired, including dialysis and cardiac surgery. It is also useful as an anticoagulant in vitro.

Dicoumarol and Warfarin

These can be taken orally for clinical use. They act by inhibiting action of vitamin K.

Edta

It acts by removing calcium from blood. It is useful both in vivo and in vitro.

Oxalates and Citrates

These also act by combining with calcium and thus removing it from blood. They are used in vitro only.

Hirudin produced by leaches, and venom of some snakes are anticoagulants.

FORMATION OF BLOOD (HAEMOPOIESIS)

In embryonic life blood cells are first formed in relation to mesenchymal cells surrounding the yolk sac. After the second month of intrauterine life blood formation starts in the liver; later in the spleen; and still later in the bone marrow. At first lymphocytes are formed along with other cells of blood in bone marrow, but later they are formed mainly in lymphoid tissues. In postnatal life blood formation is confined to bone marrow and lymphoid tissue. However, under conditions in which the bone marrow is unable to meet normal requirements, blood cell formation may start in the liver and spleen. This is referred to as ***extramedullary haemopoiesis***.

There has been considerable controversy regarding the origin of various types of blood cells. The ***monophyletic theory*** holds that all types of blood cells are derived from a common ***stem cell***; while according to the ***polyphyletic theory*** there are several independent types of stem cells. There is no doubt that in the embryo all blood forming cells are derived from mesenchyme, and that the earliest stem cells are capable of forming all types of blood cells. Subsequently the potency of stem cells becomes restricted.

We have already seen that there are embryonic stem cells that are pleuripotent. Arising from them there are the following.

a. ***Haemopoietic stem cells*** or ***haemocytoblasts***, that are present (in postnatal life) only in bone marrow and give rise to all blood cells other than lymphocytes.
b. ***Lymphopoietic stem cells*** that are present in bone marrow and in lymphoid tissues and give rise to lymphocytes. (Stages in the development of blood cells are illustrated in Figure 11.11).

Precursor cells of the erythrocyte series are called ***erythroblasts*** or ***normoblasts***. At first these cells do not contain haemoglobin and their cytoplasm is basophil. As haemoglobin begins to be formed the cytoplasm becomes acidophil. The erythroblasts become progressively smaller. Their nuclei shrink and are thrown out of the cells. The cytoplasm now has a reticular appearance (produced by RNA remaining within it): these cells are, therefore, called ***reticulocytes***. Reticulocytes leave the bone marrow and enter the blood stream. Here they lose their reticulum within a day or two and become mature erythrocytes.

Formation of Granulocytes

It is believed that neutrophil, eosinophil and basophil leucocytes arise from a common early derivative of the haemopoietic stem cell which is called a ***myeloblast***. The myeloblast matures into a larger cell called a ***promyelocyte*** which is marked by the presence of large granules (lysosomes) in its cytoplasm. The promyelocyte now gives rise to ***myelocytes*** in which the granules are smaller and ***specific*** so that at this stage neutrophil, eosinophil and basophil myelocytes can be recognized. The nucleus now undergoes transformation dividing into two or three lobes in eosinophil cells; and forming up to six lobes in neutrophils. With the nuclei assuming their distinctive appearance the myelocytes become mature granulocytes.

Formation of Monocytes

Monocytes are also formed in bone marrow from haemopoietic stem cells. Recent evidence (see below) suggests a common origin of monocytes and granulocytes. Early stages in the formation of monocytes are referred to as ***monoblasts***. The stem cells that give rise to monocytes also give rise to other cells of the mononuclear phagocyte system.

Formation of Platelets

The precursor cells of blood platelets are called ***megakaryoblasts***. The megakaryoblast enlarges to form a ***promegakaryocyte***. Still further enlargement converts it into a ***megakaryocyte***: this cell may be 50 to 100 μm in diameter, and has a multi-lobed nucleus. Platelets are formed by separation of small masses of cytoplasm from this large cell.

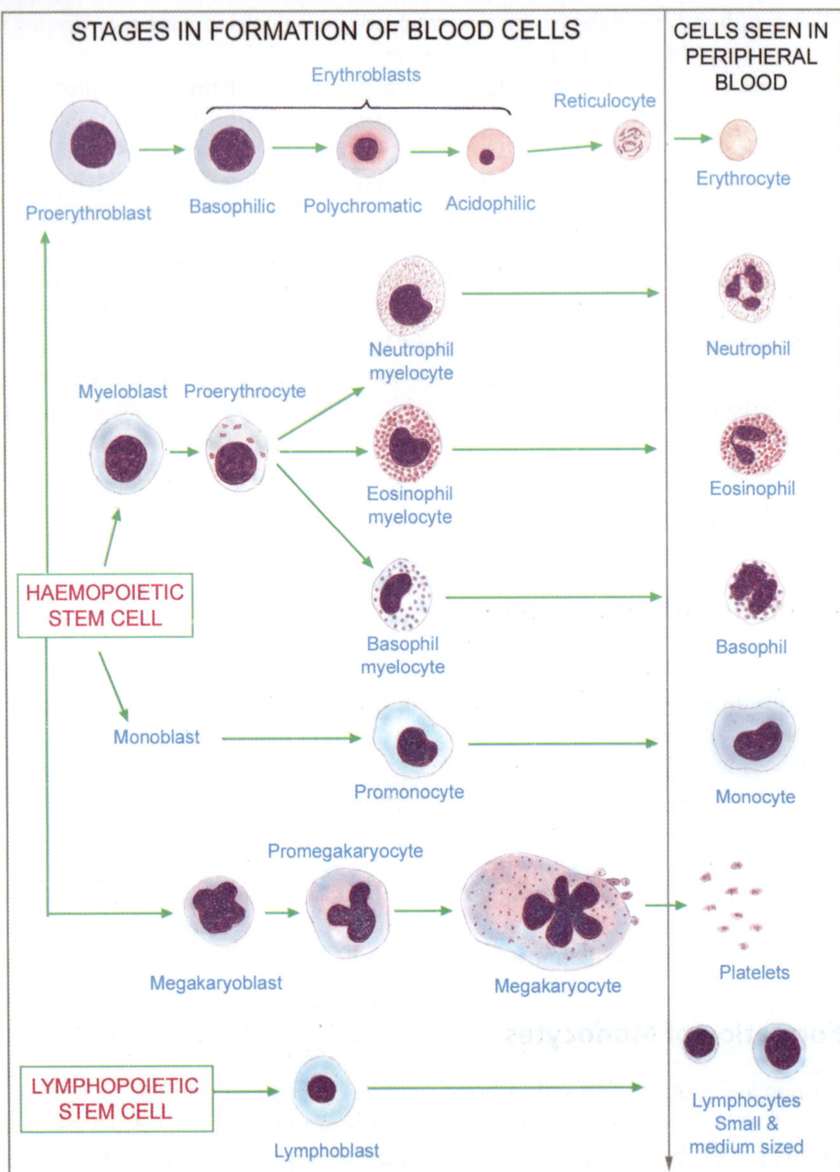

Fig. 11.11 Stages in formation of blood cells (Traditional terms used).

MONONUCLEAR PHAGOCYTE SYSTEM

Distributed widely through the body there are a series of cells that share the property of being able to phagocytose unwanted matter including bacteria and dead cells. These cells also play an important role in defence mechanisms, and in carrying out this function they act in close collaboration with lymphocytes. In the past some of the cells of this system have been included under the term ***reticulo-endothelial system***, but this term has now been discarded as it is established that most endothelial cells do not act as macrophages. The term ***macrophage system*** has also been used for cells of the system, but with the discovery of a close relationship between these cells and mononuclear leucocytes of blood the term ***mononuclear phagocyte system*** (or ***monocyte phagocyte system***) has come into common usage. It is now known that all macrophages are derived from stem cells in bone marrow that also give origin to mononuclear cells of blood.

Cells of Mononuclear Phagocyte System

The various cells that are usually included in the mononuclear phagocyte system are as follows.

1. Monocytes of blood, and their precursors in bone marrow (monoblasts, promonocytes).
2. Macrophage cells (histiocytes) of connective tissue, and macrophages present in various other tissues.

The cells of the mononuclear phagocyte system have the ability to phagocytose particulate matter, dead cells, and organisms. In the lungs, alveolar macrophages engulf inhaled particles and are seen as ***dust cells***. In the spleen and liver, macrophages destroy aged and damaged erythrocytes. The cells play an important role in the functioning of the immune system. They have the ability to stimulate T-lymphocytes.

CHAPTER

12

Lymphoid Tissues and Immunity

Introductory Remarks

When circulating blood reaches the capillaries part of its fluid content passes into the surrounding tissues as tissue fluid. Most of this fluid re-enters the capillaries at their venous ends. Some of it is, however, returned to the circulation through a separate system of ***lymphatic vessels*** (usually called ***lymphatics***). The fluid passing through the lymphatic vessels is called ***lymph***. The smallest lymphatic (or lymph) vessels are lymphatic capillaries that join together to form larger lymphatic vessels. The largest lymphatic vessel in the body is the ***thoracic duct***. It drains lymph from the greater part of the body. The thoracic duct ends by joining the left subclavian vein at its junction with the internal jugular vein. On the right side there is the ***right lymphatic duct*** that has a similar termination.

Scattered along the course of lymphatic vessels there are numerous small bean-shaped structures called ***lymph nodes*** that are usually present in groups. Lymph nodes are masses of lymphoid tissue described below. As a rule lymph from any part of the body passes through one or more lymph nodes before entering the blood stream. Lymph nodes act as filters removing bacteria and other particulate matter from lymph. Lymphocytes are added to lymph in these nodes.

Aggregations of lymphoid tissue are also found at various other sites. Two organs, the thymus and the spleen are almost entirely made up of lymphoid tissue. Prominent aggregations of lymphoid tissue are present in close relationship to the lining epithelium of the gut. Such aggregations present in the region of the pharynx constitute the ***tonsils***. Isolated nodules of lymphoid tissue, and larger aggregations called ***Peyer's patches*** are present in the mucosa and submucosa of the small intestines (specially the ileum). The mucosa of the vermiform appendix contains abundant lymphoid tissue. Lymphoid tissue is seen in the mucosa of the large intestines. Collections of lymphoid tissue are also to be seen in the walls of the trachea and larger bronchi, and in relation to the urinary tract.

Lymph

Lymph is a transudate from blood and contains the same proteins as in plasma, but in smaller amounts, and in somewhat different proportions. Suspended in lymph there are cells that are chiefly lymphocytes. Large molecules of fat (chylomicrons) that are absorbed from the intestines enter lymph vessels. After a fatty meal these fat globules may be so numerous that lymph becomes milky (and is then called ***chyle***).

LYMPHATIC VESSELS

Lymph capillaries (or lymphatic capillaries) begin blindly in tissues where they form a network (Fig. 12.1). The structure of lymph capillaries is basically similar to that of blood capillaries, but is adapted for much greater permeability. As compared to blood capillaries, much larger molecules can pass through the walls of lymph capillaries.

The structure of the thoracic duct and of other ***larger lymph vessels*** is similar to that of veins.

LYMPH NODES

Main Groups of Lymph Nodes in the Body

There are many groups of lymph nodes. From a clinical point poit of view the important ones are those that can be palpated through skin. (a) In the neck there are superficial and deep ***cervical lymph nodes***. (b) In each axilla (armpit) there are ***axillary lymph nodes***. (c) The ***inguinal lymph nodes*** lie on the front of the thigh just below the inguinal ligament.

Important groups of deep lying nodes are present in the thorax and in the abdomen.

Normal lymph nodes are not palpable. They become palpable when enlarged. They become tender when infected.

Structure of Lymph Nodes

Each lymph node consists of a connective tissue framework; and of numerous lymphocytes, and other cells, that fill the interstices of the network. The entire node is bean-shaped (Fig. 12.2).

When a section through a lymph node is examined (at low magnification) it is seen that the node has an outer zone that contains densely packed lymphocytes, and therefore stains darkly: this part is the ***cortex***.

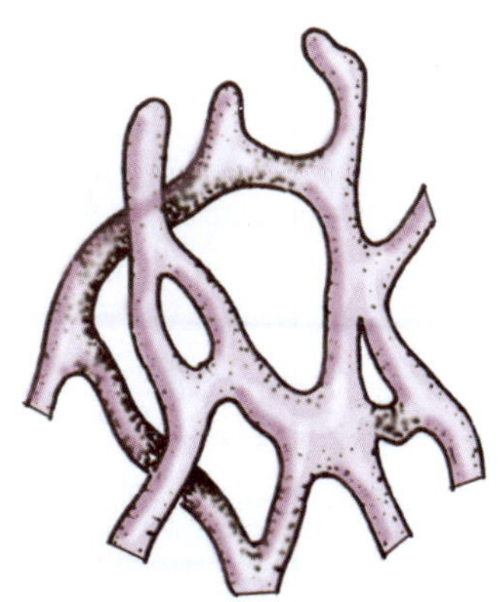

Fig. 12.1 Diagram to show part of a network of lymphatic capillaries.

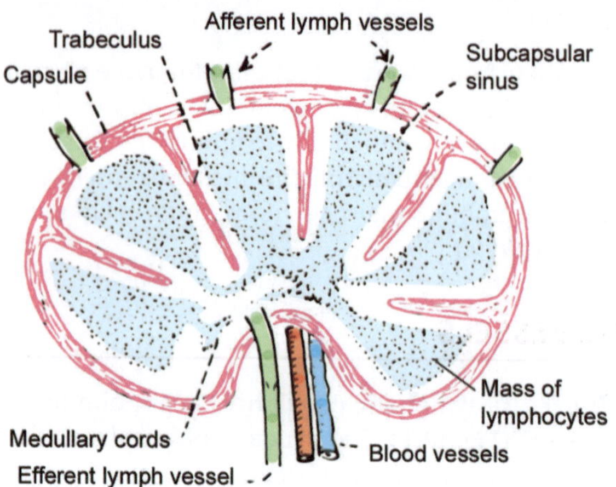

Fig. 12.2 Scheme to show some features of the structure of a lymph node.

Surrounded by the cortex, there is a lighter staining zone in which lymphocytes are fewer: this area is the ***medulla*** (Fig. 12.3).

Within the cortex there are several rounded areas that are called ***lymphatic follicles*** or ***lymphatic nodules***. Each nodule has a paler staining ***germinal centre*** surrounded by a zone of densely packed lymphocytes.

Within the medulla, the lymphocytes are arranged in the form of branching and anastomosing cords.

Each lymph node is covered by a ***capsule***. A number of ***septa*** (or ***trabeculae***) extend into the node from the capsule and divide the node into lobules. The remaining spaces within the node are filled by a delicate network of reticular fibres.

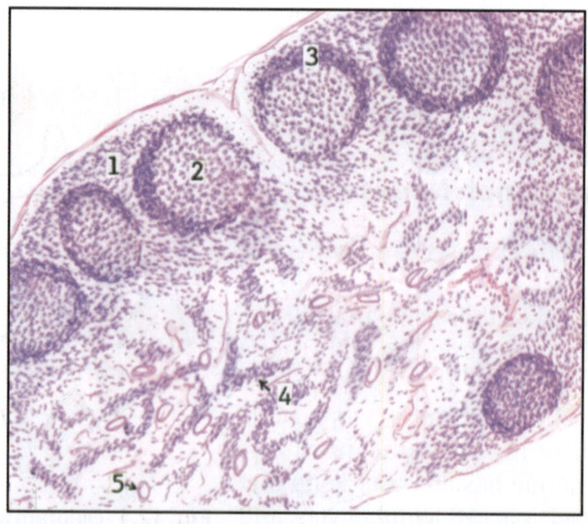

Fig.12.3 Section through a lymph node. 1-Cortex. 2, 3-Germinal center and outer zone of lymphatic follicle. 4-Medulla. 5-Blood vessel.

Cells of Lymph Nodes

Lymphocytes

Lymphocytes enter lymph nodes from blood. Some enter through lymph. Both B-lymphocytes and T-lymphocytes are present in lymph nodes. The lymphatic nodules (which constitute the ***cortex proper***) are composed of B-lymphocytes. The cells in the paler germinal centres of the nodules are mainly lymphoblasts. It is believed that they represent B-lymphocytes that have been stimulated, by antigens, to enlarge and undergo multiplication (Fig. 12.4).

The lymphocytes divide repeatedly and give rise to more B-lymphocytes aggregations of which form the dark staining 'rims' around the germinal centres. These B-lymphocytes mature into plasma cells. Plasma cells produce antibodies

The diffuse lymphoid tissue intervening between nodules is made up mainly of T-lymphocytes. T-lymphocytes are also present in medullary cords. T-cells enter lymph nodes from blood. After a few hours they leave the node via efferent lymph vessels. When activated by antigens they multiply to form a large number of activated T-cells that are sensitive to the particular antigen. These T-cells reach various tissues through the circulation.

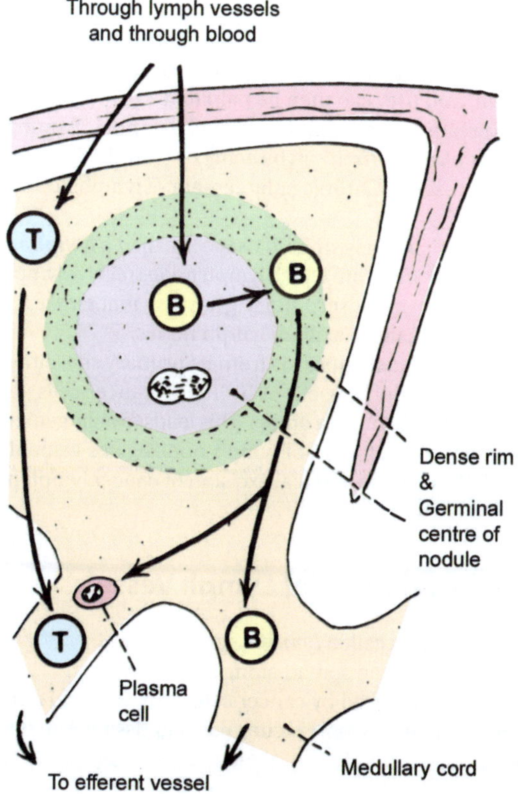

Fig. 12.4 Scheme to show the circulation of B-lymphocytes and of T-lymphocytes through a lymph node.

Apart from lymphocytes and plasma cells, fibroblasts and macrophages are also present .

Lymph entering a node passes through a system of sinuses. Here it comes into intimate contact with macrophages present in the node. Bacteria and other particulate matter are removed from lymph by these cells.

Summary of Functions of Lymph Nodes

Lymph nodes perform the following major functions.

1. They are centres of lymphocyte production. Both B-lymphocytes and T-lymphocytes are produced here by multiplication of preexisting lymphocytes. These lymphocytes pass into lymph and thus reach the blood stream.
2. Bacteria and other particulate matter are removed from lymph through phagocytosis by macrophages. Antigens thus carried into these cells are 'presented' to lymphocytes stimulating their proliferation. In this way lymph nodes play an important role in the immune response to antigens.
3. Plasma cells (representing fully mature B-lymphocytes) produce antibodies against invading antigens, while T-lymphocytes attack cells that are 'foreign' to the host body.

Some Clinical Correlations of Lymph Nodes

1. Palpation of lymph nodes is an important part of clinical examination. Normal lymph nodes are soft and cannot be felt. As a result of disease they become enlarged and firm, and they can then be palpated.
2. Infection often spreads to lymph nodes through lymph. Inflammation of lymph nodes is called ***lymphadenitis***. It can be acute or chronic. Sometimes it can lead to formation of an abscess. Chronic enlargement of lymph nodes is common in tuberculosis.
3. A malignant tumor arising in lymphoid tissue is called a ***lymphoma***. Malignant tumours, present in the area from which lymph nodes receive lymph, often spread to the lymph nodes, forming secondary growths (***metastases***). For example, cancer of the breast spreads to axillary lymph nodes.

   Carcinoma (cancer) usually spreads from its primary site, either by growth of malignant cells along lymph vessels, or by 'loose' cancer cells passing through lymph to nodes into which the area drains. This leads to enlargement of the lymph nodes of the region. Examination of lymph nodes gives valuable information about the spread of cancer. In surgical excision of cancer lymph nodes draining the region are usually removed.

Some Clinical Correlations of Lymph Vessels

1. Inflammation of vessels is called ***lymphangitis***.
2. We have seen that cancer can spread along lymph vessels.
3. Lymph vessels may be blocked by cancer cells or by surgical removal of lymph nodes. When this happens lymph accumulates in tissues and leads to swelling (***lymphoedema***).

THE SPLEEN

The spleen is an important organ located in the upper part of the abdomen, on the left side (Fig. 12.5). It is in contact with the diaphragm, the stomach, and the left kidney. Its size is approximately that of a clenched fist. The arterial supply to the spleen is through the splenic artery (a branch of the coeliac trunk). The splenic vein joins the portal vein. It follows that all blood from the spleen has to pass through the liver.

Connective Tissue Basis

The spleen is the largest lymphoid organ of the body. The surface of the spleen is covered by peritoneum (referred to as the ***serous coat***). Deep to the serous layer the organ has a ***capsule***. ***Trabeculae*** arising from the capsule extend into the substance of the spleen (Fig. 12.6).

The spaces between trabeculae are filled by a network of reticular fibres. Fibroblasts (reticular cells) and macrophages are also present in relation to the reticulum. The interstices of the reticulum are pervaded by lymphocytes, blood vessels and blood cells, and by macrophages.

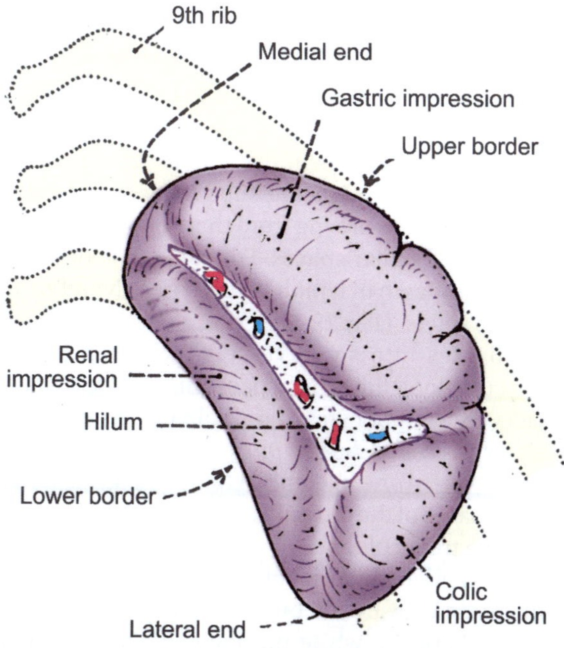

Fig. 12.5 The spleen.

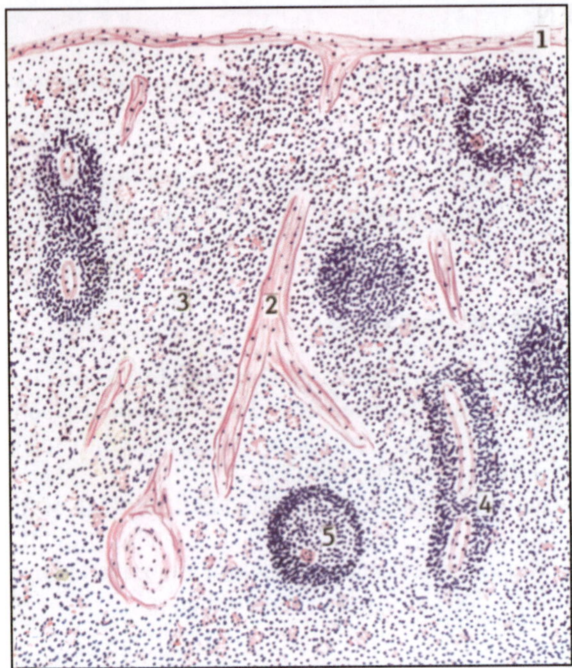

Fig. 12.6 Section through spleen. 1-Capsule. 2-Septum. 3-Red pulp. 4, 5-Cords of densely packed lymphocytes around arteriole.

Circulation through the Spleen

White Pulp and Red Pulp

On reaching the hilum of the spleen, the splenic artery divides into about five branches. Each branch divides and subdivides as it travels through the trabecular network. Arterioles arising from this network leave the trabeculae to pass into the inter-trabecular spaces. For some distance each arteriole is surrounded by a dense sheath of lymphocytes. These lymphocytes constitute the ***white pulp*** of the spleen (Fig. 12.7).

The arteriole divides into small vessels that open into the reticular framework. As a result blood flows into spaces lined by reticular cells, coming into direct contact with lymphocytes there. Splenic tissue, which is infiltrated with blood in this way, is called the ***red pulp***. The circulation in the red pulp of the spleen is thus an 'open' one in contrast to the 'closed' circulation in other organs. Blood from spaces of the red pulp is collected by wide sinusoids. These drain into veins in the trabeculae.

The spleen acts as a filter for worn out red blood cells. These are trapped in the spleen where they are destroyed by macrophages.

At places the cords of the white pulp are thicker than elsewhere and contain lymphatic nodules similar to those seen in lymph nodes. These nodules are called ***Malpighian bodies***. Each nodule has a germinal centre and a surrounding cuff of densely packed lymphocytes. The nodules are

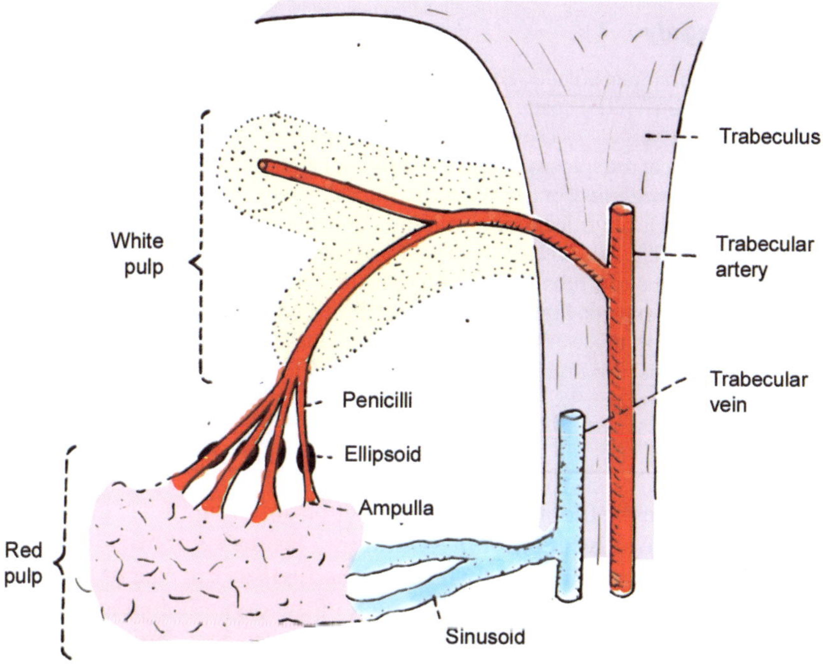

Fig. 12.7 Scheme to show some features of the splenic circulation.

easily distinguished from those of lymph nodes because of the presence of an arteriole in each of them.

The functional significance of the white pulp is similar to that of cortical tissue of lymph nodes. Most of the lymphocytes in white pulp are T-lymphocytes. Lymphatic nodules of the white pulp are aggregations of B-lymphocytes. The germinal centres are areas where B-lymphocytes are dividing.

The red pulp is like a sponge. It is permeated by spaces lined by reticular cells. The intervals between the spaces are filled by B-lymphocytes as well as T-lymphocytes, macrophages, and blood cells. These cells appear to be arranged as cords (***splenic cords***). The cords form a network.

FUNCTIONS OF THE SPLEEN

1. Like other lymphoid tissues the spleen is a centre where both B-lymphocytes and T-lymphocytes multiply, and play an important role in immune responses.
2. The spleen contains the largest aggregations of macrophages of the mononuclear phagocyte system. In the spleen the main function of these cells is the destruction of red blood corpuscles that have completed their useful life. This is facilitated by the intimate contact of blood with the macrophages because of the presence of an open circulation. Macrophages also destroy worn out leucocytes, and bacteria.
3. In fetal life the spleen is a centre for production of ***all*** blood cells. In later life only lymphocytes are produced here.

Splenomegaly

Enlargement of spleen is called ***splenomegaly***. A normal spleen cannot be palpated (as it does not reach the costal margin). It can be felt when it extend beyond this margin.

Enlargement of the spleen occurs in conditions calling for increased lymphocyte production (***leukaemias***); or conditions in which there is increased phagocytosis by macrophages (as in any infection); and in conditions involving increased destruction of erythrocytes (e.g., ***malaria***). There may be enlargement of the spleen in some infections e.g., malaria, tuberculosis and typhoid fever.

Blood from the spleen drains into the liver (through the splenic and portal veins), and passes through the liver to reach the inferior vena cava. In some diseases of the liver (e.g., cirrhosis) this drainage is interfered with. This also leads to splenomegaly.

THE THYMUS

The thymus lies in the thorax, behind the manubrium sterni, and in front of the heart. (This space is the anterior mediastinum). It consists of two lobes, right and left (Fig. 12.8). At birth the thymus weighs 10-15 g. The weight increases to 30-40 g at puberty. Subsequently, much of the organ is replaced by fat. However, the thymus is believed to produce T-lymphocytes throughout life.

The right and left lobes are joined together by fibrous tissue. Each lobe has a connective tissue capsule. Connective tissue septa passing inwards from the capsule incompletely subdivide the lobe into a large number of lobules (Figs. 12.9, 12.10).

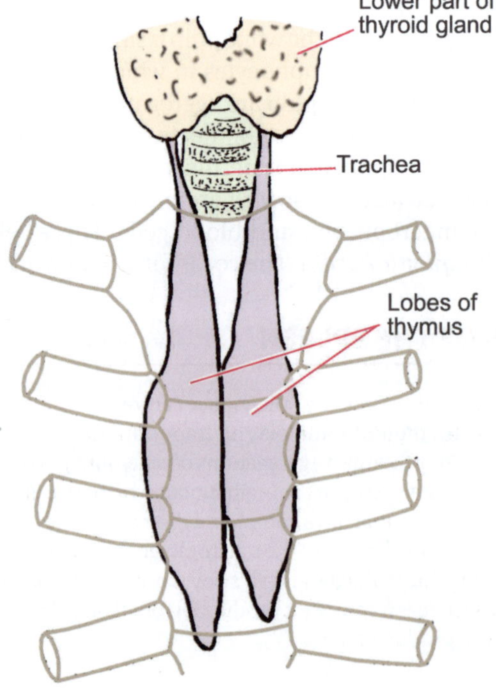

Fig. 12.8 The thymus.

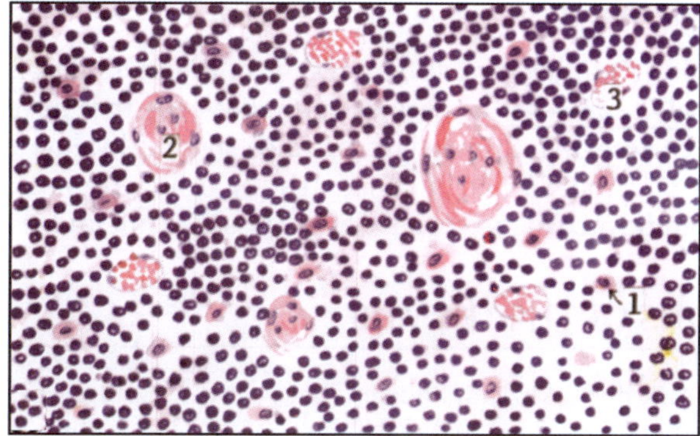

Fig. 12.9 Thymus (low power view). Note masses of lymphocytes arranged in the form of lobules. 1-Cortex. 2-Medulla. 3-Hassal's corpuscle.

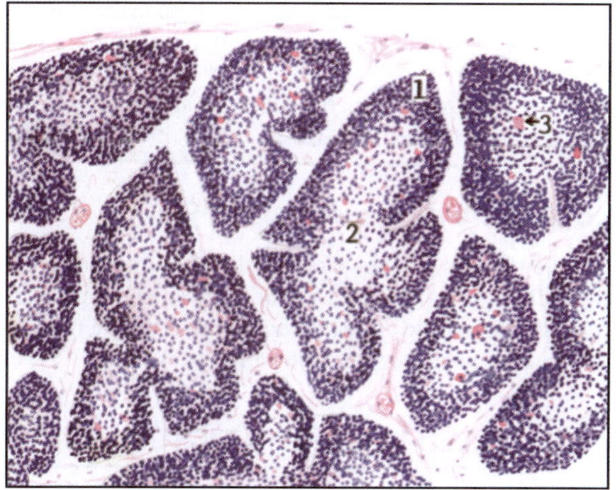

Fig. 12-10 Thymus. (High power view). 1- Epithelial cell. 2-Hassal's corpuscle. 3-Capillary.

Each lobule has an outer cortex and an inner medulla. Both the cortex and medulla contain cells of two distinct kinds of cells.

a. ***Epithelial Cells*** (epitheliocytes) are flattened. They branch and form a network.
b. ***Lymphocytes*** (also called ***thymocytes***) fill the spaces in the reticulum (formed by epithelial cells). Stem cells formed in bone marrow travel to the thymus. Here they come to lie in the superficial part of the cortex, and divide repeatedly to form small lymphocytes. Lymphatic nodules are not present in the normal thymus.

As thymocytes divide they pass deeper into the cortex, and into the medulla. Ultimately, they leave the thymus by passing into blood vessels and lymphatics.

Apart from epithelial cells and lymphocytes the thymus contains a fair number of ***macrophages*** (belonging to the mononuclear phagocyte system).

Corpuscles of Hassall

These are small rounded structures present in the medulla of the thymus. Each corpuscle represents a mass of epithelial cells that have undergone degeneration. These cells ultimately form a pink staining hyaline mass. Around this mass there is a wall formed by concentrically arranged epithelial cells. The functional significance of the corpuscles of Hassall is not understood.

FUNCTIONS OF THE THYMUS

1. The role of the thymus in lymphopoiesis has been discussed in Chapter 12. Stem cells (from bone marrow) that reach the superficial part of the cortex divide repeatedly to form smaller lymphocytes. While in the thymus, lymphocytes acquire the ability to recognize a very large number of proteins (that are foreign to the body), and to react to them. Lymphocytes passing from the thymus into the circulation react only against proteins foreign to the body. These are immunologically competent T-lymphocytes. They lodge themselves in secondary lymph organs like lymph nodes, spleen etc., where they multiply to form further T-lymphocytes of their own type when exposed to the appropriate antigen.

Because of this important role, the thymus is regarded as a ***primary lymphoid organ*** (along with bone marrow).

Thymus and Myasthenia Gravis

Enlargement of the thymus is often associated with a disease called myasthenia gravis. In this condition there is great weakness of skeletal muscle. In many such cases the thymus is enlarged and there may be a tumour in it. Removal of the thymus may result in considerable improvement in some cases.

MUCOSA ASSOCIATED LYMPHOID TISSUE

We have seen that the main masses of lymphoid tissue in the body are the lymph nodes, the spleen and the thymus. Small numbers of lymphocytes may be present almost anywhere in the body, but significant aggregations are seen in relation to the mucosa of the respiratory, alimentary and urogenital tracts. In the respiratory system the aggregations are relatively small and are present in the walls of the trachea and large bronchi.

Mucosa Associated Lymphoid Tissue in the Alimentary System

The aggregations of lymphoid tissue, present in relation to the alimentary system, are as follows.

a. Near the junction of the oral cavity with the pharynx there are a number of collections of lymphoid tissue that are referred to as ***tonsils*** (Fig. 12.11).
    1. The largest of these are the right and left ***palatine tonsils*** (Fig. 12.12), present on either side of the communication between the mouth and the pharynx. (In common usage the word tonsils refers to the palatine tonsils).

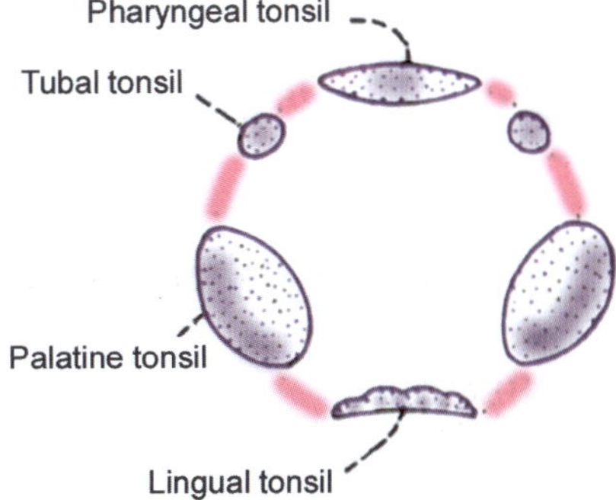

Fig. 12.11 Scheme to show various tonsils present near the junction of the oral cavity and the pharynx.

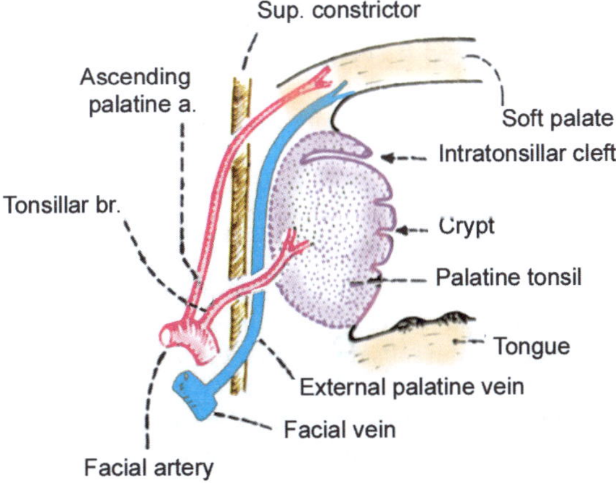

Fig. 12.12 Section through the palatine tonsil. Note its relationship to the palate and to the tongue.

The palatine tonsils are often infected (***tonsillitis***). This is a common cause of sore throat. Frequent infections can lead to considerable enlargement of the tonsils specially in children. Such enlarged tonsils may become a focus of infection and their surgical removal (***tonsillectomy***) may then become necessary.

2. Another midline collection of lymphoid tissue, the ***pharyngeal tonsil,*** is present on the posterior wall of the pharynx. In children the pharyngeal tonsil may hypertrophy and is then referred to as the ***adenoids***. The resulting swelling may be a cause of obstruction to normal breathing. The child tends to breathe through the mouth, and this may in turn lead to other abnormalities.
3. Smaller collections of lymphoid tissue are present on the dorsum of the posterior part of the tongue (***lingual tonsils***), and around the pharyngeal openings of the auditory tubes (***tubal tonsils***).

b. Small collections of lymphoid tissue, similar in structure to the follicles of lymph nodes, may be present anywhere along the length of the gut. They are called ***solitary lymphatic follicles***. Larger aggregations of lymphoid tissue, each made up of 10 to 200 follicles are also present in the small intestine. They are called ***aggregated lymphatic follicles*** or ***Peyer's patches***. These patches can be seen by naked eye.

DEFENCE MECHANISMS AND IMMUNITY

DEFENCE MECHANISMS

The animal body has to defend it self from infections, and other harmful agents. For this purpose it has developed a number of defense mechanisms. Some of these are non-specific and can take action against many substances. Others are specific and act against a specific harmful substance only.

Physical and Chemical Barriers

1. The skin and mucous membranes lining various cavities act as physical barriers to the passage of bacteria or viruses.
2. The eyelashes, hair in nostrils, wax in the external ear, and mucous over mucous membranes trap particulate matter.
3. Hydrochloric acid present in the stomach destroys most bacteria that are swallowed. Antibacterial substances are present in secretion of salivary and sebaceous glands, in nasal secretions and in lacrimal fluid.

Once bacteria or other harmful substances enter the body other mechanisms come into play.

1. Phagocytes or macrophages have the ability to surround and destroy bacteria and other substances entering the body. These include some cells present in blood and in connections tissues.
2. Some proteins present in blood and in tissues are called ***complement***. These proteins play a role in destruction of bacteria.
3. When organisms invade a tissue and damage it, an ***inflammatory reaction*** is set up. A similar reaction is also set up after physical injury to a part, or after injury by chemicals or other irritating substances.

Inflammatory Reaction

The main features of acute inflammation are:

1. Redness of the part.
2. Swelling.
3. Pain.
4. The part is warm.

Because of pain and swelling function may be lost (for example in a finger).

Most of these features are a result of increased blood flow through the region, because the local capillaries dilate. Simultaneously permeability of capillaries increases. More fluid flows into the tissue and is the cause of swelling. White blood cells (leucocytes), particularly neutrophils, leave blood vessels to enter the tissue. Here they phagocytose unwanted matter. Later, many macrophages reach the site. They remove bacteria, dead cells and other damaged tissue.

Macrophages release a substance called ***interleukin 1***. This stimulates the temperature regulating centre to raise body temperature. That is why inflammation anywhere in the body can cause fever.

In many cases destruction of tissue by inflammation leads to formation of pus (suppuration). Pus is made up of fluid in which there are cells including dead phagocytes, and bacteria, living or dead.

A small collection of pus deep to skin is called a ***boil***. A larger collection is called an ***abscess***. Generally pus in boils tries to reach the surface of the skin. Here the boil ruptures and pus flows out. Sometimes an incision has to be given to drain out the pus. If pus does not drain out fully the abscess persists and small amounts of pus can keep flowing out of a narrow channel. This is called a ***sinus***. Sometimes an abscess can drain into a cavity within the body, forming a ***fistula***.

Usually, inflammation resolves after sometime and the tissue gradually returns to normal. However, if resolution is partial the inflammation becomes chronic. An area of chronic inflammation shows large number of lymphocytes. Sometimes the defence systems of the body are unable to kill off all bacteria. In that case they may try to wall of the areas. Nodular areas, called ***granulomas*** are thus formed. One example of an infection in which this happens is tuberculosis.

LYMPHOCYTES AND THE IMMUNE SYSTEM

Numerous references have been made to the role of lymphocytes in protecting the body against foreign invaders. In this section we will briefly review their role.

Lymphocytes are an essential part of the ***immune system*** of the body that is responsible for defence against invasion by bacteria and other organisms. In contrast to granulocytes and monocytes which directly attack invading organisms, lymphocytes help to destroy them by producing substances called ***antibodies***. These are protein molecules that have the ability to recognize a 'foreign' protein (i.e., a protein not normally present in the individual). The foreign protein is usually referred to as an ***antigen***. An antigen may be part of an invading bacterium or other organism. It may be cellular (as when blood is transfused from one person to another, or when a tissue is transplanted from one person to another). It will be appreciated that there can be a very large number of such foreign proteins. The body itself also contains a very large number of proteins of its own. For any defence system to be effective it is necessary that lymphocytes should be able to distinguish between the proteins of the individual and those that are foreign to it. An antigen can be neutralized only by a specific antibody. It follows that lymphocytes must be capable of producing a very wide range of antibodies; or rather that there must be a very wide variety of lymphocytes each variety programmed to recognize a specific antigen and to produce antibodies against it.

This function of antibody production is done by B-lymphocytes. When stimulated by the presence of antigen the cells enlarge and get converted to plasma cells. The plasma cells produce antibodies. T-lymphocytes are also concerned with immune responses, but their role is somewhat different from that of B-lymphocytes. T-lymphocytes specialize in recognizing cells that are foreign to the host body. These may be fungi, virus infected cells, tumour cells, or cells of another individual. T-lymphocytes have surface receptors which recognize specific antigens (there being many varieties of T-lymphocytes each type recognizing a specific antigen). When exposed to a suitable stimulus the T-lymphocytes multiply and form large cells which can destroy abnormal cells by direct contact, or by producing cytotoxic substances called ***cytokines*** or ***lymphokines.*** From the above it will be seen that while B-lymphocytes defend the body through blood borne antibodies, T-lymphocytes are responsible for cell mediated immune responses (***cellular immunity***). T-lymphocytes can also influence the immune responses of B-lymphocytes as well as those of other T-lymphocytes; and also those of non-lymphocytic cells.

Like B-lymphocytes some T-lymphocytes also retain a memory of antigens encountered by them, and they can respond more strongly when the same antigens are encountered again.

The destruction of foreign cells by T-lymphocytes is responsible for the 'rejection' of tissues or organs grafted from one person to another. Such rejection is one of the major problems in organ transplantation.

IMMUNITY

It is a well known fact that some persons are more prone, to being affected by infectious present in the environment, than others. The power to resist an infection (when exposed to it) is called immunity.

It is important to remember that many substances that cause disease e.g., bacteria, contain proteins. The body itself also contains a very large number of proteins of its own. Proteins not present in the body itself are foreign proteins. A foreign protein is called an antigen. When a foreign protein enters the body, it can set up reactions that are harmful. Hence, it is necessary for the body to recognise the antigen and to destroy it. The ability to do is the fundamental basis of immunity. The function of recognition and destruction of antigen is performed by lymphocytes.

Two distinct methods are used for this purpose.

a. When a T- lymphocyte recognises a cell bearing an antigen the lymphocyte releases toxins that destroy the cell. As this is a cell to cell reaction, this type of immunity is called ***cell mediated immunity***.
b. When a β-lymphocyte recognises an antigen it converts itself into a plasma cell. The plasma cell produces ***antibodies*** that circulate in blood. The antibody binds with antigen. The complex formed by union of antigen and antibody is recognised by other cells (T-lymphocytes, macrophages) that destroy any cell bearing the antigen antibody complex. As antibodies circulate freely in blood, they can reach any part of the body. Immunity through antibodies is also called ***humoral immunity***.

How Immunity is Acquired

The air we breathe, the water we drink and the foods we eat are often contaminated with disease-producing bacteria or viruses (which bear antigens). When a child encounters an antigen for the first time, lymphocytes produce some antibodies against them. Some lymphocytes are able to remember that such an antigen was encountered. Such lymphocytes multiply. When the same antigen invades the body again, the quantity of antibody produced is much greater than on the first exposure. Repeated exposures strengthen the response to the antigen. The result is that if a large dose of the antigen (bacteria) happens to enter the body, there is enough antibody to destroy them, and symptoms of disease do not develop. In other words, the person has acquired immunity against the particular organisms.

Similarly immunity can also be produced artificially. Bacteria can be grown in a laboratory. There are ways in which they can be killed or weakened so much that they can no longer produce disease. However, the antigens in them remain capable of stimulating antibody production. This is how vaccines are produced. If the vaccine is injected into a person antibodies are produced and the person acquires immunity against the organism from which the vaccine was prepared. Some common diseases for which vaccines are available are cholera, typhoid, tetanus, small pox, measles, diphtheria and whooping cough.

In some cases, antigens are repeatedly injected into an animal in gradually increasing doses. When concentration of antibodies reaches its maximum, the serum of the animal is taken and used as a vaccine. Immunity acquired in this way is called ***passive immunity***. Vaccines against rabies and against snake venom are prepared in this way.

Allergy or Hypersensitivity

Many substances that are normally harmless can act as antigens, and antibodies can be produced against them. The first exposure to the antigen sensitises the individual to it. Subsequent exposure to the same antigen can produce a much stronger reaction, and this can lead to various symptoms. This is how allergic disorders are produced.

Exposure to dust, or to pollen of some plants can cause allergic rhinitis (leading to sneezing and running of nose). It can also lead to asthma. Similar reactions can be produced by some drugs (even by aspirin). In some cases the reaction can be so severe that it can result in death.

Substances (including cosmetics) applied to skin can cause symptoms which may be mild (redness, irritation), but sometimes there can be severe generalised reaction.

Autoimmune Diseases

We have seen that lymphocytes can distinguish between proteins present in the body, and those foreign to it. However, sometimes the lymphocytes may produce antibodies against one of the proteins present in the body. Lymphocytes then start attacking cells containing the protein destroying them. Some diseases caused in this way are rheumatoid arthritis, some diseases of the thyroid gland, and some disorders of blood.

AIDS (Acquired Immune Deficiency Syndrome)

This is a condition in which the immune system of the body becomes very weak. The person's ability to resist infections is lost and any infection can spread rapidly causing death.

AIDS is the result of infection by a virus (HIV or human immunodeficiency virus). The virus contains RNA. When the virus infects a cell this viral RNA produces new, (abnormal) DNA, which gets incorporated into the DNA of the cell. Because of the presence of this DNA the cell produces new copies of the virus. These spread into other cells of the body infecting them. The virus also infects blood, tissue fluids and secretions including semen. HIV infection spreads from one person to another through sexual intercourse. An infected mother passes the infection to offspring. A needle used for injection on an infected person can infect another person if reused. Transfusion of infected blood infects the recipient.

Because of easy spread, and the absence of effective drugs for cure, HIV infection is one of the most serious health problems facing the world today

CHAPTER

13

Skin and its Appendages

THE SKIN

The skin consists of a superficial layer the ***epidermis***, made up of stratified squamous epithelium; and a deeper layer, the ***dermis***, made up of connective tissue (Fig. 13.1). The dermis rests on subcutaneous tissue (***subcutis***). In sections through the skin the line of junction of the two layers is not straight, but is markedly wavy because of the presence of numerous finger-like projections of dermis upwards into the epidermis. These projections are called ***dermal papillae***. The downward projections of the epidermis (in the intervals between the dermal papillae) are sometimes called ***epidermal papillae***.

The surface of the epidermis is also often marked by elevations and depressions. These are most prominent on the palms and ventral surfaces of the fingers, and on the corresponding surfaces of the feet. Here the elevations form characteristic ***epidermal ridges*** that are responsible for the highly specific finger prints of each individual.

The Epidermis

The epidermis consists of stratified epithelium in which the following layers can be recognized (Fig. 13.2).

a. The deepest or ***basal layer*** (***stratum basale***) is made up of a single layer of columnar cells that rest on a basal lamina.

   The basal layer contains stem cells that undergo mitosis to give off cells called ***keratinocytes***. Keratinocytes form the more superficial layers of the epidermis described below. The basal layer is, therefore, also called the ***germinal layer*** (***stratum germinativum***).

b. Above the basal layer there are several layers of polygonal keratinocytes that constitute the ***stratum spinosum*** (or ***Malpighian layer***).

   Some mitoses may be seen in the deeper cells of the stratum spinosum. Because of this fact the stratum spinosum is included, along with the basal cell layer, in the ***germinative zone*** of the epidermis.

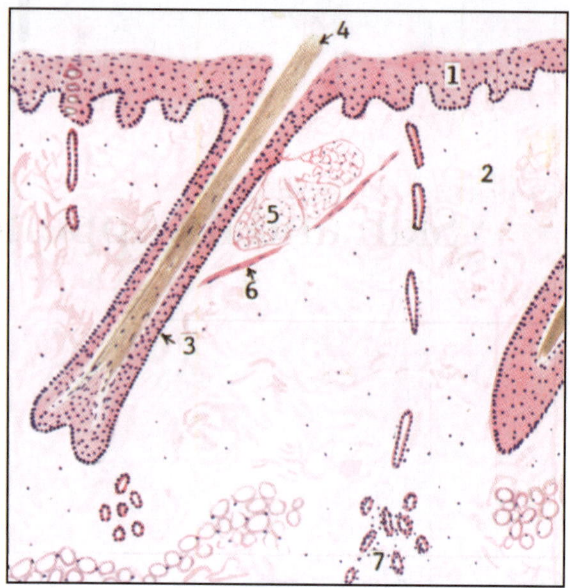

Fig. 13.1 Section through skin. 1-Epidermis. 2-Dermis. 3-Hair follicle. 4-Hair. 5-Sebaceous gland. 6- Arrector pili. 7-Sweat gland.

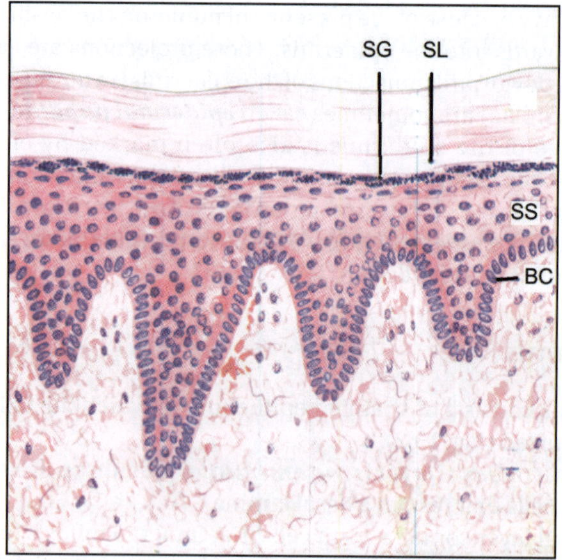

Fig. 13.2 Section through skin showing the layers of the epidermis. SC-Stratum corneum. SL-Stratum lucidum. SG-Stratum granulosum. SS-Stratum spinosum. BC-Basal cell layer.

c. Overlying the stratum spinosum there are a few layers of flattened cells that are characterized by the presence of deeply staining granules in their cytoplasm. These cells constitute the ***stratum granulosum***. The granules in them consist of a protein called ***keratohyalin***. The nuclei of cells in this layer are condensed and dark staining (pyknotic).
d. Superficial to the stratum granulosum there is the ***stratum lucidum*** (lucid = clear). This layer is so called because it appears homogeneous, the cell boundaries being extremely indistinct.
e. The most superficial layer of the epidermis is called the ***stratum corneum***. This layer is acellular. It is made up of flattened scale like elements (squames) containing keratin filaments embedded in protein. The squames are held together by glue like material containing lipids and carbohydrates. The presence of lipid makes this layer highly resistant to permeation by water.

   The thickness of the stratum corneum is greatest where the skin is exposed to maximal friction e.g., on the palms and soles. The superficial layers of the epidermis are being constantly shed off, and are replaced by proliferation of cells in deeper layers.

The Dermis

The dermis is made up of connective tissue. Just below the epidermis the connective tissue is dense and constitutes the ***papillary layer***. Deep to this there is a network of thick fibre bundles that constitute the ***reticular layer*** of the dermis.

The dermis rests on the superficial fascia through which it is attached to deeper structures.

We have seen that the dermis contains considerable amounts of elastic fibres. Atrophy of elastic fibres occurs with age and is responsible for loss of elasticity and wrinkling of the skin.

If for any reason the skin in any region of the body is rapidly stretched, fibre bundles in the dermis may rupture. Scar tissue is formed in the region and can be seen in the form of prominent white lines. Such lines may be formed on the anterior abdominal wall in pregnancy: they are known as ***linea gravidarum.***

Pigmentation of the Skin

The cells of the basal layer of the epidermis, and the adjoining cells of the stratum spinosum contain a brown pigment called ***melanin***. The pigment is much more prominent in dark skinned individuals. The cells actually responsible for synthesis of melanin are called ***melanocytes*** (See note below). Melanocytes are derived from melanoblasts. (These arise from the neural crest, present in the embryo). They may be present amongst the cells of the germinative zone, or at the junction of the epidermis and the dermis. Each melanocyte gives off many processes each of which is applied to a cell of the germinative zone. Melanin granules formed in the melanocyte are transferred to surrounding non-melanin-producing cells through these processes. Because of the presence of processes melanocytes are also called ***dendritic cells***.

The colour of skin is influenced by the amount of melanin present. It is also influenced by some other pigments present in the epidermis; and by pigments (haemoglobin and oxyhaemoglobin) present in blood circulating through the skin. The epidermis is sufficiently translucent for the colour of blood to show through, specially in light skinned individuals. That is why the skin becomes pale in anaemia; blue when oxygenation of blood is insufficient; and pink while blushing.

Blood Supply

Blood vessels do not penetrate into the epidermis. The epidermis derives nutrition entirely by diffusion from capillaries in the dermal papillae. Veins from the dermal papillae drain (through plexuses present in the dermis) into a venous plexus lying on deep fascia.

A special feature of the blood supply of the skin is the presence of numerous arterio-venous anastomoses that regulate blood flow through the capillary bed and thus help in maintaining body temperature.

Nerve Supply

The skin is richly supplied with sensory nerves. Dense networks of nerve fibres are seen in the superficial parts of the dermis. Sensory nerves end in relation to various types of specialized terminals that present in the skin.

In contrast to blood vessels some nerve fibres do penetrate into the deeper parts of the epidermis.

Apart from sensory nerves the skin receives autonomic nerves that supply smooth muscle in the walls of blood vessels; the arrectores pilorum muscles; and myoepithelial cells present in relation to sweat glands. They also provide a secretomotor supply to sweat glands. In some regions (nipple, scrotum) nerve fibres innervate smooth muscle present in the dermis.

FUNCTIONS OF THE SKIN

1. The skin provides mechanical protection to underlying tissues. In this connection we have noted that the skin is thickest over areas exposed to greatest friction.
   The skin also acts as a physical barrier against entry of microorganisms and other substances. However, the skin is not a perfect barrier and some substances, both useful (e.g., ointments) or harmful (poisons), may enter the body through the skin.
2. The skin prevents loss of water from the body. The importance of this function is seen in persons who have lost extensive areas of skin through burns. One important cause of death in such cases is water loss.
3. The pigment present in the epidermis protects tissues against harmful effects of light (specially ultraviolet light). This is to be correlated with the heavier pigmentation of skin in races living in the tropics; and with increase in pigmentation after exposure to sunlight. However, some degree of exposure to sunlight is essential for synthesis of vitamin-D. Ultraviolet light converts 7-dehydrocholesterol (present in skin) to vitamin-D.

4. The skin offers protection against damage of tissues by chemicals, by heat, and by osmotic influences.
5. The skin is a very important sensory organ, containing receptors for touch and related sensations. The presence of relatively sparse and short hair over most of the skin increases its sensitivity.
6. The skin plays an important role in regulating body temperature. Blood flow through capillaries of the skin can be controlled by numerous arterio-venous anastomoses present in it. In cold weather blood flow through capillaries is kept to a minimum to prevent heat loss. In warm weather the flow is increased to promote cooling. In extreme cold, when some peripheral parts of the body (like the digits, the nose and the ears) are in danger of being frozen the blood flow through these parts increases to keep them warm.

In warm climates cooling of the body is facilitated by secretion of sweat and its evaporation. Sweat glands also act as excretory organs.

APPENDAGES OF THE SKIN

The appendages of the skin are the hairs, nails, sebaceous glands and sweat glands.

In animals with a thick coat of hair (fur) the hair help to keep the animal warm. In man this function is performed by subcutaneous fat.

Hair

Each hair consists of a part (of variable length) that is seen on the surface of the body; and a part anchored in the thickness of the skin. The visible part is called the ***shaft***, and the embedded part is called the ***root***. The root has an expanded lower end called the ***bulb***. The bulb is invaginated from below by part of the dermis that constitutes the ***hair papilla***. The root of each hair is surrounded by a tubular sheath called the ***hair follicle***. The follicle is made up of several layers of cells that are derived from the layers of the skin (Fig. 13.3).

Hair roots are always attached to skin obliquely. As a result the emerging hair is also oblique and easily lies flat on the skin surface.

Structure of Hair Shaft

A hair may be regarded as a modified part of the stratum corneum of the skin. An outer cortex and an inner medulla can be made out in large hair, but there is no medulla in thin hair. The cortex is acellular and is made up of keratin. In thick hair the medulla consists of cornified cells of irregular shape.

The surface of the hair is covered by a thin membrane called the ***cuticle***. The cuticle is formed by flattened cornified cells. The cornified elements making up the hair contain melanin that is responsible for their colour. Both in the medulla and in the cortex of a hair minute air bubbles are present: they influence its colour. The amount of air present in a hair increases with age and, along with loss of pigment, is responsible for greying of hair.

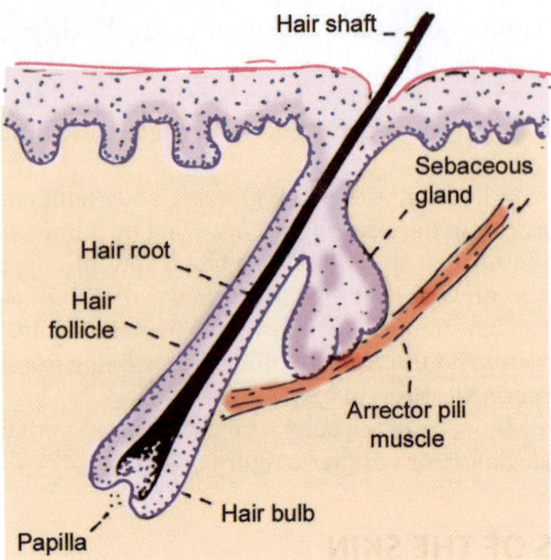

Fig. 13.3 Basic structure of a hair follicle. Also see Fig. 13.1.

Structure of Hair Follicle

The hair follicle may be regarded as a part of the epidermis that has been invaginated into the dermis around the hair root. Its innermost layer, that immediately surrounds the hair root is, therefore, continuous with the surface of the skin; while the outermost layer of the follicle is continuous with the dermis. The wall of the follicle consists of three main layers. Beginning with the innermost layer they are:

a. The ***inner root sheath*** present only in the lower part of the follicle.
b. The ***outer root sheath*** that is continuous with the stratum spinosum.
c. A connective tissue sheath derived from the dermis.

Arrector Pili Muscles

These are bands of smooth muscle attached at one end to the dermis, just below the dermal papillae; and at the other end to the connective tissue sheath of a hair follicle. A sebaceous gland lies in the angle between the hair follicle and the arrector pili. Contraction of the muscle has two effects. Firstly, the hair follicle becomes almost vertical (from its original oblique position) relative to the skin surface). Simultaneously the skin surface overlying the attachment of the muscle becomes depressed while surrounding areas become raised. These reactions are seen during exposure to cold, or during emotional excitement, when the 'hair stand on end' and the skin assumes the appearance of 'goose flesh.' The second effect of contraction of the arrector pili muscle is that the sebaceous gland is pressed upon and its secretions are squeezed out into the hair follicle. The arrector pili muscles receive a sympathetic innervation.

Sebaceous Glands

Sebaceous glands are seen most typically in relation to hair follicles. Each gland consists of a number of alveoli that are connected to a broad duct that opens into a hair follicle (Fig. 13.1). Each alveolus is pear shaped. It consists of a solid mass of polyhedral cells and has hardly any lumen. The outermost cells are small and rest on a basement membrane. The inner cells are larger, more rounded, and filled with lipid. This lipid is discharged by disintegration of the innermost cells that are replaced by proliferation of outer cells. The sebaceous glands are, therefore, examples of holocrine glands. The secretion of sebaceous glands is called ***sebum***. Its oily nature helps to keep the skin and hair soft. It helps to prevent dryness of the skin and also makes it resistant to moisture. Sebum contains various lipids including triglycerides, cholesterol, cholesterol esters and fatty acids.

Nails

Nails are present on fingers and toes. The main part of a nail is called its ***body***. The body has a free distal edge. The proximal part of the nail is implanted into a groove on the skin and is called the ***root*** (or ***radix***). The tissue on which the nail rests is called the ***nail bed***. The nail bed is highly vascular, and that is why the nails look pink in colour.

The nail represents a modified part of the zone of keratinization of the epidermis. It is usually regarded as a much thickened continuation of the stratum lucidum, but it is more like the stratum corneum in structure. The nail substance consists of several layers of dead, cornified, 'cells' filled with keratin.

When we view a nail in longitudinal section (Fig. 13.4) it is seen that the nail rests on the cells of the germinative zone (stratum spinosum and stratum basale). The germinative zone is particularly thick near the root of the nail where it forms the ***germinal matrix***. The nail substance is formed mainly by proliferation of cells in the germinal matrix. However, the superficial layers

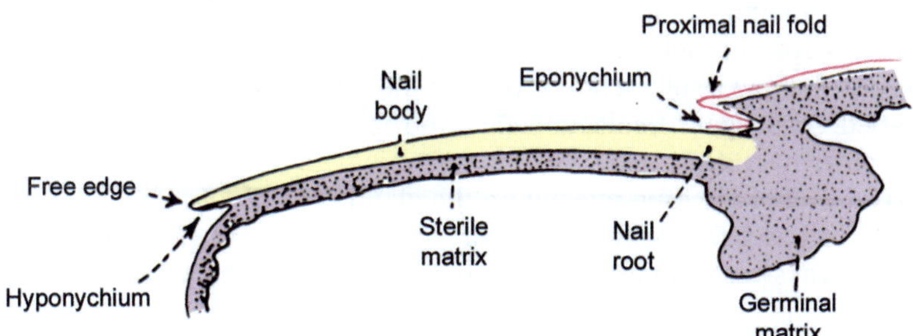

Fig. 13.4 Parts of a nail and some related structures as seen in a longitudinal section.

of the nail are derived from the proximal nail fold. When viewed from the surface (i.e., through the nail substance) the area of the germinal matrix appears white (in comparison to the pink colour of the rest of the nail). Most of this area is overlapped by the fold of skin (***proximal nail fold***) covering the root of the nail, but just distal to the nail fold a small semilunar white area called the ***lunule*** is seen. The lunule is most conspicuous in the thumb nail. The germinal matrix is connected to the underlying bone (distal phalanx) by fibrous tissue.

The germinative zone underlying the body of the nail (i.e., the nail bed) is much thinner than the germinal matrix. It does not contribute to the growth of the nail; and is, therefore, called the ***sterile matrix***. As the nail grows it slides distally over the sterile matrix. The dermis that lies deep to the sterile matrix does not show the usual dermal papillae. Instead it shows a number of parallel, longitudinal ridges. These ridges look like very regularly arranged papillae in transverse sections through a nail.

Nails undergo constant growth by proliferation of cells in the germinal matrix. Growth is faster in hot weather than in cold. Finger nails grow faster than toe nails. Nail growth can be disturbed by serious illness or by injury over the nail root, resulting in transverse grooves or white patches in the nails. These grooves or patches slowly grow towards the free edge of the nail. If a nail is lost by injury a new one grows out of the germinal matrix if the latter is intact.

Sweat Glands

Sweat glands produce sweat or perspiration. They are present in the skin over most of the body. Their number and size varies in the skin over different parts of the body. They are most numerous in the palms and soles, the forehead and scalp, and the axillae.

The entire sweat gland consists of a single long tube (Fig. 13.5). The lower end of the tube is highly coiled on itself and forms the ***body*** (or ***fundus***) or the gland. The body is made up of the secretory part of the gland. It lies in the reticular layer of the dermis, or some-times in subcutaneous tissue. The part of the tube connecting the secretory element to the skin surface is the ***duct***. It runs upwards through the dermis to reach the epidermis. Within the epidermis the duct follows a spiral course to reach the skin surface. The orifice is funnel shaped. On the palms, soles and digits the openings of sweat glands lie in rows on epidermal ridges.

The wall of the tube making up the gland consists of an inner epithelial lining, its basal lamina, and a supporting layer of connective tissue.

In larger sweat glands flattened contractile, ***myoepithelial cells*** are present between the epithelial cells and their basal lamina. They probably help in expressing secretion out of the gland.

As is well known the secretion of sweat glands has a high water content. Evaporation of this water plays an important role in cooling the body. Sweat glands are innervated by cholinergic nerves.

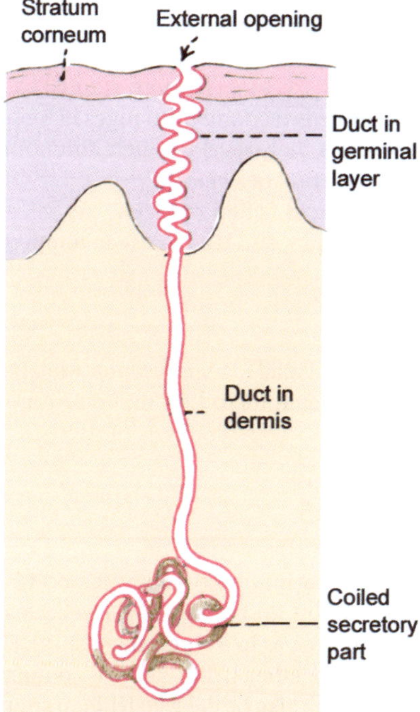

Fig. 13.5 Diagrammatic representation of the parts of a typical sweat gland.

REGULATION OF BODY TEMPERATURE

The average body temperature of a healthy person is roughly 37°C (=98.4°F). Normal variation in temperature, between individuals, and at different times of the day is about 0.5°C. The temperature is maintained within these limits by balancing heat production and heat loss.

Heat is produced by the following ways:

1. Contraction of muscles. (That is why we shiver when exposed to cold).
2. Some metabolic processes produce heat. These take place mainly in the liver, in the intestines and in adipose tissue).

Heat is lost in the following ways:

1. Evaporation of sweat (from skin) is the most important method of cooling the body. That is why we perspire so much in hot weather.
2. Some heat is lost through expired air, and through urine and faeces.

Heat generated in the body is preserved in the following manner. These measures are necessary only if environmental temperature is lower than body temperature.

a. The clothes we wear prevent loss of heat from the surface of the body.
b. Vasoconstriction of blood vessels supplying the skin reduces blood flow, and hence reduces heat loss by radiation. Reduced blood flow also reduces perspiration and its evaporation.

Mechanisms Controlling Temperature

1. A collection of nerve cells in the brain (hypothalamus) constitutes a temperature regulatory centre. These cells respond to changes in temperature of blood. This centre sends out impulses that travel through autonomic nerves, influencing vasoconstriction and secretion of sweat.
2. In some diseases, substances called pyrogens are released. These act on the temperature regulating centre, and lead to rise in temperature, as in fever.

Hypothermia

Fall of temperature below 32°C is called hypothermia. Metabolic process show down and the mechanisms that normally increase temperature are unable to act. Extreme hypothermia causes death.

HEALING OF WOUNDS

The skin is the most frequently injured tissue in the body. However, the skin has excellent powers of regeneration, and wounds heal well. Healing is better and faster if the cut is sharp and clean (e.g., as in a surgical incision). Healing is delayed if the cut edges cannot be brought together, if the wound is contaminated, and if infection supervenes. Wound healing can also be delayed if blood supply to the region is poor, if the nutrition of the individual is not adequate, or if tissue resistance is impaired by disease (e.g., diabetes) or by old age.

Healing by First Intention

If a wound has sharp edges that can be brought together, and there is no contamination, healing takes place by the process of ***first intention*** or primary healing.

1. The interval between the cut edges gets filled with blood. Clotting of this blood holds the skin edges together.
2. An inflammatory reaction sets in. Phagocytes (from blood and from connective tissue) reach the region. They engulf and remove dead tissue including the clot. The region is also infiltrated by rapidly multiplying fibroblasts. These lay down collagen fibers that bridge the gap between the cut edges and unite them.
3. Epithelial cells, and connective tissue grow and bridge the gap. New capillaries grow into the region to restore blood supply. (This new tissue growing into the region has a granular appearance and is, therefore, called ***granulation tissue***).
4. The collagen laid down by fibroblasts matures with time and firmly binds the tissue restoring it to a more or less normal condition.

Healing by Second Intention

The process of healing is more complex if some tissue has been lost and if the wound is infected.

Inflammation sets up in the region. Some tissues that are dead (slough), gradually separate from underlying healthy tissues.

Granulation tissue consisting of capillaries, phagocytes and fibroblasts gradually grows in to the region and towards the surface. In this way the depth of the wound is gradually lessened. Finally, cells of the epidermis grow into the region from all sides, and restore its continuity.

Gradually fibrous tissue, laid down to strengthen the region, increases in density. This mass of fibrous tissue is seen as a scar.

SOME DISORDERS OF SKIN

1. Inflammation of skin is called ***dermatitis***. Dermatitis is of many kinds. It can be caused by bacterial, viral or fungal infections. It can also be caused by allergy or by contact with irritant materials like acids or alkalis.
2. In old people, and in those suffering from paralysis, constant pressure over a part of skin can form ***bed sores*** (skin degenerates and gets infected).
3. ***Burns*** can damage small or extensive areas of skin. The skin may be damaged up to a partial thickness, but sometimes the full thickness of skin is destroyed. Burns can be extremely painful as nerve terminals get exposed. Infection often supervenes leading to toxaemia. Large volumes of fluid oozing out of the burnt surfaces frequently lead to dehydration. Severe toxaemia and dehydration are the main causes of death in cases with severe burns. Reduced blood volume and severe pain resulting from burns can lead to shock and renal failure.

   If the patient survives, large scars can form in the region of the burn, and these can restrict movement.
5. The skin can be the site of benign or malignant tumours (including carcinoma and malignant melanoma).

PART THREE

The Organ Systems

CHAPTER

14

Cardiovascular System

The cardiovascular system consists of the heart and of blood vessels. The blood vessels that take blood from the heart to various tissues are called ***arteries***. The smallest arteries are called ***arterioles***. Arterioles open into a network of ***capillaries*** that pervade the tissues. Exchanges of various substances between the blood and the tissues take place through the walls of capillaries. In some situations, instead of capillaries there are slightly different vessels called ***sinusoids***. Blood from capillaries (or from sinusoids) is collected by small ***venules*** that join to form ***veins***. The veins return blood to the heart (Fig. 14.1).

THE HEART

The heart is a muscular pump designed to ensure the circulation of blood through the tissues of the body. Both structurally and functionally it consists of two halves, right and left. The 'right heart' circulates blood only through the lungs for the purpose of oxygenation (i.e., through the pulmonary circulation). The 'left heart' circulates blood to tissues of the entire body (i.e., through the systemic circulation). Each half of the heart consists of an inflow chamber called the ***atrium***, and of an outflow chamber called the ***ventricle*** (Fig. 14.2). The right and left atria are separated by an ***interatrial septum***. The right and left ventricles are separated by an ***interventricular septum***. The right atrium opens into the right ventricle through the ***right atrioventricular orifice***: this orifice is guarded by the ***tricuspid valve.*** The left atrium opens into the left ventricle through the ***left atrioventricular orifice***: this orifice is guarded by the ***mitral valve.*** These valves allow flow of blood from atrium to ventricle, but not in the reverse direction.

Each chamber of the heart is connected to one or more large blood vessels (Fig. 14.2). The right atrium receives deoxygenated blood from tissues of the entire body through the ***superior and inferior venae cavae.*** This blood passes into the right ventricle. It leaves the right ventricle through a large outflow vessel called the ***pulmonary trunk.*** This trunk divides into right and left ***pulmonary***

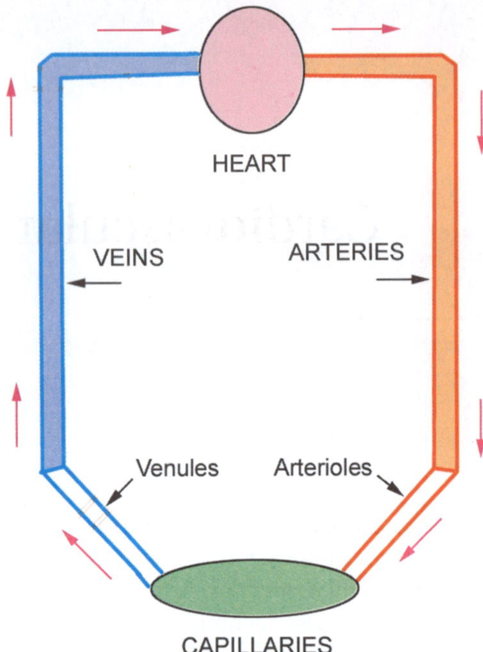

Fig. 14.1 Blood vessels of the body.

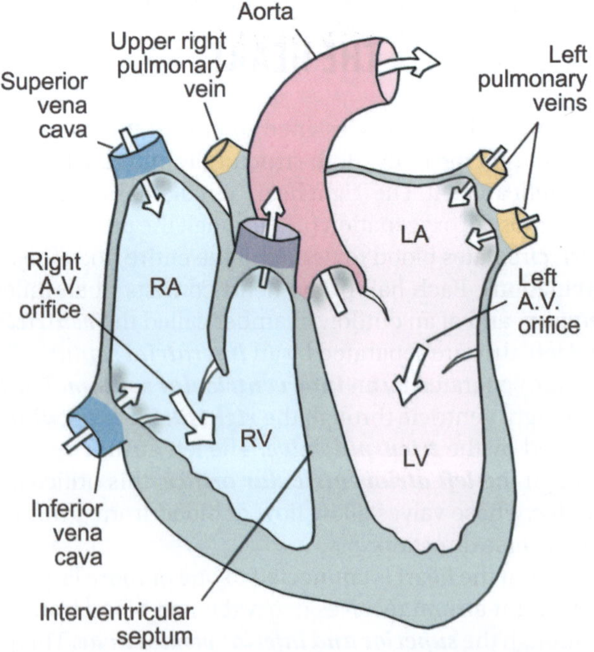

Fig. 14.2 Schematic diagram of the heart, to show its chambers and their communications.

arteries that carry blood to the lungs. Blood oxygenated in the lungs is brought back to the heart by four ***pulmonary veins*** (two right and two left) that end in the left atrium. This blood passes into the left ventricle. The left ventricle pumps this blood into a large outflow vessel called the ***aorta***: the aorta and its branches distribute blood to tissues of the entire body. It is returned to the heart (right atrium) through the venae cavae, thus completing the circuit.

Blood from many parts of the body has to return to the heart against the force of gravity. The negative intrathoracic pressure created during inspiration has a sucking effect on blood and is an important factor in facilitating venous return to the heart.

The heart is enclosed in the pericardium (Figs. 14.3 A,B,C)). The pericardium consists of an outer fibrous layer, and two layers (visceral and parietal) of serous pericardium. The visceral serous pericardium lines the external surface of the heart, while the parietal serous pericardium lines the inside of the fibrous pericardium. The two layers are separated by a thin film of fluid which prevents friction during contractions of the heart.

Some relationships of the heart can be seen in Figs. 14.3 A,B,C. In Figs. 14.3 A and B observe that anteriorly the heart is related to the body of the sternum and to costal cartilages. This aspect of the heart is, therfore, called the ***sternocostal surface***. Inferiorly, the heart is related to the diaphragm (***diaphragmatic surface***). The posterior aspect, or ***base***, of the heart is related to structures in the posterior mediastinum (aorta, oesophagus). Towards the right and left sides the heart is related to the corresponding pleura and lung.

In Fig. 14.4, note that the sternocostal surface of the heart is formed by the right atrium, the right ventricle, and the left ventricle. Note also that the apex of the heart is formed by the left ventricle. In Fig. 14.5, observe that the diaphragmatic surface is formed only by the right and left ventricles. The base of the heart is formed by the right and left atria (mainly the left).

Structure of Walls of the Heart

There are three layers in the wall of the heart.

a. The innermost layer is called the ***endocardium***. It corresponds to the tunica intima of blood vessels.

The cavities of the heart (and of all blood vessels) are lined by flattened ***endothelial cells*** or ***endotheliocytes***.

b. The main thickness of the wall of the heart is formed by cardiac muscle. This is the ***myocardium***. The structure of cardiac muscle has already been described.

c. The external surface of the myocardium is covered by ***epicardium*** (or ***visceral layer of serous pericardium***). The epicardium consists of a layer of connective tissue which is covered, on the free surface, by a layer of flattened mesothelial cells.

The ***valves of the heart*** are folds of endocardium that enclose a plate-like layer of dense fibrous tissue.

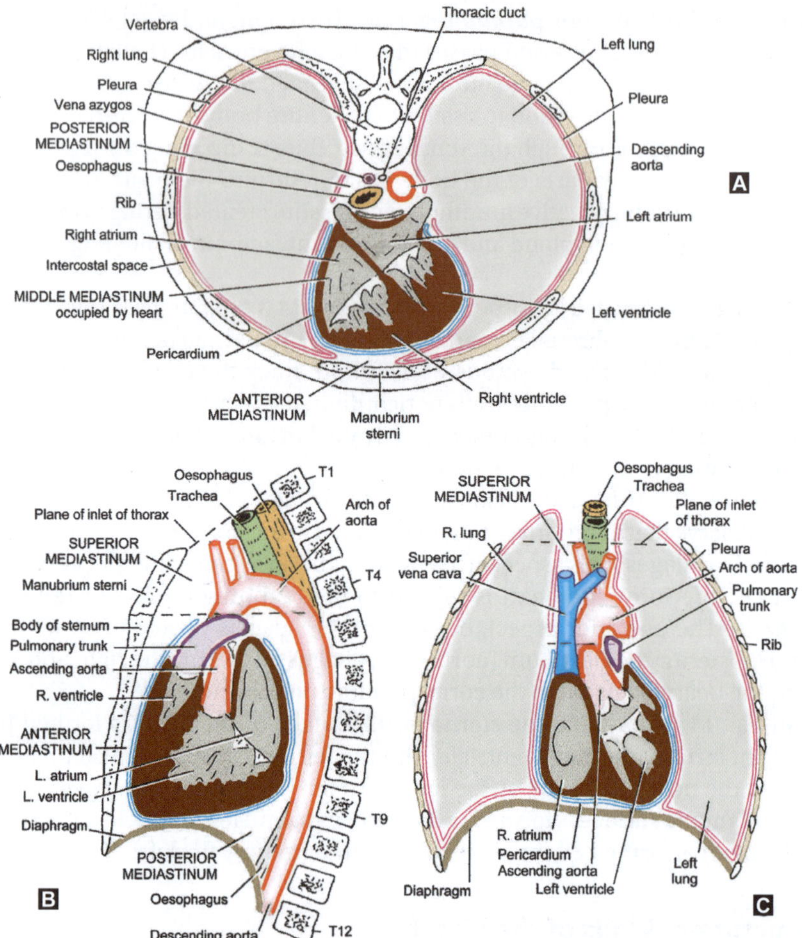

Figs14.3A to C A. Schematic transverse section through the thorax showing its important contents; B. Schematic sagittal section across the thorax to show the subdivisions of the mediastinum; C. Schematic coronal section across the thorax to show its main contents.

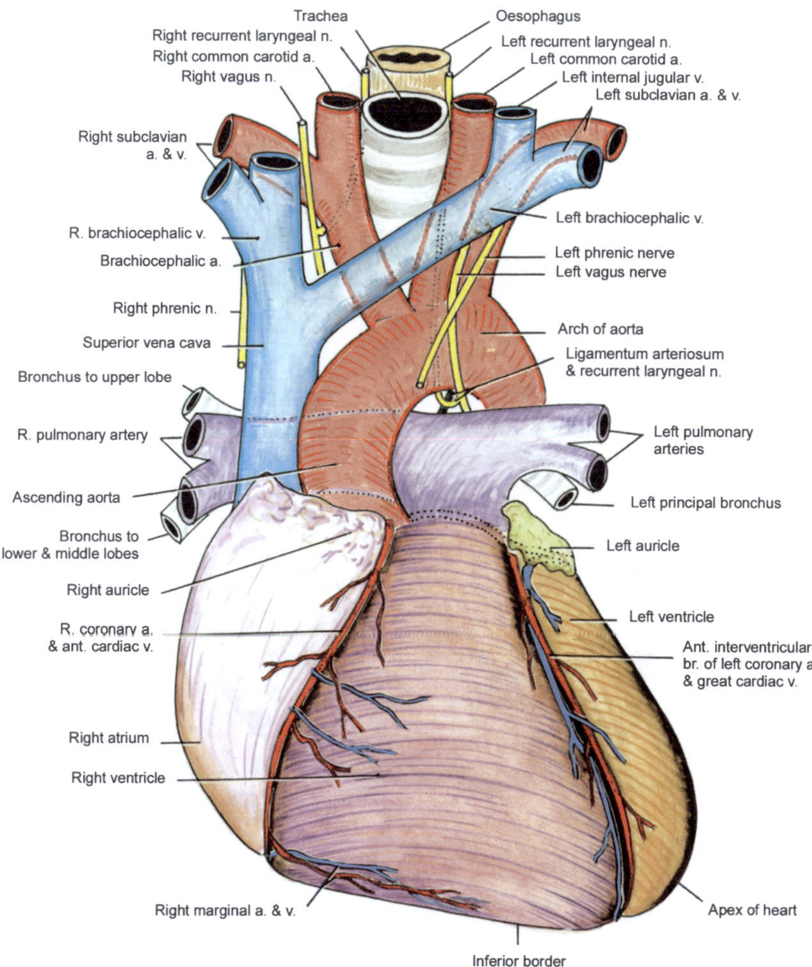

Fig. 14.4 Heart and some related structures viewed from the front.

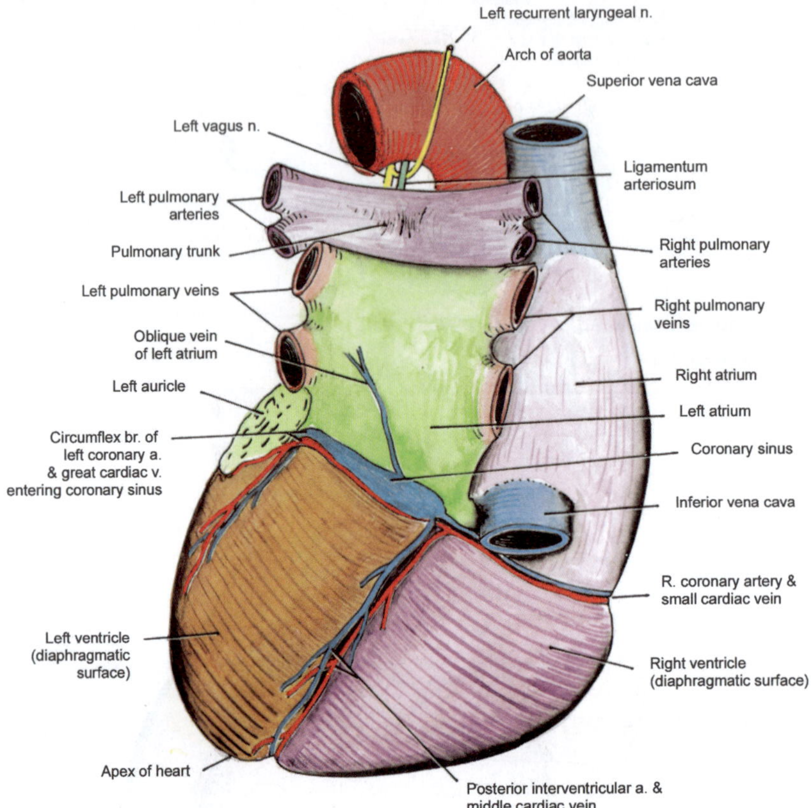

Fig. 14.5 Heart seen from behind and below.

CORONARY CIRCULATION

The heart is supplied by coronary arteries, right and left.

The ***right coronary artery*** arises from the ascending aorta (Fig. 14.6). It runs downwards on the sternocostal surface of the heart between the right atrium and right ventricle (Fig. 14.6). Reaching the inferior margin of the heart the artery curves round it to reach the diaphragmatic surface. Just before its termination it gives off the ***posterior interventricular*** branch.

The ***left coronary artery*** also arises from the ascending aorta. It is seen on the sternocostal surface of the heart (Fig. 14.6). Here the artery divides into two main branches. These are the ***circumflex*** and ***anterior interventricular*** arteries. The circumflex branch curves round the left border of the heart to reach the diaphragmatic surface. The anterior interventricular branch runs downwards between the right and left ventricles.

The right atrium and ventricle are supplied mainly by the right coronary artery, and the left atrium and ventricle by the left coronary artery. The anterior

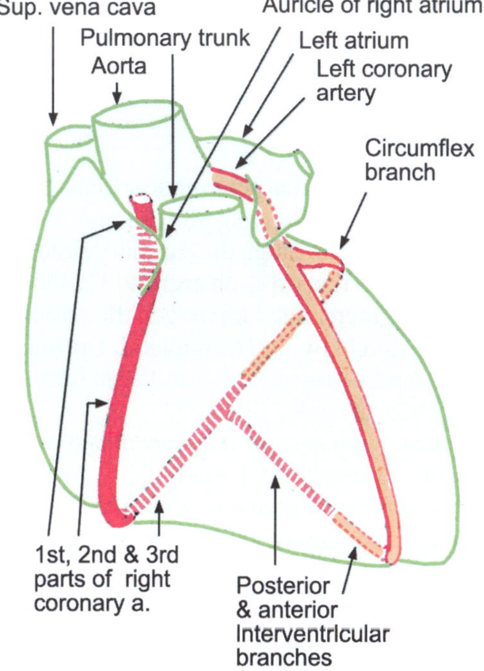

Fig. 14.6 Scheme to show the coronary arteries.

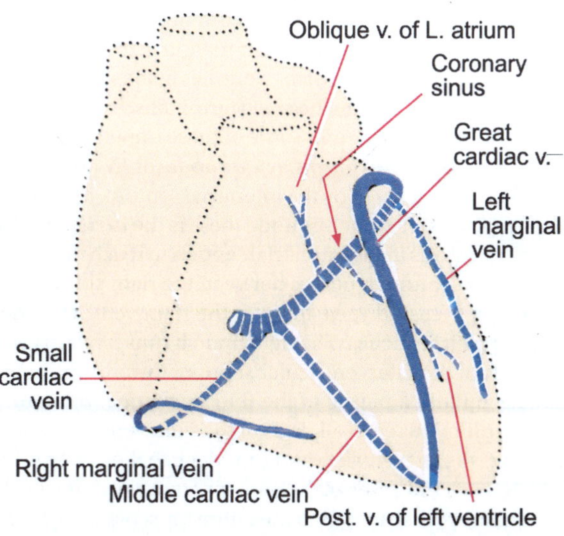

Fig. 14.7 Scheme to show the veins of the heart.

two thirds of the interventricular septum is supplied by the left coronary artery, and its posterior one third by the right coronary artery. The S.A node, the A.V node, the A.V bundle and the proximal parts of its right and left branches are supplied by the right coronary artery. The distal parts of the bundle branches are supplied by the left coronary artery.

The ***veins of the heart*** are shown in Fig. 14.7. The most important vein is the coronary sinus. It lies on the diaphragmatic surface. Its tributaries are the great cardiac vein, the small cardiac vein and the middle cardiac vein.

About 250 ml of blood flows through the coronary circulation every minute. The amount becomes much more during exercise. Cardiac muscle has a high metabolic rate and has a greater need for oxygen than other tissues. This need is met by greater extraction of oxygen from blood. During ventricular systole the coronary arteries can be pressed upon and even occluded. Their filling is mainly during ventricular diastole.

Sympathetic stimulation causes coronary vasodilatation and increased flow. With advancing age the arteries lose their elasticity. Arteriosclerotic changes can cause considerable narrowing of coronary arteries. Blood supply to the myocardium becomes insufficient, and cannot meet the requirements of exercise. When this happens the patient experiences pain in the chest during exertion, or during emotional excitement. This is called ***angina pectoris***. When a coronary artery gets blocked it leads to ***myocardial infarction*** (heart attack).

CONDUCTING SYSTEM OF THE HEART

For proper working of the heart it is essential that the chambers contract in a definite sequence. The rate at which the heart contracts is determined by a small area of specialized tissue called the ***sinuatrial node*** (commonly abbreviated to SA node). It is located in the right atrium along the anterior margin of the opening of the superior vena cava (Fig. 14.8). The greater part of the node lies in the sinus venarum part of the atrium, but anteriorly it extends into the crista terminalis. Impulses originating here spread out into the atrial musculature. Some of these impulses reach another node of specialized tissue called the ***atrioventricular node*** (or AV node). This node lies in the wall of the right atrium formed by the interatrial septum, just above the opening of the coronary sinus. Arising from this node there is the ***atrioventricular bundle***. This bundle passes forwards in the interatrial septum to reach the membranous part of the interventricular septum. It passes between the right side of this septum and the septal cusp of the tricuspid valve to enter the right ventricle. The bundle now divides into right and left branches. The right branch runs forwards on the right side of the muscular part of the interventricular septum, towards the apex of the heart. The bundle breaks up into a plexus of the fine ***Purkinje fibres*** which spread out deep to the endocardium to reach all parts of the right ventricle. The left branch of the AV bundle enters the left ventricle and runs deep to the endocardium. It divides into branches that reach the bases of the papillary muscles. Here the branches end in Purkinje fibres that are distributed to the entire musculature of the left ventricle.

The SA node, the AV node, the atrio-ventricular bundle and its branches, and the Purkinje fibres, are all made up of specialized tissue that has a partial resemblance to the structure of cardiac muscle. This tissue conducts impulses faster than cardiac muscle, but slower than nerve fibres. Impulses arising in the SA node and spreading

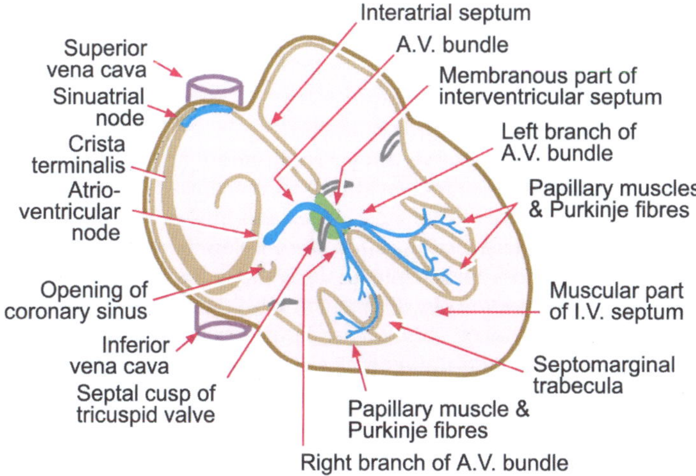

Fig. 14.8 Conducting system of the heart.

into the atrial musculature cause the atria to contract. These impulses reach the AV node, pass through the AV bundle and its branches to reach the ventricular muscle. This conduction takes time. As a result the contraction of the ventricles is not simultaneous with that of the atria, but follows after a definite interval. Within the ventricles themselves, the papillary muscles are the first to contract (as the branches of the AV bundle reach here first). This ensures closure of the mitral and tricuspid valves before the ventricles contract.

CONTROL OF HEART RATE

1. Basically heart rate is controlled by impulses arising in the SA node which is, therefore, called the pace maker. The SA node has intrinsic rhythmicity, and does not need a nerve supply for generation of impulses. However, heart rate is influenced by nerves supplying it. Sympathetic stimulation increases heart rate (positive chronotropic effect), and slowed by vagal stimulation. Sympathetic stimulation also increases force of contraction (positive ionotropic effect). The combined effect of increased heart rate and increased force of contraction causes considerable increase of cardiac output.
2. Heart rate is influenced by some hormones. The most important of these are adrenaline and noradrenaline.
3. Physical exertion and emotional stress also influence heart rate.
4. Heart rate is increased in fever.

An abnormal increase in heart rate (as in fever) is called tachycardia. Abnormal slowness is called bradycardia.

CARDIAC CYCLE

The power for flow of blood is provided by the heart, which acts as a pump. This pump like action is produced by alternate contraction and relaxation of heart muscle. Contraction is called systole. Relaxation is called diastole. The direction of flow of blood is determined by valves. The chambers of the heart contact and relax in a definite sequence.

1. First there is contraction of atria (right and left). This is ***atrial systole***. This pushes blood into the ventricles. The atria now relax.
2. Next there is contraction of ventricles (right and left). This is ***ventricular systole***. Three phases of ventricular systole are recognised. In the first phase all valves are closed. Contraction of muscle increases pressure within the ventricle (***isovolumetric ventricular contraction phase***). Now the aortic and pulmonary valves open and blood is pushed into the aorta and pulmonary trunk. The flow is at first rapid (***rapid ejection phase***) and then slows down (***slow ejection phase***).
3. Finally the ventricles relax. This is diastole. The atrioventricular valves open and blood from atria enters the ventricles. (As in systole three phases are seen: isometric relaxation, rapid filling and slow filling).

CARDIAC OUTPUT

This is the quantity of blood pumped by the left ventricle into the aorta every minute. It is about five litres. (Exactly the same quantity of blood is pumped by the right ventricle into the pulmonary trunk). The quantity pumped in one contraction of the left ventricle is ***stroke volume***. Cardiac output is equal to stroke volume multiplied by heart rate. If the stroke volume is 70ml and the heart rate is 70 cardiac output is 70x70 = 4900 ml.

Increased venous return from any cause, and resulting increase in right atrial pressure, leads to greater diastolic filling of ventricles. This causes increase in length of ventricular muscle, which in turn leads to increased stroke volume and cardiac output.

Cardiac output is increased during exercise. The effect is proportional to the severity of exercise. Cardiac output also increases during anxiety or excitement, and in later part of pregnancy.

As we have already seen sympathetic stimulation increases cardiac output both by increase of heart rate and stroke volume. Vagal stimulation decreases cardiac output, but the effect is not marked as ventricular muscle is not innervated by vagal fibres.

PULSE

When the left ventricle contracts a considerable volume of blood is forced into the initial part of the aorta. The wall of the aorta is elastic and it, therefore, undergoes dilatation. As blood flows into a more distal part of the aorta, the initial part returns to normal size, and the next part gets dilated. In this way, a wave of distention travels down the vessel, once for each heart beat. The same wave of dilatation passes into all arteries. This periodic dilatation of arteries is called the pulse. It can be felt by placing ones fingers over any artery that is superficial, specially where it lies over a bone.

The commonest artery used for feeling the pulse is the radial artery, just above the wrist. Other useful sites are the superficial temporal artery (just in front of the ear), and the dorsalis pedis artery (in the foot).

By examining the pulse we can count the heart rate. The degree of dilatation of the vessel with each heart beat is referred to as pulse volume. An experienced person can get some idea of blood pressure from pulse volume. Irregularity in the pulse can also be known.

HEART SOUNDS

Using a stethoscope we can hear two heart sounds during each heart beat. The first sound is heard at the beginning of ventricular systole and is caused by closure of atrioventricular valves. The second sound is caused by closure of aortic and pulmonary valves.

ELECTROCARDIOGRAM (ECG)

We have seen that contraction of heart muscle is preceded by a wave of depolarisation. Depolarisation is an electrical event. A depolarised area is negative with respect to a region that is not polarised. A minute electrical current flows between these regions. Tissue fluid being a good conductor of electricity, the current reaches all parts of the body. The current can be picked up by electrodes placed over skin and recorded. An instrument that records electrical changes in the heart is an electrocardiograph. The actual recording is an electrocardiogram. The parts of the body from which currents are picked up are defined as leads. These may be bipolar, or unipolar.

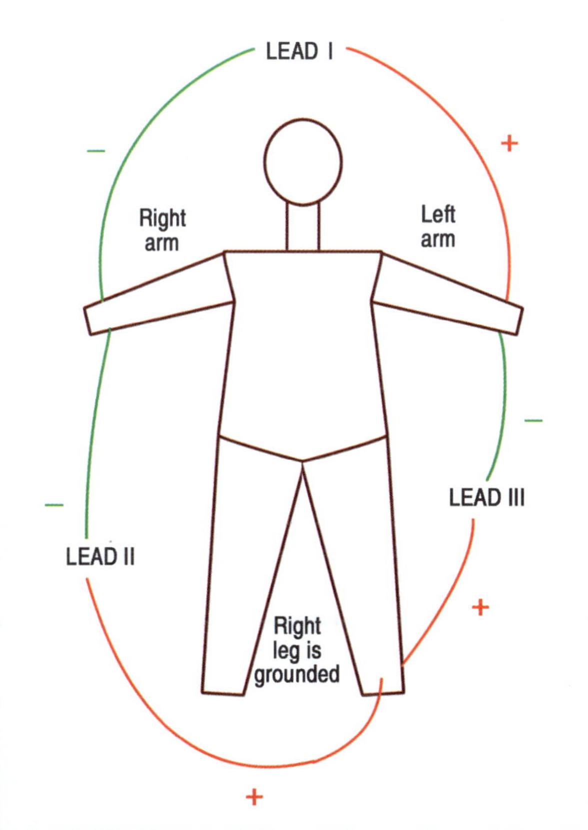

Fig. 14.9 Bipolar leads for recording an electrocardiogram.

Bipolar Leads

In lead I the positive terminal is attached to the left wrist and the negative terminal to the right wrist (Fig. 14.9). In lead II the positive terminal is on the left leg, and negative terminal on the right wrist. In lead III the positive terminal is on the left leg and the negative terminal on the left wrist. (In limb leads it does not matter to which part of the limb the terminal is attached. It is generally attached the near the wrist or ankle as this is convenient).

Unipolar Leads

Current is picked up only by one terminal that is called the ***exploring electrode***. The right arm, left arm and left leg are all connected to the negative terminal. This makes the exploring terminal positive with reference to the rest of the body. The exploring electrode may be placed on a limb, or on specific points of the chest. The pattern of recording depends only on the position of this electrode.

Normal ECG

When the two electrodes are at the same potential the recording appears as a horizontal line. A positive voltage appears as an upward deflection, and a negative voltage as a downward deflection. As the paper on which recording is done moves through the machine at constant speed, the duration of a deflection can be found by measurement. The waves (deflections) seen in a normal electrocardiogram taken with limb leads is shown in Fig.14.10. They are designated as P, Q, R, S and T waves. The Q, R and S waves are seen as the QRS complex.

The P-wave is a short upward deflection caused by atrial depolarisation.

The QRS-complex is caused by ventricular depolarisation. The Q-wave is a downward deflection. It may be absent. The R-wave is a tall upward deflection. The S-wave is a downward deflection following the R-wave.

The T-wave is a gradual upward deflection caused by ventricular repolarisation.

Between the P-wave and the QRS complex there is an isoelectric interval (seen as a straight line). The PR-interval (from beginning of P wave to beginning of QRS-

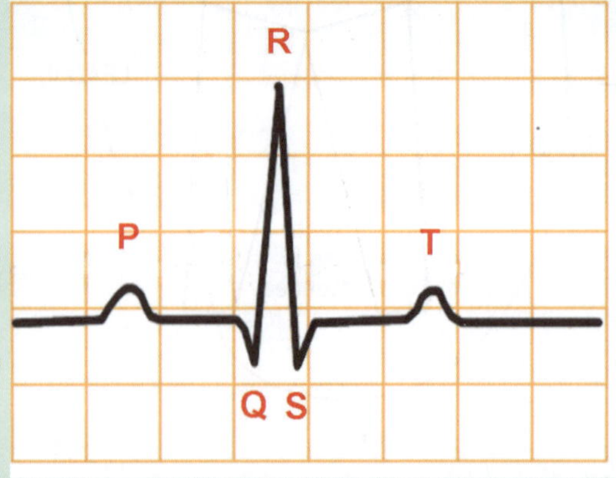

Fig. 14.10 Basic pattern of ECG tracing.

complex) indicates time taken by depolarisation to travel from the SA-node to the ventricle. The time intervening between the onset of the QRS-complex and the end of the T-wave is the QT interval. It represents ventricular depolarisation and repolarisation.

The ECG pattern changes in various diseases of the heart.

SOME DISORDERS OF THE HEART

1. ***Congenital malformations:*** Some children are born with abnormalities of the heart, or of large blood vessels arising from it. The interatrial or interventricular septa may have defects in them so that blood of the two atria or of the two ventricles gets mixed. The valves may not be formed properly.
2. When the heart is unable to pump enough blood into the circulation the condition is called ***heart failure***. The failure can be left sided or right sided.
3. We have seen that heart valves can be congenitally abnormal. They can also be damaged by infection (***endocarditis***). If the opening guarded by the valve becomes too narrow this is called ***stenosis***. ***Mitral stenosis*** is one of the commonest valvular diseases of the heart. In an effort to push blood through a narrowed atrioventricular opening, the left atrium first enlarges, and ultimately fails. When this happens, return of blood from the lungs to the heart is interfered with.
4. Changes in walls of coronary arteries, with age, lead to their narrowing. Enough blood does not reach cardiac muscle. This condition is called ***coronary insufficiency***.

At first the cardiac muscle may receive enough blood during normal activity, but not during exertion e.g, climbing stairs. When such activity in attempted the patient has pain in the chest and left shoulder. This is called ***angina pectoris***.

The state of the coronary arteries can be studied by a procedure called ***coronary angiography***, and site of narrowing or blockage can be localised. In suitable cases a segment of the blocked artery can be replaced to restore the circulation and prolong life. This procedure is called ***coronary artery bypass surgery***.

BLOOD PRESSURE

When the left ventricle contracts blood is forced into the aorta, and its branches, under pressure. This pressure provides the driving force that makes blood flow through arteries. The pressure is highest just after ventricular systole. This is called systolic blood pressure. The pressure gradually falls and is lowest during diastole. This is called diastolic blood pressure. Normal systolic blood pressure is about 120 millimeters of mercury (120 mmHg). Normal diastolic pressure is about 80 mmHg.

Blood pressure can be measured using an instrument called a sphygmomanometer (or simply blood pressure instrument).

Normal Variations in Blood Pressure

In a healthy person blood pressure increases or decreases from time to time within narrow limits. Blood pressure increases during muscular activity as more blood is required by muscles. Even mental activity can increase blood pressure. Blood pressure rises when a person is excited or angry. It is lowest when a person is resting in bed.

We have seen that activity of the heart can be expressed in terms of cardiac output (amount of blood thrown into the aorta in one minute). We have also seen that cardiac output = (stroke volume ′ heart rate). To pump blood through tissues the heart has to work against resistance to flow offered by blood vessels. This peripheral resistance is increased when smooth muscle in the walls of small arteries contracts. Conversely it falls when the vessels dilate. When peripheral resistance increases the heart has to work harder (to push the same amount of blood through tissues). Hence blood pressure rises.

Mechanisms Controlling Blood Pressure

1. Some nerve cells present in the brain (in the medulla and pons) constitute a cardiovascular centre or vasomotor centre.
2. The vasomotor centre is connected to the heart and to blood vessels through sympathetic and parasympathetic nerves.
3. Some large arteries (aorta, carotid) contain areas that are sensitive to changes in blood pressure. These areas are called ***baroreceptors.*** Nerves arising in these baroreceptors carry this information to the vasomotor centre.
4. Some small organs present close to blood vessels (carotid body and aortic body) are sensitive to concentration of oxygen or CO_2 in blood. These are called ***chemoreceptors.*** Nerves carry information from these chemoreceptors to the vasomotor centre.
5. The vasomotor centre responds to impulses from baroreceptors and chemoreceptors by sending impulses through sympathetic or parasympathetic nerves. The effect is to increase or decrease heart rate; and to cause vasoconstriction or vasodilatation. These in turn lead to variations in blood pressure.

DISORDERS OF BLOOD PRESSURE

Hypertension

In some persons blood pressure remains persistently higher than normal. This condition is referred to simply as high blood pressure, or more correctly, as hypertension. A person whose blood pressure remain persistantly above 140 / 90 mmHg is said to be hypertensive.

In hypertension the heart has to work harder than normal. Over a period of time, the left ventricle enlarges. If hypertension is untreated the heart is eventually unable to pump adequate quantity of blood. Such a condition is referred to as heart failure.

Persons with hypertension are more prone to heart attacks (myocardial infarction); and to stroke (in which an artery in the brain get blocked, leading to paralysis or death).

Persistently low blood pressure is called hypotension (see shock, below).

Shock

In some of the above sections we have seen that adequate cardiac output is essential for maintaining blood pressure, and this is in turn responsible for maintaining adequate supply of oxygen and of nutrients to cells. If the circulation is unable to maintain this supply the patient goes into a condition of ***shock***. The person becomes restless and may become unconscious. Severe shock often leads to death.

Some of the conditions that can lead to shock are as follows:

1. Reduction in volume of blood can lead to hypovolaemic shock. Reduction in volume can result from severe bleeding; loss of water from the body because of vomiting or diarrhoea; and loss of blood and plasma because of extension burns.
2. Shock can result from direct damage to the heart. This occurs if blood supply to a part of heart muscle is blocked. This muscle dies (myocardial infarction). This is what is called a heart attack.
3. Shock can occur in severe infections (bacteraemic shock or septacaemic shock); in severe allergic reactions (anaphylactic shock); or by severe disturbances in the nervous system (neurogenic shock).

If shock is mild compensatory increase in blood pressure takes place by stimulation of baroreceptors, by stimulation of adrenaline release by adrenal glands; and by increase in heart rate. The body tries to conserve water by reducing urine formation. These measures can help in recovery. However, if shock is severe, and enough fluid does not reach the brain, brain cells undergo permanent damage. Lack of oxygen and the accumulation of harmful substances (e.g. lactic acid) in blood, disrupts cellular activity and death often follows.

EFFECT OF EXERCISE ON CARDIOVASCULAR SYSTEM

1. Exercise leads to some degree of hypoxia (because of heavy demand for oxygen). This stimulates the juxtaglomerular apparatus (in the kidney) to produce erythropoietin. Erythropoietin stimulates mechanisms that result in ***release of erythrocytes from bone marrow*** into blood.
2. Muscular activity produces considerable heat. Sweating increases and fluid is lost from the body. This leads to ***reduced blood volume***.
3. ***Heart rate is increased*** by increased sympathetic tone and reduced vagal tone. In severe exercise heart rate can reach up to 250 beats per minute. Increased sympathetic tone is a result of proprioceptive impulses from muscles, increased carbon dioxide tension, raised body temperature, and increased secretion of catecholamines.
4. ***Cardiac output*** is increased.
5. ***Venous return*** to the heart is increased.
6. ***Blood flow*** through muscles increase many times.
7. In isotonic exercise, systolic ***blood pressure is raised*** but diastolic pressure remains normal. In isometric exercise both systolic and diastolic pressures are increased.

BLOOD VESSELS

ARTERIES

Basic Structure of Arteries

The histological structure of an artery varies considerably with its diameter. However, all arteries have some features in common which are as follows (Figs. 14.11, 14.12).

The wall of an artery is made up of three layers.

1. The innermost layer is called the ***tunica intima*** (tunica = coat). It is lined by endothelium. It is separated from the tunica media by the ***internal elastic lamina*** (a membrane formed by elastic fibres).
2. Outside the tunica intima there is the ***tunica media*** or middle layer. The media may consist predominantly of elastic tissue or of smooth muscle. Some connective tissue is usually present. On the outside the media is limited by a membrane formed by elastic fibres: this is the ***external elastic lamina***.
3. The outermost layer is called the ***tunica adventitia***. This coat consists of connective tissue in which collagen fibres are prominent. This layer prevents undue stretching or distension of the artery.

Elastic and Muscular Arteries

On the basis of the kind of tissue that predominates in the tunica media, arteries are often divided into elastic arteries and muscular arteries. Elastic arteries include the aorta and the large arteries supplying the head and neck (carotids) and limbs (subclavian, axillary, iliac). The remaining arteries are muscular.

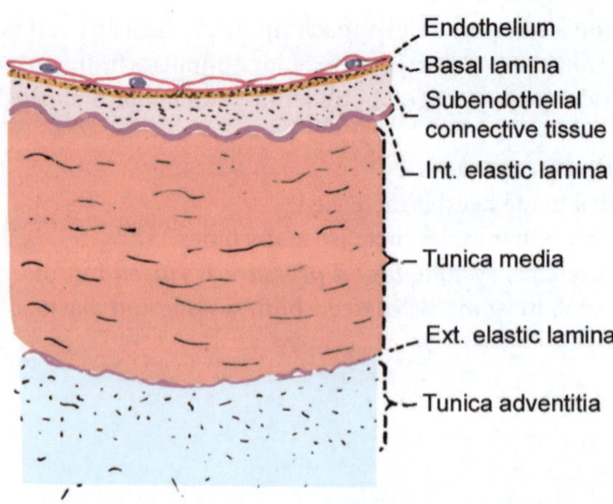

Fig. 14.11 Scheme to show the layers in the wall of a typical artery.

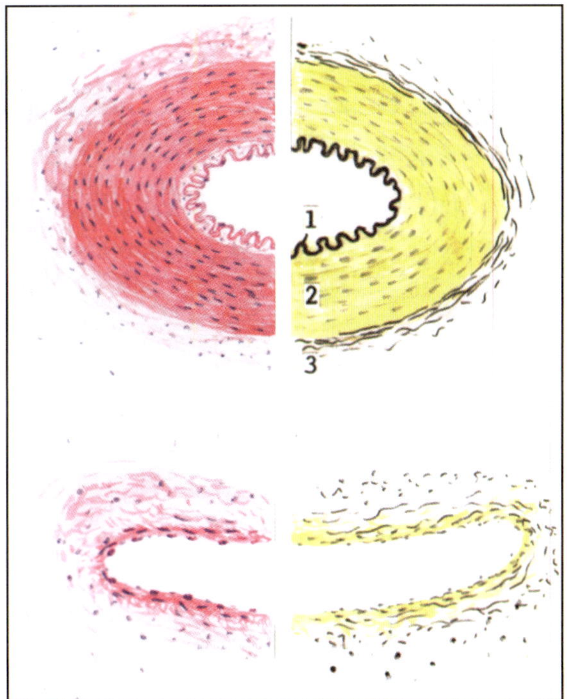

Fig. 14.12 Medium sized artery (above) and vein (below). The left half of the figure shows the appearance as seen with haematoxylin and eosin staining. The right half shows appearance when elastic fibres are stained black. 1-Internal elastic lamina. 2-Tunica media. 3-Tunica adventitia

Although all arteries carry blood to peripheral tissues, elastic and muscular arteries play differing additional roles. When the left ventricle of the heart contracts, and blood enters the large elastic arteries with considerable force, these arteries distend significantly. They are able to do so because of much elastic tissue in their walls (Fig. 14.13). During diastole (i.e., relaxation of the left ventricle) the walls of the arteries come back to their original size because of the elastic recoil of their walls. This recoil acts as an additional force that pushes the blood into smaller arteries. It is because of this fact that blood flows continuously through arteries (but with fluctuation of pressure during systole and diastole). In contrast a muscular artery has the ability to alter the size of its lumen by contraction or relaxation of smooth muscle in its wall. Muscular arteries can, therefore, regulate the amount of blood flowing into the regions supplied by them.

ARTERIOLES

When traced distally, muscular arteries progressively decrease in diameter. They then become continuous with arterioles. Arterioles have a few layers of muscle in their wall (Fig. 14.14). They are important in controlling flow of blood into the capillary bed.

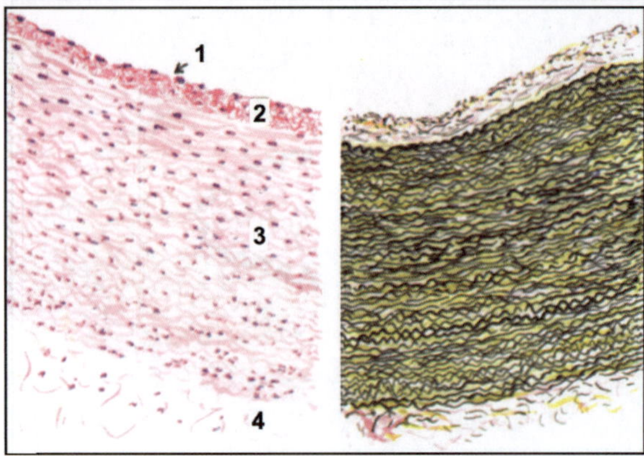

Fig. 14.13 Section through an elastic artery. Staining is as in Fig. 10.1B. 1-Endothelial lining. 2-Tunica intima. 3-Tunica media. 4-Tunica adventitia.

Arterioles having a diameter between 50 to 100 μm are called ***muscular arterioles***. Those having a diameter less than 50 μm are called ***terminal arterioles***.

VEINS

The basic structure of veins is similar to that of arteries. The tunica intima, media and adventitia can be distinguished specially in large veins. The structure of veins differs from that of arteries in the following respects (Fig. 14.12).

1. The wall of a vein is distinctly thinner than that of an artery having the same sized lumen.
2. The tunica media contains a much larger quantity of collagen than in arteries. The amount of elastic tissue or of muscle is much less.
3. Because of the differences mentioned above, the wall of a vein is easily compressed. After death veins are usually collapsed. In contrast arteries retain their patency.
4. In arteries the tunica media is usually thicker than the adventitia. In contrast the adventitia of veins is thicker than the media (specially in large veins).

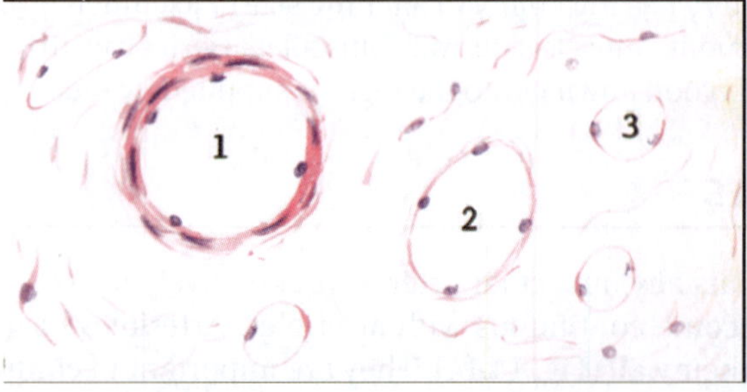

Fig. 14.14 Section showing an arteriole (1), a venule (2), and a capillary (3).

5. A clear distinction between the tunica intima, media and adventitia cannot be made out in small veins as all these layers consist predominantly of fibrous tissue.

Valves of Veins

Most veins contain valves that allow the flow of blood towards the heart, but prevent its regurgitation in the opposite direction. Typically each valve is made up of two semilunar cusps (Fig. 14.15). Each cusp is a fold of endothelium within which there is some connective tissue that is rich in elastic fibres. Valves are absent in very small veins; in veins within the cranial cavity, or within the vertebral canal; in the venae cavae; and in some other veins.

Flow of blood through veins is assisted by contractions of muscle in their walls. It is also assisted by contraction of surrounding muscles specially when the latter are enclosed in deep fascia.

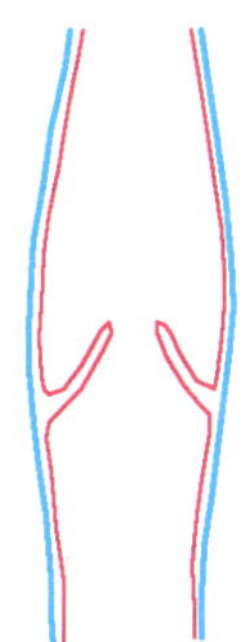

Fig. 14.15 Longitudinal section through a vein to show a valve made up of two cusps.

VENULES

The smallest veins, into which capillaries drain, are called venules (Fig. 14.14). They are 20 to 30 μm in diameter. Their walls consist of endothelium, basal lamina, and a thin adventitia consisting of longitudinally running collagen fibres. Flattened or branching cells called ***pericytes*** may be present outside the basal laminae of small venules (called ***post-capillary venules***), while some muscle may be present in larger vessels (***muscular venules***).

Functionally, venules have to be distinguished from true veins. The walls of venules (specially those of postcapillary venules) have considerable permeability and exchanges between blood and surrounding tissues can take place through them. In particular venules are the sites at which lymphocytes and other cells may pass out of (or into) the blood stream.

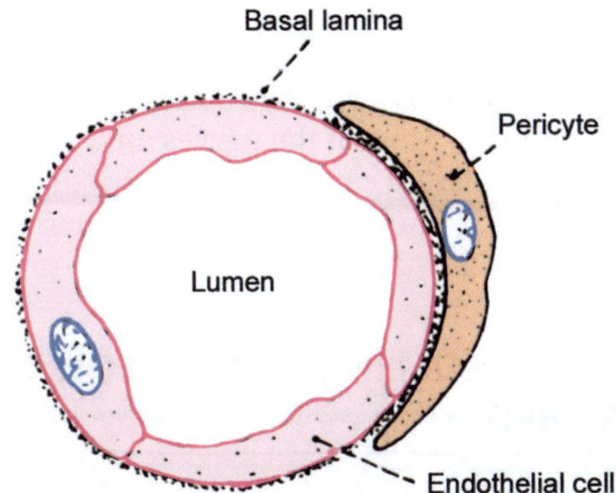

Fig. 14.16 Diagram to show the structure of a capillary.

CAPILLARIES

We have seen that terminal arterioles are continued into a capillary plexus which pervades the tissue supplied. The arrangement of the capillary plexus and its density varies from tissue to tissue, the density being greatest in tissues having high metabolic activity. Exchanges (of oxygen, carbon dioxide, fluids and various molecules) between blood and tissue take place through the walls of the capillary plexus (and through postcapillary venules).

The average diameter of a capillary is 8 μm. The wall of a capillary is formed essentially by endothelial cells which are lined on the outside by a basal lamina (glycoprotein). Overlying the basal lamina there may be isolated branching perivascular cells (pericytes), and a delicate network of reticular fibres and cells (Fig. 14.16).

SINUSOIDS

In some tissues the 'exchange' network is made up of vessels that are somewhat different from capillaries, and are called sinusoids. The main differences between capillaries and sinusoids are as follows.

1. The wall of a sinusoid consists only of endothelium supported by a thin layer of connective tissue. The wall may be incomplete at places, so that blood may come into direct contact with tissue cells.
2. Sinusoids have a broader lumen (about 20 μm) than capillaries. The lumen may be irregular. Because of this fact blood flow through them is relatively sluggish.
3. Sinusoids are found typically in organs that are made up of cords or plates of cells. These include the liver, the adrenal cortex, the hypophysis cerebri, and the parathyroid glands. Sinusoids are also present in the spleen, in the bone marrow, and in the carotid body.

Blood Vessels, Lymphatics and Nerves supplying Blood Vessels

The walls of small blood vessels receive adequate nutrition by diffusion from blood in their lumina. However, the walls of large and medium sized vessels are supplied by small arteries called ***vasa vasorum*** (literally 'vessels of vessels': singular = ***vas vasis***). These vessels supply the adventitia and the outer part of the media. These layers of the vessel wall also contain many lymphatic vessels.

Blood vessels have a fairly rich supply by autonomic nerves (sympathetic). The nerves are unmyelinated. Most of the nerves are vasomotor and supply smooth muscle. Their stimulation causes vasoconstriction in some arteries, and vasodilatation in others. Some myelinated sensory nerves are also present in the adventitia.

MECHANISMS CONTROLLING BLOOD FLOW THROUGH THE CAPILLARY BED

The requirements of blood flow through a tissue may vary considerably at different times. For example, a muscle needs much more blood when engaged in active contraction, than when relaxed. Blood flow through intestinal villi needs to be greatest when there is food to be absorbed. The mechanisms that adjust blood flow through capillaries are considered below.

Blood supply to relatively large areas of tissue is controlled by contraction or relaxation of smooth muscle in the walls of muscular arteries and arterioles. Control of supply to smaller areas is effected through arteriovenous anastomoses, and some other similar mechanisms.

Arteriovenous Anastomoses

In many parts of the body small arteries and veins are connected by direct channels that constitute arteriovenous anastomoses (Figs. 14.17, 14.18). These channels may be straight or coiled. Their walls have a thick muscular coat which is richly supplied with sympathetic nerves. When the anastomoses are patent blood is short circuited from the artery to the vein so that very little blood passes through the capillary bed. However, when the muscle in the wall of the anastomosing channel contracts its lumen is occluded so that all blood now passes through the capillaries. Arteriovenous anastomoses are found in the skin specially in that of the nose, lips and external ear; and in the mucous membrane of the alimentary canal and nose. They are also seen in the tongue, in the thyroid, in sympathetic ganglia, and in the erectile tissues of sex organs.

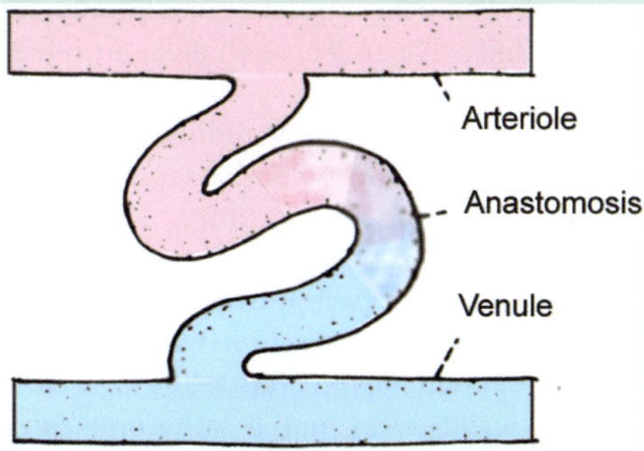

Fig. 14.17 Diagram to show an arteriovenous anastomosis (glomus).

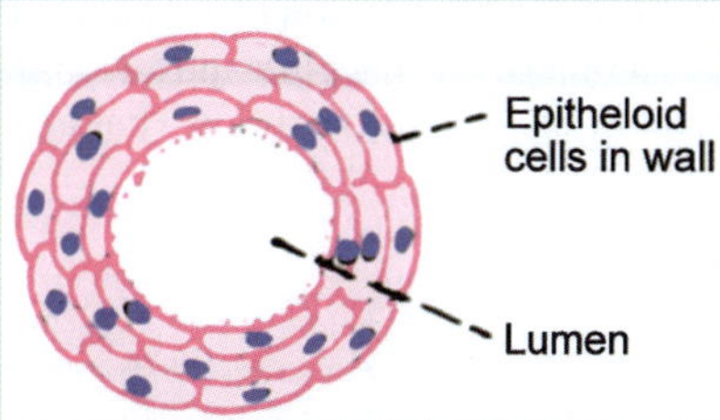

Fig. 14.18 Section across the connecting channel of an arteriovenous anastomosis.

Arteriovenous anastomoses in the skin help in regulating body temperature, by increasing blood flow through capillaries in warm weather; and decreasing it in cold weather to prevent heat loss.

FACTORS INFLUENCING BLOOD FLOW THROUGH VESSELS

Blood flow can be influenced by contraction or relaxation of muscle in the walls of arteries (specially of medium size. Contraction of muscle makes the lumen narrower (vasoconstriction) reducing flow. Relaxation makes the lumen wider (vasodilatation). Most of the time blood vessels are slightly constricted. Increased sympathetic stimulation constricts them while decreased stimulation dilates them. Vasoconstriction increases resistance (called ***peripheral resistance***) to blood flow. Therefore, the heart works harder to overcome this resistance leading to increased blood pressure. Apart from sympathetic stimulation, blood flow through tissues can be influenced by chemicals like lactic acid (produced by muscle contraction), by tissue damage, or by reduced oxygen supply.

SOME DISEASES OF BLOOD VESSELS

1. The walls of the arteries of a young person are elastic. They are soft to feel and the vessels can expand or constrict easily. With increasing age the walls gradually become harder, and elasticity is reduced. The intima (which is normally smooth) becomes rough. This occurs because of infiltration of the intima with fat (including cholesterol) and collagen. These changes are referred to as ***atheroma***. The thickenings formed are ***atheromatous plaques***. Atheroma leads to narrowing of the arterial lumen, and consequently to reduced blood flow.
2. Normally blood does not clot within a blood vessel as platelets do not adhere to the smooth vessel wall. When the wall becomes rough clots of blood can form. These can obstruct a vessel. This is called ***thrombosis***. We have seen earlier that thrombosis in a coronary artery supplying heart muscle is called ***coronary thrombosis***. It leads to ***myocardial infarction*** (which manifests as a heart attack). Thrombosis in an artery supplying the brain leads to ***stroke***.
3. An artery in which the wall is weakened by atheroma can rupture, leading to haemorrhage (bleeding). Such an event in the brain (***cerebral haemorrhage***) is another cause of stroke, which is frequently fatal.
4. Dilatation of a part of a blood vessel is called an ***aneurysm***.
5. Localised narrowing of a vessel (e.g., aorta) is called ***coarctation***.
6. Thrombosis can occur in veins (***venous thrombosis***). It can result in swelling (e.g., in a leg) and pain, and in obstruction of circulation through the part.
7. In some people (specially those who have to stand for long periods) the superficial veins of the legs become enlarged and tortuous. They are called ***varicose veins***.

CHAPTER

15

Respiratory System

INTRODUCTION

The respiratory system is meant, primarily, for the oxygenation of blood. The chief organs of the system are the right and left ***lungs***. Oxygen contained in air reaches the lungs by passing through a series of respiratory passages, which also serve for removal of carbon dioxide released from the blood.

The respiratory passages are shown in Figs. 15.1 and 15.2. Air from the outside enters the body through the right and left ***anterior nares*** (or ***external nares***) which open into the right and left ***nasal cavities.*** Apart from their respiratory function, the nasal cavities have olfactory areas that act as end organs for smell. At their posterior ends the nasal cavities have openings called the ***posterior nares*** (or ***internal nares***) through which they open into the ***pharynx.*** The pharynx is a single cavity not divided into right and left halves. It is divisible, from above downwards, into an upper part the ***nasopharynx*** (into which the nasal cavities open); a middle part the ***oropharynx*** (which is continuous with the posterior end of the oral cavity); and a lower part the ***laryngopharynx***. Air from the nose enters the nasopharynx and passes down through the oropharynx and laryngopharynx. Air can also pass through the mouth directly into the oropharynx and from there to the laryngopharynx. Air from the laryngopharynx enters a box-like structure called the ***larynx.*** The larynx is placed on the front of the upper part of the neck. Apart from being a respiratory passage it is the organ where voice is produced: it is, therefore, sometimes called the voice-box.

Inferiorly the larynx is continuous with a tube called the ***trachea.*** ⊠ The trachea passes through the lower part of the neck into the upper part of the thorax. At the level of the lower border of the manubrium sterni the trachea bifurcates into the right and left ***principal bronchi***, which carry air to the right and left lungs. Within the lung each principal bronchus divides, like the branches of a tree, into smaller and smaller ***bronchi*** that ultimately end in microscopic tubes that are called ***bronchioles.*** The bronchioles open into microscopic sac-like structures called ***alveoli.*** The walls of the alveoli contain

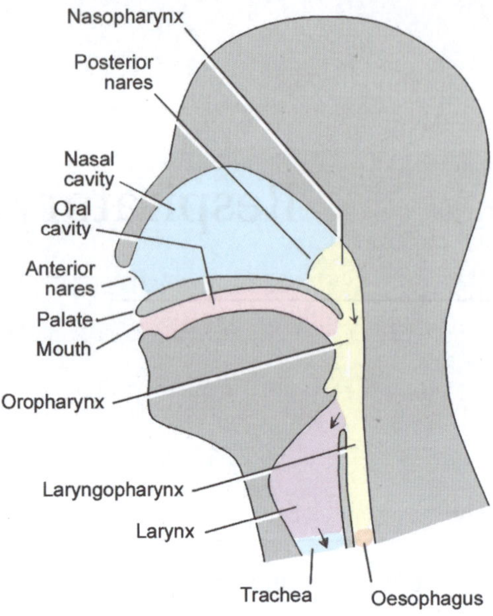

Fig. 15.1 Simplified diagram showing intercommunications between the nasal cavities, the mouth, the pharynx, the larynx and the oesophagus.

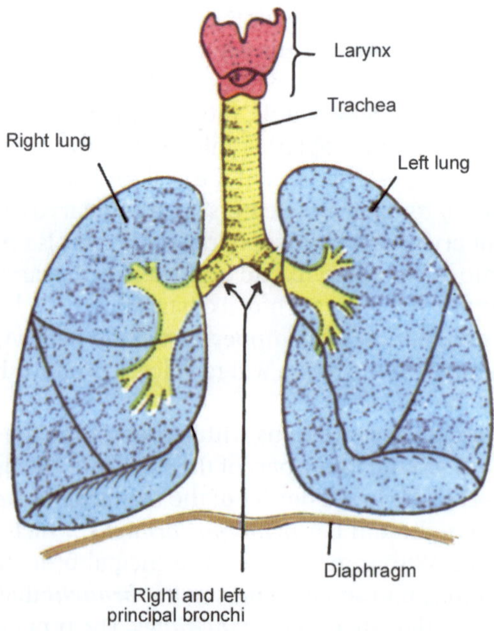

Fig. 15.2 Diagram to show the main parts of the respiratory system.

a rich network of blood capillaries. Blood in these capillaries is separated from the air in the alveoli by a very thin membrane through which oxygen can pass into the blood and carbon dioxide can pass into the alveolar air.

Mechanism of Respiration

The pumping of air in and out of the lungs is a result of respiratory movements performed by respiratory muscles. The most important of these is the ***diaphragm***. The diaphragm is so called because it forms a partition between the thorax and the abdomen. Another important set of respiratory muscles are the ***intercostal muscles*** that occupy the intercostal spaces (intervals between adjacent ribs).

When the thoracic cavity expands, a negative pressure is created within the pleural cavity. This negative pressure exerts a pull on elastic tissue within the lungs causing the lungs to expand. Expansion of the lungs draws air into them. The reverse happens in expiration.

The main force for expansion of the thoracic cavity (in inspiration) is provided by the diaphragm. When this muscle contracts its central part (which is tendinous) is pulled downwards. This increases the vertical diameter of the thorax. When the diaphragm relaxes, pressure of abdominal contents pushes it upwards.

The second force for expansion of the thorax is provided by intercostal muscles that move the ribs. These movements, along with movements of the sternum, increase the lateral and anteroposterior dimensions of the thorax.

NASAL CAVITY

The nasal cavity is divided by a median septum into right and left halves. Each half of the nasal cavity opens to the exterior through the external (or anterior) nares; and posteriorly it opens into the nasopharynx. A schematic coronal section through the nasal cavity is shown in Fig. 15.3. It is seen that each half of the cavity is triangular. It has a vertical medial wall formed by the ***nasal septum***; a sloping lateral wall; a relatively broad floor formed by the ***palate*** (which separates the nasal cavity from the oral cavity); and a narrow roof that lies at the junction of the medial and lateral walls.

These walls have a skeletal basis that is made up predominantly of bone, but is cartilaginous at some places. The skeletal basis is covered by mucous membrane. Typically the mucosa is moist and highly vascular. It serves to warm inspired air and also helps to remove dust (which sticks to the moist wall). For these reasons the mucosa is referred to as ***respiratory***. The mucosa lining the uppermost part of the septum and the adjoining part of the lateral wall differs from that present elsewhere in the nasal cavity. It is characterised by the presence of receptor cells that are sensitive to smell: the mucosa in this region is, therefore, called the ***olfactory mucosa.*** Olfactory nerves arise from this mucosa. A small area of the nasal cavity (near the anterior nares) is lined not by mucous membrane, but by skin. This skin bears hair that serve to trap dust present in inspired air.

The nasal septum is fairly often deflected to one side so that one half of the nasal cavity may be larger than the other.

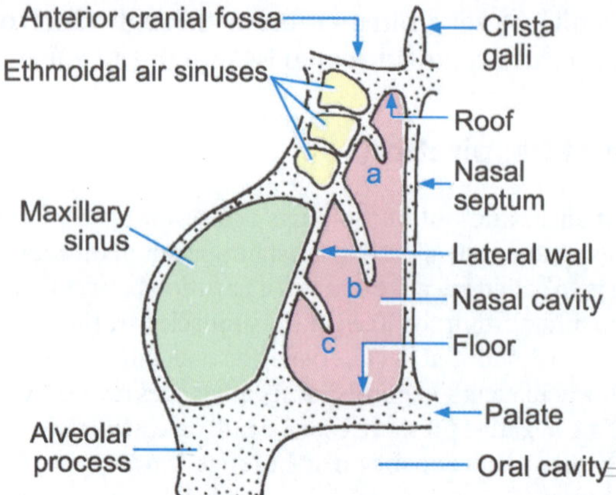

Fig. 15.3 Highly simplified coronal section through the nasal cavity. ***a, b, c:*** superior, middle and inferior conchae respectively.

The lateral wall of the nasal cavity is shown in Fig. 15.4. There are three antero-posterior elevations on the lateral wall. These are the superior, middle and inferior nasal ***conchae.*** Each concha has an upper border attached to the rest of the lateral wall and a free lower margin. The spaces deep to the superior, middle and inferior conchae are called the superior, middle and inferior ***meatuses*** respectively (2, 3, 4 in Fig. 15.5). There is a triangular space above the superior concha (1 in Fig. 15.5). This is the ***sphenoethmoidal recess***.

The part of the nasal cavity just above the anterior nares is called the ***vestibule.*** The vestibule is lined by skin.

Some additional features are labeled in Fig. 15.4.

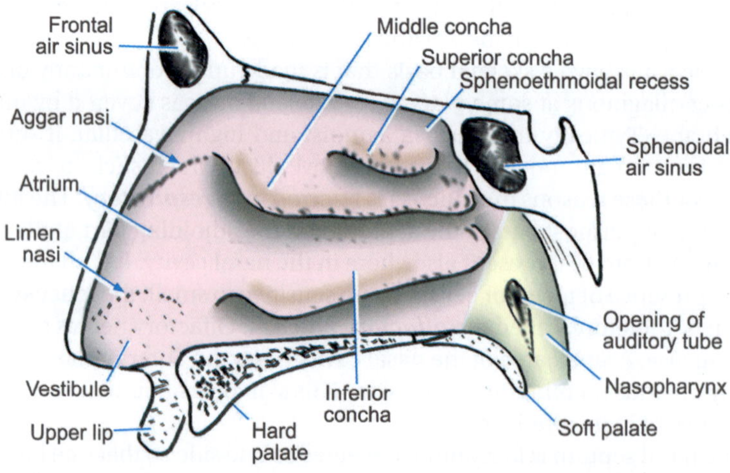

Fig. 15.4 Lateral wall of the nasal cavity with the mucous membrane intact.

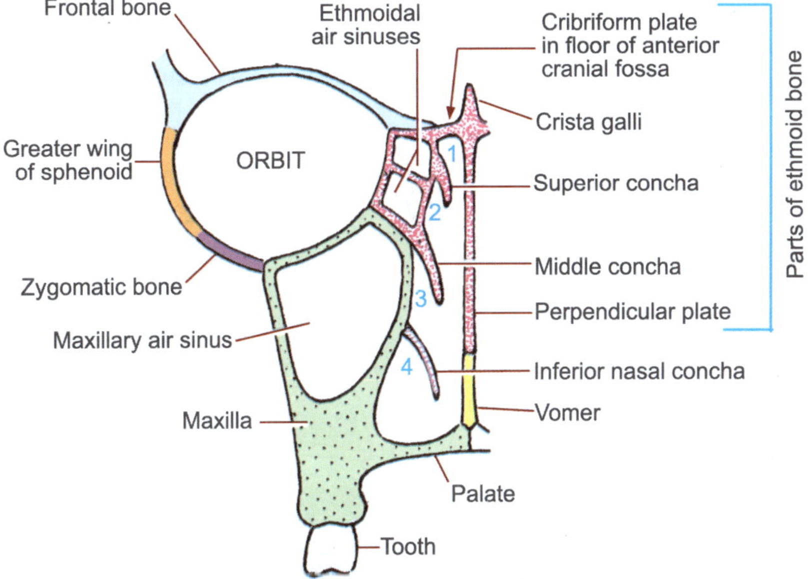

Fig. 15.5 Schematic coronal section through the nasal cavity to show some bones forming its walls. The orbit is also shown.

THE PARANASAL SINUSES

These are spaces present in the substance of bones related to the nasal cavities. Each sinus opens into the nasal cavity, and is lined by mucous membrane continuous with that of the latter. Because of this communication each sinus is normally filled with air.

The right and left ***frontal sinuses*** are present in part of the frontal bone. Each sinus opens into the middle meatus.

The right and left ***sphenoidal sinuses*** are present in the body of the sphenoid bone. Each sinus opens into the corresponding ***sphenoethmoidal recess***.

Each ***maxillary sinus*** lies within the maxilla. The sinus opens into middle meatus of the nasal cavity.

The ***ethmoidal air sinuses*** are located within the ethmoid bone. They can be divided into anterior, middle and posterior groups.

THE PHARYNX

The pharynx is a median passage that is common to the alimentary and respiratory systems (Fig. 15.6). It is divisible (from above downwards) into a nasal part (or nasopharynx) into which the nasal cavities open; an oral part (or oropharynx) which is continuous with the posterior end of the oral cavity; and a laryngeal part (or laryngopharynx) which is continuous in front with the larynx, and below with oesophagus.

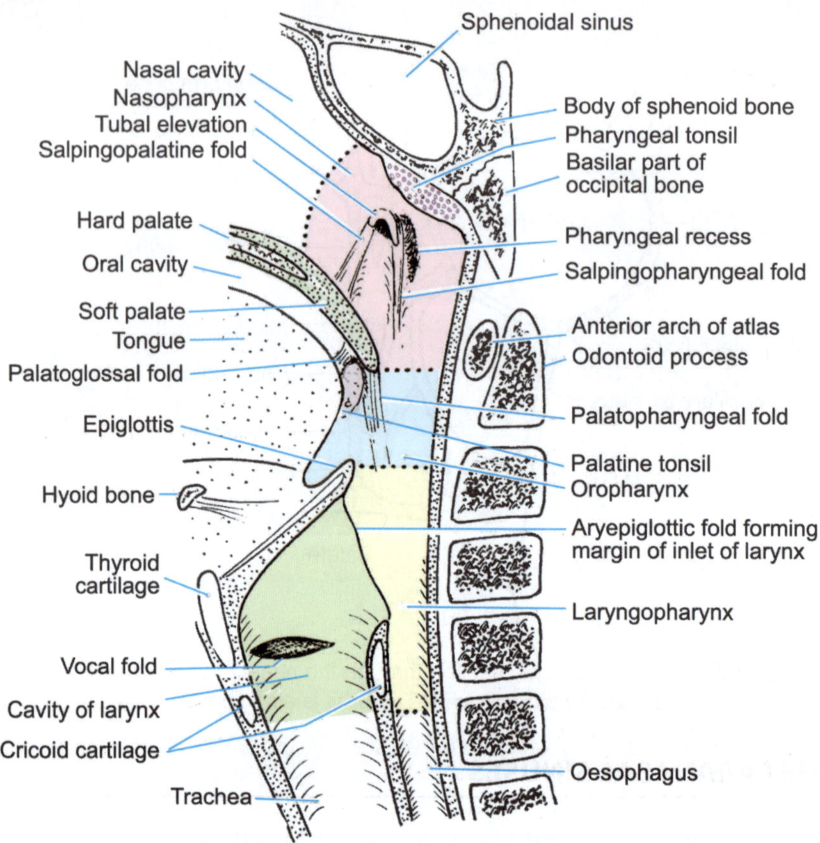

Fig. 15.6 Schematic median section through the pharynx (and neighbouring structures) to show its lateral wall. The limits of the subdivisions of the pharynx are indicated in dotted lines.

The communication between the nasopharynx and the oropharynx is called the ***pharyngeal isthmus***. This isthmus can be closed (e.g., during swallowing) by elevation of the soft palate.

The communication between the oral cavity and the pharynx is called the ***oropharyngeal isthmus*** (Fig. 15.7). It is bounded above by the soft palate, below by the posterior part of the tongue, and on either side by the palatoglossal arches. The oropharyngeal isthmus can be closed by contraction of muscles. This closure plays an important part in deglutition.

In Fig. 15.7 observe the palatine tonsil lying close to the isthmus.

The laryngopharynx lies just behind the larynx. The opening from pharynx into larynx is called the ***inlet of the larynx***.

Note the following additional features.

a. On each lateral wall of the nasopharynx there is an opening that leads into the auditory tube. This tube connects the nasopharynx to the middle ear.

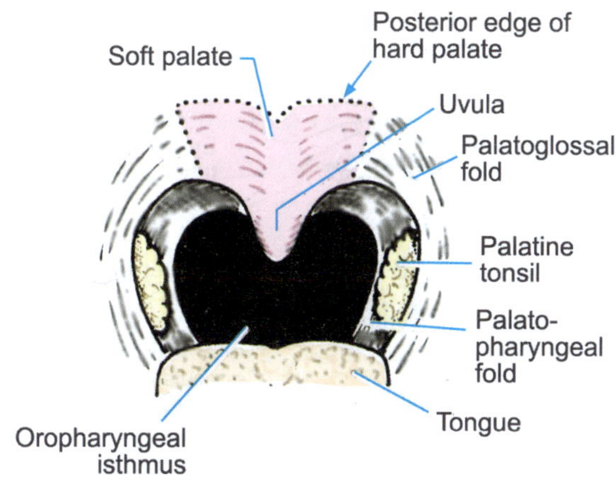

Fig. 15.7 Soft palate as seen through the mouth. The dotted line indicates its upper and lateral limits.

b. The mucosa of the median part of the roof of the nasopharynx shows a bulging produced by a mass of lymphoid tissue. This lymphoid tissue constitutes the ***pharyngeal tonsil***. (When enlarged, the pharyngeal tonsil is referred to as ***adenoids***). Some lymphoid tissue is also present behind the opening of the auditory tube. This collection of lymphoid tissue is called the ***tubal tonsil***.
c. The palatine tonsil lies in the lateral wall of the oropharynx.

THE LARYNX

The larynx is a space that communicates above with the laryngeal part of the pharynx, and below with the trachea. Apart from being a respiratory passage the larynx is the organ where voice is produced. Near the middle of the larynx there are a pair of ***vocal folds*** (one right and one left) that project into the laryngeal cavity (Fig.15.8). Between these folds there is an interval called the ***rima glottidis.*** The rima is fairly wide in ordinary breathing. When we wish to speak the two vocal folds come close together narrowing the rima glottidis. Expired air passing through the narrow gap causes the vocal folds to vibrate resulting in the production of sound. Variation in the loudness of sound is produced by the force with which air is expelled through the rima glottidis. Variation in pitch is achieved by stretching of the vocal folds to different degrees. The difference in the voice of a man and that of a woman (or of a child) is due to the fact that the vocal folds are considerably longer in the male adult.

The larynx has a rigid framework made up of cartilages. The cartilages are joined to one another by ligaments. A number of muscles are attached to the cartilages. They produce movements of the vocal folds that are necessary for speech. The cartilages, ligaments and muscles are covered on the inside by mucous membrane that is continuous above with that of the laryngeal part of the pharynx and below with that of the trachea.

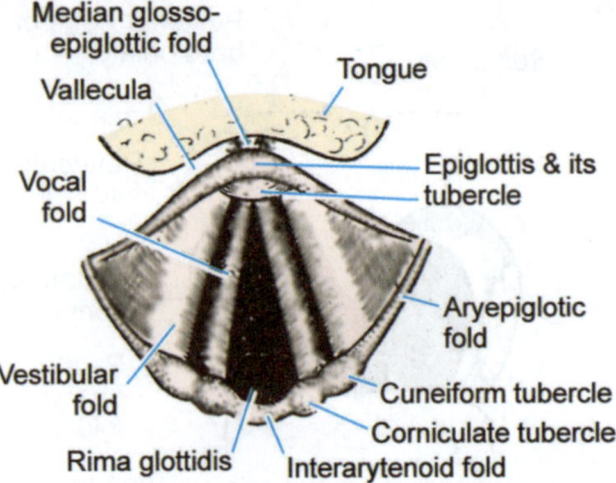

Fig. 15.8 Some features of the larynx as seen through a laryngoscope (i.e., from above). The gap between the two vestibular folds is the rima vestibuli.

Cartilages of the Larynx

These are seen from the front in Fig. 15.9 and from behind in Fig. 15.10. There are three unpaired cartilages: these are the ***thyroid cartilage***, the ***cricoid cartilage***, and the ***cartilage of the epiglottis***. The paired cartilages are the right and left ***arytenoid cartilages***; and the ***corniculate*** and ***cuneiform*** cartilages that are small nodules.

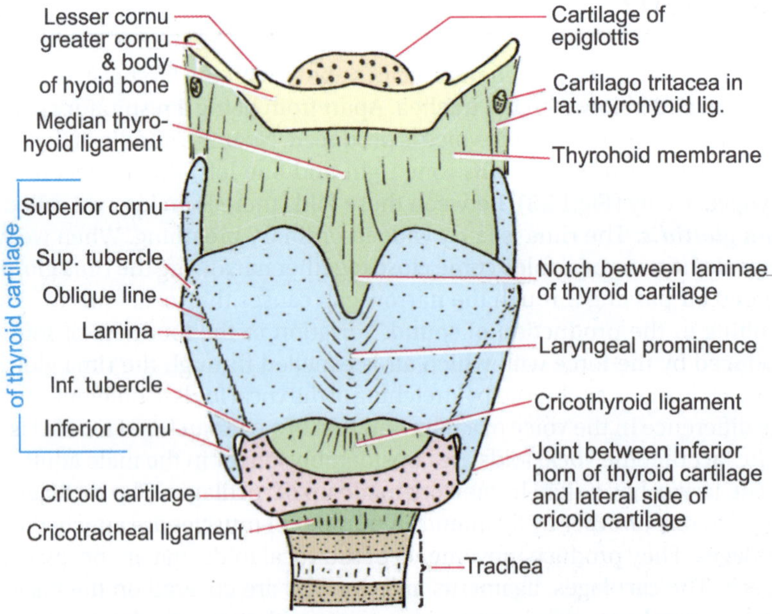

Fig. 15.9 Cartilages of the larynx as seen from the front.

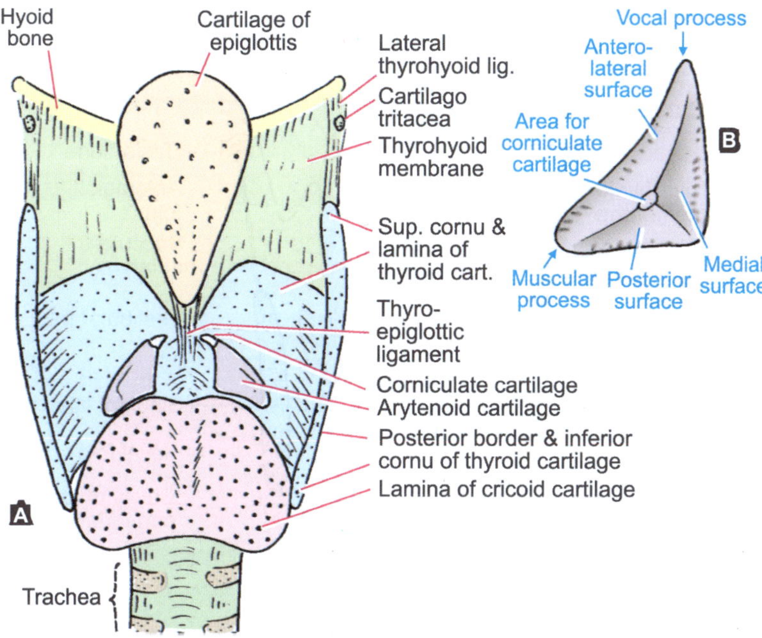

Fig. 15.10 A. Cartilages of the larynx seen from behind; B. Arytenoid cartilage of the left side seen from above.

Interior of the Larynx

The essential features to be seen in the interior of the larynx are best appreciated by examining a coronal section (Fig. 15.11).

The upper aperture of the larynx is called its ***inlet***, or ***aditus.*** Almost midway between the upper and lower ends of the larynx, two pairs of mucosal folds project into its cavity. The upper pair are the right and left ***vestibular folds.*** The lower pair are the right and left ***vocal folds.*** Each vestibular fold encloses a bundle of fibres that constitute the ***vestibular ligament.*** Each vocal fold contains a bundle of elastic fibres that constitute the ***vocal ligament***.

The right and left vocal folds are separated from each other by a fissure called the ***rima glottidis.*** The shape of the rima varies in different phases of respiration and of phonation.

The part of the laryngeal cavity lying above the vestibular folds is called the ***vestibule.*** The narrow recess between the levels of the vestibular and vocal folds (on either side) is called the ***sinus*** or ***ventricle*** of the larynx. The lower part of the cavity, below the vocal folds is not given any special name.

THE TRACHEA

The trachea is a wide tube lying on the front of the neck more or less in the middle line. The upper end of the trachea is continuous with the lower end

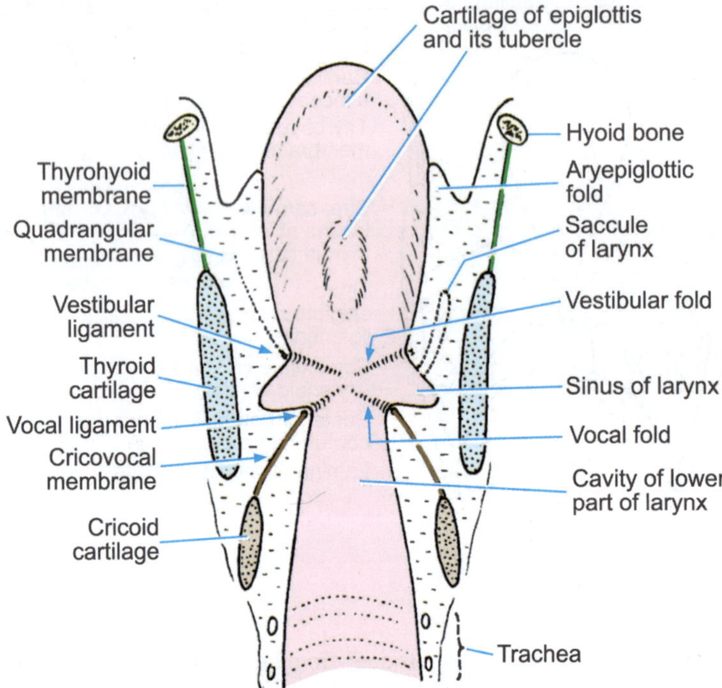

Fig. 15.11 Coronal section through the larynx viewed from behind.

of the larynx. At the root of the neck the trachea passes into the superior mediastinum.

The lumen of the trachea is kept patent because of the presence of a series of cartilaginous rings in its wall. The rings are deficient posteriorly: hence the posterior part of the wall of the trachea is flat while the rest of it is rounded (Fig. 15.12).

At its lower end the trachea ends by dividing into the right and left principal bronchi. The level of bifurcation corresponds to the lower border of the manubrium sterni.

Each principal bronchus passes downwards and laterally to enter the corresponding lung (Fig. 15.1).

THE LUNGS

The right and left lungs lie in the corresponding halves of the thorax. They are separated from each other by structures in the mediastinum (including the heart, the great vessels, the trachea, and the oesophagus). A general idea of the shape of the lungs can be had from Fig. 15.1 in which both lungs are shown as seen from the front. A basic idea of the surfaces and borders of the lungs can be obtained from Figs. 15.13 and 15.14.

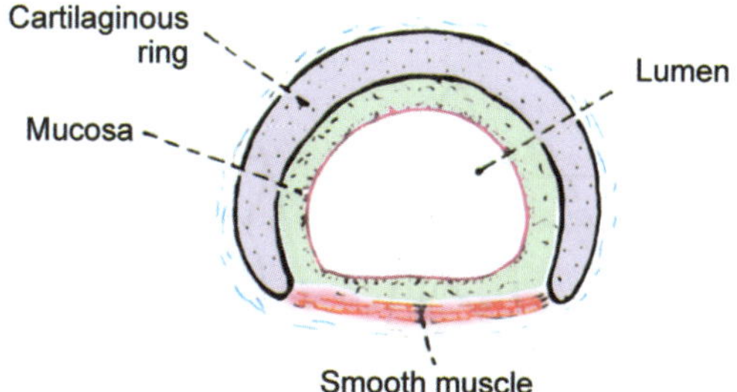

Fig. 15.12 Low power view of a section through the trachea.

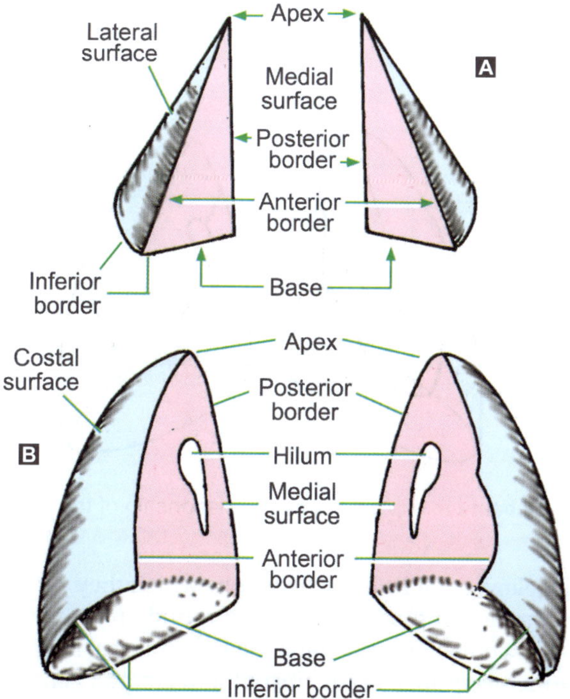

Fig. 15.13 A. Scheme to show similarity of the lungs to two halves of a cone; B. Right and left lungs seen from the anteromedial aspect.

The right and left lungs are like two halves of a cone that have been separated by a vertical cut. Each lung has a relatively narrow upper end, or ***apex***; a much broader inferior surface or ***base;*** a rounded ***lateral*** or ***costal surface;*** and a ***medial surface.*** The costal surface meets the medial surface, in front at the ***anterior border*** and behind at the ***posterior border***. The costal and medial

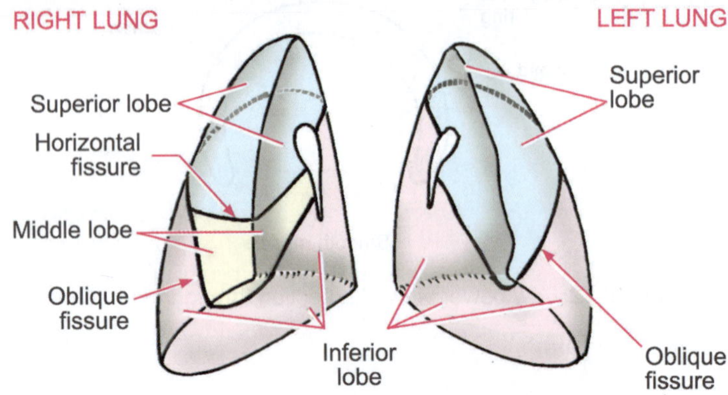

Fig. 15.14 Simplified drawings of right and left lungs as seen from the anteromedial aspect to show fissures and lobes.

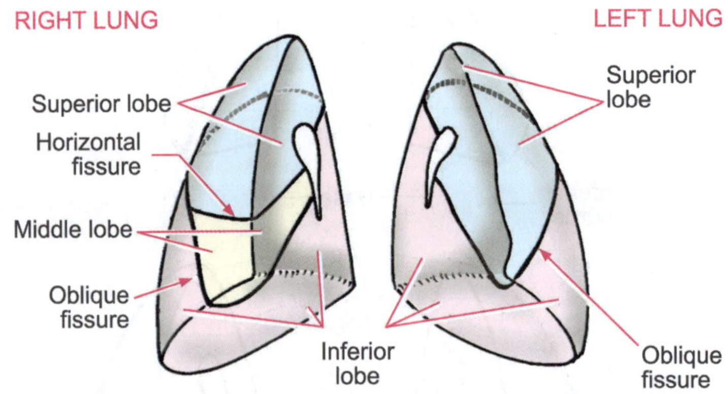

Fig. 15.15 Scheme to explain the basic relationship of the lung to pleura.

surfaces end, below, in an ***inferior border*** by which they are separated from the base. The surface of the lung is free all round and is covered by pleura (visceral layer) except at an area of the medial surface called the ***hilum*** (Fig. 15.15). The principal bronchus and the pulmonary artery enter the lung, and the pulmonary veins leave it, at the hilum.

Fissures and Lobes of the Lungs

Both the right and left lungs have a prominent ***oblique fissure***. The right lung has an additional ***horizontal fissure***. These fissures divide the left lung into ***superior*** and ***inferior lobes***. The right lung has an additional ***middle lobe***.

On entering the lung the principal bronchus divides into secondary, or ***lobar bronchi*** (one for each lobe). Each lobar bronchus divides into tertiary, or ***segmental bronchi*** (one for each segment of the lobe). The segmental bronchi

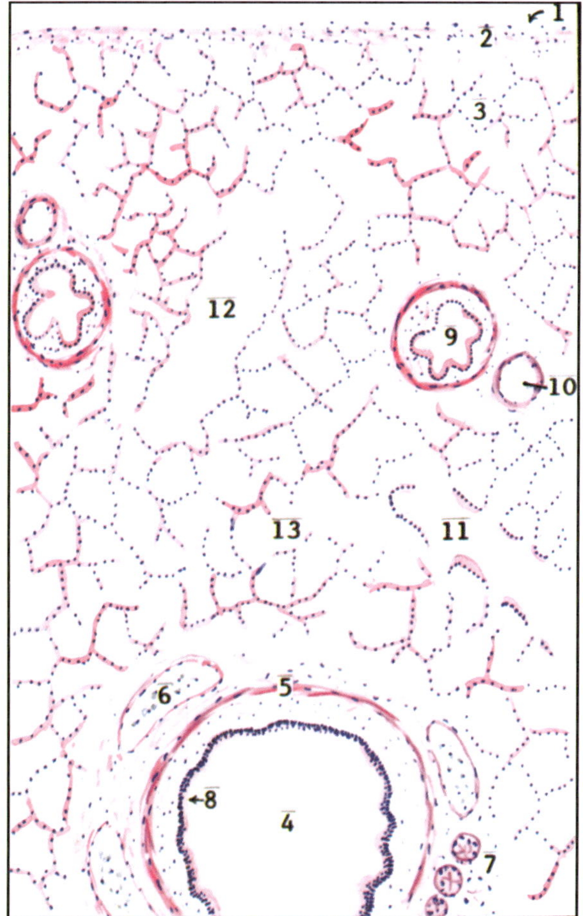

Fig. 15.16 Section through part of a lung. 1, 2-Pleura. 3-Alveolus. 4-Bronchus. 5-Smooth muscle. 6-Cartilage. 7-Glands. 8-Epithelium of bronchus. 9-Bronchiole. 10-Artery. 11-Respiratory bronchiole. 12-Alveolar duct. 13-Atrium.

divide into smaller and smaller bronchi, which ultimately end in ***bronchioles***. The lung substance is divided into numerous lobules each of which receives a ***lobular bronchiole***. The lobular bronchiole gives off a number of ***terminal bronchioles*** (Figs. 15.16, 15.17). As indicated by their name the terminal bronchioles represent the most distal parts of the conducting passage. Each terminal bronchiole ends by dividing into ***respiratory bronchioles***. Each respiratory bronchiole ends by dividing into a few ***alveolar ducts***. Each alveolar duct ends in a passage, the ***atrium***, which leads into a number of rounded ***alveolar sacs***. Each alveolar sac is studded with a number of air sacs or ***alveoli***. The alveoli are blind sacs having very thin walls through which oxygen passes from air into blood, and carbon dioxide passes from blood into air.

The structure of the larger intrapulmonary bronchi is similar to that of the trachea. As these bronchi divide into smaller ones the cartilages in the walls of

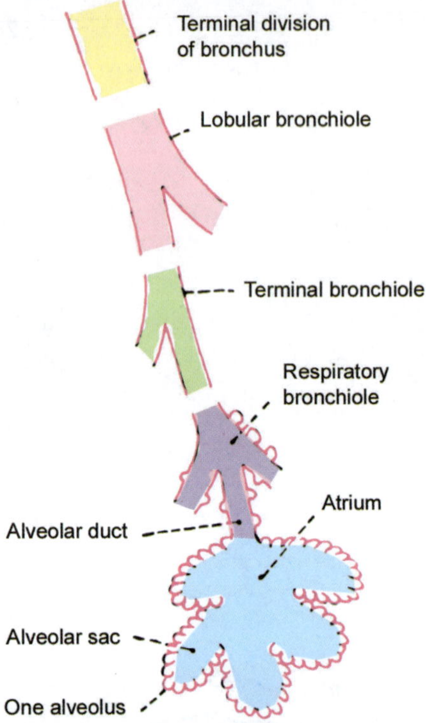

Fig. 15.17 Scheme to show some terms used to describe the terminal ramifications of the bronchial tree.

the bronchi become irregular in shape, and are progressively smaller. Cartilage is absent in the walls of bronchioles

The amount of muscle in the bronchial wall increases as the bronchi become smaller. The presence of muscle in the walls of bronchi is of considerable clinical significance. Spasm of this muscle constricts the bronchi and can cause difficulty in breathing. This is particularly likely to occur in allergic conditions and leads to a disease called ***asthma***.

Blood Vessels of the Lungs

The blood supply of the lungs is peculiar in that two sets of arteries carry blood to them.

1. The pulmonary arteries convey deoxygenated blood from the right ventricle. This blood circulates through a capillary plexus intimately related to the walls of the alveoli, and receives oxygen from the alveolar air. This blood, which is now oxygenated, is returned to the heart (left atrium) through the pulmonary veins.
2. The lungs also receive oxygenated blood like any other tissue in the body. This is conveyed through the bronchial arteries. This blood supplies the walls of the bronchi and the connective tissue of the lung.

THE PLEURA

The right and left pleurae (singular = pleura) are thin serous membranes that are closely related to the corresponding lungs and to the corresponding half of the thoracic wall. The arrangement of the pleura is best understood by thinking of it as a closed sac (Fig. 15.15A) that is invaginated (from the medial side) by the corresponding lung. As a result of this invagination the pleura of each side comes to have an inner or ***visceral layer*** that is closely adherent to the surface of the lung; and an outer, or ***parietal layer*** that lines the wall of the thoracic cavity.

SOME PHYSIOLOGICAL CONSIDERATIONS

Respiratory Cycle

Each respiratory cycle consists of:

a. ***inspiration*** in which air is taken into the lungs;
b. ***expiration*** in which air is breathed out; and
c. a short pause before the next inspiration.

Mechanism of Respiration

1. During inspiration the thoracic cavity expands because of the contraction of the diaphragm and of some intercostal muscles.
2. Expansion of the thoracic wall creates a negative pressure in the pleural cavity.
3. The negative pressure in the pleural cavity causes the lung to expand.
4. As the lungs expand air is drawn into them.
5. Expiration is caused by relaxation of the muscles that caused inspiration. The size of the thoracic cavity is reduced and air is forced out of the lungs.

For proper breathing it is necessary that the airway should be normal. In patients of asthma contraction of muscle in the walls of bronchi leads to broncho-constriction. The person has to make greater effort to breathe.

Lung Function Tests

In investigating a patient with a respiratory problem some tests are done. You should be familiar with the following terms.

1. The air taken into the lungs in one inspiration is called ***tidal volume***. It is about 500 ml.
2. In normal breathing the thoracic cavity does not expand to its full extent. Full expansion takes place when we inspire as forcefully as we can. The quantity of air then inspired is called ***inspiratory capacity***.
3. The difference between inspiratory capacity and tidal volume is ***inspiratory reserve volume***.
4. During normal expiration all air in the lungs is not expelled. The air remaining is called ***functional residual capacity***.
5. After a normal expiration, more air can be expelled by force. However some air remains in the lungs even after forceful expiration. The air that remains is ***residual volume***.

6. The maximum volume of air that can expired after maximum inspiration is called ***vital capacity***.

External and Internal Respiration

The exchange of gases between air in alveoli of the lungs, and blood is called ***external respiration***.

Exchange of gases between blood, and body cells is called ***internal respiration***. When blood circulates through tissue oxygen passes from blood to tissue fluid, and from tissue fluid to cells. Carbon dioxide passes from cells to tissue fluid, and from tissue fluid to blood. This process is the reverse of what happens in the lungs.

Transport of Blood Gases

The essential purpose of respiration is to transport oxygen present in air to blood, and to remove carbon dioxide. To understand how this happens some preliminary concepts must be considered.

1. The atmosphere is a mixture of gases. About 79% is nitrogen 21% is oxygen, and only about 0.04% is carbon dioxide. The pressure exerted by the atmosphere can be measured using a barometer. At sea level it is equal to that of a column of 760 mm of mercury.
2. Each gas exerts pressure proportional to its own concentration. The pressure of each gas is referred to as partial pressure. The partial pressure of oxygen in atmospheric air (expressed as pO_2) is (21/100) x 760 = 160 mmHg.
3. A gas exerts pressure even when it is dissolved in a liquid. Therefore, oxygen present in blood has its own pO_2 . The pressure depends on the solubility coefficient of the gas.
4. A gas can diffuse across a membrane. Diffusion always takes place from the side that has higher concentration to the side with lower concentration. Some factors that govern the rate of diffusion are the pressure difference, thickness of the membrane, solubility of the gas, and molecular weight of the gas.

Composition of Atmospheric Air and Alveolar Air

The partial pressures of gas in inspired atmospheric air, in alveolar air and in expired air are as follows

	Partial pressure mmHg			
	O_2	CO_2	N	H_2O
Atmospheric air	159	0.3	597	3.7
Alveolar air	104	40	569	47
Expired air	120	27	566	47

There is a marked difference in composition of atmospheric air and alveolar air because of the following reasons.

1. Oxygen is removed from alveolar air.
2. CO_2 is added to alveolar air.
3. Considerable water vapour is absorbed from respiratory passages.
4. About 2200 ml of air is present in alveoli at the end expiration. During inspiration only about 350 ml of air enters alveoli. Therefore, the oxygen concentration gets

diluted and pO_2 of alveolar air remains much less than in atmospheric air. For the same reason pCO_2 is more in alveolar air than in expired air.

Oxygen Uptake from Alveolar Air to Blood

The pO_2 of deoxygenated blood circulating in the walls of alveoli is about 40 mmHg. The pO_2 of alveolar air is much higher (104 mmHg). Hence oxygen diffuses easily from alveolar air to blood. The pO_2 of blood now becomes about 100 mmHg.

Oxygen absorbed in the lungs combines with haemoglobin to form oxyhaemoglobin and travels through blood in this form. One gram of haemoglobin combines with 1.34 ml of oxygen. As 100 ml of blood contains 15 g of haemoglobin the ***oxygen carrying capacity*** of blood is (15 x 1.34)=20 ml/100 ml. The capacity depends upon pO_2 of blood.

Oxygen Transport to Tissues

We have seen that pO_2 of arterial blood is about 100 mmHg. In contrast pO_2 of tissue fluid is 40 mm Hg. Hence oxygen readily diffuses from blood to tissues. When pO_2 of blood becomes 40 mmHg the blood still contains 15 ml oxygen/100ml blood. This means that out of 20 ml oxygen/100 ml taken up in lungs only 5 ml (=25%) is transferred to tissue. This is the ***oxygen utilisatioin coefficient***. This becomes much higher during exercise. Blood from tissues with pO_2 of 40 mmHg returns to the lungs for reoxygenation.

Carbon Dioxide Transport

Venous blood reaching the lungs has pCO_2 of 46 mmHg, and alveolar air has pCO_2 of 40 mmHg. Hence CO_2 readily passes into alveolar air and is expired.

Carbon dioxide is transported (in blood) in three forms.

a. Some of it is dissolved in plasma.
b. An enzyme carbonic anhydrase converts CO_2 into bicarbonate ions (HCO^-_3) and is transported in this form.
c. Carbon dioxide combines with haemoglobin to form carbaminohaemoglobin.

Control of Respiration

Respiration is controlled by the nervous system. In the medulla and pons there is a respiratory centre that influences respiration. The respiratory centre receives input from chemoreceptors (carotid body, aortic body). When CO_2 content of blood increases chemoreceptors send impulses to the respiratory centre. The respiratory centre sends impulses that increase the rate and depth of respiration, so that CO_2 levels return to normal. The respiratory centre ensures that necessary changes in respiration are made to meet the extra requirements (or altered requirements) in exercise, fever, speech, singing, or coughing. Respiration becomes faster in respiratory infections (e.g., pneumonia), and in circulatory disturbances, produced by heart failure.

Respiratory Quotient

This is an expression to show how much carbon dioxide is produced when one molecule of oxygen is used for metabolism. In a person at rest, one molecule of oxygen used for metabolism of carbohydrate produces one molecule of CO_2. Hence respiratory quotient is 1.0. (For fats the quotient is 0.7 and for proteins it is 0.8).

The respiratory quotient increases during exercise. From 1.0 it becomes 1.5 to 2.0. After termination of exercise it falls to 0.5.

Oxygen Debt

When a muscle is at rest the oxygen used by it is the ***basal consumption***.

During exertion the oxygen consumption becomes much higher, as oxygen is needed for aerobic metabolism of glucose. As intensity of exercise increases, oxygen supply falls short of demand. When this happens the muscle uses anaerobic pathways for production of ATP (See Chapter 10).

The extra oxygen used to bring the muscle back to the state that existed before beginning of exercise is called the ***oxygen debt***.

Effect of Exercise on Respiration

More oxygen is required during exercise. The factors that increase oxygen supply are as follows.

1. ***Increased pulmonary ventilation***: This is a result of increase in rate and depth of respiration. This is produced by stimulation of the respiratory centre, stimulation of chemoreceptors, by hypoxia, by increase of body temperature and by acidosis.
2. ***Increased blood flow*** through pulmonary capillaries increases the diffusion capacity for oxygen.
3. ***Increased consumption of oxygen***: The oxygen consumed by tissues, particularly by muscle, greatly increases during exercise. This is possible because of increased availability of oxygen through blood.

Hypoxia

Hypoxia is a condition in which the oxygen available to tissues is less than normal. Hypoxia can be caused by the following factors.

1. Decreased oxygen content of blood because of decreased availability of oxygen in air (e.g., at high altitude, or in some respiratory and cardiac diseases). This is called ***hypoxic hypoxia***.
2. Inability of blood to carry enough oxygen (as in anaemia). This is called ***anaemic hypoxia***.
3. Decreased flow of blood as in heart failure or shock. This is ***stagnant hypoxia***.
4. Inability of tissue to utilize oxygen (as in poisoning). This is ***histotoxic hypoxia***. Severe hypoxia can result in death. It is treated with immediate oxygen therapy.

The body reacts to hypoxia by:

1. Increased production of blood cells.
2. Increased heart rate and blood pressure.
3. Increased rate of respiration.

Effect of High Altitude

As atmospheric pressure is less, there is reduced pressure of oxygen, and this leads to hypoxia. This is the cause of mountain sickness. Breathlessness develops with mild exertion. Headache, depression and irritation are common. There is loss of appetite, nausea and vomiting.

Adaptation to high altitude takes place in a few weeks. The mechanisms for this are as follows:

1. Increase in number of erythrocytes.
2. Increased haemoglobin content of blood.
3. Increased heart rate and cardiac output.
4. Increased pulmonary ventilation because of increase in rate and force of respiration.
5. Increased flow of blood through the lungs.
6. Increased diffusing capacity of alveoli.

Artificial Respiration

This is required when breathing stops (but heart keeps beating) in cases of drowning, accidents, poisoning or electric shock. The methods used are as follows.

1. Mouth to mouth breathing.
2. Application of intermittent pressure on the back of the chest.
3. Use of machines.

ACID BASE BALANCE

Acids and Alkalis

Some naturally occurring substances have a sour taste, e.g., lemon juice and vinegar. Such substances are said to be acidic and contain acids. In contrast, some other substance are bitter in taste e.g., sodium bicarbonate used in cooking. Sodium bicarbonate is an alkali. Water is neither acidic nor alkaline.

We know that water contains two atoms of hydrogen and one of oxygen. However, these exist as two ions H^+ and OH^-. H^+ ions are responsible for making a solution acidic. The more the number of free H^+ in the solution, the stronger the acid. The OH^- ion is called a hydroxyl ion. It is responsible for alkalinity. Water is neither acid nor alkaline as it contains equal number of H^+ and OH^- ions.

The acidity of a solution is related to the number of free H^+ ions in it. This is spoken of as ***hydrogen ion concentration***. For sake of convenience hydrogen ion concentration is expressed in a scale from zero to fourteen. This is called the pH scale. Water has a pH of 7 and is neutral. The strongest acid has a pH of zero and the strongest alkali has a pH of 14.

Fluids presents within the body vary considerably in pH and most of them are mildly acidic or alkaline. For example pH of blood is about 7.4. Gastric juice, present in the stomach, is highly acidic, (about pH 2), the acidity being necessary for digestion of food. Urine is normally acidic but can sometimes be alkaline. It is very important that pH of blood and other blood fluids be maintained within narrow limits.

Acidosis and Alkalosis

If the body fluids become more acidic than normal the condition is called ***acidosis***. If the fluid is more alkaline than normal the condition is called ***alkalosis***.

Some of the factors responsible for these conditions are as follows.

1. CO_2 is produced by metabolism of carbohydrates and lipids. It is removed from the body by the lungs. Hypoventilation reduces excretion and tends to cause acidosis. Hyperventilation tends to produce alkalosis.
2. The pH of body fluids is kept within normal limits by ***buffers***. When H^+ ions are in excess, these get attached to some buffers and this prevents the fluid from becoming too acidic. In a similar manner OH^- (hydroxyl) ions get fixed to some buffers preventing the solution from becoming too alkaline.
   Some substances that act as buffers are phosphates, bicarbonates and certain proteins. The extent to which buffers can control pH is limited by the availability of buffers. Under certain circumstances all available buffer is used up, and further formation of acid leads to acidosis.
3. Various acids are produced by metabolism of amino acids, and by anaerobic metabolism of glucose. They are excreted through urine. Urine is acidic because renal tubules excrete H^+ ions and reabsorb HCO_3^- ions. Impaired renal excretion of H^+ ions leads to acidosis. Drugs that increase production of urine (diuretics) can produce alkalosis because of excessive loss of H^+ ions. Alkalosis can also be caused by vomiting.

SOME CLINICAL CONDITIONS

1. Inflammation of nasal mucosa (as in common cold) is called ***rhinitis***. It can be caused by a virus or by allergy.
2. Inflammation can occur in one of the paranasal sinuses (***sinusitis***), in the tonsil (***tonsillitis***), in the pharynx (***pharyngitis***), in the larynx (***laryngitis***), in the trachea (***tracheitis***), or in bronchi (***bronchitis***).
3. ***Asthma*** is a disease in which the lumen of bronchi becomes narrow (bronchospasm) so that respiration requires more effort than normal. Two types of asthma are recognised, one with onset in childhood and another that begins in later life. Some factors associated with asthma include (a) infection (b) allergy to substances in air such as dust or pollens, and (c) emotional disturbances.
4. ***Bronchiectasis*** is a condition in which there are abnormal dilatations in bronchi. These get filled with secretions and lead to chronic infection.
5. ***Emphysema*** is a condition in which bronchioles and alveoli are permanently dilated. It can occur in persons who have frequent coughing, which can be because of infection (chronic bronchitis) or of smoking.
6. ***Pneumonia***: In this condition there is inflammation in one or more lobes of a lung. Alveoli in the affected region fill with fluid. Accompanying infection of pleura causes pain in the chest wall. When bronchi are also affected the condition is called ***bronchopneumonia***. In the absence of treatment there can be destruction of lung tissue and formation of pus. A collection of pus in the lung is called a ***lung abscess***.
7. ***Tuberculosis*** (in the lungs) is one of the most serious health problems of the world. In poor countries it is a major cause of early death. However, if the disease

is recognised at an early stage, and adequate treatment given the disease is treatable in most cases.

Typically a patient complains of weakness, gradual loss of weight, persistent cough, and fever (specially in the evening). With cough, the patient brings out expectoration, and in later stages sputum contains blood. Such patients throw the germs causing tuberculosis into air, every time they cough. Other persons can get infected by inhaling infected air.

Almost all persons in India are exposed to tubercular infection in childhood. However, in most cases this primary infection is overcome by defence mechanisms of the body, and in this process the person acquires resistance to fight further exposure to infection. However, if resistance is weak, or if the person is malnourished, secondary infection can develop.

A person who has not had a primary infection has no resistance to tuberculosis. A child can be given resistance artificially by injection of BCG vaccine.

In tuberculosis, the bacilli frequently lodge themselves in the apical parts of the lung and rounded nodules, or tubercles, are formed. From here infection spreads to lymph nodes near the hilum of the lung. Infection can extend to pleura causing pleural effusion (See below). The infection can spread to the other lung, to the abdomen, and to bones (specially vertebrae). There is one form of tuberculosis that occurs in cows (bovine tuberculosis). The cow's milk can get infected and a person can get infection by drinking this milk. The Indian custom of boiling milk before use is a good preventive measure.

8. Carcinoma arising in bronchi is called ***bronchial carcinoma***.
9. Inhalation of toxic substances (e.g., sand particles, asbestos) can cause chronic disease of the lungs.
10. Obstruction of one of the large bronchi can lead to collapse of the part of the lung supplied by the bronchus.
11. The normal pleural cavity contains only a thin film of fluid that lubricates the adjacent pleural surfaces and prevents friction when the lungs expand or contract. An abnormal collection of serous fluid in the pleural cavity is called ***pleural effusion***. The pleural cavity can also contain pus (***empyema***); blood (=***haemothorax***); or air (=***pneumothorax***).

CHAPTER
16
The Alimentary Canal

The alimentary (or digestive) system includes all those structures that are concerned with eating, and the digestion and absorption of food. The system consists of an alimentary canal that starts at the ***mouth*** and ends at the ***anus***.

The external opening of the mouth is the ***oral fissure*** bounded by the upper and lower lips. Within the mouth cavity (or ***oral cavity***) there are the ***teeth*** with which food is chewed; and the ***tongue*** that helps the processes of chewing and swallowing in addition to being an organ of taste. The roof of the mouth is formed by the ***palate*** (that separates the mouth from the nasal cavities). Posteriorly, the mouth opens into the ***oral part of the pharynx***. This part of the pharynx is continuous, below, with the ***laryngeal part of the pharynx***. The latter becomes continuous with the ***oesophagus***. The oesophagus is a tube that descends through the lower part of the neck, and then through the entire length of the thorax, to pierce the diaphragm and reach the abdomen. Here the oesophagus ends by joining the ***stomach***. The stomach is a large sac-like organ that acts as a store of swallowed food. After this food is partially digested in the stomach it passes into the ***small intestine***. The small intestine is in the form of a tube about 5 meters long. It is divided, into three parts. These are the ***duodenum***, the ***jejunum*** and the ***ileum***. The small intestine is followed by the ***large intestine***. The large intestine is about one and a half meters long. Its main subdivisions are the ***caecum***, the ***ascending colon***, the ***transverse colon***, the ***descending colon***, the ***sigmoid*** (or ***pelvic***) ***colon***, the ***rectum*** and the ***anal canal***. The anal canal opens to the exterior at the ***anus***.

Closely related to the alimentary canal there are several accessory organs. In the region of the mouth there are three pairs of ***salivary glands.*** In the abdomen we have two large glands: the ***liver*** and the ***pancreas.*** These are considered in Chapter 17.

THE ORAL CAVITY & PHARYNX

A layperson uses the word 'mouth' loosely both for the external opening and for the cavity it leads to. Strictly speaking, the term mouth should be applied only to the external opening that is also called the ***oral fissure.*** The cavity (containing the tongue and teeth) is the mouth cavity or ***oral cavity***.

A basic idea of the boundaries of the oral cavity can be had from Fig. 16.1 that is a coronal section through it. Laterally the cavity is bounded by the cheeks; above by the palate (which separates it from the nasal cavity); and below it has a floor to which the tongue is attached. Projecting into the cavity (from above and below), just medial to the each cheek, there are the alveolar processes of the upper and lower jaws that bear the teeth. When the mouth is closed bringing the upper and lower teeth into apposition, the oral cavity is seen to consist of a part between the teeth of the two sides (the ***oral cavity proper***); and a part between the alveolar processes and the cheeks. The latter is called the ***vestibule***. In Fig. 16.1 the vestibule is seen in two halves right and left, but when traced anteriorly the two halves become continuous in the middle line in front of the teeth. Here the vestibule communicates with the exterior; and this part lies deep to the upper and lower lips. When the teeth are in apposition the vestibule communicates with the oral cavity proper through a space behind the last tooth. (This is a point of practical importance. It means that any liquid put into the vestibule will find its way into the mouth even if the jaws are kept closed).

The oral cavity proper communicates posteriorly with the oral part of the pharynx. The communication between the two is called the ***oropharyngeal isthmus*** (Fig. 15.7). The roof of the oral cavity is formed by the palate (described below). The chief structure in the floor is the tongue. The rest of the floor is formed by mucous membrane passing from the sides of the tongue to the gum. The anterior part of the tongue is not attached to the floor and that is why it can be protruded out of the mouth. This part of the tongue is attached to the floor by a median fold of mucosa called the ***frenulum linguae***.

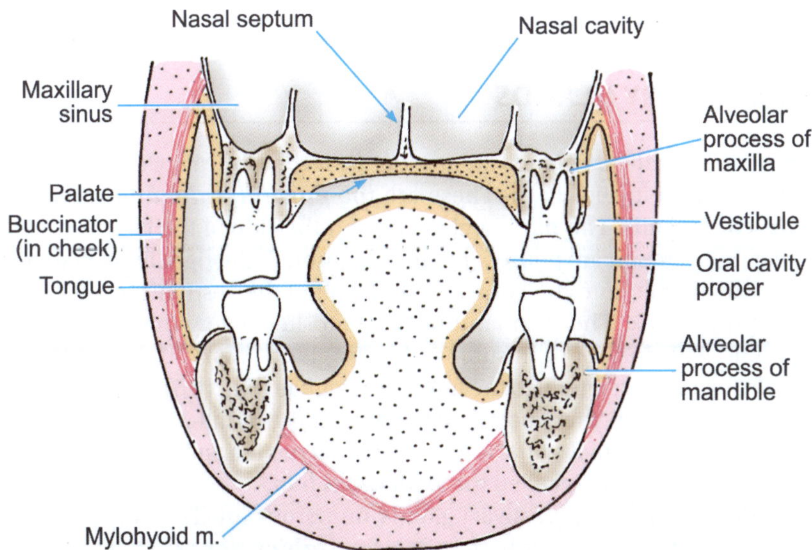

Fig. 16.1 Schematic coronal section through the oral cavity.

Lips and Cheeks

Some facts worth noting about the lips and cheeks are as follows.

The ***lips***, upper and lower, are lined on the outside by skin and on the inside by mucous membrane. The junction between the two forms the 'edge' of each lip. The substance of the lip is formed by the orbicularis oris muscle and by numerous smaller muscles that blend with it. The points, on either side, where the upper and lower lips meet are called the ***angles of the mouth***. The deep surface of each lip is connected to the gum by a median fold of mucous membrane called the ***frenulum***.

The ***cheeks*** are, like the lips, made up of an outer layer of skin, an inner layer of mucous membrane and an intervening layer of muscle, connective tissue and fat. The muscle layer is formed chiefly by the buccinator. The fat is specially prominent in infants and is responsible for the rounded appearance of the cheeks. Numerous glands are present in relationship to the lips and cheeks. They open into the vestibule of the mouth.

The Palate

The palate separates the oral cavity from the nasal cavity. It is divisible into an anterior, larger part the ***hard palate***, and a posterior part the ***soft palate***. The median part of the soft palate is prolonged downwards as a conical projection called the ***uvula***.

The lateral margins of the soft palate are continuous with two folds of mucous membrane. The anterior of these connects the palate to the lateral margin of the posterior part of the tongue and is called the ***palatoglossal fold.*** The posterior fold connects the palate to the wall of the pharynx and is called the ***palatopharyngeal fold*** (Fig. 15.7). The palatine tonsil is lodged in the interval between these folds.

THE SALIVARY GLANDS

Three pairs of salivary glands are present near the oral cavity and pour their secretions into it (Fig. 16.2). These are the ***parotid***, ***submandibular*** and ***sublingual*** glands. The parotid gland lies on the side of the face just below the ear. Its secretion are poured into mouth through the right and left parotid ducts which open into the corresponding half of the vestibule, on the inner side of the cheek. The submandibular gland lies below the ramus of the mandible. The duct for each submandibular gland opens on the ***sublingual papilla*** located just lateral to the frenulum linguae (Fig. 16.5). The sublingual glands lie just below the mucosa on the floor of the mouth. Each gland raises a ridge of mucosa which starts at the sublingual papilla and runs laterally and backwards. This ridge is called the ***sublingual fold***.

In addition to the main salivary glands, numerous small salivary glands are situated in the mucous membrane of the lips (***labial glands***), cheeks (***buccal glands***), tongue (***lingual glands***), and palate (***palatine glands***).

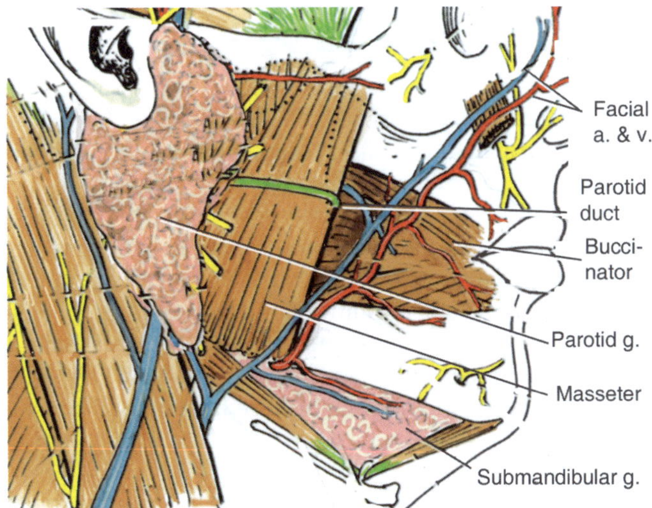

Fig. 16.2 Diagram of side of face showing the location of the parotid and submandibular salivary glands.

Histology of Salivary Glands

Salivary glands are compound tubulo-alveolar glands (racemose glands). Their secretory elements may be rounded (acini), pear shaped (alveoli), tubular, or a mixture of these (tubulo-acinar, tubulo-alveolar). The secretory elements lead into a series of ducts through which their secretions are poured into the oral cavity. In sections through salivary glands we see a large number of closely packed acini (or alveoli) with ducts scattered between them (Fig. 16.3). These elements are supported by connective tissue that also divides the glands into lobules, and forms capsules around them. Blood vessels, lymphatics and nerves run in the connective tissue.

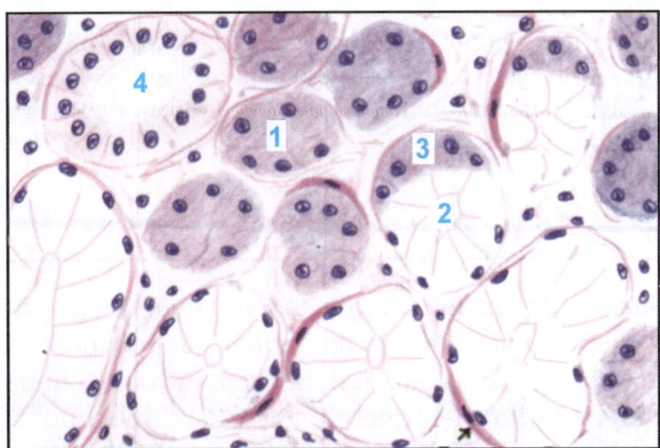

Fig. 16.3 Section through submandibular gland. 1-Serous acinus. 2-Mucous acinus. 3. Demilune. 4. Duct.

The cells lining the alveoli of salivary glands are usually described either as ***serous*** or ***mucous***. In sections serous cells stain darkly. They have rounded nuclei that lie towards the base. In contrast mucous cells stain very lightly and, therefore, appear empty. The cells are in fact almost completely filled in by a mucoid material that stains very poorly (Fig. 16.3). This material pushes the nuclei towards the basement membrane.

An alveolus is typically made up entirely of serous cells or of mucous cells. However, in some cases mucous alveoli are covered (on one or more sides) by groups of serous cells that are arranged in the form of ***crescents*** or ***demilunes***. In the parotid gland the alveoli are almost entirely serous, only an occasional mucous alveolus being present. In the submandibular gland some alveoli are serous and some are mucous, the latter being frequently capped by serous crescents. The sublingual glands are made up predominantly of mucous alveoli.

Saliva

Saliva is secreted by salivary glands. About 1.5 litres of saliva is produced every day. Saliva consists of water (98%), mineral salts and mucous. The proportion of these is variable. Secretion of the parotid glands is serous. That of the sublingual glands is mucous, and that of the submandibular glands is mixed. The main function of saliva is to keep the mouth moist. This helps in chewing of food and formation of a bolus. By dissolving food it makes the appreciation of taste possible. Moisture in the mouth is essential for speech. Saliva is the natural way to keep the mouth clean by washing away particles of food. If some irritating substance enters the mouth, thick saliva rich in mucous is produced to counter the irritation.

Saliva contains an enzyme ***amylase*** that acts on polysaccharides and breaks them down to maltose. Action of this enzyme continues till food enters the stomach.

Saliva also contains lysozyme, immunoglobulin, and clotting factors that act against bacteria.

Secretion of Saliva

A small quantity of saliva is secreted constantly. The quantity increases considerably when there is food in the mouth. Impulses arising from receptors in the mouth travel to salivatory nuclei in the brainstem. Parasympathetic nerve fibres arising in these nuclei reach the salivary glands through the facial and glossopharyngeal nerves, and stimulate secretion. The sight and smell of good food can produce salivary secretion through a conditioned reflex.

THE TEETH

As the teeth can be seen and felt some facts about them are commonly known. We know that the newborn have no teeth; that the first tooth appears when the infant is about six months old; that the teeth in young children gradually fall off and are replaced by new ones that can last throughout life. The teeth that appear in children and fall off with time are called ***deciduous*** (or milk) teeth. The teeth of the second set that gradually replace the deciduous teeth constitute the ***permanent*** teeth.

The teeth, both deciduous and permanent, have varying shapes. Some have sharp cutting edges and are, therefore, called ***incisors***. Others are sharp and pointed: these are called ***canines*** as they form the most prominent teeth in canine species (e.g., dogs). Still others have edges suitable for a grinding function: these are called ***molars***. In the permanent set we also have grinding teeth that are somewhat smaller than the molars and are called the ***premolars*** (as they lie in front of the molars).

A set of deciduous teeth consists of the following. Beginning from the middle line (in front) there is a central incisor, a lateral incisor (i.e., two incisors); one canine; and two molars (distinguished from each other by being called the first and second molars). There are, thus, five teeth in each half of each jaw i.e., twenty in all.

A set of permanent teeth consists of the following. Beginning from the middle line there is a central incisor, a lateral incisor, a canine, two premolars (first and second, that replace the deciduous molars), and three molars (first, second and third). Thus in each half of each jaw there are eight teeth, or thirty two in all.

Structure of a Typical Tooth

A tooth consists of an upper part, the ***crown***, which is seen in the mouth; and of one or more ***roots*** that are embedded in sockets in the jaw bone (mandible or maxilla). The greater part of the tooth is made up of a bone like material called ***dentine***. Dentine lying in the crown is covered by a much harder white material called the ***enamel***. Dentine forming the root is covered by a thin layer of ***cement***. The cement is united to the wall of the bony socket in the jaw through a layer of fibrous tissue called the ***periodontal ligament***. The soft tissue covering the external surface of the alveolar process is the gum. The gum normally overlaps the lower edge of the crown. Within the dentine there is a ***pulp canal*** that contains a mass of cells, blood vessels and nerves that constitute the pulp. The blood vessels and nerves enter the pulp canal at the apex of the root through an ***apical foramen***.

THE TONGUE

The tongue lies in the oral cavity. The anterior part of the tongue (or ***apex***) can be protruded out of the mouth. It has free upper and lower surfaces. The greater part of the tongue is attached below to the floor of the mouth. The attached part is called the ***root*** of the tongue. This part of the tongue has a free upper surface or ***dorsum***. On either side, the tongue has ***lateral edges*** that are also free. The free surfaces of the tongue are lined by mucous membrane. The substance of the tongue is made up mainly of muscle.

The tongue helps in mastication by pushing food between the upper and lower teeth. It converts chewed food into a rounded bolus. It plays an essential role in swallowing (see below). Because of the presence of taste buds it acts as the main organ of taste.

Features on the Dorsum of the Tongue

The features seen when the tongue is viewed from above, are shown in Fig. 16.4. Some features present on the lower aspect of the anterior part of the tongue are shown in Fig. 16.5.

The upper surface (or ***dorsum***) is seen in Fig. 16.4. Identify the anterior end or ***apex***, and the lateral edges. Near its posterior end the dorsum of the tongue is marked by a V-shaped groove called the ***sulcus terminalis***. The apex of the 'V' points backwards and is marked by a depression called the ***foramen caecum***. The limbs of the sulcus terminalis runs forwards and laterally to the lateral margin of the tongue. The sulcus terminalis divides the dorsum into an anterior larger part (two thirds) and a posterior smaller part (one third). The anterior part lies in the oral cavity and is, therefore, called the ***oral part.*** It faces upwards and comes into contact with the palate. The posterior one third faces backwards and is called the ***pharyngeal part***.

The mucous membrane covering the oral part of the dorsum of the tongue is rough because of the presence of numerous finger like projections or ***papillae***. The largest of these papillae are seen in a row just in front of the sulcus limitans. These are the ***vallate*** papillae. Other papillae present on the tongue are described as ***fungiform***. They are present at the apex and along the sides of the tongue. The most numerous papillae are small and conical in shape. They are called ***filiform*** papillae (Fig. 16.6).

The ***pharyngeal part of the tongue*** faces backwards and forms part of the anterior wall of the oropharynx. Its surface is not covered by papillae. However,

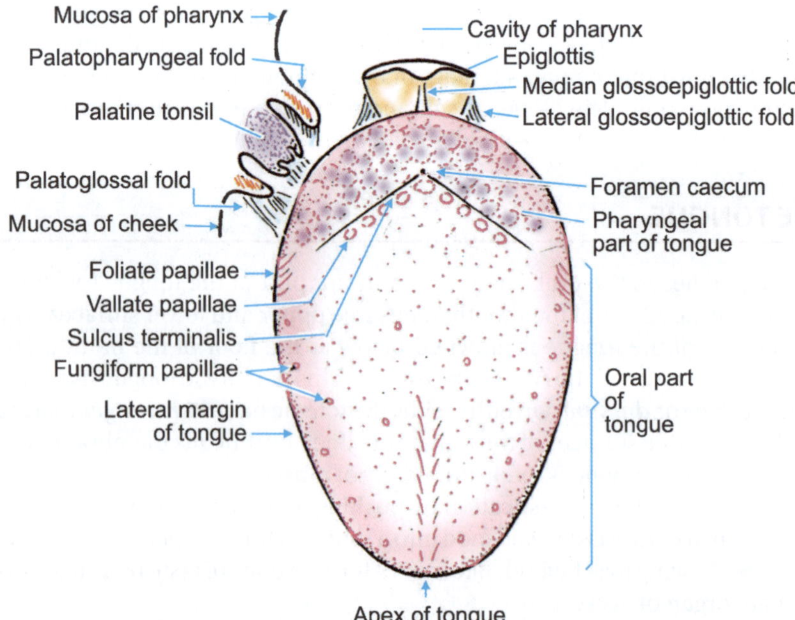

Fig. 16.4 Tongue and some related structures seen from above.

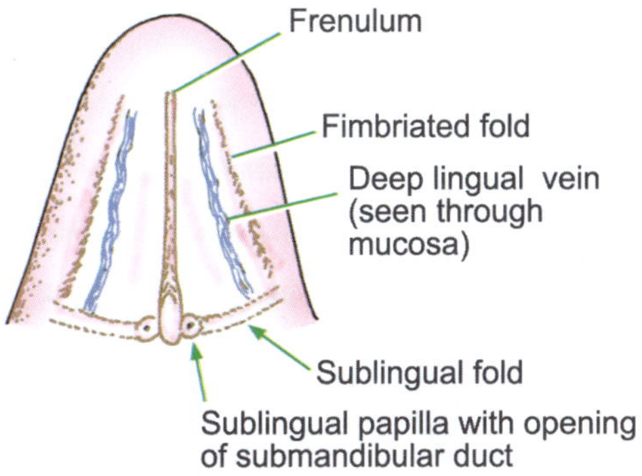

Fig. 16.5 Some structures seen on the undersurface of the anterior part of the tongue.

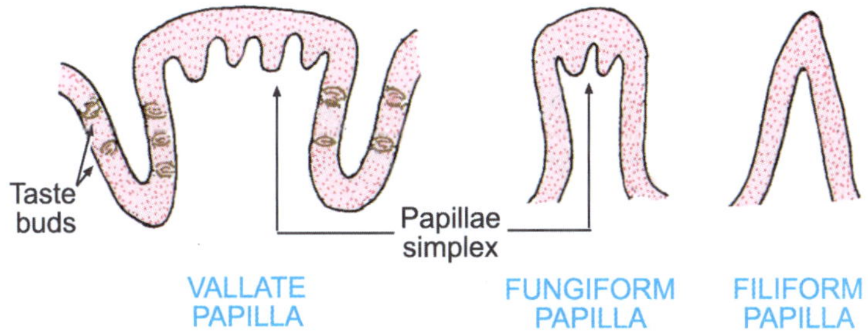

Fig. 16.6 Various kinds of papillae to be seen on the surface of the tongue.

it shows a number of rounded elevations which are produced by collections of lymphoid tissue lying deep to the mucosa. This lymphoid tissue is referred to, collectively, as the ***lingual tonsil***.

The tongue bears ***taste buds*** that are end organs for taste. Sensations of taste from the anterior two-thirds of the tongue travel through the lingual nerve. Those for the posterior one third of the tongue pass through the glossopharyngeal nerve.

The movements of the tongue are produced by a number of muscles (Fig. 16.7). Some of these are intrinsic: they lie entirely within the tongue. In addition, there are extrinsic muscles that enter the tongue from outside. These muscles are responsible for various movements of the tongue. They are supplied by the hypoglossal nerve.

THE PHARYNX

The pharynx is a median passage that is common to the alimentary and respiratory systems (Fig. 15.1). It is divisible (from above downwards) into a

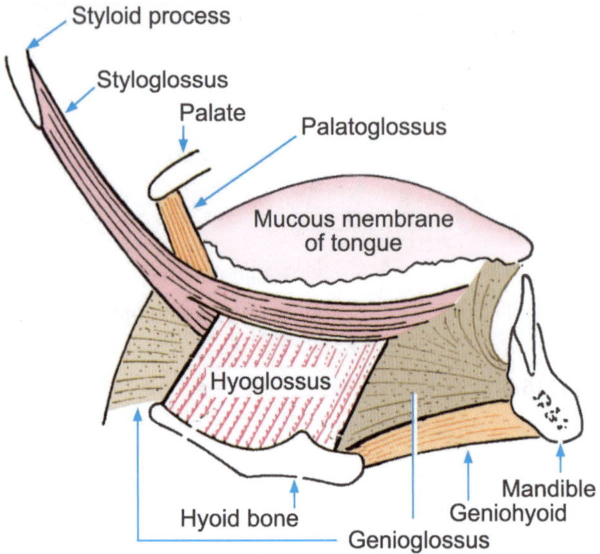

Fig. 16.7 Some muscles of the tongue.

nasal part (or ***nasopharynx***) into which the nasal cavities open; an ***oral part*** (or ***oropharynx***) which is continuous with the posterior end of the oral cavity; and a ***laryngeal part*** (or ***laryngopharynx***) which is continuous in front with the larynx, and below with oesophagus. The pharynx has been described in Chapter 15.

Swallowing or Deglutition

1. After food has been adequately chewed, and moistened by saliva, it is shaped (by pressure of tongue and cheeks) into a rounded mass or bolus.
2. The mouth closes and the tongue pushes the bolus into the pharynx.
3. Food entering the oropharynx is carried downwards by contraction of constrictor muscles present in the wall of the pharynx. Other muscles running longitudinally help by pulling the pharynx upwards and by shortening it.
   The communication between oropharynx and nasopharynx is called the ***pharyngeal isthmus***. This opening can be closed by the soft palate helped by the action of a ***palatopharyngeal sphincter***. Closure of the pharyngeal isthmus presents food from entering the nasopharynx. Food is also prevented from going into the larynx, or back into the mouth, by the actions of muscles that close these communications.
4. Contractions of pharyngeal muscles push food into the oesophagus. Once food enters the oesophagus, peristaltic contractions of muscle in its wall move food along its length until it reaches the stomach.
   Circular muscle present at the junction of pharynx and oesophagus, acts as a sphincter and prevents air from entering the oesophagus. However, some air does enter along with food.

BASIC PATTERN OF THE STRUCTURE OF THE ALIMENTARY CANAL

The structure of the alimentary canal, from the oesophagus up to the anal canal, shows several features that are common to all these parts. We shall consider these common features before examining the individual parts of the canal.

The walls of the oral cavity, and of the pharynx are partly bony, and partly muscular. However, from the upper end of the oesophagus up to the lower end of the anal canal the alimentary canal has the form of a fibro-muscular tube. The wall of the tube is made up of the following layers (from inner to outer side) (Fig. 16.8).

A. The innermost layer is the ***mucous membrane*** that is made up of:
   a. A lining epithelium.
   b. A layer of connective tissue, the ***lamina propria***, that supports the epithelium.
   c. A thin layer of smooth muscle called the ***muscularis mucosae***.
B. The mucous membrane rests on a layer of loose areolar tissue called the ***submucosa***.
C. The gut wall derives its main strength and form because of a thick layer of muscle (***muscularis externa***) that surrounds the submucosa.
D. Covering the muscularis externa there is a ***serous layer*** or (alternatively) an ***adventitial layer***.

Some general features of these layers are briefly considered below.

It may be noted at the outset that the oesophagus and anal canal are merely transport passages. The part of the alimentary canal from the stomach to the rectum is the proper digestive tract, responsible for digestion and absorption of food. Reabsorption of secreted fluids is an important function of the large intestine.

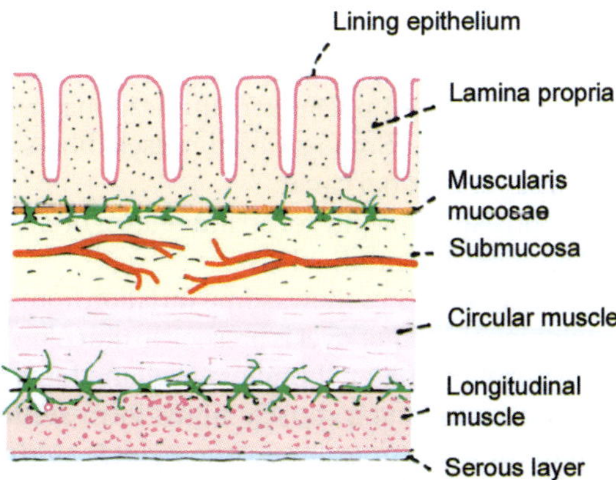

Fig. 16.8 Scheme to show the layers of the gut. Note the large blood vessels in the submucosa; the myenteric nerve plexus between the longitudinal and circular layers of muscle; and the subcutaneous nerve plexus near the muscularis mucosae.

The Lining Epithelium

The lining epithelium is columnar all over the gut; except in the oesophagus, and in the lower part of the anal canal, where it is stratified squamous. This stratified squamous epithelium has a protective function in these situations. The cells of the more typical columnar epithelium are either absorptive or secretory.

The epithelium of the gut presents an extensive absorptive surface. The factors contributing to the extent of the surface are as follows.

1. The ***considerable length*** of the alimentary canal, and specially that of the small intestine.
2. The presence of ***numerous folds*** involving the entire thickness of the mucous membrane. These folds can be seen by naked eye.
3. At numerous places the epithelium dips into the lamina propria forming ***crypts*** (see below).
4. In the small intestine the mucosa bears numerous finger-like processes that project into the lumen. These processes are called ***villi***. Each villus has a surface lining of epithelium and a core formed by connective tissue.
5. The luminal surfaces of the epithelial cells bear numerous microvilli.

The epithelium of the gut also performs a very important secretory function. The secretory cells are arranged in the form of numerous glands as follows.

a. Some glands are unicellular, the secretory cells being scattered among the cells of the lining epithelium.
b. In many situations, the epithelium dips into the lamina propria forming simple tubular glands. (These are the crypts referred to above).
c. In other situations (e.g., in the duodenum) there are glands lying in the submucosa. They open into the lumen of the gut through ducts traversing the mucosa.

The Muscularis Externa

Over the greater part of the gut the muscularis externa consists of smooth muscle. The only exception is the upper part of the oesophagus where this layer contains striated muscle fibres. Some striated muscle fibres are also closely associated with the wall of the anal canal.

The muscle layer consists (typically) of an inner layer of circularly arranged muscle fibres, and an outer longitudinal layer.

The arrangement of muscle fibres shows some variation from region to region. In the stomach an additional oblique layer is present. In the colon the longitudinal fibres are gathered to form prominent bundles called the ***taenia coli***.

Localised thickenings of circular muscle fibres form ***sphincters*** that can occlude the lumen of the gut. For example, the ***pyloric sphincter*** is present around the pyloric end of the stomach, and the ***internal anal sphincter*** surrounds the anal canal. A functional sphincter is seen at the junction of the oesophagus with the stomach. A valvular arrangement at the ileocaecal junction (ileocaecal valve) prevents regurgitation of caecal contents into the ileum.

Nerve Plexuses

The gut is richly supplied with nerves. A number of nerve plexuses are present as follows.

a. The ***myenteric plexus*** (***of Auerbach***) lies between the circular and longitudinal coats of muscle.
b. The ***submucosal plexus*** (***of Meissner***) lies in the submucosa (near its junction with the circular muscle layer).

INDIVIDUAL PARTS OF THE ALIMENTARY CANAL

THE OESOPHAGUS

The oesophagus is a tubular structure that starts at the lower end of the oropharynx. It descends through the lower part of the neck, and enters the thorax through its inlet. After passing through the thorax the oesophagus enters the abdomen. After a very short course through the abdomen it ends by joining the cardiac end of the stomach.

Histology of Oesophagus

The ***mucosa*** is lined by stratified squamous epithelium (Fig. 16.9). The ***muscle layer*** consists of the usual circular and longitudinal layers. However, it is unusual in that the muscle fibres are partly striated and partly smooth. In the upper one third (or so) of the oesophagus the muscle fibres are entirely of the striated variety, while in the lower one third all the fibres are of the smooth variety. Both types of fibres are present in the middle one third of the oesophagus.

The circular muscle fibres present at the lower end of the oesophagus possibly act as a sphincter guarding the cardiooesophageal junction.

THE STOMACH

The stomach is a sac like structure that serves as a reservoir of swallowed food, and plays an important part in digesting it. It has a capacity of about one litre. It is the most dilated part of the alimentary canal. Its shape varies considerably depending upon whether it is full or empty; and is also influenced by posture. However, for purposes of description we can presume it to have the form shown in Fig. 16.10. The cranial end of the stomach is continuous with the oesophagus. As this end lies close to the heart it is named the ***cardiac end***.

The caudal end of the stomach is continuous with the duodenum. This end is called the ***pyloric end***, or simply the ***pylorus***. The stomach has two surfaces, anterior and posterior. These surfaces meet at a concave upper border, and at

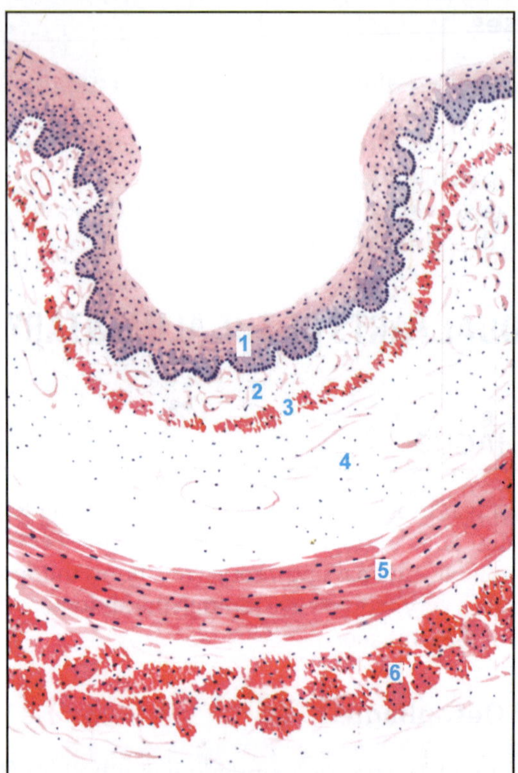

Fig. 16.9 Section through oesophagus. 1-Stratified squamous epithelium. 2-Lamina propria. 3-Muscularis mucosae. 4-Submucosa. 5-Circular muscle. 6-Longitudinal muscle.

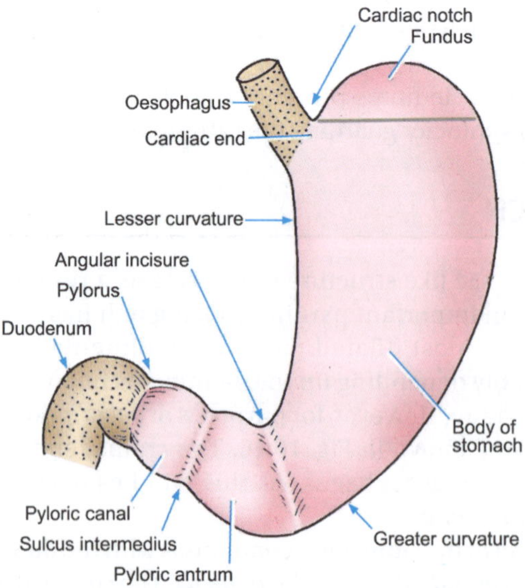

Fig. 16.10 Subdivisions of the stomach.

a lower border that is convex. The concave upper border is called the ***lesser curvature***, and the convex lower border is called the ***greater curvature***.

The stomach is divided into a number of parts as follows (Fig. 16.10).

a. At the junction of the left margin of the oesophagus with the greater curvature of the stomach there is a deep ***cardiac notch***. Because of the upward convexity of the adjoining part of the greater curvature a part of the stomach lies above the level of the cardio-oesophageal junction. This part of the stomach is called the ***fundus***.
b. We have seen that the upper part of the lesser curvature faces to the right, while its lower part faces upwards. The junction of these two parts of the curvature is often marked by a notch called the ***angular incisure***. The part of the stomach to the left of the incisure is more or less rounded and is called the ***body*** (excluding the part already defined as the fundus).
c. The part of the stomach to the right of the angular incisure is the ***pyloric part***. It consists of a relatively dilated left part (continuous with the body) called the ***pyloric antrum***; and a narrower right part called the ***pyloric canal***.

The position of the stomach relative to the surface of the body is shown in Fig. 16.11. The cardiac end (or orifice) is situated to the left of the median plane, behind the left seventh costal cartilage. The pylorus (or pyloric orifice) lies to the right of the midline. The highest part of the stomach is the fundus. It reaches the left fifth intercostal space, just below the nipple. The lowest part of the stomach is formed by the pyloric antrum. In the full stomach it may lie below the level of the umbilicus.

The shape of the stomach can be studied in the living by taking skiagrams after giving a meal containing barium sulphate (***barium meal***). Commonly the stomach is J-shaped having a long vertical part (above and to the left) and a shorter horizontal part (below and to the right) (Fig. 16.12B).

Sometimes the stomach may be orientated almost transversely. This is described as a ***steer-horn*** type of stomach (Fig. 16.12A).

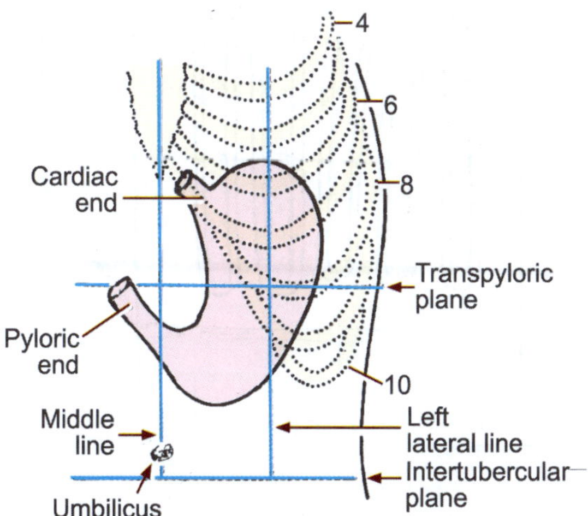

Fig. 16.11 Surface projection of the stomach.

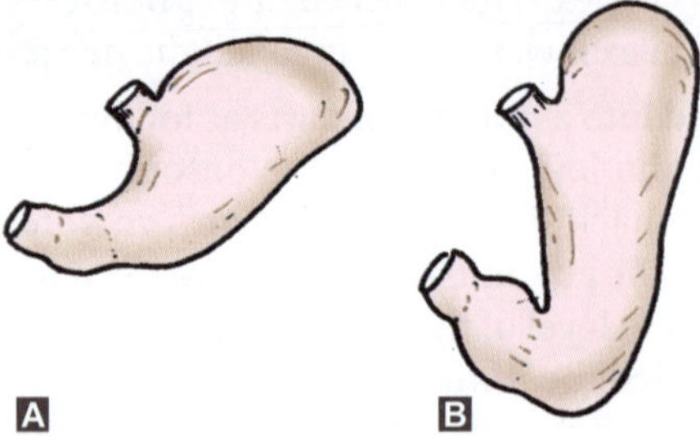

Fig. 16.12 A. Steerhorn stomach; B. J-shaped stomach.

Histology of Stomach

The wall of the stomach has the four basic layers described above: a mucous membrane, a submucosa, a muscularis externa, and a serous layer (Fig. 16.13). The mucous membrane and the muscularis externa have some special features that are described below.

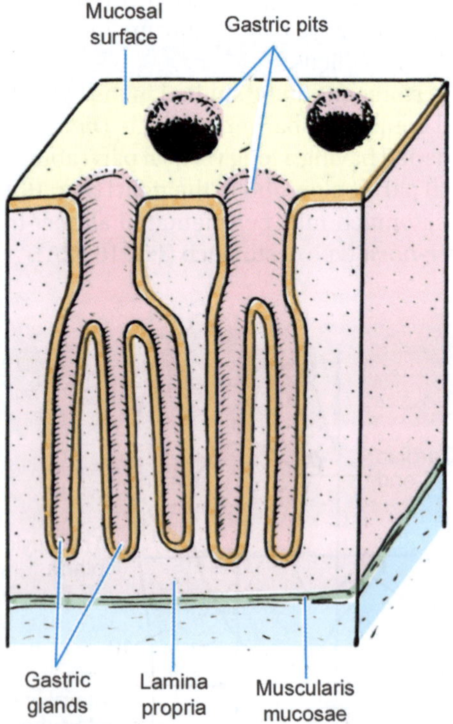

Fig. 16.13 Scheme to show the basic structure of the mucous membrane of the stomach.

As seen with the naked eye the mucous membrane shows numerous folds (or ***rugae***) that disappear when the stomach is distended. The lining epithelium is columnar and mucous secreting. The apical parts of the lining cells are filled by mucin. Mucous secreted by cells of the lining epithelium protects the gastric mucosa against acid and enzymes produced by the mucosa itself.

At numerous places the lining epithelium dips into the lamina propria to form the walls of depressions called ***gastric pits***. These pits extend for a variable distance into the thickness of the mucosa. Deep to the gastric pits the mucous membrane is packed with numerous ***gastric glands***. These glands are of three types: main gastric, cardiac and pyloric.

The ***main gastric glands*** are present over most of the stomach, but not in the pyloric region and in a small area near the cardiac end. The main gastric glands open into gastric pits, each pit receiving the openings of several glands. Here the gastric pits occupy the superficial one fourth or less of the mucosa, the remaining thickness being closely packed with gastric glands. The following varieties of cells are present in the epithelium lining the glands (Fig. 16.14).

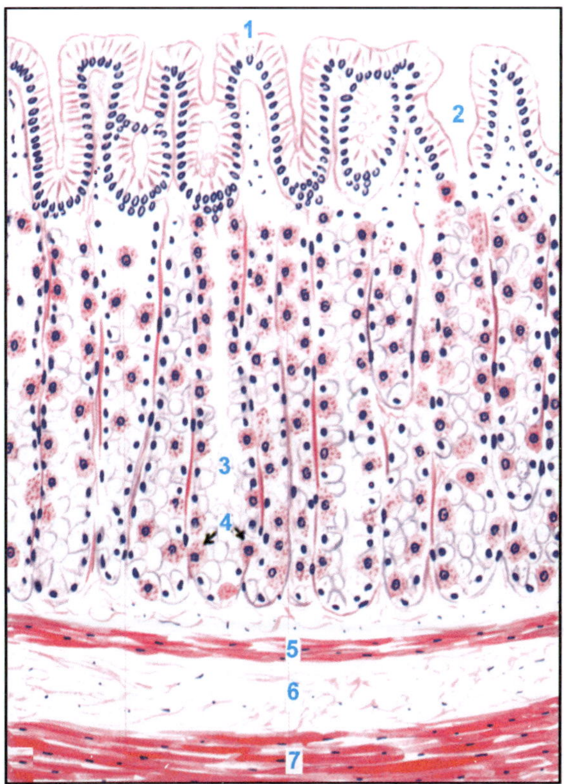

Fig. 16.14 Section through body of the stomach. 1-Lining by columnar epithelium. 2-Gastric pit. 3-Gastric glands. 4-Oxyntic cells. 5-Muscularis mucosae. 6-Submucosa. 7-Circular muscle.

a. The most numerous cells are called ***chief cells***, ***peptic cells***, or ***zymogen cells***. Chief cells secrete the digestive enzymes of the stomach including pepsin. Pepsin is produced by action of gastric acid on pepsinogen. Pepsin breaks down proteins into small peptides. It is mainly through the action of pepsin that solid food is liquefied.

b. The ***oxyntic*** or ***parietal cells*** are large, with a large central nucleus. They are present singly, amongst the peptic cells. Oxyntic cells are responsible for the secretion of hydrochloric acid. They also produce an ***intrinsic factor*** that combines with vitamin B_{12} (present in ingested food and constituting an ***extrinsic factor***) to form a complex necessary for normal formation of erythrocytes.

c. Near the upper end (or 'neck') of the glands there are mucous secreting cells that are called ***mucous neck cells***.

d. Near the basal parts of the gastric glands there are ***endocrine cells.*** These cells probably secrete the hormone ***gastrin***. Some of the cells can be shown to contain serotonin (5HT).

The ***cardiac glands*** are confined to a small area near the opening of the oesophagus. They are mucous secreting. An occasional oxyntic or peptic cell may be present (Fig. 16.15).

In the pyloric region of the stomach the gastric pits are deep and occupy two thirds of the depth of the mucosa (Fig. 16.16). The ***pyloric glands*** that open into these pits are short and occupy the deeper one third of the mucosa. The

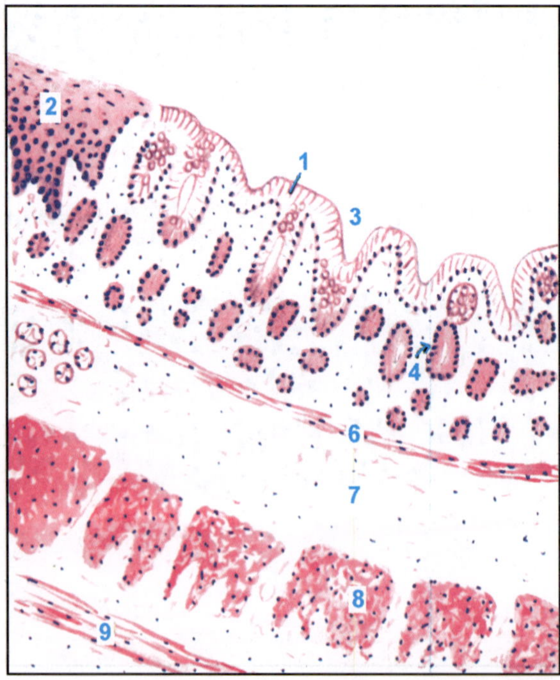

Fig. 16.15 Stomach, cardiac end. 1-Columnar epithelium. 2-Stratified squamus lining of lower end of oesophagus. 3-Gastric pit. 4-Cardiac gland. 5-Oesophageal gland. 6-Muscularis mucosae. 7-Submucosa. 8-Circular muscle. 9-Longitudinal muscle.

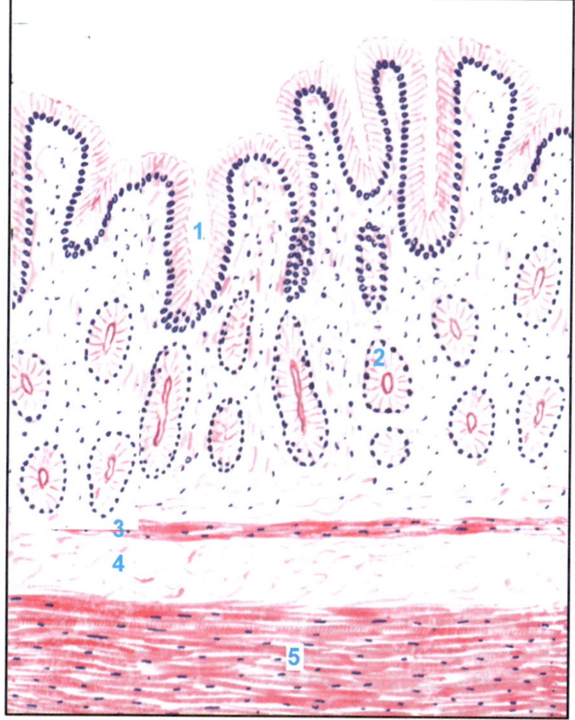

Fig. 16.16 Stomach, pyloric part. 1-Gastric pit. 2-Pyloric gland. 3-Muscularis mucosae. 4-Submucosa. 5. Circular muscle.

glands are lined by mucous secreting cells. Occasional oxyntic and endocrine cells may be present. In addition to other substances, pyloric glands secrete the hormone gastrin.

The ***muscularis externa*** of the stomach is well developed. Three layers, oblique, circular and longitudinal (from inside out) are usually described. The circular fibres are greatly thickened at the pylorus where they form the pyloric sphincter.

Functions of the Stomach

The stomach is a reservoir for food. Its average capacity is between 1-1.5 litres.

Contractions of stomach muscle churn up the food and thoroughly mix it up with gastric juice secreted by the stomach, and thus liquefy it. The enzyme ***pepsin*** present in gastric juice is useful in digestion of proteins, which are broken down into polypeptides.

Gastric juice is highly acidic. The acid helps in digestion. It also kills microorganisms that enter the stomach.

The stomach plays an important role in digestion and absorption of iron. Hydrochloric acid dissolves iron salts.

After food is thoroughly liquefied, and has been acidified, it passes into the duodenum.

Gastric juice also contains ***intrinsic factor***, which is necessary for absorption of vitamin B_{12}. Some mineral salts are also present.

Mucous protects the wall of the stomach from mechanical injury and from harmful effects of hydrochloric acid.

Gastric Secretion

Glands present in gastric mucosa produce about 2.5 litres of gastric juice every day. The composition of gastric juice is as follows.

1. Water.
2. Mucous.
3. Hydrochloric acid.
4. Pepsinogen, a proteolytic enzyme precursor.
5. Inorganic ions.
6. Intrinsic factor essential for absorption of vitamin B_{12}.

Mucous is secreted by surface epithelium, and by cells lining the gastric pits. These cells also produce bicarbonate. Alkaline mucous protects gastric mucosa from the corrosive effect of hydrochloric acid.

Hydrochloric acid is secreted by the parietal (or oxyntic) cells of gastric glands. In production of HCl water is dissociated into H^+ and OH^- ions. The H^+ ions pass out of the cells by active transport. Chloride ions are also added by active transport. Acid secretion is increased by histamine, by acetyl choline, by gastrin and by vagal stimulation.

Intrinsic factor produced by parietal cells is a glycoprotein. Its presence is essential for absorption of vitamin B_{12}. Absence of this factor leads to perniceous anaemia.

Secretion of Pepsinogen

Pepsinogen is secreted by chief cells (peptic cells). It is stored in zymogen granules of these cells. Secretion is increased by vagal stimulation, by gastrin, and by histamine. Hydrochloric acids acts on pepsinogen and converts it into pepsin. Pepsin is a proteolytic enzyme. It splits proteins into proteoses, peptones and polypeptides.

Control of Gastric Secretion

1. Vagal stimulation (acting through nerve plexuses in the wall of the stomach) increases secretion of HCl, and of pepsin.
2. Vagal stimulation also acts indirectly by release of gastrin. Gastrin is also released by presence of partially digested proteins (peptides and amino acids) in the stomach. Gastrin is released by gastrin producing cells into blood and reaches the gastric mucosa through arterial blood. It stimulates secretion of HCl and of pepsin.
3. Presence of food, and gastric distension, stimulate secretion through stretch receptors present in the wall of the stomach.
4. Secretion of gastric juice is inhibited by some hormones, produced by the intestine. These are secretin, cholecystokinin, and gastric inhibitor peptide.

Apart from secretion of gastric juice the stomach acts as a store of ingested food. Peristaltic movements of the stomach mix food thoroughly with gastric juice. They empty the stomach after digestion of food has been completed.

THE SMALL INTESTINE

The small intestine is a tube about five meters long. It is divided into three parts. These are (in craniocaudal sequence) the ***duodenum*** (about 25 cm long); the ***jejunum*** (about 2 meters long); and the ***ileum*** (about 3 meters long). We will first consider the gross anatomy of these parts and then consider the histology of the small intestine.

The Duodenum

The duodenum forms the first 25 cm (10 inches) of the small intestine. It is in the form of a roughly C-shaped loop which is retroperitoneal and, therefore, fixed to the posterior abdominal wall. It is continuous at its cranial end with the stomach. The junction between the two is called the ***pyloroduodenal junction***. At its caudal end, the duodenum becomes continuous with the jejunum at the ***duodenojejunal flexure***.

The duodenum is subdivided into four parts as follows (Fig. 16.17). The ***first*** or ***superior part*** begins at the pylorus and passes backwards, upwards and to the right. It is about 5 cm long. The ***second or descending part*** is about 8 cm long. It passes downwards (with a slight convexity to the right). The ***third*** or ***horizontal part*** is about 10 cm long. It passes from right to left (with a slight downward convexity) and crosses the midline at the level of the third lumbar vertebra. The ***fourth*** or ***ascending part*** is about 2 cm long. It runs upwards and to the left and ends by joining the jejunum at the duodenojejunal flexure. The junction of the superior and descending parts of the duodenum is called the ***superior duodenal flexure***; while that between the descending and horizontal part is called the ***inferior duodenal flexure***.

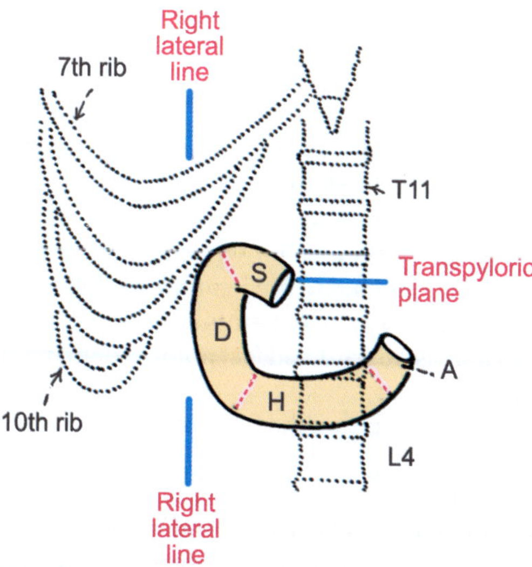

Fig. 16.17 Parts of the duodenum and their surface projection. S= superior part; D= descending part; H= horizontal part; A= ascending part.

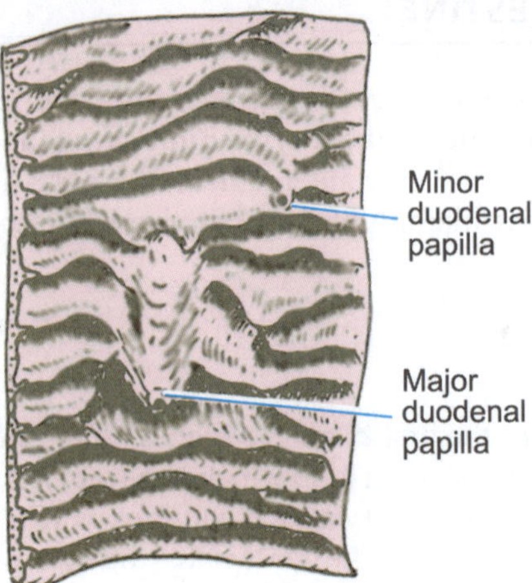

Fig. 16.18 Interior of the descending part of the duodenum showing the major and minor papillae. Note the transverse folds of the mucous membrane.

Features on Interior of Duodenum

As in the rest of the small intestine the mucous membrane of the duodenum is marked by transverse folds (Fig. 16.18). In the posterolateral portion of the descending part the mucous membrane also shows a prominent vertical fold. The lower part of this fold is marked by a projection called the ***major duodenal papilla***. The papilla bears an opening of a common channel, the ***hepatopancreatic ampulla***, into which the bile duct and the main pancreatic duct open. A short distance cranial to, and in front of, the major duodenal papilla there is a smaller projection called the ***minor duodenal papilla***. The minor papilla has an opening for the accessory pancreatic duct.

The Jejunum and Ileum

The jejunum and ileum are in the form of a long coiled tube suspended from the posterior abdominal wall by ***the*** mesentery (Note: Any fold of peritoneum attaching an organ to the abdominal wall is a mesentery, and such folds are given different names. However, when we refer only to the mesentery the reference is to the fold connected to the jejunum and ileum). The jejunum is proximal to the ileum. It is about two meters long, whereas the ileum is about three meters long. There is no hard and fast point of demarcation between the jejunum and ileum.

They are distinguished mainly on the basis of the structure of their walls. The mucous membrane of the jejunum is marked by the presence of numerous, large, transverse, folds (Figs. 16.19, 16.20). These are few or absent in the ileum. The submucosa of the ileum contains large aggregations of lymphoid tissue that can be seen with the naked eye and are called the ***aggregated lymphatic follicles*** or ***Peyer's patches***. There are no such patches in the proximal jejunum. The distal jejunum has some patches, but these are smaller and fewer than those in the ileum.

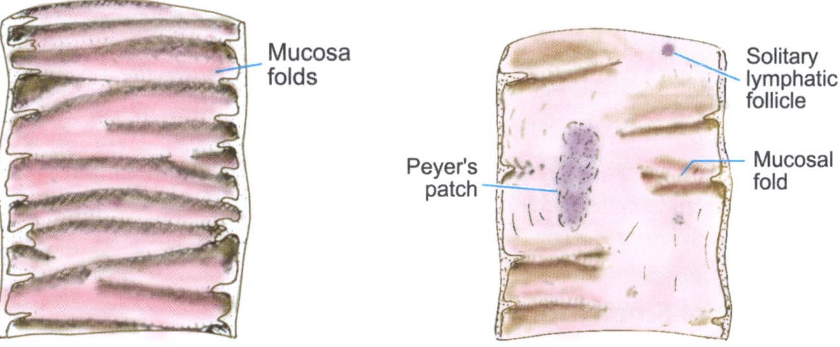

Fig. 16.19 Internal surface of part of jejunum.

Fig. 16.20 Internal surface of part of ileum.

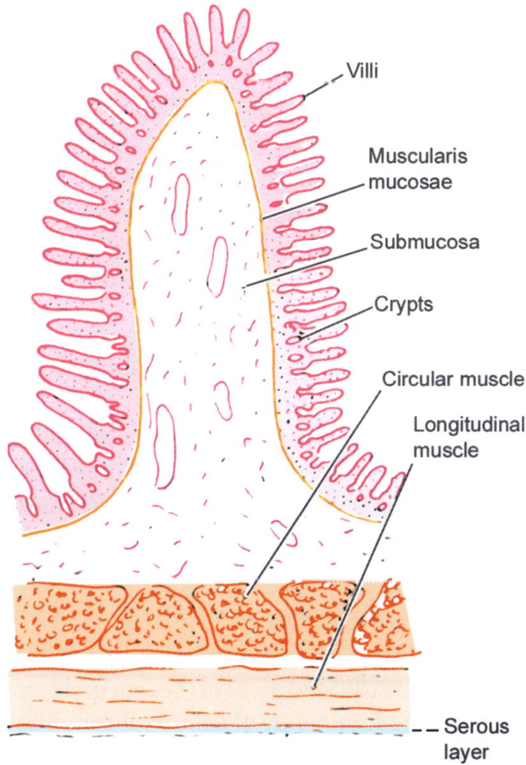

Fig. 16.21 Longitudinal section through a part of the small intestine seen at a very low magnification to show a mucosal fold.

The Mesentery

We have seen that the fold of peritoneum through which coils of jejunum and ileum are suspended from the posterior abdominal wall is called ***the*** mesentery. The attachment of the mesentery to the posterior abdominal wall is referred to as the ***root*** of the mesentery. The root is about 15 cm long. When traced towards the gut the mesentery increases very greatly in length so that it can give attachment to the entire length of the jejunum and ileum (which we have seen is about five meters).

Histology of Small Intestine

The wall of the small intestine is made up of the usual four layers: serous, muscular, submucous, and mucous. The mucous membrane exhibits several special features that are described below.

The Mucous Membrane

The surface area of the mucous membrane of the small intestine is extensive (to allow adequate absorption of food). This is achieved by virtue of the following.

a. The considerable length of the intestine.
b. The presence of numerous circular folds in the mucosa (Figs. 16.21, 16.22).
c. The presence of numerous finger-like processes, or ***villi***, that project from the surface of the mucosa into the lumen.
d. The presence of numerous depressions or ***crypts*** that invade the lamina propria.
e. The presence of microvilli on the luminal surfaces of the cells lining the mucosa.

The ***villi*** are, typically, finger like projections consisting of a core of reticular tissue covered by a surface epithelium. The connective tissue core contains numerous blood capillaries. Each villus contains a central lymphatic vessel called a lacteal. It has been estimated that the presence of villi increases the surface area of the epithelial lining of the small intestine about eight times.

The crypts are tubular invaginations of the epithelium into the lamina propria. They are really simple tubular ***intestinal glands*** that are lined by epithelium.

The Epithelial Lining

The epithelium covering the villi, and areas of the mucosal surface intervening between them, consists predominantly of columnar cells that are specialised for absorption. These are called ***enterocytes.*** Scattered amongst the columnar cells there are mucous secreting goblet cells. Most of the cells lining the crypts (intestinal glands) are undifferentiated cells that multiply to give rise to absorptive columnar cells and to goblet cells. Near the bases of the crypts there are ***Paneth cells*** that secrete enzymes. Endocrine cells (***enterochromaffin cells***) are also present.

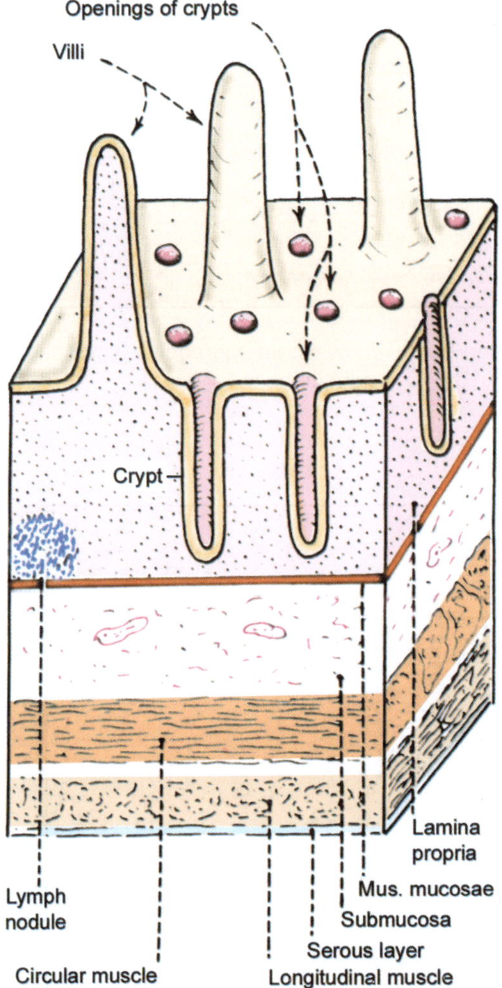

Fig. 16.22 Scheme to show the basic structure of the small intestine.

Lymphoid Tissue of the Small Intestine

Solitary and aggregated lymphatic follicles (***Peyer's patches***) are present in the lamina propria of the small intestine (Fig. 16.23). The solitary follicles become more numerous, and the aggregated follicles larger, in proceeding caudally along the small intestine. They are most prominent in the terminal ileum.

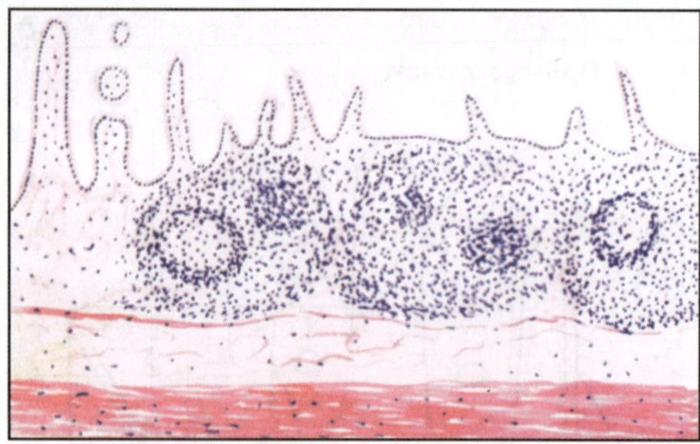

Fig. 16.23 Terminal ileum showing an aggregated lymphatic follicle (Peyer's patch) in the submucosa.

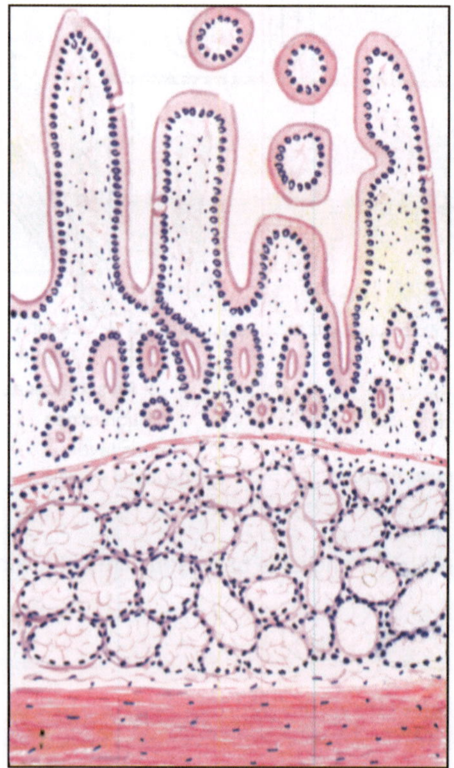

Fig. 16.24 Duodenum. Note that the submucosa is packed with mucous secreting glands (of Brunner).

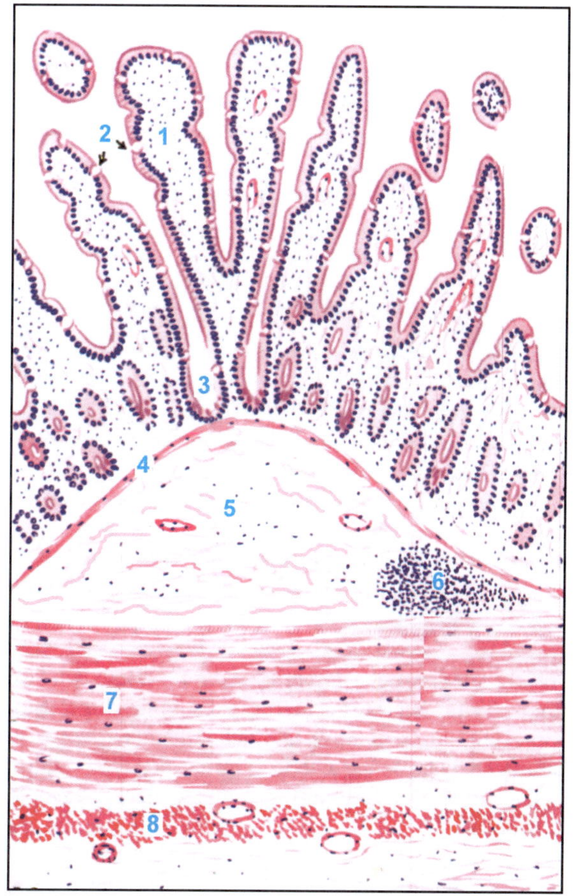

Fig. 16.25 Jejunum. 1-Villus. 2-Goblet cells. 3-Crypt. 4-♥Muscularis mucosae. 5-Submucosa. Note the solitary lymphatic nodule(6) seen towards the right side. 7-Circular muscle. 8. Longitudinal muscle.

Distinguishing Features of Duodenum, Jejunum, and Ileum

1. Sections through the small intestine are readily distinguished from those of other parts of the gut because of the presence of villi.
2. The duodenum is easily distinguished from the jejunum or ileum because of the presence in it of glands in the submucosa. (No glands are present in the submucosa of the jejunum or ileum). These ***duodenal glands*** (of Brunner) are compound tubulo-alveolar glands (Fig. 16.24). Their ducts pass through the muscularis mucosae to open into the intestinal crypts (of Lieberkuhn). The alveoli of the duodenal glands are lined, predominantly, by mucous secreting columnar cells. The secretions of the duodenal glands contain mucous, bicarbonate ions (to neutralize gastric acid entering the duodenum) and an enzyme that activates trypsinogen produced by the pancreas.

3. As compared to the ileum the jejunum shows the following features (Fig. 16.25).
   a. A larger diameter.
   b. A thicker wall.
   c. Larger and more numerous circular folds.
   d. Larger villi.
   e. Fewer solitary lymphatic follicles. Aggreated lymphatic follicles are absent in the proximal jejunum, and small in the distal jejunum.

Functioning of the Small Intestine

Muscle in the wall of the small intestine produces peristaltic movements that move intestinal contents onwards.

Intestinal juice, secreted by mucosal cells, helps in digestion of carbohydrates, proteins and fats. Digested food is absorbed into the circulation. Absorption is facilitated by the large surface area of the mucosa provided by the presence of villi.

Pancreatic juice produced by the pancreas, and bile produced by the liver are poured into the duodenum and play an important role in digestion. These juices are alkaline and neutralise the acid entering the intestine from the stomach.

Secretions of Small Intestine

The crypts of Lieberkuhn produce a watery secretion. About two litres are poured into the intestine every day. Most of the fluid is reabsorbed. This constant circulation of water keeps intestinal contents liquid and facilitates absorption of nutrients. This secretion is stimulated by presence of food. A hormone, VIP (vasoactive intestinal polypeptide), also increases secretion. (It is a local hormone produced by some cells in the epithelium).

Enzymes responsible for digestion are not present in this secretion. The enzymes are located in lining cells of the intestine (in their brush border). They are as follows.

1. Disaccharidase. Three types, one each for the sugars sucrose, maltose and lactose are present. Maltase splits maltose into two molecules of glucose. Sucrase splits sucrose into glucose and fructose. Lactase splits lactose into glucose and galactose.
2. Peptidase. This splits polypeptides into amino acids.
3. Lipase. It is responsible for breakdown of triglycerides (into fatty acids and glycerol).

Goblet cells of the intestine secrete mucous that serves as lubricant.

The glands of Brunner, present in the duodenum, produce a secretion that is thick because of the presence abundant mucous. It protects the duodenum from erosion by acid entering it from the stomach. This secretion is increased by vagal stimulation, by secretin, and by presence of any irritant. In spite of the protective effect of this secretion the duodenum is a common site of peptic ulcer.

THE LARGE INTESTINE

Introductory Remarks

The large intestine is about one and a half meters long. The main subdivisions of the large intestine are shown in Fig. 16.26. These are the ***caecum,*** the ***ascending***

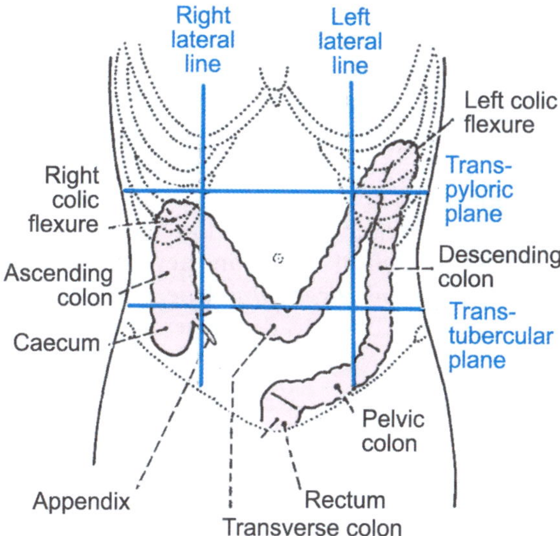

Fig. 16.26 Surface projection of the large intestine. Note that the position of the transverse colon, and of the pelvic (sigmoid) colon is highly variable.

colon, the ***transverse colon***, the ***descending colon,*** the ***sigmoid*** (or ***pelvic***) ***colon***, the ***rectum*** and the ***anal canal***. The terminal part of the ileum becomes continuous with the large intestine at the ***ileocaecal junction***. At this junction the caecum is also joined by a short, narrow, blind tube called the ***vermiform appendix***. The ascending colon meets the transverse colon at the ***right colic flexure***. The junction of the transverse colon with the descending colon is called the ***left colic flexure***.

We have already seen that the ascending colon, and the descending colon are retroperitoneal. They are in direct contact with the abdominal wall and do not have a mesentery. The transverse colon is suspended from the posterior abdominal wall by the ***transverse mesocolon***; and the sigmoid colon by the ***sigmoid mesocolon***. The caecum is usually surrounded all round by peritoneum and, therefore, has considerable mobility. Its posterior aspect is separated from the posterior abdominal wall by a recess of the peritoneal cavity called the ***retrocaecal recess***. The vermiform appendix often lies in this recess. The rectum is partially covered by peritoneum, while the anal canal does not come in contact with peritoneum at all.

The following differences enable a segment of the colon to be easily distinguished from a segment of small intestine.

a. The colon is much wider than the small intestine. That is why it is called the 'large' intestine.
b. The outer diameter of a segment of small intestine is more or less uniform. In contrast a segment of the colon shows a series of ***sacculations*** (also called ***haustrations***).

c. In the case of the small intestine the layer of longitudinal muscle is of uniform thickness all round its circumference. In the caecum and colon, however, the longitudinal muscle layer shows thickenings at three places on the circumference. These thickenings of muscle form three prominent bands that run along the length of the colon, approximately equidistant from each other. These bands are called the ***taenia coli***. The taenia coli appear to be shorter than the rest of the wall of the colon. This may be one reason for presence of sacculations in the wall of the colon.
d. Attached to the outer wall of the colon there are numerous irregular projections called the ***appendices epiploicae***. Each of these consists of a small mass of fat enclosed by a covering of peritoneum.

Parts of the Colon

Ascending Colon

The ascending colon lies vertically in the right lateral region of the abdomen. It is about 15 cm long. Its lower end is continuous with the caecum. Its upper end meets the transverse colon at the right colic flexure.

Transverse Colon

The transverse colon is the longest subdivision of the large intestine. It begins at the right colic flexure and ends at the left colic flexure. Between the two flexures the transverse colon forms a downward loop of varying size. Its lowest part frequently descends to a level below the umbilicus and may even descend into the pelvis. Its total length is about 50 cm.

Descending Colon

The descending colon begins at the left colic flexure. Its upper end, therefore, lies in the left hypochondrium. From here it descends to reach the left side of the brim of the true pelvis. It ends by becoming continuous with the sigmoid colon.

Sigmoid Colon

The sigmoid colon, or pelvic colon is continuous at one end with the descending colon, and at the other end with the rectum. The junction with the descending colon lies over the pelvic brim (left half). The junction with the rectum is more or less in the middle line.

Histology of the Colon

The structure of the colon conforms to the general description of the structure of the gut (Figs. 16.27, 16.28). The mucous membrane of the colon shows numerous crescent-shaped folds. There are no villi. The mucosa shows numerous closely arranged tubular glands or crypts similar to those in the small intestine. The mucosal surface, and the glands, are lined by an epithelium

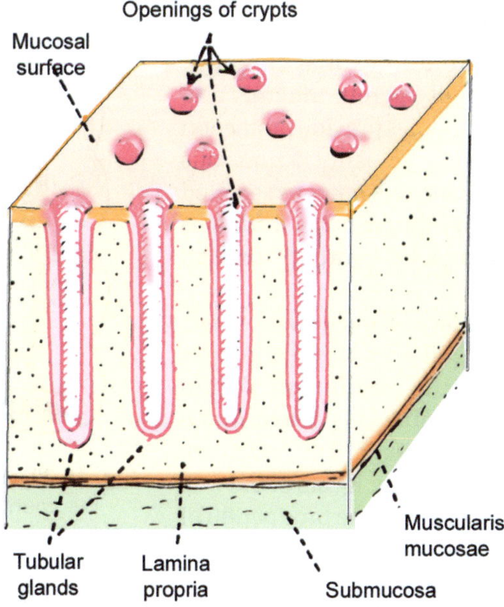

Fig. 16.27 Scheme to show the basic features of the structure of the mucous membrane of the large intestine.

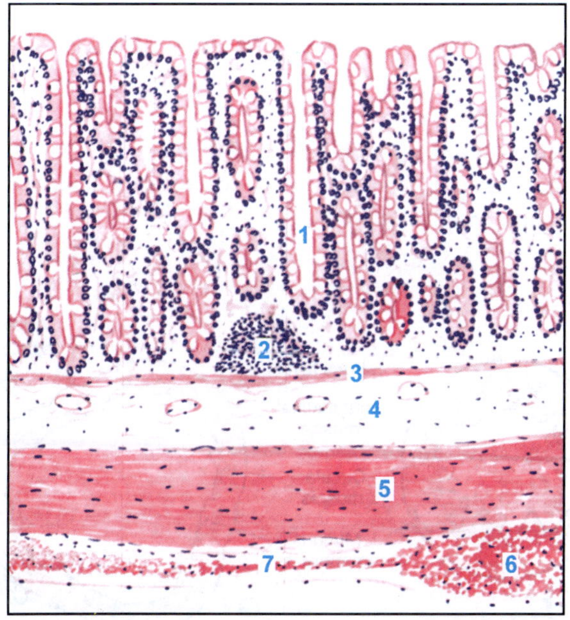

Fig. 16.28 Section through a part of the large intestine. 1-Crypt. 2-Lymphatic nodule. 3-Muscularis mucosae. 4-Submucosa. 5-Muscle coat. 6-Taenia coli. 7-Longitudinal muscle.

made up predominantly of columnar cells. Their main function is to absorb excess water and electrolytes from intestinal contents. Many columnar cells secrete mucous and antibodies. The antibodies provide protection against pathogenic organisms. Numerous goblet cells are present. The mucous secreted by them serves as a lubricant that facilitates the passage of semisolid contents through the colon.

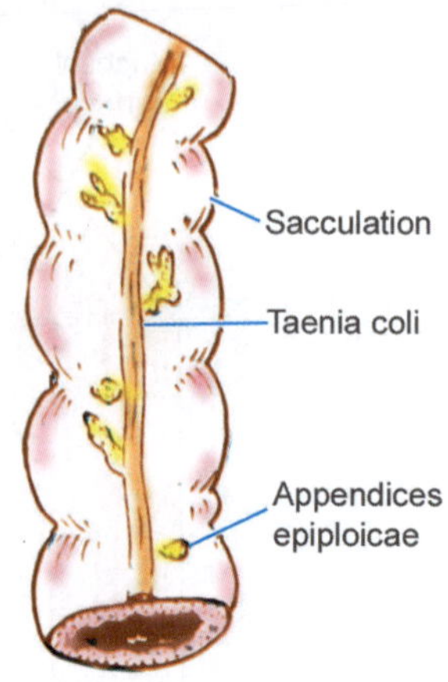

Fig. 16.29 Diagram to show a segment of the colon.

The longitudinal layer of muscle is unusual. Most of the fibres in it are collected to form three thick bands, the ***taenia coli***. A thin layer of longitudinal fibres is present in the intervals between the taenia. The taenia are shorter in length than other layers of the wall of the colon. This results in the production of ***sacculations*** (also called ***haustrations***) on the wall of the colon (Figs. 16.29, 16.30).

In many situations peritoneum forms small pouch-like processes that are filled with fat. These yellow masses are called the ***appendices epiploicae***.

Secretions of Large Intestine

These are mucoid and alkaline. Mucous lubricates faecal matter. Secretion is increased by stimulation of mucosa.

Caecum

The terminal ileum joins the large intestine in the right iliac fossa. The part of the large intestine lying (here) below the level of the ileocaecal junction is called the caecum.

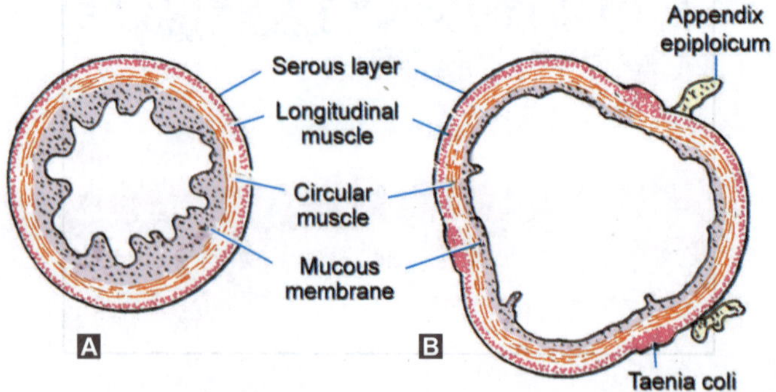

Fig. 16.30 Transverse sections through the small intestine (A) and large intestine (B) to show differences in basic structure.

Vermiform Appendix

The vermiform appendix looks very much like a round worm: hence the name vermiform. It is a tube only a few millimeters wide, and about 9 cm in length. At one end (the apex), the appendix is blind; and at the other end (the base), it opens into the caecum. The appendix is mobile and highly variable in position.

Histology of the Vermiform Appendix

The structure of the vermiform appendix resembles that of the colon (described above) with the following differences:
1. The appendix is the narrowest part of the gut.
2. The crypts are poorly formed.
3. The longitudinal muscle coat is complete and equally thick all round. Taenia coli are not present.
4. The submucosa contains abundant lymphoid tissue that may completely fill the submucosa.

Rectum

The rectum lies in the true pelvis. Above it is continuous with the sigmoid colon, and inferiorly with the anal canal.

Histology of the Rectum

The structure of the rectum is similar to that of the colon except for the following.
1. A continuous coat of longitudinal muscle is present. There are no taenia.
2. Peritoneum covers the front and sides of the upper one-third of the rectum; and only the front of the middle third. The rest of the rectum is devoid of a serous covering.
3. There are no appendices epiploicae.

The Anal Canal

The anal canal is about 4 cm long. The upper 3 cm are lined by mucous membrane, and the lower 1 cm by skin (Fig. 16.31). The area lined by mucous membrane can be further divided into an upper part (15 mm) and a lower part (15 mm).

The mucous membrane of the upper 15 mm of the canal is lined by columnar epithelium. The mucous membrane of this part shows six to twelve longitudinal folds that are called the ***anal columns***. The lower ends of the anal columns are joined to each other by short transverse folds called the ***anal valves***. The anal valves together form a transverse line that runs all round the anal canal: this is the ***pectinate line***. The mucous membrane of the next 15 mm of the canal is lined by nonkeratinized stratified squamous epithelium. This region does not have anal columns. The mucosa has a bluish appearance

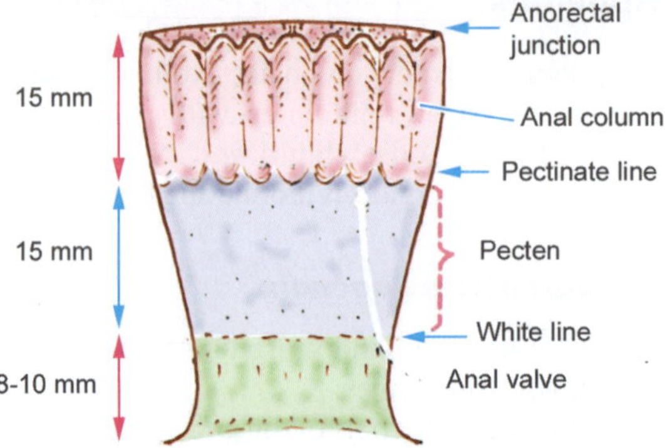

Fig. 16.31 Diagram to show some features in the interior of the anal canal.

because of the presence of a dense venous plexus between it and the muscle coat. This region is called the ***pecten*** or ***transitional zone***. The lower limit of the pecten forms the ***white line*** (***of Hilton***).

The lowest 8 to 10 mm of the anal canal are lined by true skin in which hair follicles, sebaceous glands and sweat glands are present.

Above each anal valve there is a depression called the ***anal sinus***. Atypical (apocrine) sweat glands open into each sinus. They are called the ***anal*** (or ***circumanal***) ***glands***.

The anal canal is surrounded by two layers of muscle (circular and longitudinal) that are continuous with those of the rectum. The circular muscle is thickened to form the ***internal anal sphincter***. Outside the layer of smooth muscle, there is the ***external anal sphincter*** that is made up of striated muscle.

Prominent venous plexuses are present in the submucosa of the anal canal. The internal haemorrhoidal plexus lies above the level of the pectinate line, while the external haemorrhoidal plexus lies near the lower end of the canal.

Intestinal Motility

Movements of small intestine are of two types. In segmentation movements there is alternate contraction and relaxation of short segments of intestine. These movements do not propel food down the intestine. They move it back and forth ensuring thorough mixing and absorption of food.

Peristaltic movements propel intestinal contents. A ring of contraction passes down the intestine for a short distance. A new wave, starting distal to the previous wave, carries food down the intestine. A series of such waves result in peristalsis.

These movements of small intestine are increased by vagal stimulation, by 5-hydroxytryptamine (secreted by endocrine cells of the gut), and by thyroxine. Emotions influence intestinal movements. Fear decreases motility, and anger increases it.

When food reaches the terminal ileum, it is held up for some time as the ileocaecal sphincter is normally closed. Ingestion of food causes increased peristaltic movements in the terminal ileum. This constitutes the ***gastro-ileal reflex.*** The ileocaecal sphincter relaxes and intestinal contents enter the caecum.

As in the small intestine, segmentation movements take place in the large intestine as well. They help in resorption of water and salts from the contents. In the large intestine peristaltic waves occur in the form of a ***mass movement***. There is a marked increase of pressure and this results in movement of colonic contents. These movements are stimulated by entry of food into the stomach. This is the ***gastro-colic reflex***.

Normally, contents of the colon accumulate in the sigmoid colon. They remain there till a strong mass movement forces them into the rectum. This produces an urge for defaecation. In actual defaecation there is strong parasympathetic stimulation by neurons located in the sacral part of the spinal cord (sacral outflow) resulting in a strong mass movement. Simultaneously, the glottis is closed and the diaphragm contracts. Abdominal muscles also contract. This greatly increases intra-abdominal pressure. The combined effect of mass movement and increased abdominal pressure causes defaecation. The sigmoid colon and descending colon are emptied of their contents.

CHAPTER

17

Liver and Pancreas

THE LIVER

The liver is one of the largest organs in the body weighing about 1.5 kg. It is by far the largest gland. It is included amongst the accessory organs of the alimentary system because it produces a secretion, the bile, which is poured into the duodenum (through the bile duct) and assists in the digestive process. All the blood circulating through the capillary bed of the abdominal part of the alimentary canal (excepting the lower part of the anal canal) reaches the liver through the portal vein and its tributaries. In this way all substances absorbed into the blood from the stomach and intestines are filtered through the liver, where some of them are stored; and some toxic substances may be destroyed. Numerous other functions essential to the well being of the individual are performed in the liver. It is, therefore, regarded as one of the vital organs.

The liver lies in the upper, right part of the abdominal cavity (Fig. 17.1). It lies immediately below the diaphragm. When seen from the front (Fig. 17.1) the liver is roughly triangular and appears to have upper, lower and right borders. Most of the liver is placed deep to the costal margin and only a small part of it comes in contact with the anterior abdominal wall. A liver extending below the level of the lateral part of the right costal margin is regarded as enlarged.

Fig. 17.2 is a schematic parasagittal section through the liver. It shows that the liver has basically two surfaces. Above it has a convex ***diaphragmatic surface***, and below it has an inferior or ***visceral surface***. The diaphragmatic surface is extensive. Part of it faces forwards, part of it upwards, and part of it backwards. The diaphragmatic and visceral surfaces meet in front at a sharp ***inferior border***.

Almost the entire surface of the liver is covered by peritoneum. At many places this peritoneum is reflected on to the diaphragm in the form of so-called ligaments. These ligaments keep the liver in place.

The visceral surface of the liver shows a depression called the ***porta hepatis***. Blood vessels enter the liver here, and the hepatic ducts leave it. The margins of the porta hepatis give attachment to a double-layered fold of peritoneum

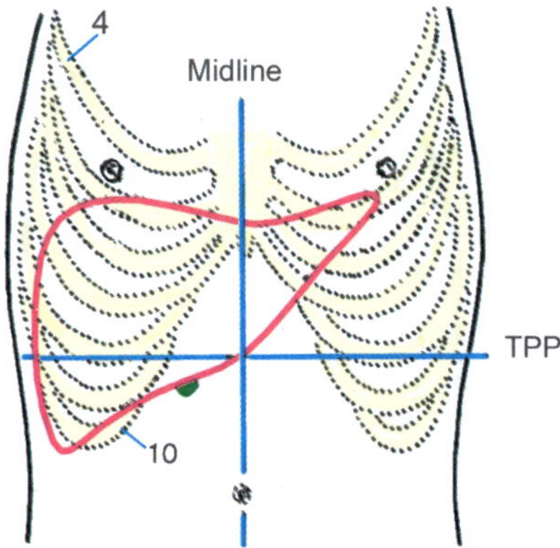

Fig. 17.1 Surface projection of the liver as seen from the front.

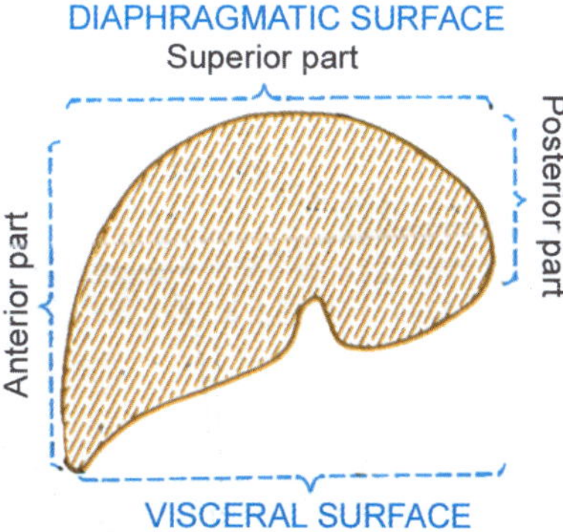

Fig. 17.2 Schematic sagittal section through the liver to show its surfaces.

called the ***lesser omentum***. The lesser omentum connects the liver to the lesser curvature of the stomach.

The liver is shown as seen from the front in Fig. 17.4. We see the anterior and superior parts of the diaphragmatic surface. Note that the anterior part of the diaphragmatic surface is lined by peritoneum except along a line near the median plane. Along this line the peritoneum is reflected off from the liver to the diaphragm, and to the upper part of the anterior abdominal wall as the ***falciform ligament***. The line of attachment of the falciform ligament is used to divide the liver into a larger right lobe and a much smaller left lobe. However, most authorities agree that the division of the liver into right and left lobes should be based on the areas drained by the right and left hepatic ducts. This plane of division is shown in Fig. 17.4 in red line.

The posterior aspect of the liver shows a deep notch for the vertebral column. To the right of this notch there is a deep groove in which the inferior vena cava is lodged.

The liver is shown as seen from behind in Fig. 17.5. The upper part of this figure shows the posterior part of the diaphragmatic surface. The lower part

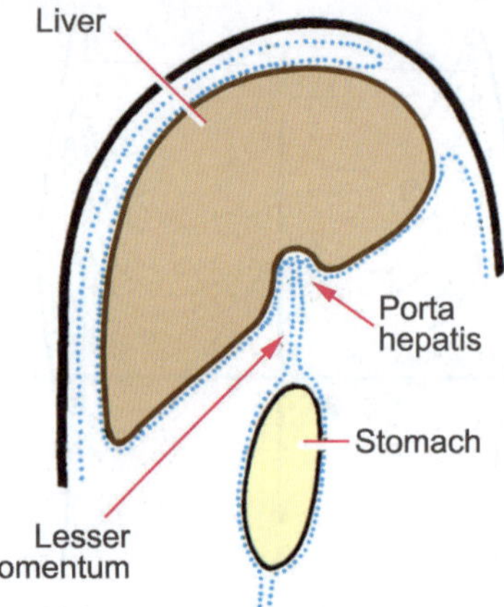

Fig. 17.3 Schematic parasagittal section through the liver to show its basic peritoneal relations.

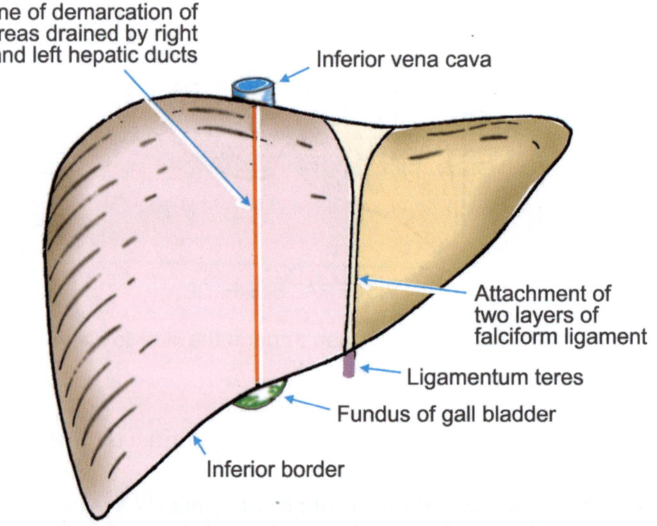

Fig. 17.4 Liver viewed from the front.

of the figure shows the visceral surface. Note that a considerable area on the posterior part of the diaphragmatic surface of the liver is not covered by peritoneum and is, therefore, called the ***bare area***.

To the left of the groove for the inferior vena cava there is a circumscribed part of the posterior surface that is called the ***caudate lobe***.

The most conspicuous feature on the visceral surface of the liver is the ***gall bladder***. It lies in a depression on the liver surface called the fossa for the gall bladder. Starting near the right end of the porta hepatis the gall bladder runs downwards and forwards across the visceral surface.

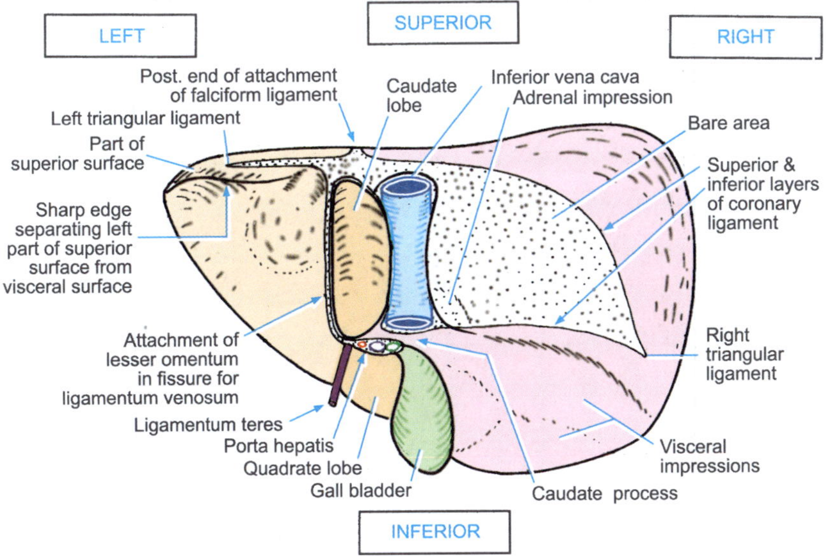

Fig. 17.5 Liver viewed from behind.

The part of the visceral surface immediately to the left of the gall is called the ***quadrate lobe*** (because of its quadrangular shape).

Blood Vessels of the Liver

The liver receives oxygenated blood through the hepatic artery. This artery is a branch of the coeliac trunk. Entering the liver at the porta hepatis it divides into two main branches that are distributed to the 'true' right and left lobes.

The liver receives blood from the gastrointestinal tract through the portal vein. At the porta hepatis the portal vein divides into right and left branches that accompany branches of the hepatic artery. Blood from the liver is drained by a number of hepatic veins that open directly into the inferior vena cava. They do not pass through the porta hepatis.

The liver is separated only by peritoneum from a number of important organs. These include the oesophagus, the stomach, the duodenum, the transverse colon, and the right kidney. The peritoneal space around the liver is divided into a number of pockets. These pockets can become sites of infection.

HISTOLOGY OF THE LIVER

The liver substance is divisible into a large number of large lobes, each of which consists of numerous lobules (Figs. 17.6, 17.7). The exocrine secretion of the liver cells is called ***bile***. Bile is poured out from liver cells into very delicate ***bile canaliculi*** that are present in intimate relationship to the cells (Fig. 17.8). From the canaliculi bile drains into progressively larger ducts that end in the ***bile duct***. This duct conveys bile into the duodenum where bile plays a role in digestion of fat.

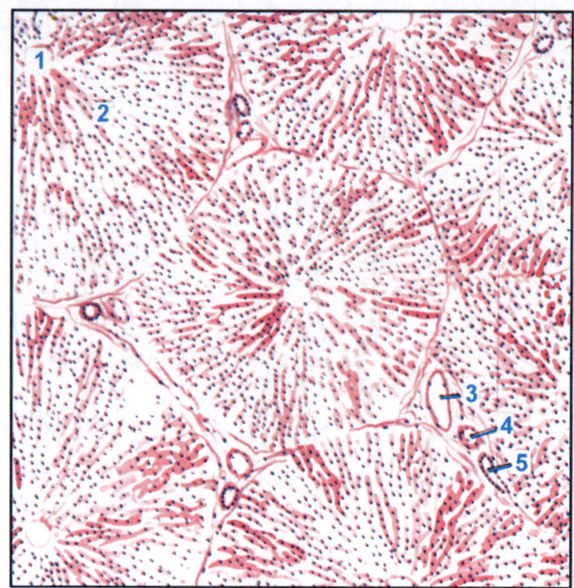

Fig. 17.6 Section through liver (low power view). 1-Central vein. 2-Liver cells arranged as radiating cords or plates that form hexagonal lobules.. 3-Branch of portal vein. 4-Branch of hepatic artery. 5-Interlobular duct. 3, 4 and 5 form a portal triad.

All blood draining from the stomach and intestines (and containing absorbed food materials) reaches the liver through the portal vein and its branches. Within the liver this blood passes through sinusoids and comes into very intimate relationship with liver cells. The liver is thus able to 'screen' all substances entering the body through the gut. Some of them (e.g., amino acids) are used for synthesis of new proteins needed by the body. Others (e.g., glucose, lipids) are stored in liver cells for subsequent use; while harmful substances (e.g., drugs, alcohol) are detoxified. The need for intimate contact between blood in the sinusoids, and liver cells, thus becomes obvious. The portal vein also brings blood from the spleen to the liver. This blood contains high concentrations of products formed by breakdown of erythrocytes in the spleen. Some of these products (e.g., bilirubin) are excreted in bile, while some (e.g., iron) are stored for re-use in new erythrocytes.

In addition to deoxygenated blood reaching the liver through the portal vein, the organ also receives oxygenated blood through the ***hepatic artery*** and its branches. The blood entering the liver from both these sources passes through the hepatic sinusoids and is collected by tributaries of hepatic veins. One such tributary runs through the centre of each lobule of the liver where it is called the ***central vein*** (see below).

The liver may be regarded as a modified exocrine gland that also has other functions. It is made up, predominantly, of liver cells or ***hepatocytes.*** Each hepatocyte is a large cell with a round open faced nucleus, with prominent nucleoli (Figs. 17.6 to 17.8).

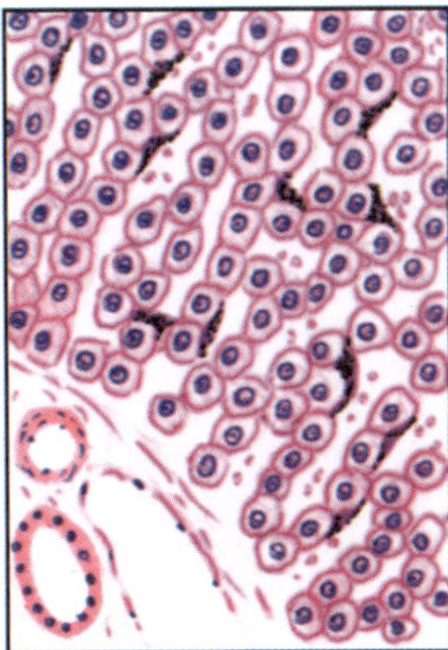

Fig. 17.7 High power view of the liver. Note cords of cells separated by sinusoids. Phagocytic cells (of Kupffer) (containing dark ingested material) are seen scattered along the walls of sinusoids.

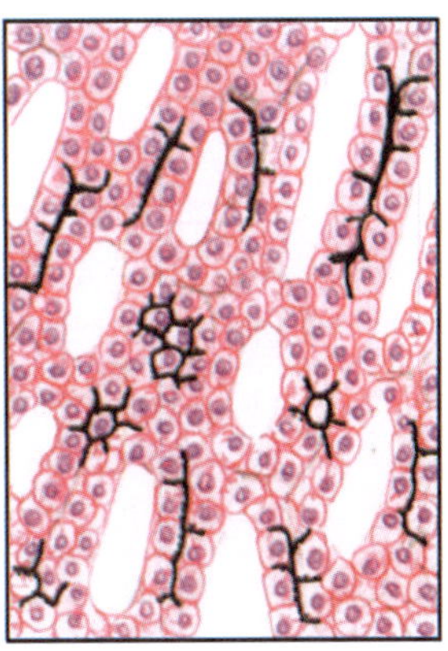

Fig. 17.8 High power view of the liver. Note the bile capillaries (black) intervening between liver cells.

In sections through the liver, the substance of the organ appears to be made up of hexagonal areas that constitute the ***hepatic lobules***. In transverse sections each lobule appears to be made up of cords of liver cells that are separated by sinusoids. However, the cells are really arranged in the form of plates (one cell thick) that branch and anastomose with one another to form a network. Spaces within the network are occupied by sinusoids.

Along the periphery of each lobule there are angular intervals filled by connective tissue. These intervals are called ***portal canals***, the 'canals' forming a connective tissue network permeating the entire liver substance. Each 'canal' contains (a) a branch of the portal vein; (b) a branch of the hepatic artery, and (c) an interlobular bile duct. These three structures collectively form a ***portal triad***. Blood from the branch of the portal vein, and from the branch of the hepatic artery, enters the sinusoids at the periphery of the lobule and passes towards its centre. Here the sinusoids open into a ***central vein*** that occupies the centre of the lobule. We have already seen that the central vein drains into hepatic veins (which leave the liver to end in the inferior vena cava).

Bile is secreted into ***bile canaliculi*** by liver cells (Fig. 17.9). These canaliculi have no walls of their own. They are merely spaces present between plasma membranes of adjacent liver cells. At the periphery of a lobule the canaliculi become continuous with delicate ***intralobular ductules***, which in turn become continuous with larger ***interlobular ductules*** of portal triads. The interlobular ductules are lined by cuboidal epithelium. Some smooth muscle is present in the walls of larger ducts.

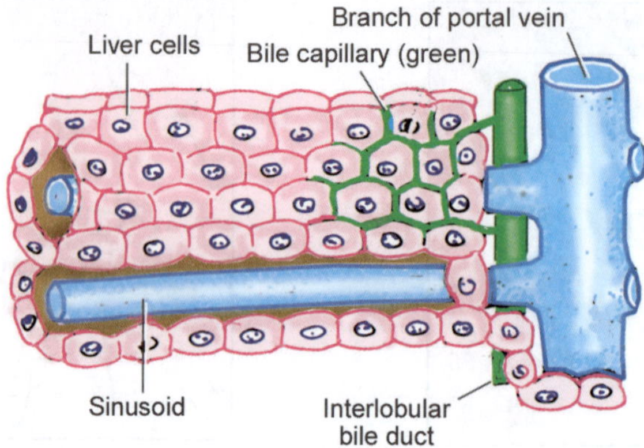

Fig. 17.9 Diagram to show relationship of bile capillaries to liver cells.

FUNCTIONS OF THE LIVER

The liver performs numerous functions. Some of these are as follows.

1. We have seen that the liver acts as an exocrine gland for the ***secretion of bile***. However, the architecture of the liver has greater resemblance to that of an endocrine gland, the cells being in intimate relationship to blood in sinusoids. This is to be correlated with the fact that liver cells take up numerous substances from the blood, and also pour many substances back into it.
2. The liver plays a prominent role in metabolism of carbohydrates, proteins and fats.
   a. ***Carbohydrate metabolism***: The liver is a store of glycogen. It helps to regulate blood glucose. When necessary it can convert lipids and amino acids to glucose (***neoglucogenesis*** or ***gluconeogenesis***).
   b. ***Lipid metabolism***: The liver synthesizes fatty acids, cholesterol and ketone bodies. The role of bile in digestion and absorption of fats is discussed in Chapter 18.
   c. ***Protein metabolism***: The liver is responsible for synthesis of plasma proteins. It is also responsible for breakdown (transamination and deamination) of proteins and the production of urea.
3. The liver acts as a store for various substances including glucose (as glycogen), proteins, lipids, vitamins and iron.
4. The liver plays a protective role by detoxifying substances (including drugs and alcohol) that enter the body. Removal of bile pigments from blood (and their excretion through bile) is part of this process.
5. The macrophage cells (of Kupffer) lining the sinusoids of the liver have a role similar to that of other cells of the mononuclear phagocyte system. They are of particular importance as they are the first cells of this system that come in contact with materials absorbed through the gut. They also remove damaged erythrocytes from blood.
6. During fetal life, the liver is a centre for haemopoiesis.
7. The liver converts vitamin D_3 to a more active form that promotes absorption of calcium.

Composition and Functions of Bile

Bile, secreted by liver cells, consists of water, inorganic salts, bile salts, bile pigments, cholesterol, lecithin and fatty acids. In the gall bladder most of the water and inorganic salts are reabsorbed so that bile is concentrated five to six times. Bile is alkaline.

Bile acids are derived from cholesterol. ***Bile salts*** (sodium taurocholate and sodium glycocholate) are formed by combination of a bile acid with sodium or potassium. Bile salts excreted into bile are almost completely reabsorbed into blood, and go back to the liver, to be re-excreted.

Bile salts are essential for emulsification of fat. This greatly facilitates the digestion and absrption of fat as described in Chapter 18.

Bile pigments (bilirubin and biliverdin) present in bile are responsible for colour of bile. When erythrocytes finish their useful life they are destroyed (mainly in the spleen, and also by Kupffer cells of the liver)). One of the by products of their destruction is the pigment bilirubin. Bilirubin is excreted by the liver through bile, and reaches the intestine. In the large intestine, bilirubin is converted into stercobilin, which is responsible for the brownish colour of faeces. Some bilirubin is converted into urobilinogen, which is absorbed into blood and is excreted through urine.

In diseases of the liver, in which the liver is unable to excrete bilirubin, this pigment accumulates in blood resulting in jaundice. Jaundice also results from obstruction to flow of bile into the intestine for any reason.

Cholesterol, present in bile, is needed for production of bile salts. It has no direct role in digestion. Cholesterol can give rise to gall stones.

Secretion of bile is stimulated by vagal stimulation, by secretin and by bile salts themselves.

Some Disorders of the Liver

1. Inflammation in the liver is called hepatitis. It is frequently caused by viruses (***viral hepatitis***), and by a protozoan parasite ***entamoeba histolytica*** (***amoebic hepatitis***). An abscess may form in the liver as a sequel of amoebic hepatitis.
2. ***Cirrhosis*** of the liver is a disease in which many hepatocytes are destroyed, the areas being filled by fibrous tissue. This gradually leads to collapse of the normal architecture of the liver.
3. One effect of cirrhosis of the liver is to disrupt the flow of blood through the liver. As a result of increased resistance to blood flow there is increased blood pressure in the portal circulation (***portal hypertension***). In portal hypertension anastomoses between the portal and systemic veins dilate to form varices (e.g., at the lower end of the oesophagus). Rupture of these varices can result in fatal bleeding.
4. We have seen above that inability of liver cells to remove bilirubin from blood results in jaundice.
5. When a large number of hepatocytes are destroyed this leads to liver failure. The various functions (listed above) are interfered with. Hepatic failure may be acute or chronic. Accumulation of waste products in blood (due to lack of detoxification by the liver) ultimately leads to unconsciousness (***hepatic coma***) and death.

   The degree of hepatic cell dysfunction can be determined by estimation of some enzymes released by damaged liver cells. The enzymes usually tested for are SGOT (serum glutamic oxaloacetic transaminase) and SGPT (serum glutamic pyruvic transaminase).

EXTRAHEPATIC BILIARY APPARATUS

The passages through which bile, produced in the liver, passes before entering the duodenum are seen in Fig. 17.10. The ***right*** and ***left hepatic ducts*** emerge at the porta hepatis and join to form the ***common hepatic duct***. At its lower end the common hepatic duct is joined by the ***cystic duct*** (from the ***gall bladder***) to form the ***bile duct***. The bile duct opens into the duodenum.

THE GALL BLADDER

The gall bladder is a small sac attached to the visceral surface of the liver (Fig. 17.15). It is held in place by peritoneum that covers its inferior (or posterior) surface. Its superior (or anterior) aspect is in direct contact with liver tissue. However, the lowest part of the gall bladder, which is called the ***fundus***, projects beyond the inferior border of the liver (Fig. 17.4) and is, therefore, surrounded all round by peritoneum. The central part of the gall bladder is called the ***body***. The narrow part succeeding the body is called the ***neck***. The neck is connected to the ***cystic duct*** through which the gall bladder drains into the bile duct.

The wall of the gall bladder is made up of a mucous membrane, a fibromuscular coat, and a serous layer that covers part of the organ.

The mucous membrane of the gall bladder is lined by a tall columnar epithelium with a striated border (Fig. 17.11). The mucosa is highly folded. The folds are called ***rugae***. The folds may branch and anastomose with one another to give a reticular appearance.

The fibromuscular coat is made up mainly of connective tissue. Smooth muscle fibres are present and run in various directions.

The gall bladder stores and concentrates bile. This bile is discharged into the duodenum when required. In between meals the sphincter of Oddi

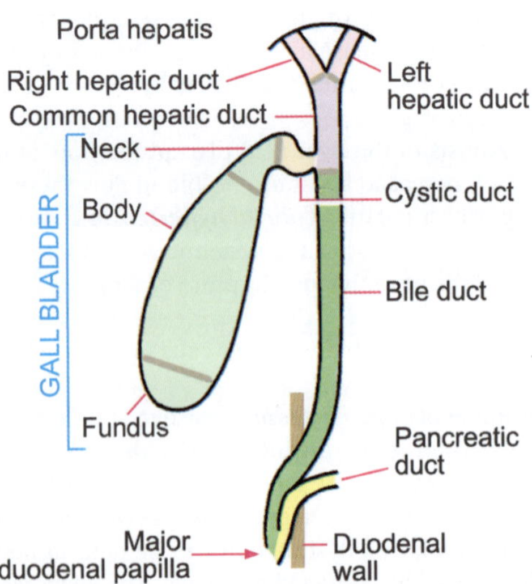

Fig. 17.10 Scheme to show the parts of the extrahepatic biliary apparatus.

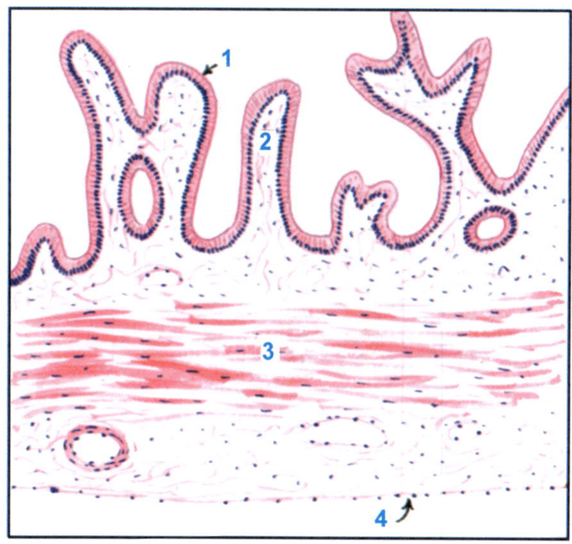

Fig. 17.11 Structure of the gall bladder. 1- Mucous membrane lined by columnar epithelium. 2-Mucosal fold. 3-Muscle coat. 4-Serous layer (peritoneum) lined by flattened mesothelium.

remains closed so that bile cannot flow into the duodenum. So it enters the gall bladder and keeps getting concentrated. When food enters the duodenum, the sphincter relaxes, the gall bladder contracts, and concentrated bile flows into the duodenum. Entry of food into the duodenum stimulates the production of the hormone CCK that stimulates strong contractions of the gall bladder.

As bile is alkaline it helps to neutralize acid entering the duodenum from the stomach.

Inflammation of the gall bladder is called ***cholecystitis***. We have seen that cholesterol may form gall stones (***cholelithiasis***). The gall bladder can be visualised in the living by administration of radio-opaque dyes. The procedure is called ***cholecystography***. The gall bladder can also be studied by ultrasound examination.

THE BILE DUCT

The bile duct extends from just below the porta hepatis to the middle of the descending part of the duodenum. It is about 7 cm long. It descends through the lesser omentum, passes behind the first part of the duodenum and behind the head of the pancreas. Part of the duct may be embedded in pancreatic tissue.

Just outside the duodenal wall, the bile duct is joined by the pancreatic duct. The bile and pancreatic ducts may open separately on the major duodenal papilla, or may join to form a common passage called the ***hepatopancreatic ampulla*** (Fig. 17.12).

The hepatic ducts, the cystic duct, and the bile duct have a common structure. They have a mucosa surrounded by a wall made up of connective tissue, in which some smooth muscle may be present.

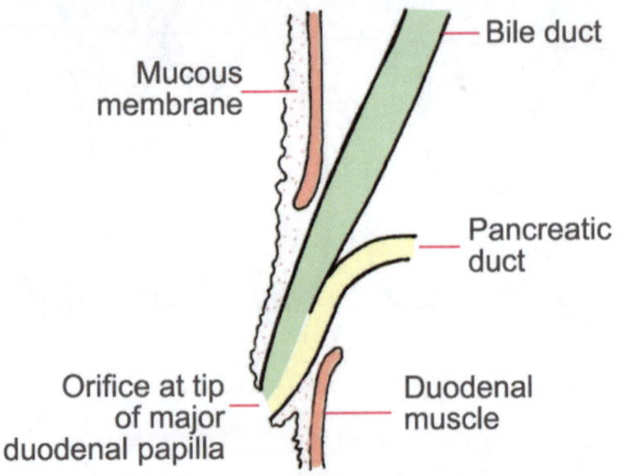

Fig. 17.12 Terminal parts of the bile and pancreatic ducts.

The mucosa is lined by a tall columnar epithelium with a striated border.

Blockage of the bile duct (by inflammation, by a gall stone, or by carcinoma) leads to accumulation of bile in the biliary duct system, and within the bile capillaries. As pressure in the passages increases bile passes into blood leading to ***jaundice***. The sclera, the skin, and the nails appear to be yellow in colour, and bile salts and pigments are excreted in urine. Jaundice occurring as a result of such obstruction is called ***obstructive jaundice***. Jaundice is seen in the absence of obstruction in cases of hepatitis.

A gallstone passing through the bile duct can cause severe pain. This pain is ***biliary colic***.

Sphincters related to the Bile and Pancreatic Ducts

The terminal part of the bile duct is surrounded) by a ring of smooth muscle that forms the ***sphincter choledochus*** (choledochus = bile duct) (Fig. 17.13). It normally keeps the lower end of the bile duct closed. As a result, bile formed in the liver keeps accumulating in the gall bladder (and also undergoes considerable concentration). When food enters the duodenum (specially a fatty meal) the sphincter opens and bile stored in the gall bladder is poured into the

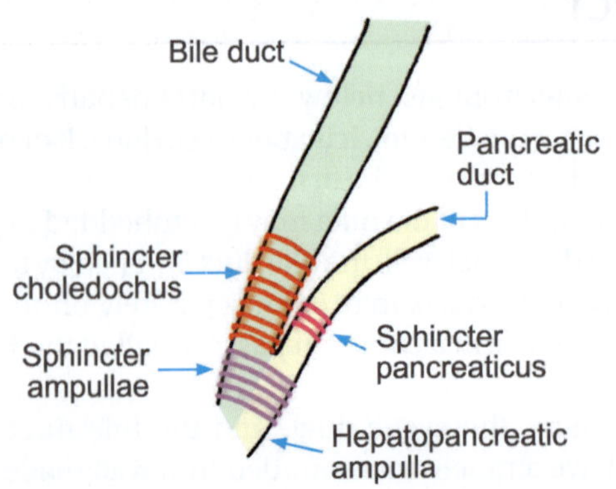

Fig. 17.13 Sphincters around the terminal parts of the bile and pancreatic ducts.

duodenum. The sphincter choledochus is, therefore, essential for filling of the gall bladder. Another less developed sphincter is usually present around the terminal part of the pancreatic duct. This is the ***sphincter pancreaticus***. A third sphincter surrounds the hepatopancreatic ampulla and is called the ***sphincter ampullae***. The sphincters named above are often referred to collectively as the ***sphincter of Oddi***.

THE PANCREAS

The pancreas is a large gland present in close relationship to the duodenum and stomach (Fig. 17.14). It lies obliquely on the posterior abdominal wall, partly to the right of the median plane, and partly to the left. Its right end is enlarged and is called the ***head***. Next to the head there is a short, somewhat constricted part called the ***neck***. The neck is continuous with the main part of the gland that is called the ***body***. The left extremity of the pancreas is thin and is called the ***tail.***

The head lies in the C-shaped space bounded by the duodenum. The neck is placed behind the pylorus, and the body of the pancreas lies behind the body of the stomach. The tip of the tail comes in contact with the spleen.

The pancreas is in intimate contact with a number of abdominal structures. These include the duodenum, the stomach, the spleen, the inferior vena cava, the abdominal aorta, and the left kidney.

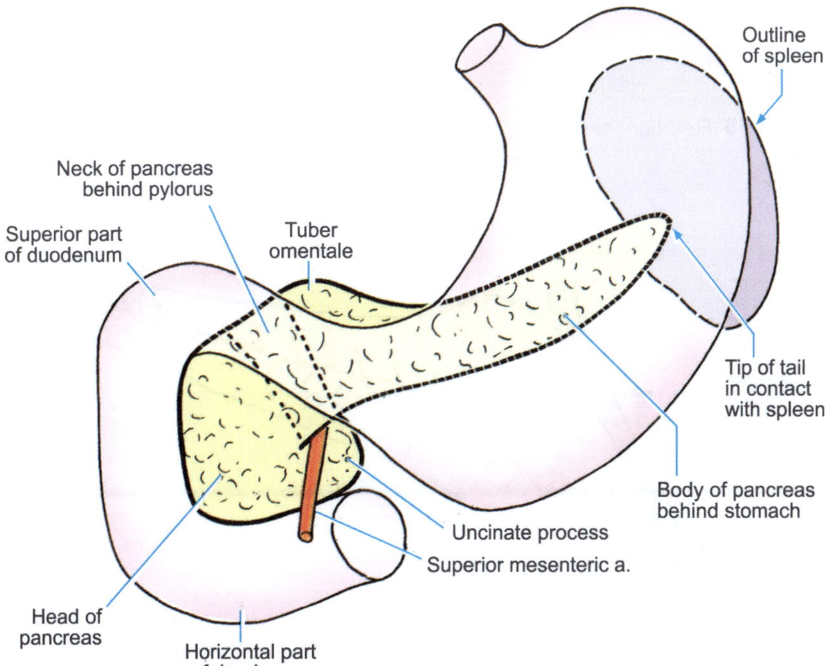

Fig. 17.14 Parts of the pancreas and their relationship to the stomach, the duodenum and the spleen.

In Fig. 17.15 observe that the splenic vein joins the superior mesenteric vein to form the portal vein, just behind the pancreas. The portal vein lies behind the neck of the pancreas. The splenic vein lies behind the body of the pancreas.

Ducts of the Pancreas

Secretions of the pancreas are poured into the duodenum through two ducts (Fig. 17.16).

a. The ***main pancreatic duct*** begins in the tail of the pancreas, and passes to the right through the body. It ends by joining the bile duct just outside the duodenal wall. We have already seen that usually the two ducts unite a short

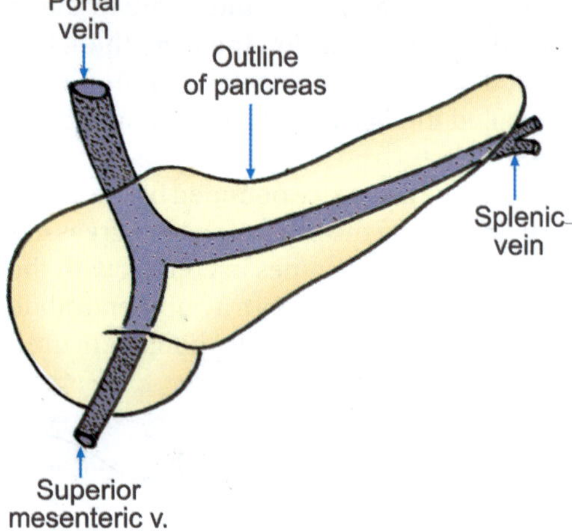

Fig. 17.15 Relationship of portal vein, superior mesenteric vein and splenic vein to the pancreas.

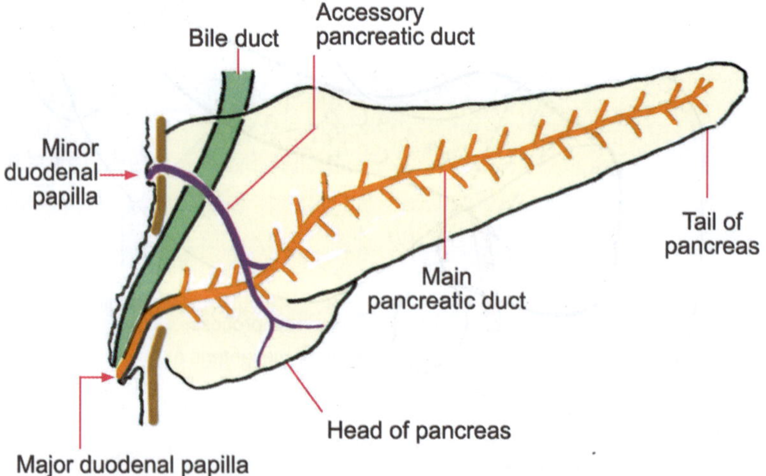

Fig. 17.16 Schematic diagram of the ducts of the pancreas.

distance above the major duodenal papilla to form the hepatopancreatic ampulla. The terminal part of the main pancreatic duct is surrounded by the sphincter pancreaticus.

b. The ***accessory pancreatic duct*** opens into the duodenum at the minor duodenal papilla.

HISTOLOGY OF THE PANCREAS

The pancreas is a gland that is partly exocrine, and partly endocrine, the main bulk of the gland being constituted by its exocrine part (Fig. 17.17). The exocrine pancreas secretes enzymes that play a very important role in the digestion of carbohydrates, proteins and fats. We have seen that after digestion, and absorption through the gut, these products are carried to the liver through the portal vein. The endocrine part of the pancreas produces two very important hormones, ***insulin*** and ***glucagon***. These two hormones are also carried through the portal vein to the liver where they have a profound influence on the metabolism of carbohydrates, proteins and fats. The functions of the exocrine and endocrine parts of the pancreas are thus linked.

The Exocrine Part

The exocrine part of the pancreas is in the form of a serous, compound tubulo-alveolar gland. The pancreas is enveloped by a delicate capsule. Septa extend from the capsule into the gland and divide it into lobules.

The secretory elements of the exocrine pancreas are long and tubular (but they are usually described as alveoli as they appear rounded or oval in sections). The lining cells contain numerous secretory (or zymogen) granules.

Secretions produced in the alveoli are poured into ***intercalated ducts*** (also called ***intralobular ducts***). From the intercalated ducts the secretions pass into larger, ***interlobular ducts***. They finally pass into the duodenum through the ***main pancreatic duct*** and the ***accessory pancreatic duct.*** The cells lining the pancreatic ducts control the bicarbonate and water content of pancreatic secretion. These actions are under hormonal and neural control.

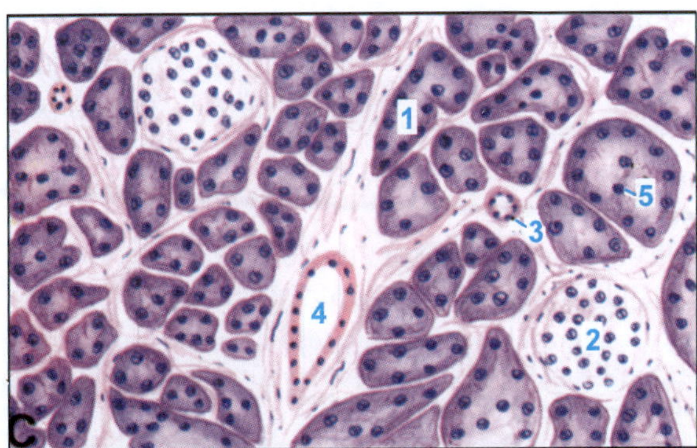

Fig. 17.17 Structure of pancreas. 1-Serous acini. 2-Pancreatic islet. 3-Intralobular duct. 4-Interlobular duct.

The Endocrine Part

The endocrine part of the pancreas is in the form of numerous rounded collections of cells that are embedded within the exocrine part. These collections of cells are called the ***pancreatic islets***, or the ***islets of Langerhans*** (Fig. 17.18). The human pancreas has about one million islets. They are most numerous in the tail of the pancreas.

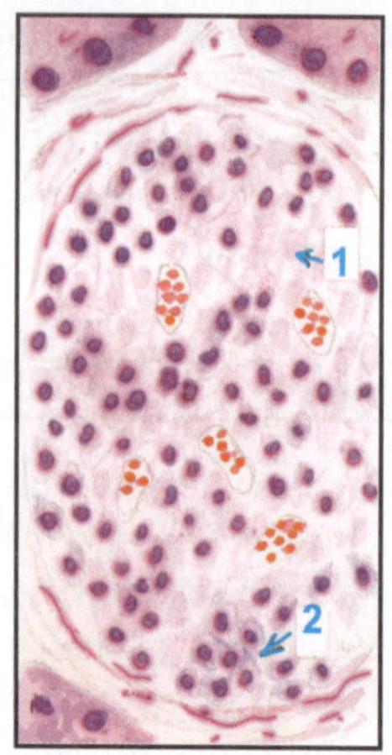

Fig. 17.18 Pancreatic islet. 1-Alpha cells. 2-Beta cells. 3-Capillary.

The islets are very richly supplied with blood through a dense capillary plexus. The intervals between the capillaries are occupied by cells that are arranged in groups or as cords. In ordinary preparations stained with haematoxylin and eosin, all the cells appear similar, but with the use of special procedures three main types of cells can be distinguished as follows.

a. The ***alpha cells*** (or ***A-cells***) secrete the hormone ***glucagon***. They form about 20% of the islet cells.
b. The ***beta cells*** (or ***B-cells***) secrete the hormone ***insulin***. About 70% of the cells are of this type.
c. The ***delta cells*** (or ***D-cells***) probably produce the hormones ***gastrin*** and ***somatostatin***. Somatostatin inhibits the secretion of glucagon by alpha cells, and (to a lesser extent) that of insulin by beta cells. It also inhibits actions of secretin and gastrin.

The functional role of the pancreatic hormones will be considered in Chapter 22 along with functions of other endocrine glands and their hormones.

Pancreatic Juice

Pancreatic juice contains the following.

1. Water.
2. Inorganic constituents are ions of sodium, potassium, chloride and bicarbonate. Because of the presence of bicarbonate pancreatic juice is alkaline (pH 8.0). Bicarbonate ions are added to pancreatic juice while passing through intercalated ducts. They are added by active transport. Bicarbonate neutralises hydrochloric acid entering the duodenum from the stomach.
3. The digestive enzymes present are the following.

    a. Amylase helps in digestion of carbohydrates. Polysaccharides are broken down to dissacharides, mainly maltose. (Conversion of dissacharides to monosaccharides takes place under the influence of enzymes located in the brush border of intestinal epithelium).
    b. Lipase helps in digestion of fats. It splits triglycerides into fatty acids and monoglyceride. This action is greatly promoted by emulsification of fat.

c. The pancreas produces a number of inactive precursors of proteolytic enzymes. This is to ensure that the enzymes do not break down the proteins of the pancreas itself.

Trypsinogen produced in the pancreas is acted upon enterokinase (produced in the small intestine) to form trypsin. Trypsin has the power to activate all the other proteolytic enzymes produced in the pancreas. These include chymotrypsin, carboxy-peptidase, elastase, ribonuclease, and deoxyribonuclease.

Proteins are broken down first into peptones and proteoses and then into small polypeptides. RNA and DNA are broken into nucleotides. Further breakdown of polypeptides into amino acids takes place in the brush border of intestinal epithelial cells.

Regulation of Pancreatic Secretion

When food enters the duodenum, the latter produces two hormones secretin and cholecystokinin (CCK). These hormones reach the pancreas through blood and stimulate production of a large quantity of pancreatic juice. Gastrin, secreted by cells in the stomach, also increases pancreatic secretion. Somatostatin produced by some cells in the stomach and intestine, and by pancreatic islets inhibits secretion of secretin and gastrin.

CHAPTER

18

Nutrition, Digestion and Metabolism

NUTRITION

The energy required by the body for performing various functions is obtained from food. Food is also required for growth, for repair of tissues after injury or disease, and for replacement of tissues that have a limited life. The food taken by a person constitutes his diet.

Substances in food that can be utilised by the body are called nutrients, and the use of nutrients is called nutrition. Any food contains one or more of the following.

a. Carbohydrates
b. Proteins
c. Fats
d. Vitamins
e. Mineral salts
f. Water

The body requires all these in appropriate proportion. The greater part of the diet of most persons is made up of carbohydrates (in the form of *chappatis*, bread or rice). Protein requirements are met through milk, eggs, or the flesh of animals. In vegetarians, lentils (*dal*) and beans are important sources of protein. Fats are obtained through milk and milk products (butter or *ghee*), or from vegetable oils (mustard oil, groundnut oil, sunflower oil, etc.).

Fresh vegetables and fruits are important constituents of diet. Apart from carbohydrates, they provide vitamins and mineral salts which are essential for the body.

An adequate intake of water is essential, more so in a hot country like India.

A diet containing all necessary constituents in appropriate amount is called a balanced diet. A person not receiving such a diet shows signs of deficiency of one or more substances.

CARBOHYDRATES

Food grains such as wheat and rice are made up predominantly of starch, which is a complex form of carbohydrate. Another form of carbohydrate, which is well known to us, is sugar.

Carbohydrates are so called because they contain carbon, oxygen and hydrogen.

The simplest form in which carbohydrates exist is that of glucose. Carbohydrates in food are ultimately broken down (by the process of digestion) to glucose. Glucose is absorbed into blood and reaches all part of the body. The chemical structure of glucose is shown in Fig. 18.1. The carbon atoms are arranged in the form of a ring. Atoms of hydrogen and oxygen are attached to the carbon atoms.

Sugars, like glucose, which exist as single molecules, are called monosaccharides. Another example of a monosaccharide is fructose (fruit sugar). Sugars made up of two molecules are called disaccharides. The sugar we use in homes is a disaccharide called sucrose. It is made up of one molecule of glucose plus one of fructose.

Carbohydrates, derived from food, constitute the must important source of energy required for various needs. When available in excess, glucose is converted to glycogen, which is stored in the body. Excess carbohydrate is also converted into fat.

PROTEINS

Animal flesh is made up mainly of proteins. Egg white (albumin) is also a common form of protein. Proteins are also present in many plant foods specially beans and lentils.

Proteins in food are broken down by digestion, into amino acids. Each amino acid contains carbon, hydrogen, oxygen, and nitrogen. Some of them contain sulphur. The simplest amino acid is glycine. Its structure is shown in Fig. 18.2.

Amino acids join together to form proteins. Proteins exist in various forms. Some proteins form the structural basis of cells and tissues, while others serve as enzymes, hormones, antibodies and many other biologically active substances.

Proteins are essential for growth and repair of tissues. When available in excess, proteins can be used to provide energy, or for storage as fat, but normally carbohydrates are used for this purpose.

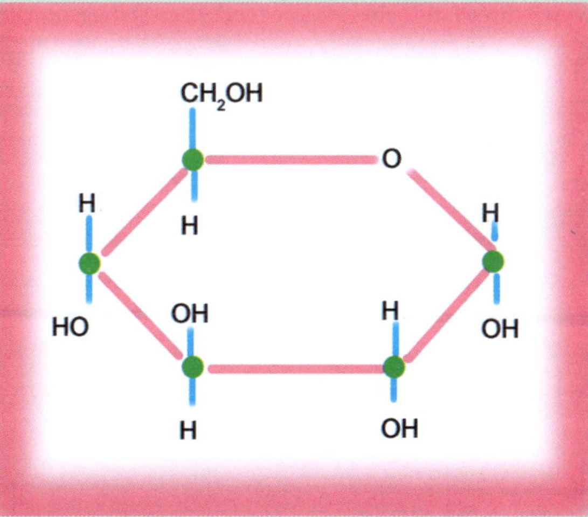

Fig. 18.1 Structure of glucose.

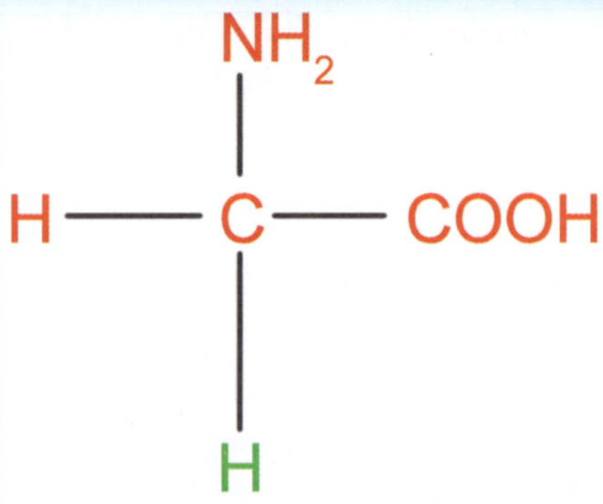

Fig. 18.2 Basic structure of an aminoacid.

FATS OR LIPIDS

Lipids are important constituents of cells and tissues. We obtain fats through milk and milk products (butter, cheese, ghee, cream) and also through vegetable oils (groundnut oil, mustard oil, sunflower oil and many others). Considerable fat is also present in many non-vegetarian foods.

Like carbohydrates, fats also contain carbon, hydrogen and oxygen. Some lipids contain phosphorus (phospholipids).

The basic structure of a molecule of fat is shown in Fig. 18.3. It consists of a core of glycerol to which three fatty acids are attached. During digestion, fats are broken down into fatty acids and glycerol. Fats present in food are absorbed in the form of these end products.

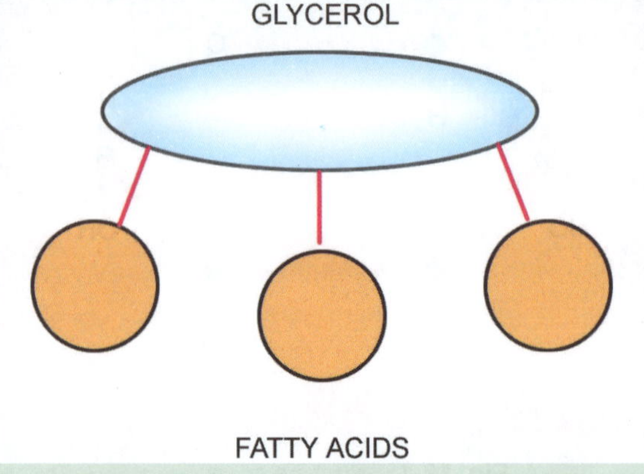

Fig. 18.3 Basic structure of a molecule of fat.

Like carbohydrates, lipids are a source of energy for the body. When available in excess, fat is stored in the body. Fats are essential constituents of many tissues e.g., of cell membranes and of myelin sheaths of nerves.

VITAMINS

Vitamins are substances (present in some foods) that are essential for health. They are needed in small amounts. Vitamins are of two types (1) water soluble, (2) fat soluble. The fat-soluble vitamins are vitamins A, D, E and K. Water-soluble vitamins, are B (made up of several components), and C. The fat-soluble vitamins are present in fatty foods like milk, cheese and eggs. They are also present in some vegetables and fruits. Water-soluble vitamins are present in vegetables, liver, meat, etc. Some vitamins are stable but many are destroyed by heat or by exposure to light.

Vitamin A is necessary for vision, specially in poor light. When this vitamin is deficient the patient suffers from ***night blindness***. The vitamin is also important for growth (specially in bone and in epithelia) and for resistance to infection.

Vitamin B complex consists of the following components.

Vitamin B1, (thiamine) is necessary for utilization of carbohydrate. It is also necessary for functioning of the nervous system. Deficiency of this vitamin causes a disease called ***beri beri***. The person becomes very weak, and does not grow normally. The person may develop oedema and degeneration of nerves.

Vitamin B2 (riboflavine) is necessary to keep the eyes and vision normal. In deficiency there is blurred vision and cataract may form. Cracks appear in skin at the angles of the mouth (***angular stomatitis***).

Folic acid is synthesised by bacteria in the colon. Deficiency can occur if these bacteria are destroyed by antibiotics. Folic acid is essential for synthesis of DNA and cell multiplication (specially in bone marrow). Deficiency leads to megaloblastic anaemia.

Niacin (or nicotinic acid) is important in fat metabolism. Deficiency causes a disease called pellagra. There are disturbances in skin, mouth and nervous system.

Vitamin B6 (or pyridoxine) plays a role in amino acid metabolism.

Vitamin B12 (or cyanacobalamin) is required in DNA synthesis. Deficiency leads to megaloblastic anaemia and to degenerative changes in the nervous system.

Other components of vitamin B-complex are pantothenic acid and biotin.

Vitamin C

This is needed in protein metabolism and in production of collagen. It is an antioxidant. It is therefore, useful in wound repair and in resistance to infections. In vitamin C deficiency (***scurvy***) the gums get swollen and bleed easily.

Vitamin D

This vitamin is essential for metabolism of calcium and phosphorus, and for maintaining strength of bones. Deficiency in children causes rickets. Deficiency in adults causes osteomalacia. The bones become soft and deformities develop, e.g., in the pelvis.

Vitamin E

This vitamin is an antioxidant. It protects the body from infections by improving immunity.

Vitamin K

This vitamin is required for production of various factors that are important for normal clotting of blood. This vitamin is synthesised by bacteria in the colon.

Mineral Salts

In addition to vitamins, the body requires adequate intake of several inorganic chemical salts.

Calcium and phosphorus are essential for normal bone growth. Calcium is obtained mainly from milk.

Sodium and potassium play an essential role in contraction of muscle, transmission of nerve impulse, and for maintaining electrolyte balance of the body.

Iron is essential for normal formation of blood. Deficiency leads to anaemia.

Iodine is essential for production of hormones by the thyroid gland.

Fibre

After food has been digested and nutrients in it absorbed, some residue is left. This residue is referred to as fibre. Fibre increases the bulk of food eaten and this bulk increases the feeling of satisfaction that comes after eating. Fibre also adds to the bulk of faeces and helps to soften them, thus preventing constipation. Vegetables are rich in fibre.

Water

Water is essential for life. About 70% of body weight is made up of water. All tissues, including blood and lymph contain water. Cell function is impossible without water. Adequate intake of water is essential to replace water lost through perspiration, urine, faeces and expired air. Excessive water loss through vomiting or diarrhoea, through loss of blood or through oozing of fluid in extensive burns, leads to dehydration. Severe dehydration is a life-threatening condition that has to be treated or prevented by intravenous administration of fluids.

DIGESTION AND ABSORPTION

Digestion of Carbohydrates

1. Salive contains the enzyme amylase that acts on polysaccharides and breaks them down to the disaccharide maltose. Action of this enzyme continues till food enters the stomach.

2. Pancreatic juice also contains amylase that breaks down polysaccharides to disaccharides, chiefly maltose.
3. Breakdown of disaccharides into monosaccharides takes place under the influence of disaccharidases present in the lining cells of the small intestine, in their brush border. There are three enzymes.
   a. Maltase breaks down maltose into two molecules of glucose.
   b. Sucrase splits sucrose into glucose and fuctose.
   c. Lactase splits lactose into glucose and galactose.

Digestion of Proteins

1. In the stomach proteins are broken down to polypeptides (peptones) by action of pepsin.
2. Several proteolytic enzymes are produced in the pancreas (trypsin, carboxypeptidase, elastase etc.), but these are stored in inactive form. (Trypsin is stored in the pancreas as tyrpsinogen). Enterokinase, an enzyme in intestinal cells converts trypsinogen into trypsin. In turn trypsin activates other enzymes.

Under the influence of these enzymes proteins are broken down, first into peptones and proteoses, and then into small polypeptides. Further breakdown into small peptides and amino acids occurs through the action of peptidases present in the brush border of intestinal cells, and in their cytoplasm. Small peptides and aminoacids are absorbed into blood by active transport, and also by diffusion.

Digestion and Absorption of Fats

Fat ingested through food is mostly in the form of neutral fat (triglycerides). Cholesterol esters and phospholipids are also present. Almost all digestion takes place in intestines.

1. ***Pancreatic lipase*** splits triglycerides into fatty acids and monoglyceride. ***Cholesterol esterase*** breaks up cholesterol esters to cholesterol and fatty acids. Phospholipids are broken down by ***phospholipase***.
2. The action of pancreatic lipases is increased several thousand times by emulsification of fat. In the process of emulsification, droplets of fat are broken down into much smaller particles. This greatly increases the surface area available for action of lipase.

   To enable emulsification, presence of a detergent is required. This function is performed by bile salts. They lower the surface tension of the fat globule. Once surface tension is reduced, segmentation movements of the intestine readily break up the fat globule into fine droplets. Lecithin present in bile also facilitates emulsification.
3. Apart from promoting emulsification of fat bile salts play an important role in absorption of fatty acids and monoglycerides. They surround newly formed fatty acids and monoglycerides to form small globules called ***micelles***. Molecules of bile salts have one end that is mixable with water (hydrophilic) and another end that is mixable with fat. These molecules surround fatty acids in such a way that the fat component is in the centre and is in contact with the fat-soluble part of bile salt molecules. The surface of the micelle is formed by hydrophilic ends, and can therefore mix with water easily.

Micelles, formed in this way, reach the brush border of intestinal cells. Here they release the fatty acid and monoglycerides into the cytoplasm of the cell, and the bile salts go back into the intestinal lumen and are reused.

4. Fatty acids entering the cytoplasm of intestinal cells pass into blood. Larger fatty acids recombine to form triglycerides. These cannot enter blood capillaries. Instead they pass into lymphatic capillaries (lacteals) present in villi. They travel to larger lymph vessels and reach blood through the thoracic duct.

METABOLISM

In simple terms, metabolism tells us what happens to nutrients that are absorbed. It consists of numerous chemical reactions. These reactions release energy, which is utilised for various purposes. Metabolism also includes a study of chemical reactions through which various molecules required for repair and growth of tissues are produced.

ATP

Adenosine triphosphate (usually abbreviated to ATP) is one of the most important molecules in the body. ATP serves as a source of energy. When energy is available it is stored in the form of ATP. When energy is required ATP is converted into energy (Figs. 18.4, 18.5).

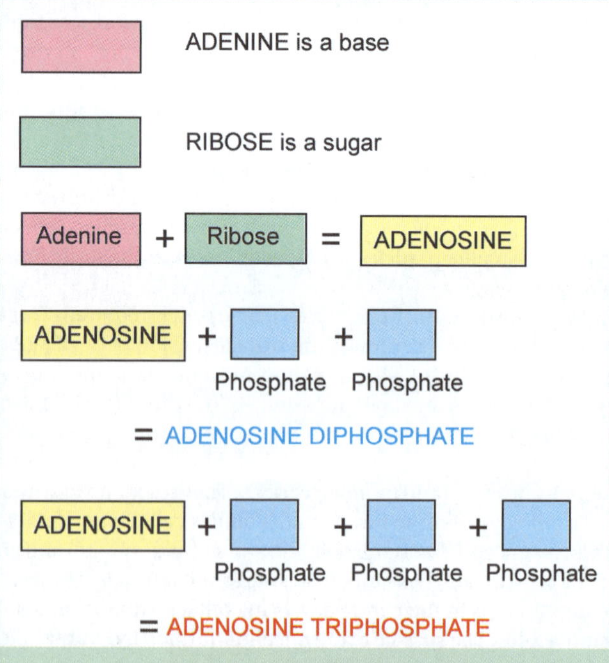

Fig. 18.4 Structure of ATP.

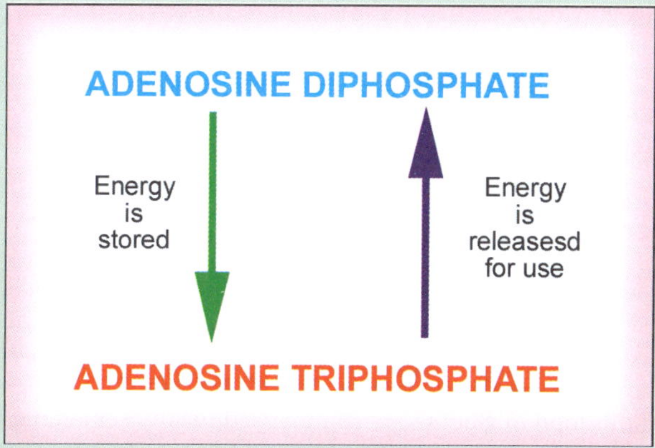

Fig. 18.5 Role of ATP in metabolism.

Catabolism and Anabolism

Metabolism consists of two basic processes. In catabolism large molecules are broken down into smaller ones. Energy is released and is stored as ATP.

In anabolism small molecules are joined together to form large molecules. Energy is needed for this, and is taken from stored ATP.

A proper balance of catabolism and anabolism is necessary for good health.

The energy that a food can generate is usually expressed in calories, or kilocalories (kcal).

Basal Metabolic Rate

The breaking down of large molecules for release of energy requires the presence of oxygen (Compare with the need of oxygen, present in air, for burning fuel). In the process oxygen combines with carbon (e.g., in carbohydrate) to form carbon dioxide. The speed at which oxygen is utilised, and carbon dioxide produced, tells us how fast metabolism is taking place. This is referred to as metabolic rate.

The metabolic rate is lowest when a person is at rest (so that no energy is being used by muscles); when the body is warm (so that energy is not needed for producing heat); and when the person has not had anything to eat for several hours (so that energy is not being used for digestion or absorption of food). This level of metabolism is called the basal metabolic rate (BMR). BMR is higher in the young (as compared to the old), higher in men than in women. Some diseases (e.g., hyperactivity of the thyroid gland) raise BMR.

CARBOHYDRATE METABOLISM

We have seen that carbohydrates ingested in food, are ultimately broken down into glucose. Glucose is the most important source of energy. When glucose is not available amino acids, fatty acids and glycerol can also be converted into glucose. This is called gluconeogenesis. Glucose absorbed into blood (in the intestine) reaches the liver. When available in excess glucose is converted to glycogen, and is stored in that form. When required glycogen is reconverted into glucose. Apart from the liver, glycogen is also stored in skeletal muscle. If availability of glucose is more than what can be stored as glycogen, it is converted into fat, which gets deposited at various sites in the body.

How Glucose is Used to Release Energy

Energy is generated by breakdown of glucose. The process is efficient when oxygen is available in adequate quantity. Utilization of glucose in the presence of oxygen is called aerobic catabolism. Some utilization of glucose can also take place in the absence of oxygen (anaerobic catabolism) but this process is not efficient. The steps involved in utilization of glucose are summarised below. Remember that energy released is stored in the form of ATP.

Glucolysis

Step 1. Glucose (from the circulation) enters the cytoplasm of a cell. Each molecule of glucose forms two molecules of pyruvic acid. Energy is released in the form of two molecules of ATP. Glucolysis is an anaerobic process (Fig. 18.6).

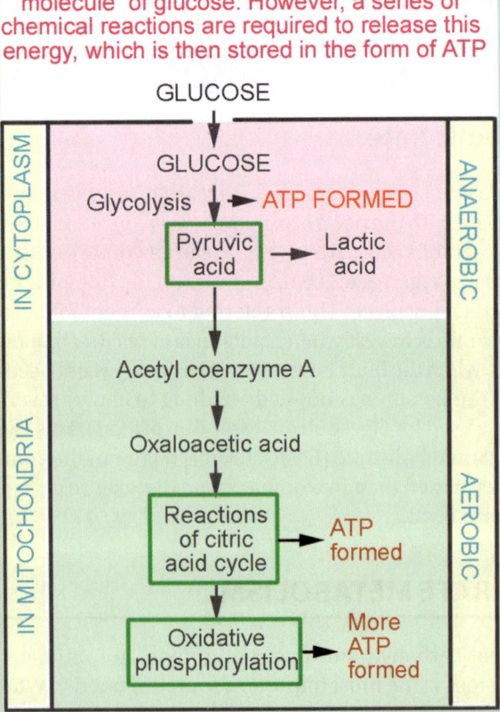

Fig. 18.6 Deriving energy from glucose.

Step 2. The two molecules of pyruvic acid enter mitochondria and undergo a series of reactions that are known as the citric acid cycle or Krebs' cycle. In this process two more molecules of ATP are generated. Oxygen is required for this reaction.

Step 3. Some substances produced in the citric acid cycle undergo oxidative phosphorylation to produce several more molecules of ATP. This takes place within mitochrondria and requires adequate supply of oxygen.

Step 4. When adequate supply of oxygen is not available (e.g., during heavy exercise) the two molecules of pyruvic acid formed by glucolysis (see step 1 above) remain in the cytoplasm and are converted to lactic acid. Accumulation of lactic acid in muscles, leads to pain and cramps (that athletes often complain of). Later when adequate blood supply (oxygen supply) is restored accumulated lactic acid is removed as follows.

Some of it is reconverted into pyruvic acid. Pyruvic acid is oxidized to form CO_2 and water. CO_2 enters blood and is removed through the lungs. Water (if in excess) is removed from the body through urine.

PROTEIN METABOLISM

We have seen that in the process of digestion, proteins are broken down into amino acids. Conversely, when a protein is required in the body (e.g., for growth or repair of tissue), it is synthesised by joining together amino acids.

There are about twenty amino acids in the body. We obtain them through proteins present in diet. Some of these can also be synthesised in the body. However, there are some that cannot be synthesised and their presence in diet is essential. That is why they are called essential amino acids.

Each protein is made up of polypeptides. Each polypeptide is made up of amino acids joined to form chains. One protein differs from another because of the amino acids present, and the sequence in which they are arranged.

We have seen that amino acids are used to synthesise proteins required for cell growth and replacement. Many hormones, antibodies and enzymes are also proteins.

The body maintains a small reserve of amino acids for use as required. This is called the amino acid pool. Amino acids released by protein breakdown are added to the pool and those required for synthesis are removed. However, the amino acid pool can hold only a small quantity of amino acids. When in excess amino acids are disposed off as follows.

1. When other sources are not available, amino acids can be converted to glucose for obtaining energy. Other amino acids form products used in glucose metabolism (acetyl coenzyme A, oxaloacetic acid).
2. Amino acid can be broken down by the process of deamination. As a result, urea is formed and is excreted through urine.
3. Some proteins are lost in faeces.

FAT METABOLISM

We have seen that fat present in food is broken down into fatty acids and glycerol. These are absorbed into lacteals (in villi). They pass into larger lymph vessels to ultimately reach the thoracic duct. This duct opens into large veins in the neck. In this way fatty acids and glycerol reach the bloodstream. Their fate is as follows.

1. Some fatty acids and glycerol are used by cells to provide energy (see below).
2. Some are used in synthesis of some secretions.
3. In the liver fatty acids combine with glycerol to form triglycerides (a form in which fat can be stored). When required triglycerides can be broken down into glycerol and fatty acids and these can be used to provide energy.

How Fatty Acids are Used to Provide Energy

While discussing the production of energy from glucose we have seen that one intermediate product of glucose utilization is acetyl coenzyme A which is then used in reactions involving the citric acid cycle. Fatty acids can be converted into acetyl coenzyme A, which can be used to provide ATP (just as in glucose metabolism).

Sometimes (as in a fasting individual) acetyl coenzyme A produced from fatty acids may be more than can be utilised. The enzyme is then converted into ketone bodies (in the liver). Ketone bodies can be excreted through lungs and kidneys. High concentrations of ketone bodies are toxic.

CHAPTER

19

The Urinary System

The organs of the body that are concerned with the formation of urine and its elimination from the body are referred to as urinary organs. They consist (Fig. 19.1) of the right and left ***kidneys***, in which urine is formed; the right and left ***ureters***; the ***urinary bladder***, in which urine is stored temporarily and is also concentrated; and the ***urethra*** that carries urine from the urinary bladder to the exterior.

Urine production, and its composition, is controlled exclusively by the kidneys. The urinary bladder is responsible for storage of urine until it is voided. The ureter and urethra are simple passages for transport of urine.

THE KIDNEYS

FUNCTIONS OF THE KIDNEYS

Before considering the structure and functioning of the kidney in detail it is useful to briefly summarise the functions of the kidneys.

Functions Concerned with Homeostasis

1. The chief function of the kidney is the excretion of waste products produced in the body through urine. These substances include urea, creatinine, uric acid, and bilirubin.
2. Excretion of harmful substances entering the body. These include drugs, toxins, heavy metals, and pesticides.
3. The kidneys maintain the water balance of the body, by excreting it when it is in excess, and conserving it when there is substantial loss of water (e.g., from perspiration in hot weather). In this way the water content of plasma and of tissue fluid is kept fairly constant.
4. The kidneys maintain electrolyte balance specially that of sodium.

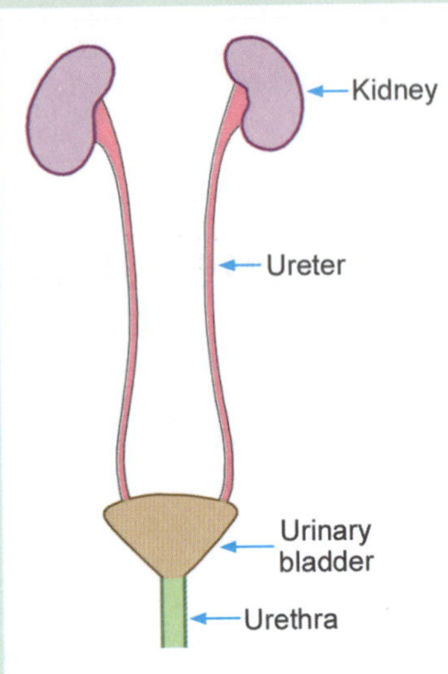

Fig. 19.1 The urinary organs.

5. The kidneys regulate the acid-base balance so that the pH of blood and of body fluids is maintained within narrow limits.

Other Functions of Kidneys

6. The kidneys play an important role in control of blood pressure (through the renin-angiotensin mechanism).
7. Erythropoietin secreted by the kidneys stimulates production of erythrocytes.
8. The kidneys play a role in regulation of blood calcium through vitamin D.
9. The kidneys produce a number of hormones including renin, erythropoietin, thrombopoietin, and prostaglandins.

BASIC STRUCTURE OF THE KIDNEY

The structure of the kidney is complex. Understanding is facilitated if the main facts are studied first before going in to details.

Each kidney has a characteristic bean-like shape (Fig. 19.2). It has a convex lateral margin; and a concavity on the medial side that is called the ***hilum***. It has upper and lower ends and anterior and posterior surfaces. Terminal branches of the renal artery enter the kidney at the hilum, and the veins emerge from it. The hilum also gives attachment to the upper expanded end of the ureter (miscalled the ***renal pelvis***).

The position of the kidneys relative to the anterior abdominal wall is shown in Fig. 19.3. Note the following. Because of the presence of the liver on the right side, the right kidney lies slightly lower than the left kidney. The hilum of each kidney lies more or less in the transpyloric plane, a little medial to the tip of the ninth costal cartilage. The vertical axis of the kidney is placed obliquely (Figs.

19.2 and 19.3) so that its upper end is nearer the median plane than the lower end. Note the dimensions of the kidney shown in Fig. 19.2.

The upper end is about 2.5 cm (one inch) from the median plane, while the lower end is about 7.5 cm (three inches) from it.

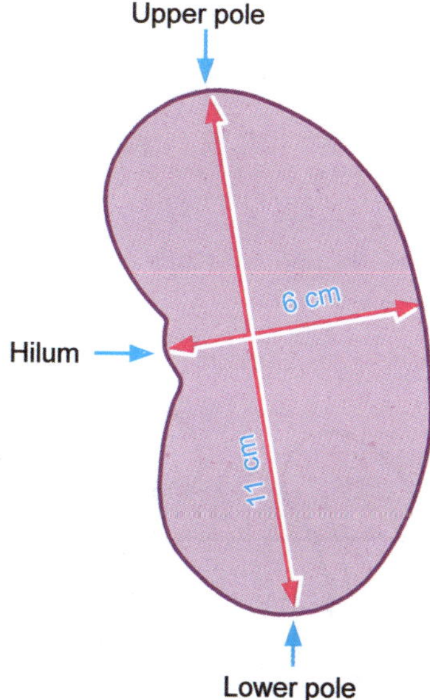

Fig. 19.2 Approximate dimensions of a kidney. The antero-posterior diameter is about 3 cm.

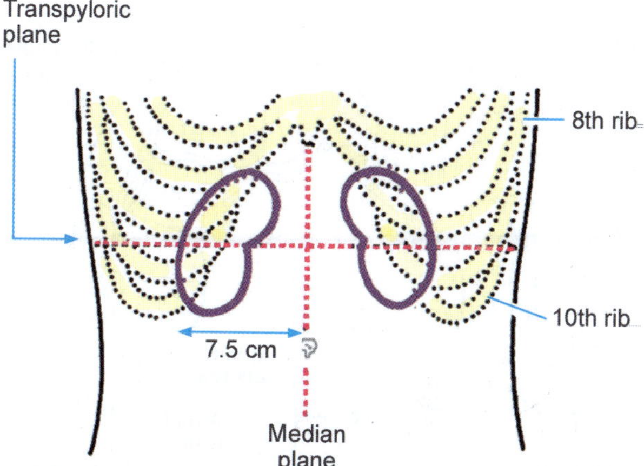

Fig. 19.3 Projection of the kidney to the front of the body.

In relation to the posterior surface of the body the hilum of the kidney lies at the level of the first lumbar spine (Fig. 19.4), the upper pole at the level of the 11th thoracic spine, and the lower pole at the level of the third lumbar spine. In Fig. 19.4 note that the area in which the kidney lies can be represented as a parallelogram (***Morrison's parallelogram***).

The kidneys are closely related to a number of important structures. These are shown in Figs. 19.5. and 19.6.

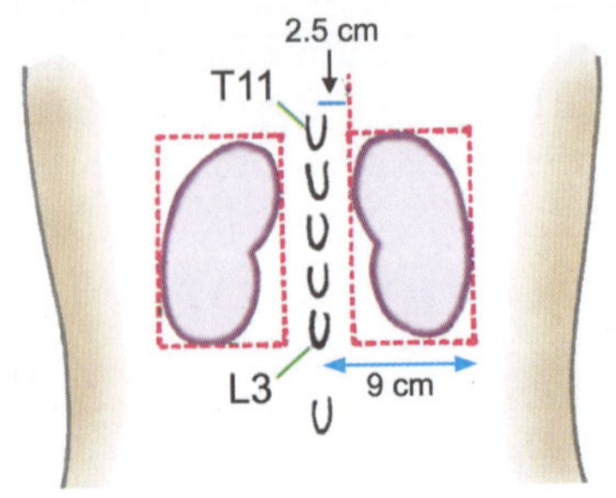

Fig. 19.4 Surface projection of the kidney on the back of the body.

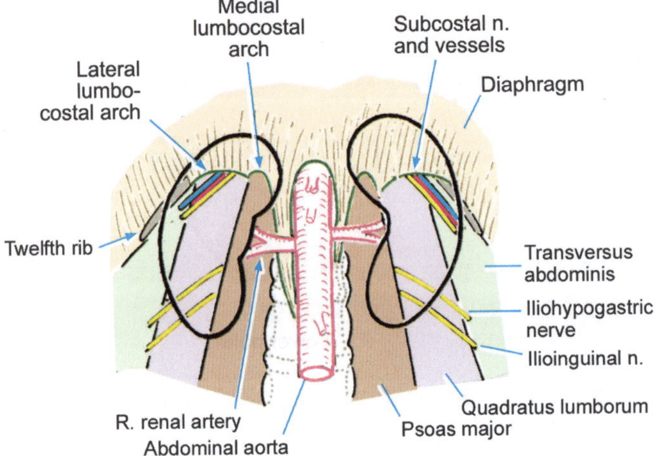

Fig. 19.5 Posterior relations of kidneys.

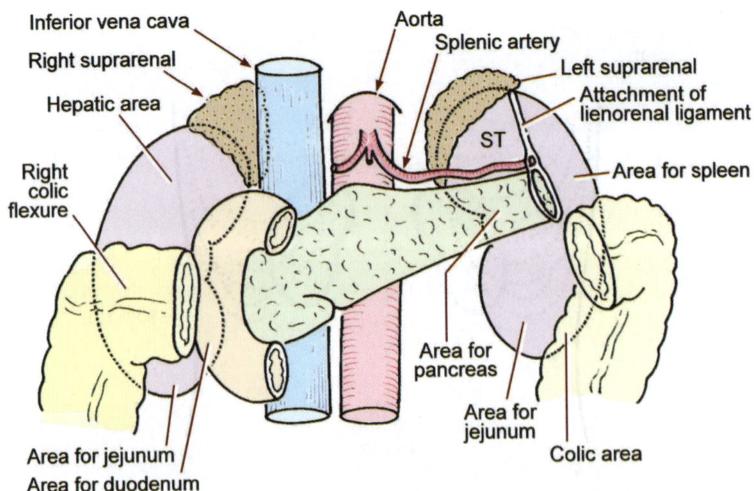

Fig. 19.6 Scheme to show the anterior relations of the right and left kidneys.

Gross Internal Structure

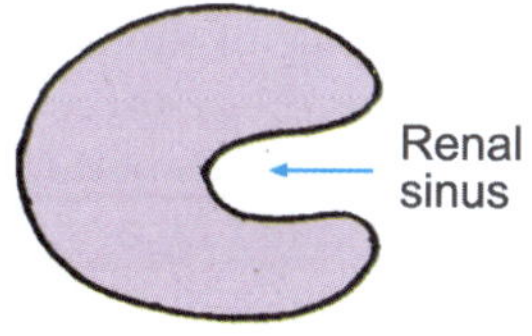

Fig. 19.7 Transverse section through a kidney to show the hilum and the renal sinus.

When we examine a transverse section across a kidney it is seen that the hilum leads into a space called the ***renal sinus*** (Fig. 19.7). The renal sinus is occupied by the upper expanded part of the ureter that is called the ***renal pelvis***; by renal vessels, and by some fat. Within the renal sinus the pelvis divides into two (or three) parts called ***major calices*** (singular = calyx) (Fig. 19.8). Each major calyx divides into a number of minor calices (Fig. 19.9). The end of each minor calyx is shaped like a cup. A projection of kidney tissue called a ***papilla*** fits into the cup.

Some features of the internal structure of the kidney can be seen when we examine a coronal section through the organ (Fig.19.8). Kidney tissue consists of an outer part called the ***cortex***, and an inner part called the ***medulla***.

The medulla is made up of triangular areas of renal tissue that are called the ***renal pyramids***. Each pyramid has a base directed towards the cortex; and an apex (or papilla) that is directed towards the renal pelvis, and fits into a minor calyx. Pyramids show striations that pass radially towards the apex.

The renal cortex consists of the following:

a. Tissue lying between the bases of the pyramids and the surface of the kidney, forming the ***cortical arches*** or ***cortical lobules***. This part of the cortex shows light and dark striations. The light lines are called ***medullary rays***.

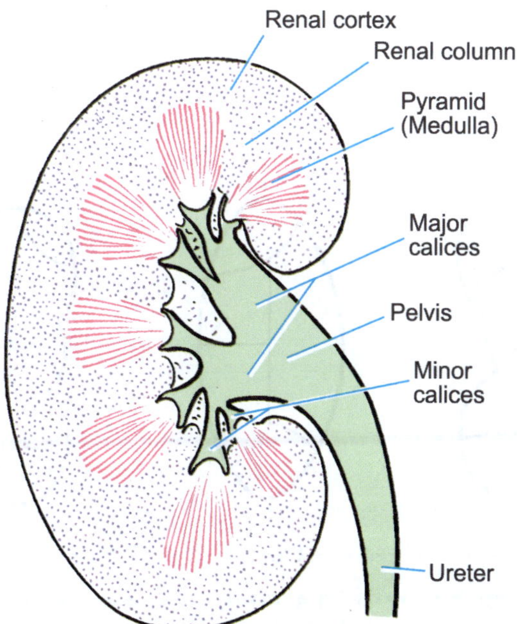

Fig. 19.8 Some features to be seen in a coronal section through the kidney.

b. Tissue lying between adjacent pyramids is also a part of the cortex. This part constitutes the ***renal columns***.
c. In this way each pyramid comes to be surrounded by a 'shell' of cortex. The pyramid and the cortex around it constitute a lobe of the kidney. This lobulation is obvious in the fetal kidney.

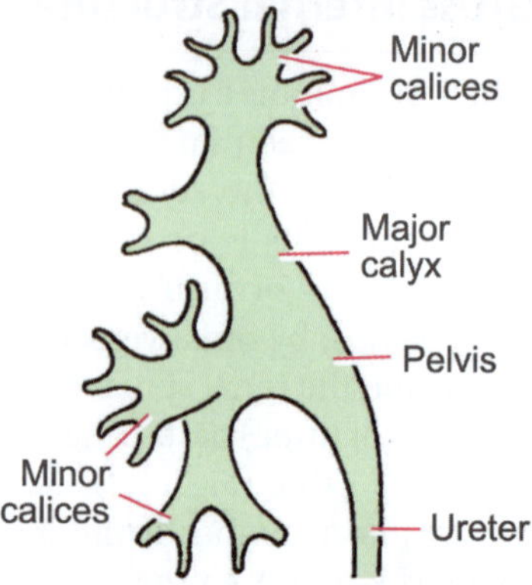

Fig. 19.9 Scheme to show the major and minor calices.

Renal Capsule

The kidney tissue is intimately covered by a thin layer of fibrous tissue that is named the capsule. In the healthy kidney the capsule can be easily stripped off; but it become adherent in some diseases.

Renal Fascia

Outside the capsule the kidney is surrounded by a layer of ***perirenal fat*** (also called ***perinephric fat***). Some of this fat extends into the renal sinus.

Renal Segments

The kidneys are supplied by the renal arteries and are drained by the renal veins. Near the hilum of the kidney the renal artery divides into anterior and

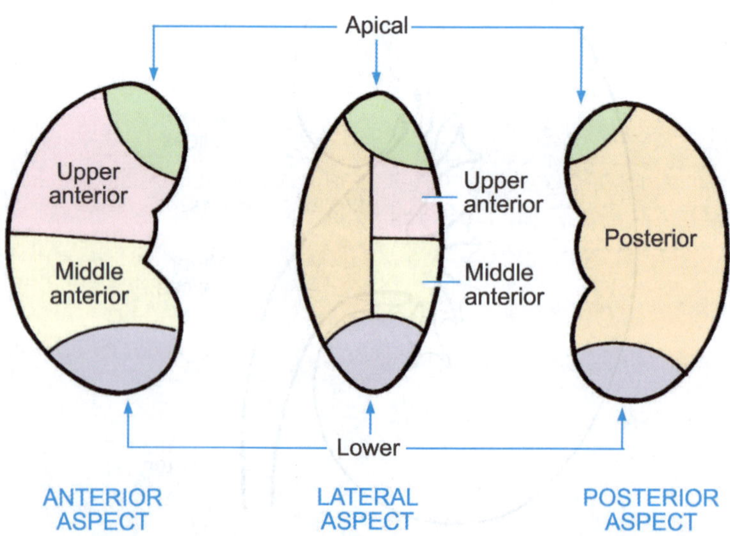

Fig. 19.10 Scheme to show the segments of the kidney.

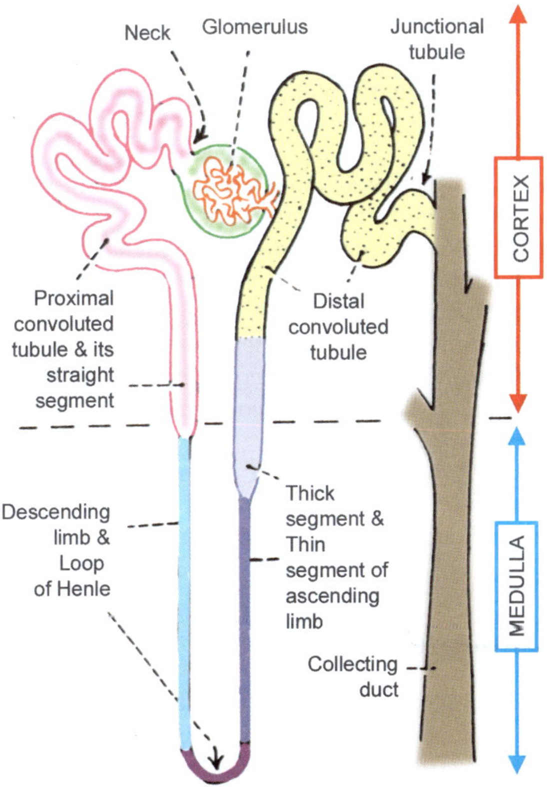

Fig. 19.11 Parts of a nephron. A collecting duct is also shown.

posterior divisions. Within the renal sinus these divide further into primary branches each of which supplies a specific region of renal tissue, there being no anastomoses between arteries to adjoining regions. These primary branches are called ***segmental arteries***. Based on their distribution the kidney can be divided into five segments as shown in Fig. 19.10. These segments are of surgical importance.

THE URINIFEROUS TUBULES

From a functional point of view the kidney may be regarded as a collection of numerous ***uriniferous tubules*** that are specialised for the excretion of urine. Each uriniferous tubule consists of an excretory part called the ***nephron***, and of a ***collecting tubule***. The collecting tubules draining different nephrons join to form larger tubules called ***papillary ducts***, each of which opens into a minor calyx at the apex of a renal papilla. Each kidney contains one to two million nephrons.

Urinary tubules are held together by scanty connective tissue. Blood vessels, lymphatics and nerves lie in this connective tissue.

Parts of the Nephron

The nephron consists of a ***renal corpuscle*** (or ***Malpighian corpuscle***), and a long complicated ***renal tubule*** (Fig. 19.11). The renal corpuscle is a rounded structure consisting of (a) a rounded tuft of blood capillaries called the ***glomerulus***; and (b) a cup-like, double layered covering for the glomerulus called the ***glomerular capsule*** (or ***Bowman's capsule***). The glomerular capsule represents the cup-shaped blind beginning of the renal tubule. Between the two layers of the capsule there is a ***urinary space*** that is continuous with the lumen of the renal tubule.

The renal tubule is divisible into several parts that are shown in Fig. 19.11. Starting from the glomerular capsule there are: (**a**) the ***proximal convoluted tubule***; (**b**) the ***loop of Henle*** consisting of a ***descending limb***, a ***loop***, and an ***ascending limb***; and (**c**) the ***distal convoluted tubule***, which ends by joining a collecting tubule.

Renal corpuscles, and (the greater parts of) the proximal and distal convoluted tubules are located in the cortex of the kidney. The loops of Henle and the collecting ducts lie in the medullary rays and in the substance of the pyramids.

The Renal Corpuscle

We have seen that the glomerulus is a rounded tuft of anastomosing capillaries (Figs. 19.12, 19.13). Blood enters the tuft through an afferent arteriole and leaves it through an efferent arteriole (Fig. 19.17). (Note that the efferent vessel is an arteriole, and not a venule. It again breaks up into capillaries as described below). The afferent and efferent arterioles lie close together at a point that is referred to as the ***vascular pole*** of the renal corpuscle.

We have seen that the glomerular capsule is a double-layered cup, the two layers of which are separated by the urinary space. The urinary space becomes continuous with the lumen of the renal tubule at the ***urinary pole*** of the renal corpuscle.

The Renal Tubule

We have seen that the renal tubule is made up (in proximo-distal sequence) of the proximal convoluted tubule, the loop of Henle, and the distal convoluted tubule. The distal convoluted tubule ends by opening into a collecting tubule.

The following additional details may be noted.

a. The junction of the proximal convoluted tubule with the glomerular capsule is narrow and is referred to as the ***neck***.
b. The proximal convoluted tubule is made up of an initial part having many convolutions (lying in the cortex), and of a terminal straight part that descends into the medulla to become continuous with the descending limb of the loop of Henle.
c. The descending limb, the loop itself, and part of the ascending limb of the

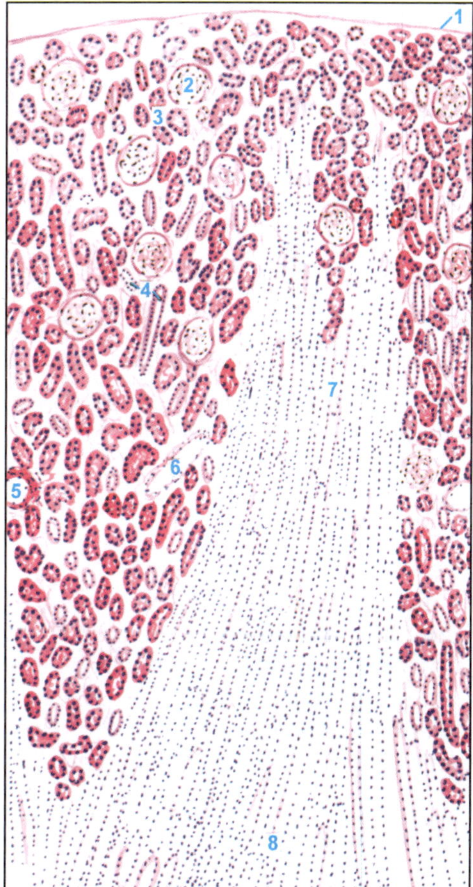

Fig. 19.12 Kidney (low power view). 1-Capsule, 2-Renal corpuscle. 3-Proximal convoluted tubule. 4-Distal convoluted tubule. 5-Artery. 6-Vein. 7-Medullary ray. 8-Collecting duct.

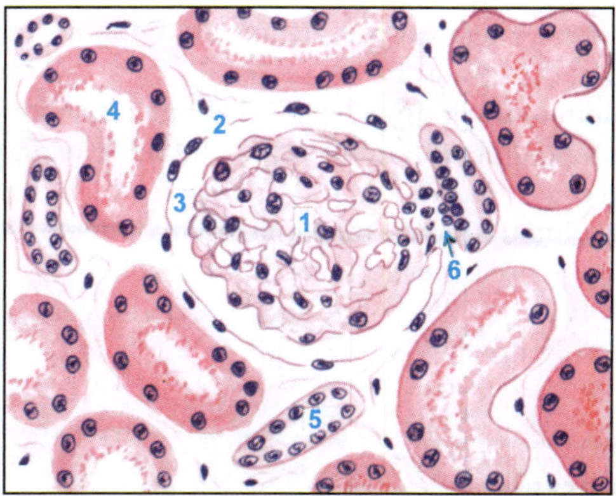

Fig. 19.13 Renal cortex (high power view). 1-Glomerulus. 2-Urinary space. 3-Proximal convoluted tubule. 5-Distal convoluted tubule. 6-Macula densa.

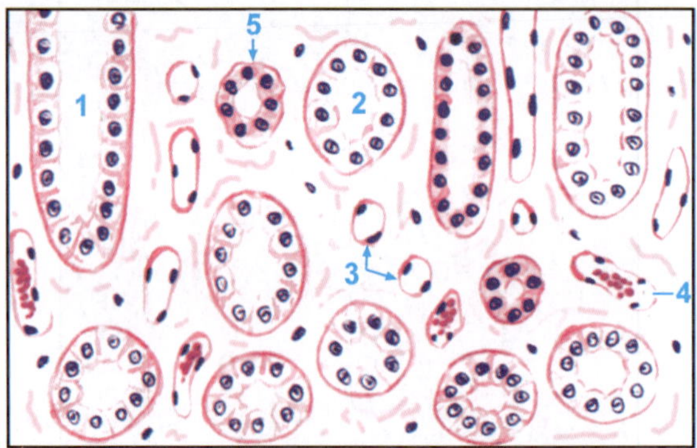

Fig. 19.14 Renal medulla (high power view). 1, 2-Collecting duct (L.S & T.S). 3, 5-Loop of Henle (thin and thick segments). 4-Capillary.

loop of Henle are narrow and thin walled. They constitute the ***thin segment*** of the loop. The upper part of the ascending limb has a larger diameter and thicker wall and is called the ***thick segment***.

d. The distal convoluted tubule has a straight part continuous with the ascending limb of the loop of Henle, and a convoluted part lying in the cortex. At the junction between the two parts, the distal tubule lies very close to the renal corpuscle of the nephron to which it belongs. The terminal part of the distal convoluted tubule is again straight. This part is called the ***junctional tubule*** or ***connecting tubule***, and ends by joining a collecting duct.

Epithelium Lining the Renal Tubule

The renal tubule is lined by a single layer of epithelial cells that are supported on a basal lamina. The features of the lining cells, as seen with the light microscope in different parts of the renal tubule, are described below.

The ***neck*** is lined by simple squamous epithelium continuous with that of the glomerular capsule.

The ***proximal convoluted tubules*** are 40-60 μm in diameter. They have a relatively small lumen. These tubules are lined by cuboidal (or columnar) cells having a prominent brush border.

The thin segment of the loop of Henle is about 15-30 μm in diameter. It is lined by a low cuboidal or squamous cells. The thick segment of the loop is lined by cuboidal cells.

The distal convoluted tubules are 20-50 μm in diameter. They are lined by cuboidal cells that do not have a brush border.

The smallest collecting tubules are 40-50 μm in diameter, and the largest as much as 200 μm. They are lined by a simple cuboidal or columnar epithelium (Fig. 19.14).

Renal Blood Vessels

Knowledge of some features of the arrangement of blood vessels within the kidney is essential to the understanding of renal function.

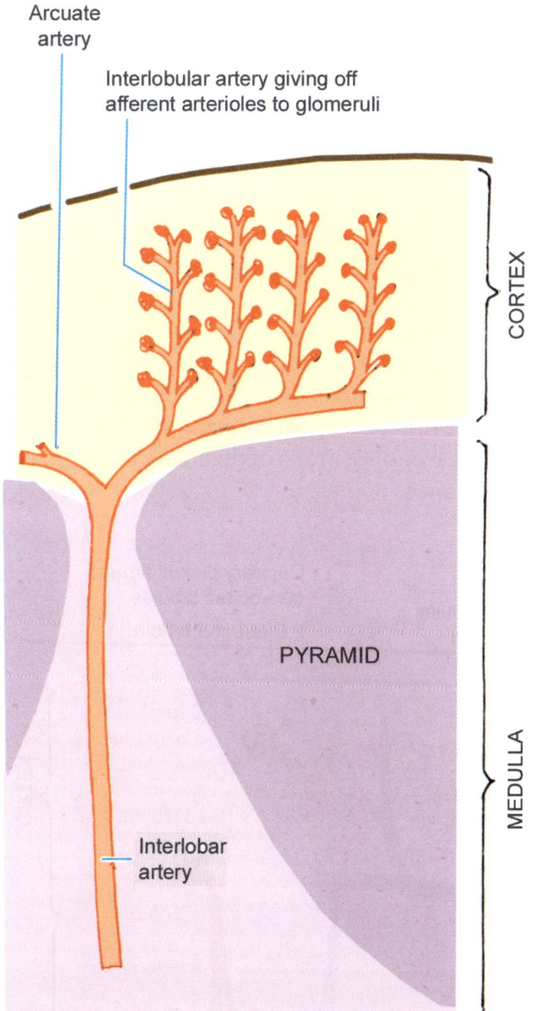

Fig. 19.15 Scheme to show the arrangement of arteries within the kidney.

At the hilum of the kidney each renal artery divides into a number of ***lobar arteries*** (one for each pyramid) (Fig. 19.15). Each lobar artery divides into two (or more) ***interlobar arteries*** that enter the tissue of the renal columns and run towards the surface of the kidney. Reaching the level of the bases of the pyramids, the interlobar arteries divide into ***arcuate arteries***. The arcuate arteries run at right angles to the parent interlobar arteries. They lie parallel to the renal surface at the junction of the pyramid and the cortex. The arcuate arteries give off a series of ***interlobular arteries***. Each interlobular artery gives off a series of arterioles that enter glomeruli as ***afferent arterioles***.

Blood from these arterioles circulates through glomerular capillaries that join to form ***efferent arterioles*** that emerge from glomeruli.

The behaviour of efferent arterioles leaving the glomeruli differs in case of glomeruli located more superficially in the cortex and those lying near the pyramids.

Efferent arterioles arising from the majority of glomeruli (superficial) divide into capillaries that surround the proximal and distal convoluted tubules. These capillaries drain into ***interlobular veins***, and through them into ***arcuate veins*** and ***interlobar veins***. Efferent arterioles arising from glomeruli nearer the medulla (***juxtamedullary glomeruli***) divide into several straight vessels that descend into the medulla. These are the ***descending vasa recta*** (Figs. 19.16, 19.17). These form a capillary plexus that surrounds the descending and ascending limbs of the loop of Henle. This plexus is drained by ***ascending vasa recta*** that run upwards parallel to the descending vasa recta to reach the cortex. Here they drain into interlobular or arcuate veins. The parallel orientation of the ascending and descending vasa recta and their close relationship to the ascending and descending limbs of the loops of Henle is of considerable physiological importance.

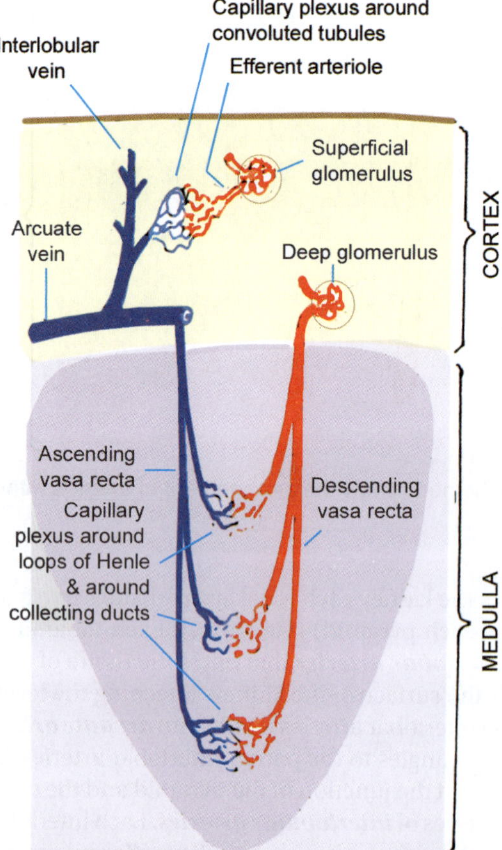

Fig. 19.16 Scheme to show behaviour of efferent arterioles of glomeruli in the superficial and deeper parts of the renal cortex.

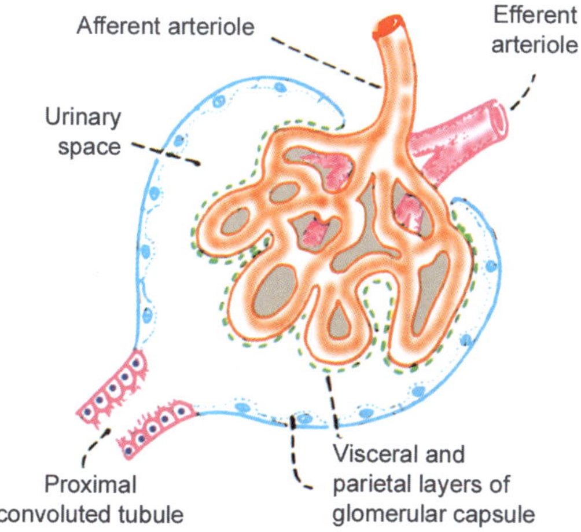

Fig. 19.17 Scheme to show the basic structure of a renal corpuscle.

From this account of the renal blood vessels it will be clear that two sets of arterioles and capillaries intervene between the renal artery and vein. The first capillary system, present in glomeruli, is concerned exclusively with the removal of waste products from blood. It does not supply oxygen to renal tissues. Exchange of gases (oxygen, carbon dioxide) between blood and renal tissue is entirely through the second capillary system (present around tubules).

It has been said that in most tissues the blood supply exists to provide service to the parenchyma (in the form of the supply of oxygen and nutrients, and the removal of carbon dioxide and other waste products). In the kidney, on the other hand, the parenchyma exists to provide service to blood (by removal of waste products in it).

It has also been held that interlobular arteries divide the renal cortex into small lobules. Each lobule is defined as the region of cortex lying between two adjacent interlobular arteries. A medullary ray, containing a collecting duct, runs vertically through the middle of the lobule (midway between the two arteries) (Fig. 17.9). Glomeruli lie in a zone adjacent to the arteries while other parts of the nephron lie nearer the centre of the lobule.

Renal Blood Flow

The amount of blood flowing through the kidney every minute is 1.2 litres. This is 20% of cardiac output. Blood flow is not affected by variation in blood pressure between 70 mmHg and 200 mmHg. This is called ***autoregulation of renal blood flow***. Constant blood flow maintains a constant glomerular filtration rate. However, about 90% of this blood flow passes through the cortex only. The medulla receives only 10% of it.

Further details about the Renal Corpuscle

Glomerular Filtration Barrier

In the renal corpuscle water and various small molecules pass, by filtration, from blood (in the glomerular capillaries) to the urinary space of the glomerular capsule. Theoretically the barrier across which the filtration would have to occur is constituted by (a) the capillary endothelium, (b) by the cells (podocytes) forming the glomerular (or visceral) layer of the glomerular capsule, and (c) by a ***glomerular basement membrane*** that intervenes between the two layers of cells named above, and represents the fused basal laminae of the two layers. In fact, however, the barrier is modified as follows.

1. Firstly, the endothelial cells of glomerular capillaries show numerous fenestrae or pores that are larger than pores in many other situations. The fenestrae are not closed by membrane. As a result filtrate passes easily through the pores, and the endothelial cells do not form an effective barrier.
2. The ***podocytes*** are so called because they possess foot-like processes. Each podocyte has a few ***primary processes*** that give the cell a star shaped appearance. These processes are wrapped around glomerular capillaries and interdigitate with those of neighbouring podocytes. Each primary process terminates in numerous ***secondary processes*** also called ***pedicels*** (or end feet) that rest on the basal lamina. The cell body of the podocyte comes in contact with the basal lamina only through the pedicels. Between the areas of attachment of individual pedicels there are gaps in which the basal lamina is not covered by podocyte cytoplasm. Filtration takes place through the basal lamina at these gaps that are, therefore, called ***filtration slits*** or ***slit pores***. These slits are filled by a layer of fine filaments that constitute the ***glomerular slit diaphragm***. From what has been said above it will be clear that the filtrate does not have to pass through podocyte cytoplasm.

It follows, therefore, that the only real barrier across which filtration occurs is the basal lamina (or the glomerular basement membrane) that is thickened at the filtration slits by the glomerular slit diaphragm. The efficacy of the barrier is greatly enhanced by the presence of a high negative charge in the basement membrane and in podocyte processes. [Loss of this charge, in some diseases, leads to excessive leakage of protein through the barrier].

Glomerular Basement Membrane

As compared to typical membranes the glomerular basement membrane is very thick (about 300 nm). It contains glycosaminoglycan heparan sulphate which bears a strong negative charge. The glomerular basement membrane is, therefore, both a physical barrier and an electrical barrier to the passage of large molecules.

The glomerular basement membrane (and overlying podocyte cytoplasm) does not go all round a glomerular capillary. The gap is filled in by mesangium described below. Also note that in the interval between capillaries the basement membrane is in contact with mesangium.

Defects in the glomerular basement membrane are responsible for the nephrotic syndrome in which large amounts of protein are lost through urine. The regular arrangement of podocyte processes is also disorganized in this condition.

The Mesangium

On entering the glomerulus the afferent arteriole divides (usually) into five branches, each branch leading into an independent capillary network. The glomerular circulation can, therefore, be divided into a number of lobules or segments.

Glomerular capillaries are supported by the ***mesangium*** that is made up of mesangial cells surrounded by a non-cellular mesangial matrix. Mesangial cells give off processes that run through the matrix. Mesangium intervenes between the capillaries of the glomerulus.

Mesangial cells contain filaments similar to myosin. They bear angiotensin II receptors. It is believed that stimulation by angiotensin causes the fibrils to contract. In this way mesangial cells may play a role in controlling blood flow through the glomerulus. Other functions attributed to mesangial cells include phagocytosis, and maintenance of glomerular basement membrane. The mesangium becomes prominent in a disease called glomerulonephritis.

Further details about the Renal Tubule

With the EM the lining cells of the proximal convoluted tubules show microvilli on their luminal surfaces. Near the base of each cell the plasma membrane shows numerous infoldings. Numerous mitochondria lie longitudinally in the cytoplasm intervening between the folds. The presence of microvilli, and of the basal infoldings greatly increases the surface area available for transport. Numerous enzymes associated with ionic transport are present in the cytoplasm.

The loop of Henle is also called the ***ansa nephroni***. With the EM the flat cells lining the thin segment of the loop of Henle show very few organelles indicating that the cells play only a passive role in ionic movements across them.

The length of the thin segment of the loop of Henle is variable. In the case of nephrons starting from glomeruli lying deep in the cortex (juxtamedullary glomeruli) the loops of Henle pass deep into the medulla. In the case of nephrons starting from glomeruli lying in the middle of the cortical thickness part of the loop of Henle lies in the cortex. Some loops (associated with glomeruli placed in the superficial part of the cortex) may lie entirely within the cortex.

The structure of the (ascending) thick segment of the loop of Henle is similar to that of distal convoluted tubules. The cells of the distal convoluted tubules resemble those of the proximal convoluted tubules with the following differences.

a. They have only a few small microvilli.
b. The basal infoldings of plasma membrane are very prominent and reach almost to the luminal surface of the cell. This feature is characteristic of

cells involved in the active transport of ions. Enzymes concerned with active transport of ions are present in the cells. At the junction of the straight and convoluted parts of the distal convoluted tubules, the cells show specializations that are described below in connection with the juxtaglomerular apparatus.

In the proximal part of the collecting system the collecting tubules are lined by two types of cells. The majority of cells (called ***clear cells***) have very few organelles, a few microvilli and some basal infoldings. The lining epithelium also contains some ***dark cells*** (or ***intercalated cells***). These have microvilli, but basal infoldings are not seen. They contain numerous mitochondria.

The cells of the collecting ducts do not have microvilli, or lateral infoldings of plasma membrane. Very few organelles are present in the cytoplasm.

PRODUCTION OF URINE

Blood circulating through glomeruli is separated from the cavity of the glomerular capsule by the glomerular filtration barrier described above. Water and many types of molecules pass through this barrier by the simple process of filtration. This fluid has a composition similar to that of plasma except that it does not contain plasma proteins. The fluid is called the ***glomerular filtrate***.

Although the glomerular membrane is highly permeable, the permeability is selective. Plasma proteins do not pass through, but haemoglobin, if present in free form in plasma, passes through. The electrical charge of the molecule is also important. Positively charged particles pass through more easily than negatively charged ones.

The volume of filtrate formed every minute (by both kidneys) is the ***glomerular filtration rate (GFR)***. This is about 125 ml per minute. Note that this works out to about 180 litres per day. An average person passes only about 1.0 to 1.5 litres of urine per day. It follows that most of the water in the glomerular filtrate has to be reabsorbed.

A more or less constant glomerular filtration rate is maintained. It is not influenced by variations in blood present (unless systolic blood pressure falls below 80 mmHg, as in shock), or by nervous influences. The fact that glomerular capillaries intervene between two arterioles (not an arteriole and a venule) ensures that the pressure in the capillaries is high. This facilitates glomerular filtration.

The maintenance of the glomerular filtration rate depends on blood flow through glomeruli. The total blood flow through the kidney (every minute) is 1250 ml. Of this 650 ml is plasma. We have seen that the glomerular filtration rate is 125 ml.

Filtration fraction is the proportion of plasma flow per minute to glomerular filtration rate. In other words it is 125/650 = 0.2 approximately.

Glomerular filtration coefficient: This is the product of *Glomerular permeability* and *effective surface area* of glomerular membrane. This is decreased by angiotensin II, vasopressin, norepinephrine and histamine. It is increased by renal prostaglandins and by dopamine.

Factors Influencing GFR

These are :

a. Hydrostatic pressure.
b. Osmotic pressure gradient.
c. Area of the capillary bed.
d. Permeability of capillaries.

GFR is increased during pregnancy as metabolites produced in the fetus have also to be excreted.

It is decreased in hypotention and in advanced renal diseases.

Estimation of GFR

The creatinine clearance test is used as a measure of GFR because (a) rate of production of creatinine in the body is constant, (b) it is completely filtered through glomeruli and (c) it is not reabsorbed or secreted by tubules.

Effect of Tubules on Glomerular Filtrate

As the glomerular filtrate pass through the convoluted tubules substances in it may behave in three ways.

a. They may pass into urine unchanged.
b. They may be reabsorbed, partially or completely.
c. Their quantity may be increased as a result of secretion by tubules.

The ultimate composition of urine leaving the kidneys depends upon these three processes of filtration, reabsorption, and secretion.

Substances that are completely reabsorbed by active transport are glucose (see below), amino acids, vitamins and electrolytes (sodium, potassium, chloride, bicarbonate). Parathyroid hormone, and calcitonin (produced by the thyroid gland) control reabsorption of calcium. Aldosterone (produced by the adrenal cortex) controls reabsorption of sodium.

A very small quantity of protein that passed into the filtrate is reabsorbed by pinocytosis and is broken down into amino acids by cells of the proximal convoluted tubules.

Most of the water in filtrate is reabsorbed by passive diffusion. Reabsorption of water is influenced by the antidiuretic hormones (ADH) produced by the posterior lobe of the hypophysis cerebri. One function of the kidney is to maintain osmolarity of body fluids. The normal urine output is about 1.5 litres per day. When plasma osmolarity is high the water content of urine decreases and urine becomes more concentrated (Further details are given below).

Substances that are partially reabsorbed include urea, uric acid, sulphates and phosphates.

Substances secreted into the filtrate are potassium and hydrogen ions (by active transport). Maintenance of the pH of blood is helped secretion of hydrogen ions by tubules (Correlate this with the fact that urine is normally acidic). Some drugs e.g., penicillin are also secreted.

When plasma glucose level is normal all glucose is reabsorbed. When plasma glucose goes above a certain level (known as the renal threshold) (normal value 180 mg%) glucose appears in urine (as in diabetes). In a congenital defect called renal glycosuria glucose appears in urine even when plasma glucose level is normal (ie., the renal threshold is lowered).

Role of Proximal Convoluted Tubules

These tubules play a vital role in selective reabsorption of many substances from the glomerular filtrate. The substances reabsorbed include water, glucose, amino acids, proteins of small molecular size, and various ions including sodium, chloride, phosphate, bicarbonate and calcium.

Reabsorption is facilitated by the presence of microvilli and foldings of the lateral and basal plasma membranes. Energy for the process is provided by the numerous mitochondria present.

Role of Loop of Henle (Thin Segment)

The main role of the loop of Henle is to create a hypertonic environment in the medulla. This environment plays a very important part in reabsorption of large quantities of water by collecting ducts. The creation of this hypertonic environment is a complex process, various aspects of which are considered below.

Medullary Gradient

The concentration of NaCl (osmolarity) in interstitial fluid surrounding the tubules varies in different parts of the kidney. In the cortex osmolarity is 300 units (which is the same as in plasma). As we proceed deeper into the medulla osmolarity gradually increases to a maximum of 1200 units. This increase in osmolarity is the medullary gradient. Urine passing through collecting ducts is exposed to the medullary gradient. As the collecting ducts are permeable, water diffuses out of the ducts and urine becomes more and more concentrated.

Countercurrent Multiplier System

The medullary gradient is created by the counter current multiplier system formed by loops of Henle.

a. The descending and ascending limbs of the loop of Henle lie close to each other. However flow of fluid through the two limbs is in opposite direction. (This is the meaning of 'countercurrent').
b. Fluid entering the descending limb of the loop has lower osmolarity as compared to the surrounding interstitium. Hence water passively diffuses out of the tube making the fluid in the descending limb more and more concentrated. The concentration becomes maximum at the apex of the loop (1200 units).
c. This fluid very rich in NaCl now enters the ascending limb of the loop of Henle. NaCl is actively transported out of the tube into the interstitium. As a result high osmolarity of the medullary interstitium is maintained. Another result is that filtrate leaving the loop of Henle is hypotonic.

Countercurrent Exchange System

Normally blood flow through a part tends to remove NaCl from regions of high osmolarity. This does not happen in the renal medulla because the descending and ascending vasa recta are arranged in the form of U-shaped tube (just like the loop of Henle). Water that diffuses out of the descending vessel, (because of an osmolarity gradient), is taken up by the ascending vessel. Solutes diffusing out of the ascending vessel are taken up by the descending vessel. This diffusion is facilitated by the close approximation of the ascending and descending vasa recta. As a result the medullary gradient is maintained.

Role of Distal Convoluted Tubules

a. Like the proximal convoluted tubules, the distal tubules are involved in selective reabsorption of ions (chiefly sodium and bicarbonate).
b. The tubules secrete hydrogen ions into the filtrate. This, combined with the reabsorption of bicarbonate, makes the urine acidic. This process is controlled by aldosterone (produced in the adrenal cortex).
c. We have seen that filtrate entering the distal convoluted tubules (from the loop of Henle) is hypotonic (osmolarity about 100). In the presence of ADH (antidiuretic hormone produced by the pars posterior of the hypophysis cerebri) the distal convoluted tubules become highly permeable to water. Water diffuses out and the osmolarity of fluid leaving the tubules is about 300.

The convoluted tubules add various substances to the glomerular filtrate. These include hydrogen ions (that make the urine acid), ammonia, creatinine and para-amino-hippuric acid. Various drugs, or their breakdown products, are also excreted in this way.

Role of Collecting Ducts

The collecting tubules and ducts play a very important role is final concentration of urine. As the filtrate passes through the collecting ducts, it once more enters the hypertonic environment of the medulla. This hypertonic environment, combined with the high permeability of the collecting ducts to water, forces water out of the ducts (into the interstitial space, and from there into blood). The urinary volume is greatly reduced and the urine becomes concentrated.

However, the permeability of the collecting ducts is variable and is controlled by antidiuretic hormone (ADH). This hormone can thus regulate the dilution of urine depending upon functional requirements. Absence or deficiency of ADH is marked by excretion of very large volumes of dilute urine (***diabetes insipidus***).

The efficacy of the mechanism for resorption of water from the glomerular filtrate is shown by the fact that the filtrate is reduced from an original volume of about 200 litres a day to an average urine output of 1.5 litres per day.

Juxtaglomerular Apparatus

A part of the distal convoluted tubule (at the junction of its straight and convoluted parts) lies close to the vascular pole of the renal corpuscle, between the afferent and efferent arterioles. In this region the muscle cells in the wall of the afferent arteriole are modified. They are large and rounded (epitheloid) and have spherical nuclei. Their cytoplasm contains granules that can be stained with special methods. These are ***juxtaglomerular cells***. They are innervated by unmyelinated adrenergic nerve fibres.

The wall of the distal convoluted tubule is also modified at the site of contact with the arteriole. Here the cells lining it are densely packed together, and are columnar (rather than cuboidal as in the rest of the tubule). These cells form the ***macula densa*** (Fig. 17.4). The cells of the macula densa lie in close contact with the juxtaglomerular cells, the two together forming the ***juxtaglomerular apparatus*** or complex.

The granules of the juxtaglomerular cells contain an enzyme called ***renin***. Renin acts on ***angiotensinogen*** present in blood and converts it into ***angiotensin I***. Another enzyme (present mainly in the lungs) converts angiotensin I into ***angiotensin II***. Angiotensin II increases blood pressure. It also stimulates the secretion of aldosterone by the adrenal cortex, thus influencing the reabsorption of sodium ions by the distal convoluted tubules, and that of water through the collecting ducts.

The juxtaglomerular apparatus is a mechanism that controls the degree of resorption of ions by the renal tubule. It appears likely that cells of the macula densa monitor the ionic constitution of the fluid passing across them (within the tubule). The cells of the macula densa act as chemo receptors. They are stimulated by decreased level of sodium in the distal convoluted tubules. They appear to influence the release of renin by the juxtaglomerular cells. Renin influences aldosterone production (through angiotensin II) and hence controls tubular resorption. In this way it helps to regulate plasma volume and blood pressure. Secretion of renin is also stimulated by sympathetic stimulation.

The juxtaglomerular cells also act as baroreceptors reacting to a fall in blood pressure, or hypovolaemia, by release of renin.

Composition of Urine

Ninety-six per cent of urine is water. The remaining four per cent is made up of salts dissolved in water. The main salt is urea (formed by protein break down). Other substances present are sodium, potassium, uric acid, creatinine, ammonia, chlorides, phosphates, sulphates, and oxalates.

SOME OTHER FUNCTIONS OF THE KIDNEY

Maintenance of Water Balance

The body has to maintain a balance between water intake and water loss. Water intake is for all practical purposes equal to the water contained in what we eat and drink. (A small quantity called metabolic water is released during chemical reactions within the body).

Some water is excreted through expired air and some in faeces. In hot weather considerable water is lost through perspiration (sweating). However, the most important water loss is through the kidneys.

Nature tries to maintain a more or less constant concentration of water within the body. Some cells in the brain (hypothalamus) are sensitive to osmotic pressure of blood (which is in turn a reflection of its water content). These cells are osmoreceptors. When water content of plasma is less than normal, these cells send impulses to the posterior lobe of the hypophysis cerebri (pituitary). These impulses lead to increased secretion of antidiuretic hormone (ADH). This hormone acts or renal tubules, increasing reabsorption of water.

In some diseases urine output is increased (polyurea). This happens in diabetes, but water loss is compensated for by increased thirst and drinking of water.

Maintenance of Sodium and Potassium Ion Concentrations

Sodium and potassium ions are essential for the body and their concentration has to be maintained at proper level. Intake of sodium takes place through food. Excess sodium is excreted in urine, and through sweat (when environmental temperature is high). Excretion of sodium is controlled though the hormone aldosterone that is secreted by the adrenal cortex.

Role of Kidney in Control of Blood Pressure

Juxtaglomerular cells produce renin. Renin enters the blood stream. Here it interacts with angiotensinogen to form angiotensin-1. Other enzymes convert angiotensin-1 to angiotensin-2. The action of angiotension is to increase blood pressure.

When blood pressure is low the production of renin and of angiotensin is stimulated and this increases blood pressure. Low blood volume stimulates secretion of aldosterone, which increases reabsorption of sodium and of water, to restore blood volume.

Synthesis of Erythropoietin

The kidney secretes erythropoietin. It stimulates production of erythrocytes.

Maintenance of pH

Role of kidney in maintaining pH has already been mentioned. The distal convoluted tubules secrete hydrogen ions into the filtrate. This, combined with the reabsorption of bicarbonate, makes the urine acidic. This process is controlled by aldosterone (produced in the adrenal cortex).

SOME DISEASES OF THE KIDNEYS

Inflammation of the kidney (by infection or other cause) is called ***nephritis***. When glomeruli are chiefly involved the condition is called ***glomerulonephritis***. Infections in the renal pelvis and calyces is called ***pyelonephritis*** (acute or chronic). From here infection can spread into renal tissue, and abscesses can form.

Glomerulonephritis

Inflammation in kidneys is usually produced by immune reactions. Various types of glomerulonephritis are recognised. The patient may pass blood in urine (haematuria). Plasma proteins are lost through urine (because of damage to glomeruli). Symptoms of acute nephritis or of renal failure may occur.

Nephrotic Syndrome

This can occur in any disease in which glomeruli are damaged.

Marked protein loss leads to oedema all over the body. Apart from glomerulonephritis, nephrotic syndrome can occur after some infections (hepatitis, malaria) or after use of some drugs.

Renal Failure

Renal failure is a state in which the kidneys are unable to maintain enough urine flow to remove waste products from the body. Acute renal failure can occur in shock as enough blood does not flow through the kidney. It can be produced by any cause that obstructs flow of urine e.g., a large calculus in the renal pelvis, or a tumour of the bladder (or of a surrounding organ like the cervix of the uterus). Acute renal failure can also be due to severe damage to the kidney itself. Such damage can be caused by reduced blood supply, or by ingestion of drugs (or chemicals) toxic to the kidneys.

Chronic renal failure occurs in diseases in which there is slowly progressing damage to renal tissue. Symptoms appear when about 75% of renal function is lost. Retention of urea in blood leads to ***uraemia***. As reabsorption of water is interfered with, volume of urine increases, but it has a low specific gravity. Acidosis, and electrolyte imbalance are seen. Anaemia and hypertension are important side effects.

Causes of renal damage that can land to renal failure include diabetes mellitus, chronic glomerulonephritis and chronic pyelonephritis. Arteriosclerotic changes and hypertension can damage the kidney.

Association of Kidney with Hypertension

1. The kidneys can be damaged in hypertension. There is damage to glomeruli, and this can lead to renal failure. Damage to renal tissue itself becomes a cause for further increase in blood pressure.
2. Damage to kidneys, through chronic glomerulonephritis or pyelonephritis, can be a cause of hypertension. Damage to kidneys reduces blood flow through glomeruli. This increases production of renin, which leads to elevation of blood pressure.

Calculi (Stones)

In many individuals stones are formed in the renal pelvis. The factors that lead to formation of calculi are not truly understood. Their formation is greater in people with inadequate water intake, alkaline pH of urine, presence of infection, etc.

A stone formed in the renal pelvis may remain there and gradually enlarge. Progressive pressure on renal tissue can damage it.

A small stone can pass into the ureter. Passage of a store through the ureter can cause severe spasmodic pain (***renal colic***).

A stone can reach the urinary bladder. It can remain there, gradually increasing in size, and can become quite large. Sometimes small stones can pass through the urethra to the exterior. A stone can get impacted (stuck) at any site in the urinary passages, and can become a cause of urinary obstruction.

Other Diseases

1. In case of urinary obstruction, the pelvis of the kidney can undergo dilatation (***hydronephrosis***). Pressure leads to gradual destruction of renal tissue.
2. Infection in the ureter (***ureteritis***), urinary bladder (***cystitis***) or in the urethra (***urethritis***) can occur.
3. ***Tumours*** can form in the kidney or in the urinary bladder.

KIDNEY FUNCTION TESTS

In clinical work kidney function can be evaluated by a number of tests.

Endogenous Creatinine Clearance

Urine passed over a 24 hour period (sometimes over a 4 hour period) is collected and the concentration of creatinine in it is estimated. Simultaneously, creatinine content of plasma is also measured.

$$\text{Creatinine clearance (ml/min)} = \frac{\text{Urinary creatinine concentration} \times \text{Urinary volume}}{\text{Plasma creatinin concentration}}$$

Creatinine clearance is a measure of glomerular filtration rate.

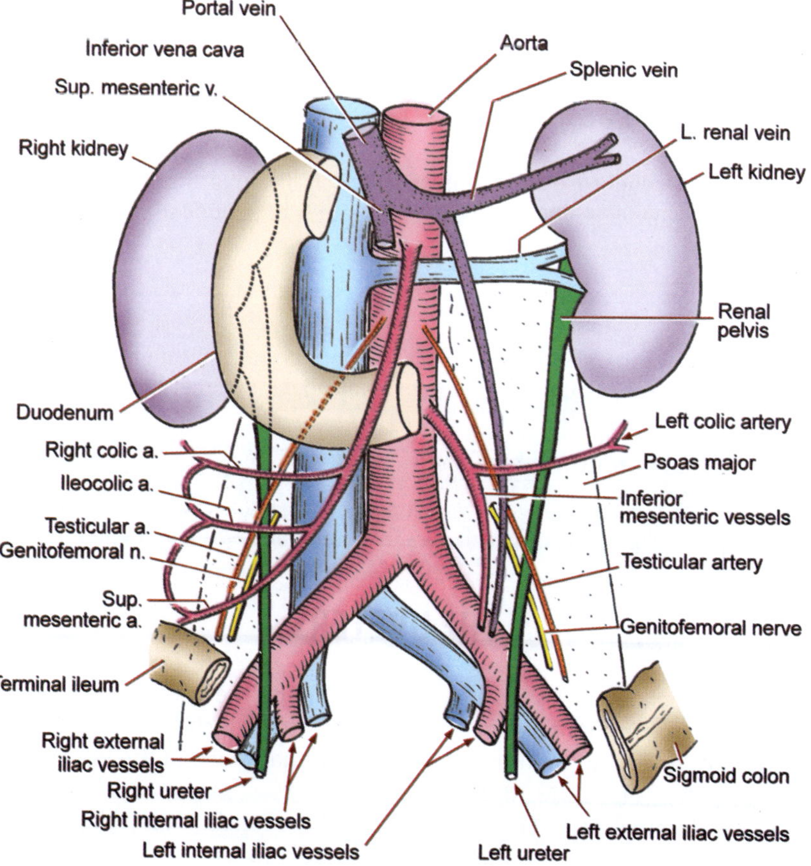

Fig. 19.18 Relations of abdominal parts of right and left ureters.

Plasma Creatinine Concentration

The normal value is 0.2 to 1.4 mg%. Increase of this value indicates that there is fairly advanced renal damage.

Blood Urea

Normal value is 15 to 40 mg%. The value increases in advanced renal damage.

Urine Examination for Albumin and Blood Cells

Presence of albumin, or of blood cells in urine occurs in some diseases of the kidneys.

Urinary Concentration Test

Ability of tubules to concentrate urine is found out by testing the specific gravity of urine. Specific gravity below 1.02 indicates that urine is not being concentrated.

Urinary Dilution Test

Specific gravity is measured by making the patient drink one litre of water. Normally 75% (750 ml) is excreted within four hours and specific gravity can fall up to 1.004.

Urinary pH

The ability of kidneys to excrete hydrogen ions is tested by giving the patient 0.1 g/kg body weight ammonium chloride. After six hours the urine pH should be less than 5.3.

Glycosuria

Presence of glycosuria when blood glucose is normal is an indication of inability of tubules to reabsorb glucose. It is a sign of renal tubular dysfunction.

Intravenous Pyelography

A radiograph is taken after giving an intravenous injection of a radio-opaque dye (urographin). The renal pelvis, calyces and ureters can be visualised.

THE URETERS

The ureter (right or left) is a long tube that connects the lower end of the renal pelvis with the urinary bladder. It is about 25 cm (10 inches) long. The upper half of this length lies on the posterior abdominal wall and the lower half in the true pelvis (Figs. 19.18, 19.19).

The abdominal part of each ureter runs downwards (with a slight medial inclination). At the brim of the pelvis the ureter crosses the upper end of the external iliac artery (and vein), and comes to lie on the lateral wall of the pelvis. Finally it leaves the pelvic wall and turns forwards to reach the urinary bladder.

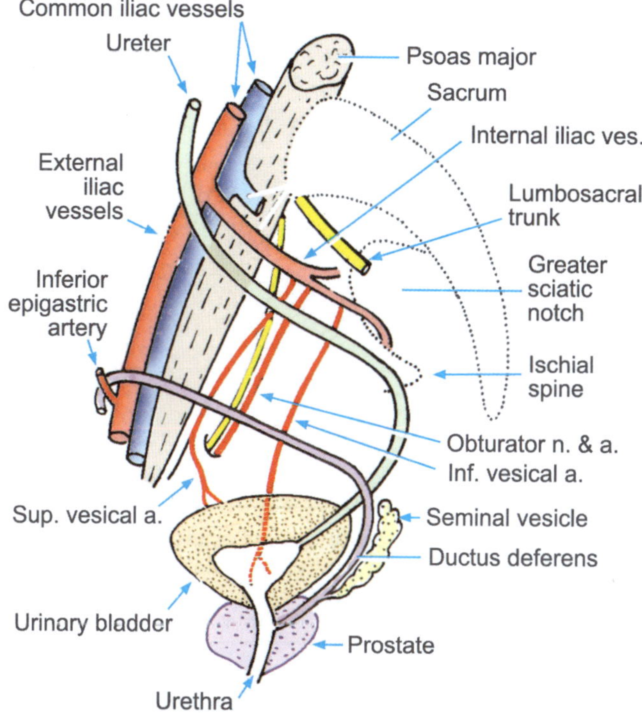

Fig. 19.19 Scheme to show the course and relations of the pelvic part of the ureter in the male.

The wall of the ureter has three layers: an outer fibrous coat, a middle layer of smooth muscle, and an inner lining of mucous membrane (Fig. 19.20).

The mucous membrane has a lining of transitional epithelium. The mucosa (consisting of epithelium and the underlying connective tissue) shows a number of longitudinal folds that give the lumen a star-shaped appearance in transverse section. The folds disappear when the ureter is distended.

The muscle coat has an inner longitudinal layer and an outer circular layer of smooth muscle.

Reflux of urine from the urinary bladder into the ureters is prevented by the oblique path followed by the terminal part of the ureter, through the bladder wall. When the musculature of the bladder contracts this part of the ureter is compressed. This mechanism constitutes a physiological sphincter.

The renal pelvis and the ureters are frequently visualised in the living by taking skiagrams after injecting radio-opaque dye into a vein. The dye is excreted by the kidney into urine rendering the pelves, ureters and urinary bladder visible. The procedure is called ***excretion urography*** (also called intravenous or descending pyelography or urography. The ureters can also be visualised by direct injection of radio-opaque dyes into them by using an instrument introduced through the urethra and urinary bladder: this procedure is called ***ascending or retrograde pyelography*** (or urography).

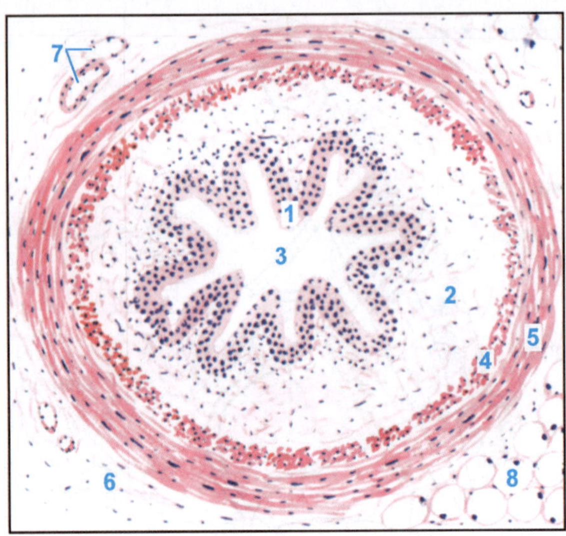

Fig. 19.20 Ureter. 1-Mucosa lined by transitional epithelium. 2-Connective tissue. 3-Lumen (star shaped). 4, 5-Muscle coat (inner longitudinal, and outer circular). 6-Connective tissue. 7-Blood vessel.

THE URINARY BLADDER

In the adult, the urinary bladder lies in the pelvis. However, when distended with urine, part of it extends above the level of the pubic symphysis and comes in contact with the anterior abdominal wall. In the infant the bladder lies above the level of the pubic symphysis i.e., it is an abdominal organ rather than a pelvic one.

Urine is formed continuously in the kidneys and is conveyed to the urinary bladder through the ureters. The urinary bladder acts as a reservoir. When it is distended beyond a certain limit the desire for passing urine is felt. This limit is usually reached when the bladder contains about 300 ml of urine. The maximum capacity of the urinary bladder is about 500 ml.

The empty urinary bladder has four surfaces each of which is triangular (Fig. 19.21). In other words the bladder is shaped like a tetrahedron. The ***posterior surface*** is also called the ***base*** or ***fundus***. It is broad above and pointed below. The ***superior surface*** faces upwards. Its posterior end is broad. Anteriorly it narrows to form the ***apex*** of the bladder. The right and left ***inferolateral surfaces*** face downwards, laterally and forwards. They meet the superior surface at the right and left ***lateral borders.*** Posteriorly they meet the lateral margins of the base.

The right and left ureters join the urinary bladder at its posterolateral angles. The lowest part of the bladder is called the neck. The urethra emerges from the bladder here (Fig. 19.22). The apex of the bladder gives attachment to the lower end of the median umbilical ligament.

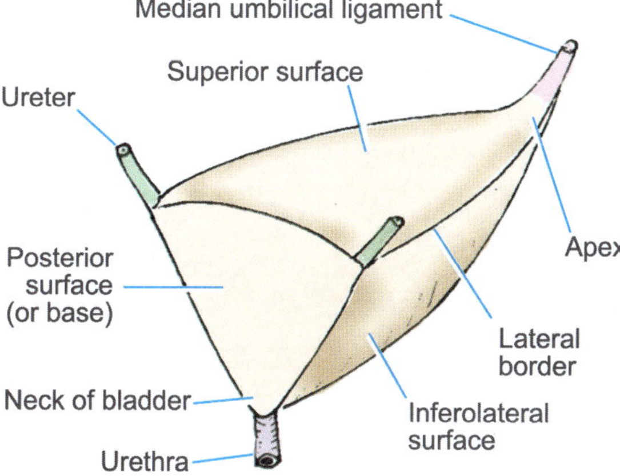

Fig. 19.21 Scheme to show the surfaces of the urinary bladder.

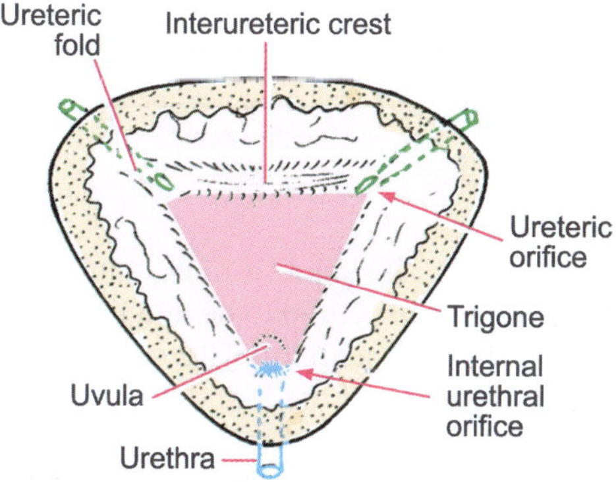

Fig. 19.22 Some features to be seen in the interior of the urinary bladder.

The wall of the urinary bladder consists of an outer serous layer, a thick coat of smooth muscle, and a mucous membrane (Fig. 19.23).

The mucous membrane is lined by transitional epithelium. When the bladder is distended (with urine) the lining epithelium becomes thinner. This results from the ability of the epithelial cells to change shape and move over one another.

The transitional epithelium lining the urinary bladder (and the rest of the urinary passages) is capable of withstanding osmotic changes caused by variations in concentrations of urine. It is also resistant to toxic substances present in urine.

In the empty bladder the mucous membrane is thrown into numerous folds (or rugae) that disappear when the bladder is distended. Some mucous glands may be present in the mucosa specially near the internal urethral orifice.

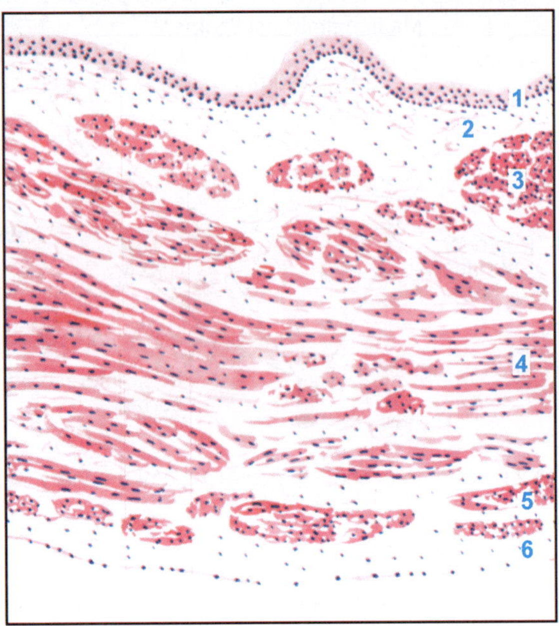

Fig. 19.23 Urinary bladder. 1-Transitional epithelium. 2-Connective tissue. 3, 4, 5-Muscle layers.

The muscle layer is thick. The smooth muscle in it forms a meshwork. Internally and externally the fibres tend to be longitudinal. In between them there is a thicker layer of circular (or oblique) fibres. Contraction of this muscle coat is responsible for emptying of the bladder. That is why it is called the ***detrusor muscle***. Just above the junction of the bladder with the urethra the circular fibres are thickened to form the ***sphincter vesicae***.

THE URETHRA

The urethra is a tube that connects the lower end (or neck) of the urinary bladder to the exterior: urine stored in the bladder is passed out through it. The urethra is much longer in the male (about 20 cm) as compared to the female (4 cm). In both sexes its average diameter is about 6 mm.

THE MALE URETHRA

The male urethra is divisible into three parts (Fig. 19.24).

1. The first part starts at the internal urethral orifice and descends through the prostate to reach the urogenital diaphragm. This part of the urethra is embedded within the prostate gland and is, therefore, called the ***prostatic part***. It is about 3 cm long.

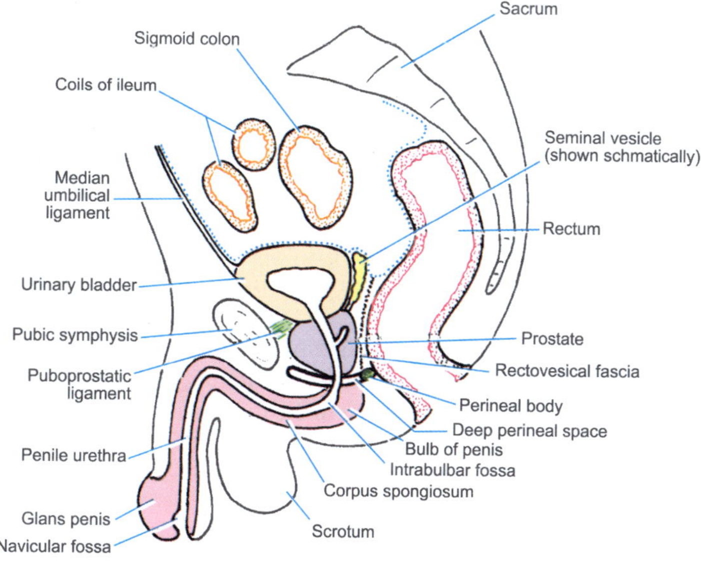

Fig. 19.24 Sagittal section through the male pelvis.

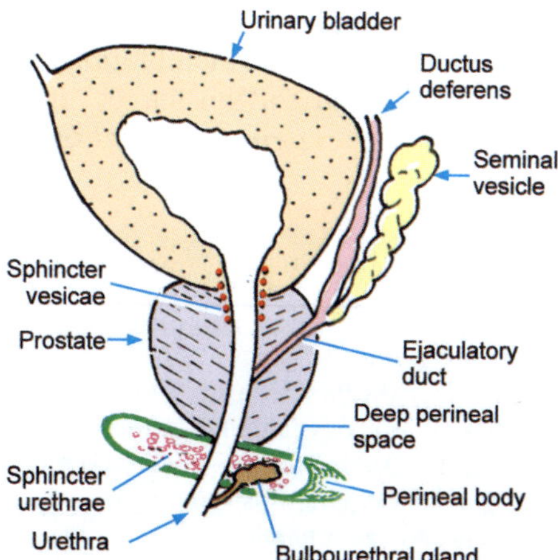

Fig. 19.25 Diagram showing the sphincters of the urethra, and the bulbourethral glands.

2. The next part passes through the deep perineal space, present in the perineum. This part is called the membranous urethra. It is about 1.5 cm long. It is surrounded by the sphincter urethrae externus.
3. The part of the urethra passes through the penis, and opens to the exterior at the tip of the penis. This is called the penile or spongiose part.

THE FEMALE URETHRA

The female urethra corresponds (topographically) to the prostatic and membranous parts of the male urethra, and is about 4 cm long. Throughout its length the urethra is closely related to the anterior wall of the vagina. It opens to the exterior in the perineum.

Although the male urethra is much longer than the female urethra the structure of the two is the same. The wall of the urethra is composed of mucous, submucous and muscular layers. In the case of the male, the prostatic urethra is surrounded by prostatic tissue; and the penile urethra by erectile tissue of the corpus spongiosum.

The mucous membrane consists of a lining epithelium that rests on connective tissue. The epithelium varies in different parts of the urethra. Both in the male and female the greater part of the urethra is lined by pseudostratified columnar epithelium. A short part adjoining the urinary bladder is lined by transitional epithelium, while the part near the external orifice is lined by stratified squamous epithelium.

The mucosa shows invaginations or recesses into which mucous glands open.

The submucosa consists of loose connective tissue. The muscle coat consists of an inner longitudinal layer and an outer circular layer of smooth muscle. This coat is better defined in the female urethra. In the male urethra it is well defined only in the membranous and prostatic parts, the penile part being surrounded by occasional fibres only.

In addition to this smooth muscle the membranous part of the male urethra, and the corresponding part of the female urethra are surrounded by striated muscle that forms the ***external urethral sphincter*** (or ***sphincter urethrae***) (Fig. 19.25).

MICTURITION

Emptying of the urinary bladder leads to passing of urine, or micturition. For this purpose the detrusor muscle in the bladder wall contracts, and sphincters (internal and external) relax. Urine produced by kidneys travels down the ureters and gets stored in the urinary bladder. As the volume of urine increases the walls of the bladder are gradually stretched. When this stretching reaches a certain limit nerve endings present in the walls are stimulated.

In infants, emptying of the bladder takes place automatically in response to stimuli from the bladder wall. It is not under voluntary control. Nerve impulses from the bladder reach the lower part of the spinal cord. Here nerve cells are stimulated and impulses pass down from them to the bladder muscle, causing it to contract. This is an example of a spinal reflex.

As the child grown up, and the nervous system matures, nervous inputs reaching the spinal cord (from the bladder wall) are relayed to the brain. They make the person conscious of the desire to urinate. If the time and place are not convenient, urination can be postponed for sometime. When the time is convenient, suitable signals pass from the brain to the spinal cord, and from there to the bladder, leading to micturition.

Inability to delay micturition is called ***urinary incontinence***. Apart from infants, emptying of the urinary bladder can become automatic in unconscious persons, and in those with injury to the spinal cord.

CHAPTER

20

Male Reproductive Organs

The Reproductive System

Both in the male and in the female the reproductive system consists of genital organs that are concerned with the function of reproduction. These organs may be divided into the ***primary sex organs,*** or ***gonads,*** which are responsible for the production of gametes; and the ***accessory sex organs,*** which play a supporting role. The genital organs are also divided into the ***internal genital organs*** (or ***internal genitalia***) which include the gonads and those supporting organs that cannot be seen from the outside of the body; and the ***external genital organs*** (or ***external genitalia***) which are visible on the outside. In human beings (as in many other animal groups) fertilization takes place within the female body. This requires that male gametes be introduced into the female body through the process of ***copulation*** or ***coitus*** (commonly referred to as sexual intercourse). The male and female organs that are concerned with copulation are referred to as ***copulatory organs***. The region of the body where the external genitalia (and anus) are located is referred to as the ***perineum***.

In this chapter we will consider the male genital organs. The female genital organs will be considered in the next chapter.

Male Reproductive Organs

The male gonads are the right and left ***testes*** (singular = testis) (Fig. 20.1). They produce the male gametes, which are called ***spermatozoa*** (singular = ***spermatozoon***). From each testis the spermatozoa pass through a complicated system of genital ducts. The most obvious of these are the ***epididymis*** and the ***ductus deferens***. At its termination, the ductus deferens is joined by the duct of the ***seminal vesicle*** (a sac like structure), to form the ***ejaculatory duct.*** The right and left ejaculatory ducts open into the urethra.

The testis, epididymis and the initial part of the ductus deferens of both sides lie in a sac like structure covered by skin: this sac is called the ***scrotum***. From here the ductus deferens passes upwards and enters the abdomen by passing

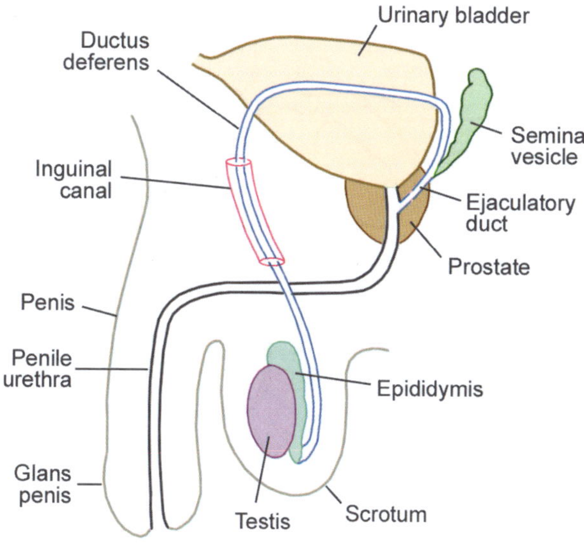

Fig. 20.1 Diagram to show the male reproductive organs.

through an oblique passage in the anterior abdominal wall: this passage is called the ***inguinal canal***. Here the ductus deferens is surrounded by several structures that collectively form the ***spermatic cord***.

As spermatozoa pass through the genital ducts, named above, they undergo maturation. They get mixed up with secretions produced by the seminal vesicle and the prostate to form the ***seminal fluid*** or ***semen.*** The process of ejection of semen from the body is called ***ejaculation***. In this process semen is poured into the urethra and passes through it to the exterior. The male urethra is, therefore, both a urinary and a genital passage.

The ***penis*** is the male organ of copulation. Because it is capable of becoming rigid it can be introduced into the vagina of the female, and semen can be injected into the vaginal cavity.

THE PERINEUM

As seen on the surface of the body the perineum is the region where the external genitalia and the anus are located. Some knowledge of the perineum is necessary for understanding the reproductive organs.

In relation to the skeleton, the boundaries of the perineum correspond to those of the pelvic outlet (Fig. 20.2). This outlet is rhomboid in shape, and can be divided into anterior and posterior triangular areas. These are the ***urogenital triangle*** placed anteriorly, and the ***anal triangle*** placed posteriorly.

Some genital organs are located in the urogenital triangle. In the male these are the scrotum (containing the right and left testis and epididymis), and the penis. In the female we see the external genitalia that are present around the external openings of the urethra and the vagina.

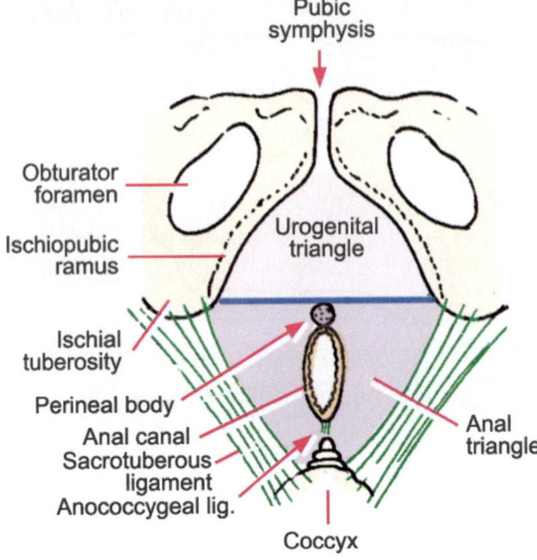

Fig. 20.2 Boundaries of the perineum.

The anal canal passes through the ***anal triangle***. The anal canal opens to the exterior at the anus.

Urogenital Triangle

The ***urogenital triangle*** is placed between the right and left ischiopubic rami. Stretching transversely across the rami there are three membranes between which are enclosed two spaces as shown in Fig. 20.3. From above downwards the membranes are as follows:

a. Part of the pelvic fascia, that is continuous laterally with the fascia on the obturator internus, constitutes the ***superior fascia of the urogenital diaphragm.***

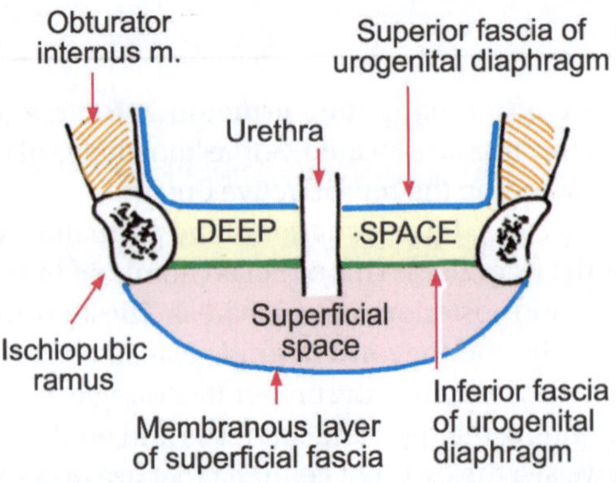

Fig. 20.3 Schematic coronal section through urogenital triangle to show formation of superficial and deep perineal spaces.

b. The second membrane is the ***inferior fascia of the urogenital diaphragm.*** It is thick and is also called the ***perineal membrane.***

c. The most superficial membrane is the membranous layer of superficial fascia.

Between the upper and middle membranes there is the ***deep perineal space*** (or pouch); and between the middle and lower membranes there is the ***superficial perineal space (or pouch).***

Anal Triangle and Ischiorectal Fossa

To understand the arrangement of structures in the anal triangle it is essential to have a clear picture of two muscles present in relation to the true pelvis. One of these is the ***obturator internus.*** The second muscle is the ***levator ani*** (Fig. 20.4)

The lateral wall of the true pelvis is covered by the obturator internus muscle. The levator ani takes origin from the fascia covering the obturator internus, and runs downwards and medially towards the midline. The levator ani muscles of the right and left sides meet in the midline and form the ***pelvic diaphragm.***

The anal canal passes through the anal triangle to reach the exterior. It is surrounded by two sphincters, internal and external. On either side of the anal canal there is a triangular space called the ***ischiorectal fossa.*** Its importance is that it is often the site of infection. An abscess or fistula may form.

The Scrotum

The scrotum is a sac that has a wall made up of by skin. Closely united to the skin there is a layer of smooth muscle, which constitutes the ***dartos muscle.*** The scrotum consists of two halves, right and left that are separated from each other by a septum. Each half of the scrotum is lined by a number of membranes. These are the coverings of the testis (Fig. 20.13). Each half of the scrotum contains the corresponding testis, epididymis, and the initial part of the ductus deferens.

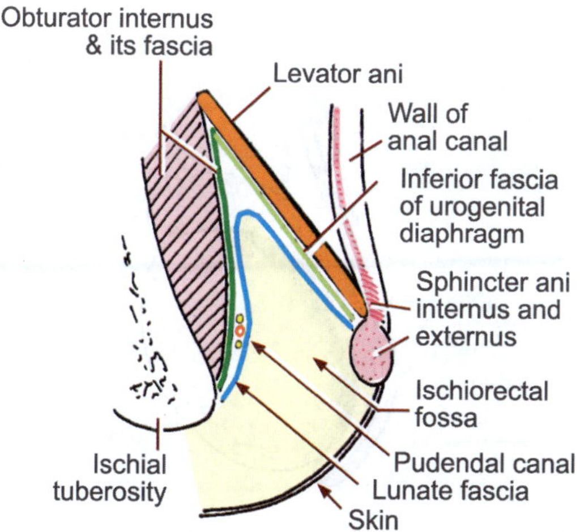

Fig. 20.4 Coronal section through ischiorectal fossa.

THE TESTIS AND EPIDIDYMIS

Each testis (right or left) is an oval shaped structure about 4 cm in its longest (vertical) diameter. It is about 2.5 cm broad and about 3 cm in anteroposterior diameter. The two testes lie in the scrotum (Figs. 20.5, 20.6).

The epididymis is a mass formed by tortuous tubules (Fig. 20.7). Its upper end lies near the upper pole of the testis: it is enlarged and is called the ***head***. The middle part of the epididymis is of medium size and called the ***body***. Its lower part is thin and is called the ***tail*** (Fig. 20.6).

On each side the testis and epididymis lie in a closed sac that is called the ***tunica vaginalis*** (Fig. 20.7). The walls of the sac are formed by a thin membrane (similar in structure to peritoneum). It has a visceral layer lining the testis and a parietal layer. The two layers are separated by a potential space.

Deep to the visceral layer of the tunica vaginalis, we see a dense fibrous membrane, the ***tunica albuginea***. In the posterior part of the testis the connective tissue forming the tunica albuginea is thicker than elsewhere

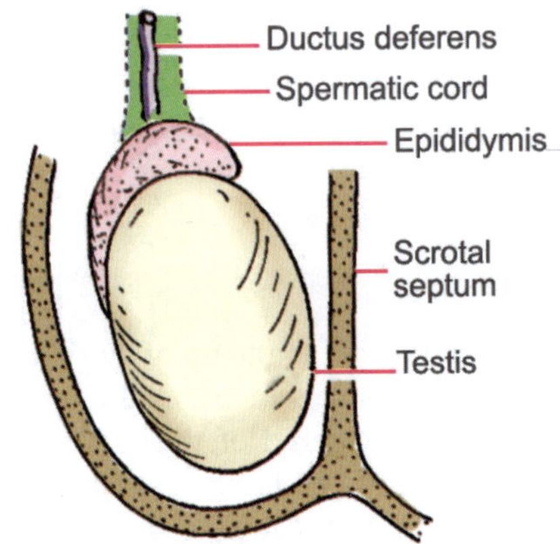

Fig. 20.5 Right testis seen from the front.

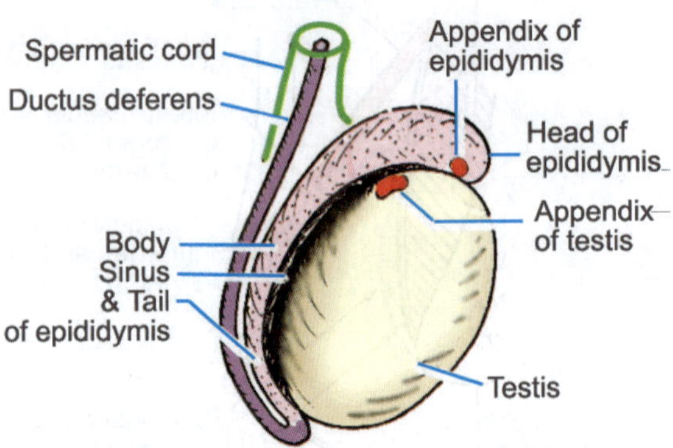

Fig. 20.6 Right testis seen from the lateral side.

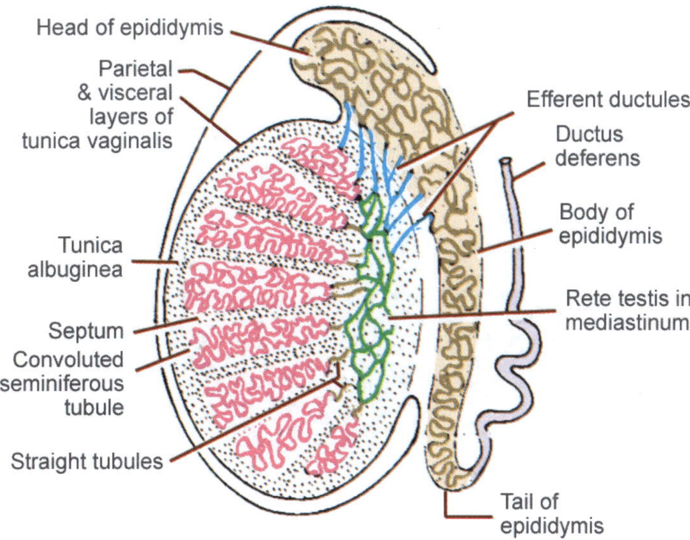

Fig. 20.7 Schematic coronal section through testis.

and projects into the substance of the testis: this projection is called the ***mediastinum testis***. Numerous septa pass from the mediastinum testis to the tunica albuginea, and divide the substance of the testis into a large number of lobules. Each lobule contains one or more highly convoluted ***seminiferous tubules***. These tubules are lined by an epithelium the cells of which are concerned with the production of spermatozoa. From Fig. 20.7 it will be seen that each lobule is roughly conical, the apex of the cone being directed towards the mediastinum testis. Near the apex of the lobule the seminiferous tubules lose their convolutions and join one another to form about twenty to thirty larger ***straight tubules***. These enter the fibrous tissue of the mediastinum testis and unite to form a network called the ***rete testis***. The rete testis gives off twelve to twenty ***efferent ductules***. These ductules pass from the upper part of the testis into the head of the epididymis. Within the head these tubules become highly convoluted. The ***head of the epididymis*** is in fact nothing but a mass of these convoluted tubules. At the lower end of the head of the epididymis these tubules end in a single tube called the ***duct of the epididymis***. The body and tail of the epididymis are formed by convolutions of this duct. At the lower end of the tail the duct of the epididymis becomes continuous with the ductus deferens.

SEMINIFEROUS TUBULES

Each tubule is lined by several layers of cells that represent stages in the formation of spermatozoa (Fig. 20.8). They are therefore called ***germ cells***. The process of formation of spermatozoa is called ***spermatogenesis***. Seminiferous tubules also contain cells that perform a supporting function. These are the Sertoli cells.

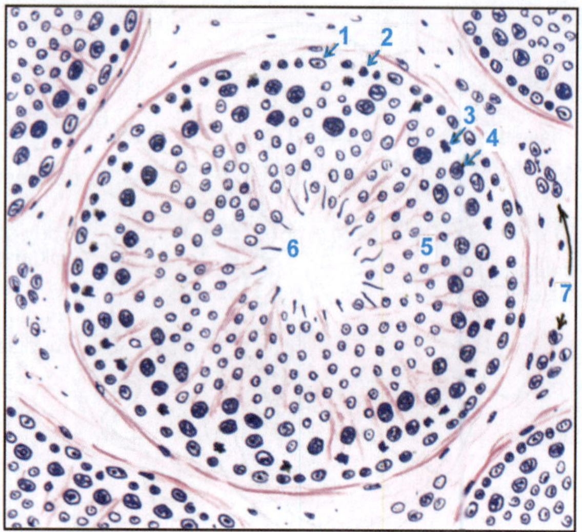

Fig. 20.8 Testis, high power view. 1-Sustentacular cells. 2-Spermatogonia. 3-Dividing spermatogonia. 4-Spermatocyte. 5-Spermatid. 6-Spermatozoa.7-Interstitial cells.

Stages of Spermatogenesis

The main steps of spermatogenesis are as follows. To understand the process you must know the basic steps of mitosis and meiosis (Chapter 6).

1. ***Spermatogonia*** or germ cells divide mitotically, to give rise to more spermatogonia, and also to form ***primary spermatocytes***. Spermatogonia and primary spermato-cytes contain the normal number of chromosomes (44+X+Y).
2. ***Primary spermatocytes*** now divide so that each of them forms two ***secondary spermatocytes***. This is the first meiotic division. It reduces the number of chromosomes to half the normal number (22+X) or (22+Y).
3. Each ***secondary spermatocyte*** divides to form two ***spermatids***. This is the second meiotic division, and this time there is no reduction in chromosome number.
4. Each spermatid (22+X or 22+Y) gradually changes its shape to become a spermatozoon. This process of transformation of a circular spermatid to a spermatozoon is called ***spermiogenesis***.

Structure of Spermatozoon

The spermatozoon is an elongated thread-like structure with an enlarged end. The enlarged end is called the ***head***. It is followed, in that order, by a ***neck***, a ***middle piece*** and a ***principal piece*** or ***tail***. An axial filament passes through the middle piece and extends into the tail. Most of the length of the spermatozoon is constituted by the tail (Fig. 20.9). Movements of the tail make the spermatozoon motile.

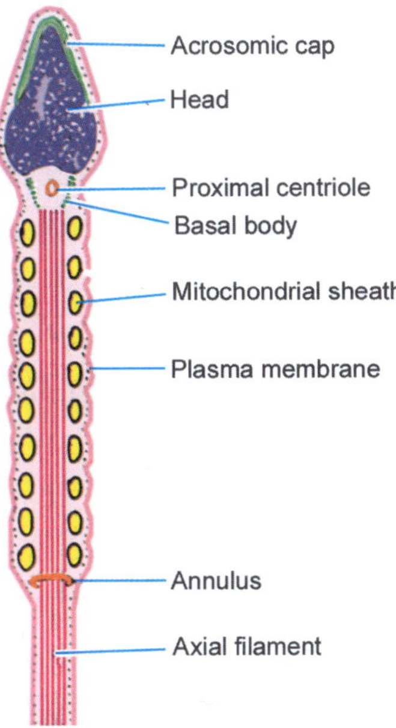

Fig. 20.9 Structure of a spermatozoon as seen by EM.

During the process of spermiogenesis the head of the spermatozoon is derived from the nucleus of the spermatid. The mitochondria of the spermatid collect in the middle piece of the spermatozoon and form a sheath round the axial filament.

The axial filament grows out of centrioles.

Interstitial Cells of the Testis

These cells lie in the connective tissue that intervenes between seminiferous tubules. Interstitial cells secrete male sex hormone (testicular androgens). This hormone is responsible for development of genital organs, and for sex desire, in the male.

Microscopic Structure of Epididymis

The highly convoluted tubules of the head of the epididymis are lined by ciliated columnar epithelium. The distal part of the epididymis is made up of the duct of the epididymis which is greatly coiled on itself. It is lined by pseudostratified columnar epithelium (Fig. 20.10).

Spermatozoa produced in the testis undergo maturation and become motile in the epididymis.

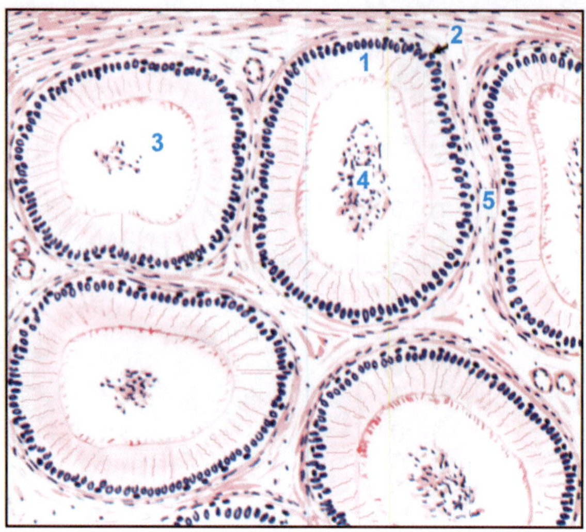

Fig. 20.10 Epidydimis. 1-Lining of tall columnar cells. 2-Basal cell. 3-Stereocilia. 4-Clump of spermatozoa.

THE DUCTUS DEFERENS

A good idea of the path followed by the ductus deferens can be had by examining Fig. 20.1. It is seen that beginning in the scrotum (as a continuation of the epididymis) the ductus deferens passes through the inguinal canal to enter the abdomen. It reaches the posterior aspect of the urinary bladder. Here the ductus deferens terminates by joining the duct of the seminal vesicle to form the ejaculatory duct (Fig. 20.11). The part of the ductus deferens that lies in the inguinal canal forms part of the spermatic cord.

Near the seminal vesicle the ductus bears a dilatation called the ***ampulla;*** but the terminal part of the ductus again narrows down before joining the duct of the seminal vesicle (Fig. 20.11).

The wall of the ductus deferens has a thick muscular wall. The mucous membrane shows a number of folds so that the lumen appears star shaped. It is lined by columnar epithelium (Fig. 20.12).

The vas deferens and its ampulla store spermatozoa.

THE SPERMATIC CORD

The spermatic cord extends from the upper pole of the testis, through the inguinal canal, to the deep inguinal ring. Apart from the ductus deferens it contains blood vessels, lymphatics and nerves.

The spermatic cord has a number of coverings that are described below.

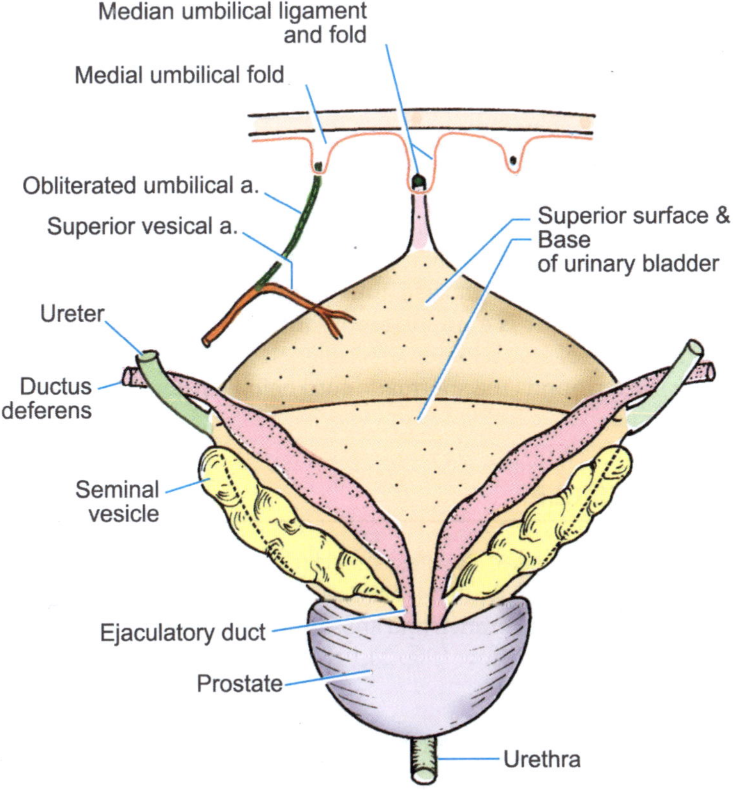

Fig. 20.11 Male urinary bladder and some related structures seen from behind.

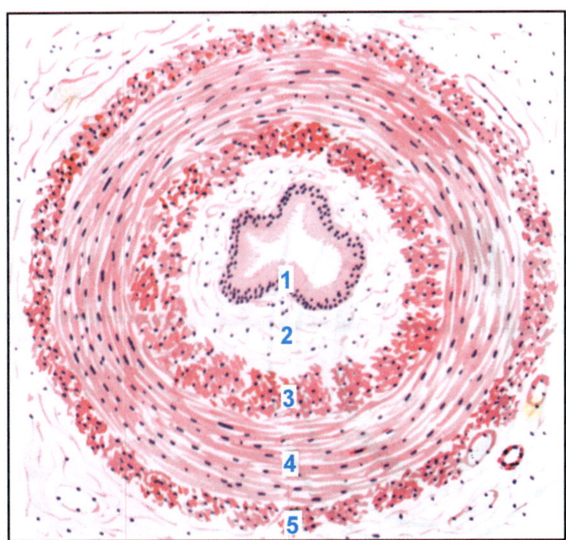

Fig. 20.12 Ductus deferens. 1-Pseudostratified columnar epithelium. 2-Lamina propria. 3, 4, 5-Muscle layers (inner longitudinal, middle circular, outer longitudinal).

Coverings of Spermatic Cord and of Testis

When the testis descends through the inguinal canal during development, it carries with it prolongations from various layers of the abdominal wall. These provide a series of coverings for the testis and for the spermatic cord (Fig. 20.13). These are as follows:

a. The innermost covering is derived from the fascia transversalis and is called the ***internal spermatic fascia.*** It starts at the deep inguinal ring.
b. The next covering is derived from the internal oblique muscle of the abdomen. This layer is partly muscular and partly fibrous: it is called the ***cremasteric fascia***. The muscle fibres constitute the ***cremaster muscle***.
c. The outermost layer is a prolongation of the aponeurosis of the external oblique muscle of the abdomen. It is called the ***external spermatic fascia.*** This fascia surrounds the spermatic cord below the level of the superficial inguinal ring.

SEMINAL VESICLE

The seminal vesicle is a sac like mass that is really a convoluted tube. The tube has an outer covering of connective tissue. The mucosal lining is thrown into numerous thin folds that branch and anastomose thus forming a network. The lining epithelium is columnar (Fig. 20.14).

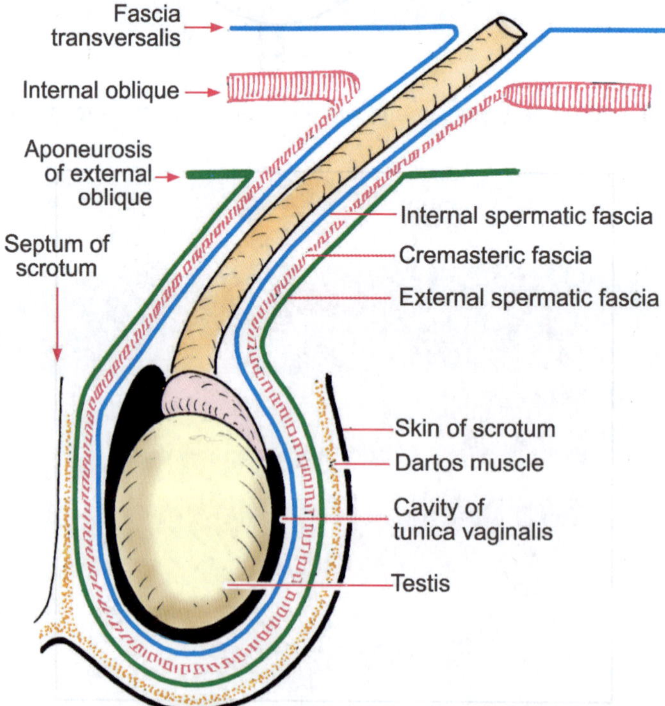

Fig. 20.13 Scheme to show the coverings of the spermatic cord and testis.

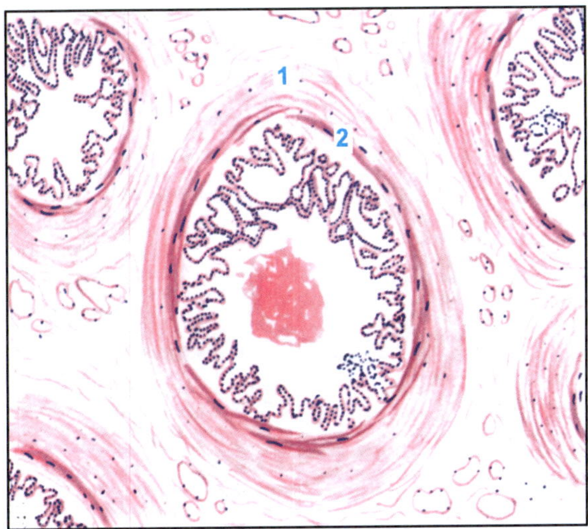

Fig. 20.14 Seminal vesicle (low power). It is made up of a convoluted tubule that is cut up several times. 1-Connective tissue. 2-Smooth muscle.

The seminal vesicles produce a thick secretion, which forms sixty percent of semen. The secretion contains fructose, fibrinogen and prostaglandins.

THE PENIS

The penis consists of a ***root*** that is fixed to the perineum, and of a free part, which is called the ***corpus*** (or body) (Figs. 20.15, 20.16). The free part is lined all round by skin. The apical part of the penis is enlarged and conical: this part is called the ***glans penis*** (Fig. 20.16).

The skin covering the penis is loosely attached except over the glans. Here it is firmly attached to underlying tissues. The glans is also covered by a fold of skin, which extends from the neck of the penis towards the tip. This fold is called the ***prepuce*** (Fig. 20.16). The prepuce normally covers the greater part of the glans, but can be retracted to expose the latter. The space between the surface of the glans and the prepuce is called the ***preputial sac***.

A transverse section through the free part of the penis is shown in Fig. 20.15. The substance of the penis is made up of three masses of spongy tissue, two dorsal and one ventral. The dorsal masses are the right and left ***corpora cavernosa*** (singular = corpus cavernosum). They lie side by side and are separated only by a median fibrous septum. The ***corpus spongiosum*** is placed in the midline ventral to the corpora cavernosa. It is traversed by the penile part of the urethra.

The substance of the corpora cavernosa and of the corpus spongiosum contains numerous small spaces separated by delicate partitions. These spaces are in communication with blood vessels. Most of them are normally empty, but during erection of the penis the spaces become filled with blood leading to enlargement and rigidity of the penis.

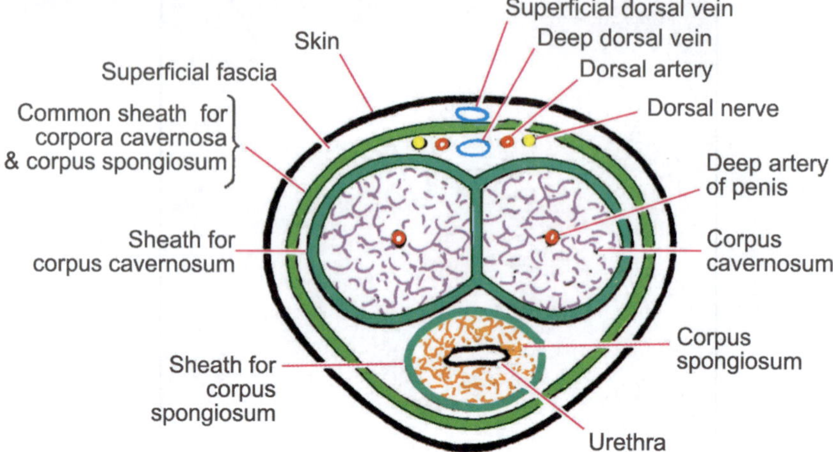

Fig. 20.15 Schematic cross section through the free part of the penis.

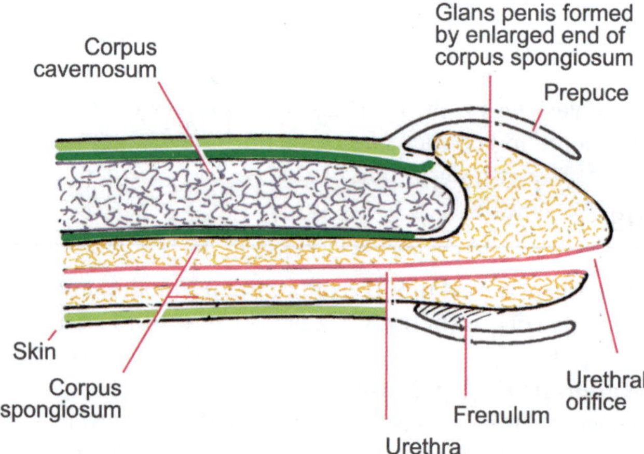

Fig. 20.16 Schematic parasagittal section through the penis.

A longitudinal section through the penis, a little to one side of the midline is shown in Fig. 20.16. From this figure it is seen that the distal part of the corpus spongiosum is greatly enlarged to form the substance of the glans penis.

When traced into the perineum (i.e., into the root of the penis) the right and left corpora cavernosa separate to form the right and left ***crura*** (singular= crus) of the penis. The crura lie in the superficial perineal space.

The corpus spongiosum also extends into the superficial perineal space. Its proximal end is enlarged to form the ***bulb*** of the penis.

THE PROSTATE

The prostate is a glandular organ. It lies just below the urinary bladder and is traversed by the prostatic part of the urethra (Figs. 19.25, 20.11). The prostate is divided into a number of lobes. The substance of the prostate consists of glandular tissue. The secretions are poured into prostatic part of the urethra.

The prostate is made up of numerous glands that are embedded in a framework of fibromuscular tissue. The follicles of glandular tissue are lined by columnar epithelium (Fig. 20.17).

The prostate lies immediately in front of the rectum. It can be examined by a finger inserted into the rectum (PR or per-rectal examination).

Prostatic secretion is thin, milky and acidic. It contains various ions, acid phosphatase, and enzymes. It constitutes about 20% of semen.

Inflammation in the prostate is called ***prostatitis***. In many old men the prostate undergoes enlargement (***benign hypertrophy***). It is also a common site of cancer.

SEMEN

Semen is made up of the following.

1. Spermatozoa produced in the testis.
2. Secretions of seminal vesicle, of prostate and of bulbourethral gland.

Fructose, present in semen gives nutrition to spermatozoa. Alkalinity of semen increases vaginal pH to about six. Spermatozoa are most motile at this pH.

Fibrinogen added to semen in the seminal vesicle causes clotting of semen after ejaculation. This helps to retain semen in the vagina. About 15 minutes later fibrinolysins, present in semen, dissolve the clot and allow free movement of spermatozoa.

The average quantity of semen ejaculated is about 3 ml. Each ml contains about 100 million spermatozoa.

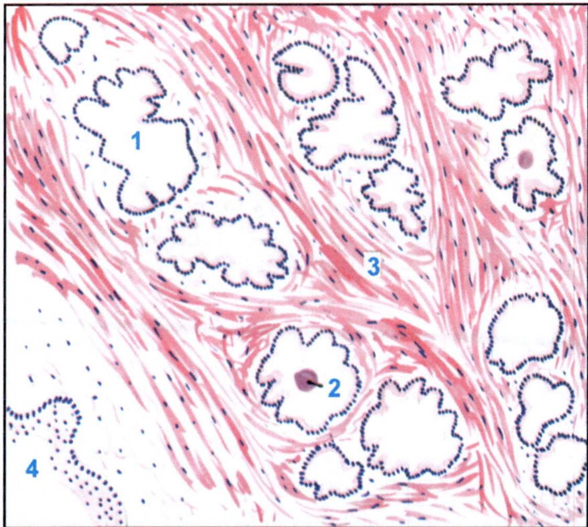

Fig. 20.17 Prostate (low power view). 1-Follicle of irregular shape. 2-Amyloid body. 3-Fibromuscular tissue. 4-Prostatic urethra lined by transitional epithelium.

TESTOSTERONE

Testosterone is the most important male sex hormone (or androgen). Testosterone is secreted by interstitial cells (cells of Leydig) of the testis. The effects of testosterone are as follows.

1. It is responsible for growth of male sex organs (testis, scrotum, penis) particularly at puberty.
2. It is responsible for appearance of secondary sex characters of the male. These are:
   a. Characteristic male pattern of growth of hair on the face and on other parts of the body.
   b. Growth of larynx and of vocal cords leading to lower pitch of the voice (heavier voice).
   c. Growth of muscles, particularly of the shoulders. The shoulders become broad.
3. Testosterone is responsible for male sexual desire. This action takes place through the hypothalamus.
4. Testosterone caused increased development of muscles all over the body. This is referred to as ***anabolic effect***. There is increased synthesis and decreased breakdown of proteins. For this reason atheletes use androgens to improve their performance.
5. There is increased bone growth, both in length and in thickness. This is responsible for sudden increase in height of children at puberty.
6. Testosterone stimulates production of erythropoietin leading to greater haemoglobin concentration and RBC count.
7. Production of testosterone starts in fetal life and leads to development of sex organs as in the male.

Regulation of Testicular Activity

1. The hypothalamus produces the gonadotropin releasing hormone (GnRH). This hormone passes through the hypothalamo-hypophyseal portal vessels and reaches the pars anterior of the hypophysis cerebri.
2. Under the influence of GnRH the hypophysis cerebri produces two hormones FSH and LH. (These hormones are produced both in the male and female, but the actions are different in the two). In the male FSH acts on seminiferous tubules and stimulates spermatogenesis. LH acts on interstitial cells of the testis and stimulates production of testosterone. A polypeptide, inhibin, produced by seminiferous tubules, inhibits secretion of FSH by the hypophysis cerebri.

Other Androgens

Dehydroepiandrosterone is an androgen produced by the adrenal cortex. It does not have significant effect in males. In females it has considerable anabolic effect. Some tumours of the adrenal gland produce large amounts of dehydroepiandrosterone. This has a masculinising effect in the female and early onset of puberty in the male.

Dihydrotestosterone is derived from testosterone. Other substances formed by degradation of testosterone are androsterone, epiandrosterone and etiocholanolone.

These three are collectively referred to as 17-ketosteroids. They are mostly produced by the adrenal gland. Their urinary excretion is increased in some tumours of the adrenal cortex.

SOME DISEASES OF REPRODUCTIVE ORGANS

Diseases transmitted through sexual intercourse

Many diseases can be transmitted from one person to another through sexual intercourse. These are referred to as sexually transmitted diseases, or as venereal diseases. Some of them are as follows.

Gonorrhea

This is a bacterial disease. In men it causes urethritis. It can spread to other organs of the male genital tract. In women it can involve all reproduction organs including the ovaries. In the male it can cause urethral strictures. In the female it can lead to obstruction of uterine tubes and infertility.

Syphilis

This is a chronic infection that leads to widespread damage. Soon after infection, a sore appears on the penis, or on female external genitalia. After a few weeks rashes appear on the skin. After a few years, lesions (called gamma) appear in various organs of the body including the brain. The infection can pass from mother to child during childbirth.

HIV Infection or AIDS

HIV infection or AIDS spreads through sexual intercourse. Various other viral, fungal or protozoal infections can be transmitted through sex.

DISORDERS OF MALE GENITAL TRACT

1. Infection of the glans penis is called ***balanitis***. ***Urethritis***, ***epididymitis*** and ***prostatitis*** can occur.
2. The testis may be undesended at birth. Tumours may arise in the testis.
3. The prostate is a common site of cancer. In many old persons there is benign enlargement of the prostate. It leads to difficulty in micturition, and eventually to urinary retention. It is treated by surgical removal of the prostate (***prostatectomy***).
4. Accumulation of fluid in the scrotum is called ***hydrocoele***. In some cases of ***hernia***, coils of intestine can reach the scrotum.

CHAPTER

21

Female Reproductive Organs

GROSS ANATOMY AND HISTOLOGY OF FEMALE REPRODUCTIVE ORGANS

The female reproductive organs are shown in Fig. 21.1. The female gonads are the right and left ***ovaries***. The female internal genital organs are the ***uterus***, the ***uterine tubes*** and the ***vagina***. The vagina is the female organ of copulation. It opens to the exterior through a depression in the perineum called the ***vestibule***. The female external genital organs are present around the vestibule. They are the ***labia majora,*** the ***labia minora*** and the ***clitoris***; and some deeper structures that are associated with them. The ***mammary glands*** are accessory organs of reproduction.

In a mature female one ovum is produced every month (in the right or left ovary). It travels into the uterine tube towards the uterus. Spermatozoa introduced into the vagina can travel from the vagina into the uterus to reach the uterine tube. If a spermatozoon encounters an ovum fertilization can take place. (Fertilization normally takes place in the uterine tube). The fertilized ovum then travels to the uterus where it gets lodged and starts developing into a fetus (unborn child in the process of development).

The uterus provides the fetus with nutrition and with a suitable environment for its growth. The period during which a fetus is growing in the uterus is called ***pregnancy***. During pregnancy a fetus receives nutrition and oxygen from the mothers' blood. Transfer of these from mother to fetus takes place through an organ called the ***placenta***. The uterus enlarges greatly during pregnancy. At the end of pregnancy the fetus is expelled out of the uterus. It passes through the vagina to the exterior as a new born infant. The process of childbirth is called ***parturition***. The mammary glands provide the newborn baby with nourishment in the form of milk.

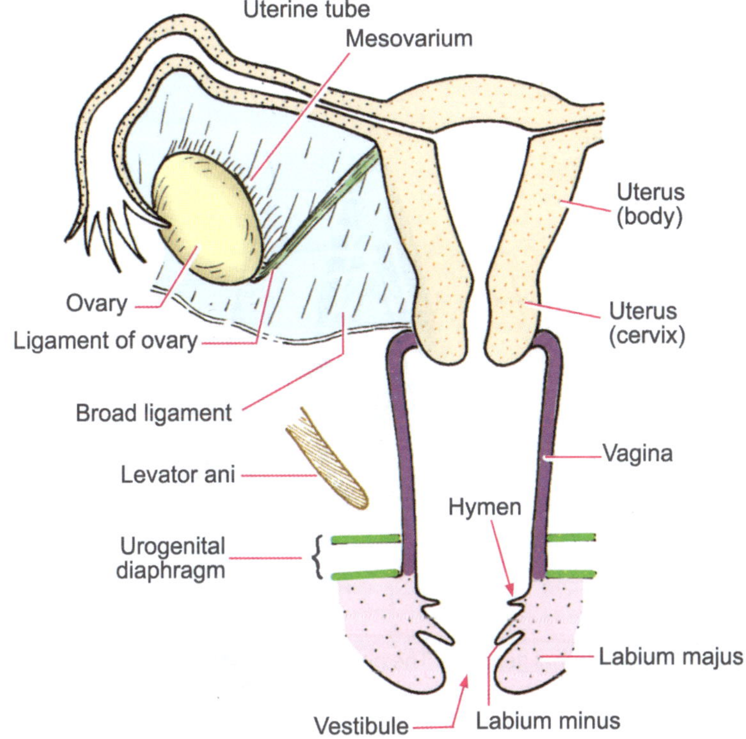

Fig. 21.1 Scheme to show the female reproductive organs.

Female External Genitalia

The region of the female external genitalia is referred to as the ***vulva*** or the ***pudendum.*** It is seen in surface view in Fig. 21.2. When viewed from the surface we see a midline ***pudendal cleft.*** The vagina and the urethra open to the exterior through this cleft.

The cleft is bounded on either side by an elevation called the ***labium majus.*** The labia majora are folds of skin. The space between the anterior and posterior layers of skin is filled by connective tissue and fat. The labia majora are developmentally equivalent to the scrotum. This explains the termination of the round ligaments of the uterus in them. Like the scrotum the superficial fascia in the labia majora has some smooth muscle in it. The right and left labia majora are joined anteriorly by a fold called the ***anterior labial commissure***; and posteriorly by the ***posterior labial commissure.***

When the labia majora are separated we see two smaller and thinner folds of skin deep to them. These are the ***labia minora*** placed on either side of the vaginal orifice (Fig. 21.2). Posteriorly, the two labia minora are joined together by a fold called the ***frenulum***: this fold is conspicuous only in a virgin. Anteriorly, the labia minora join each other near the clitoris. The space between the right and left labia minora is called the ***vestibule.***

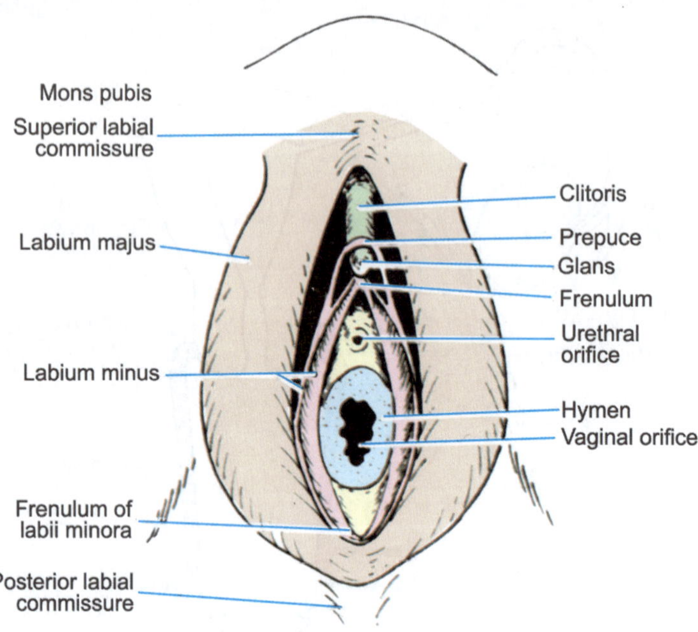

Fig. 21.2 Female external genitalia. The pubic hair are not drawn for sake of clarity.

The ***clitoris*** is a small median rod-like structure placed between the anterior parts of the labia majora. In structure it resembles a miniature penis with the exception that the urethra does not pass through it. Like the penis it has a ***glans***, a ***body*** and a ***root.*** The body is made up of ***corpora cavernosa*** which extend into the perineum as the crura of the clitoris. The bulb and corpus spongiosum (of the penis) are represented in the female by two masses of erectile tissue placed on either side of the vaginal orifice. These are called the ***bulbs of the vestibule.***

The crura of the clitoris and the bulbs of the vestibule are placed in the superficial perineal space (Fig. 21.3).

Deep to the labia minora the vaginal orifice is partially closed by a circular fold of mucous membrane called the ***hymen.*** It is well defined only in the virgin. In married women its position is marked by rounded elevations called the ***carunculae hymenales.***

The external orifice of the female urethra is located a short distance in front of the vaginal opening.

The ***mons pubis*** is a surface elevation overlying the pubic symphysis: it is produced by a mass of fat present just under the skin. The mons pubis is included in the female external genitalia.

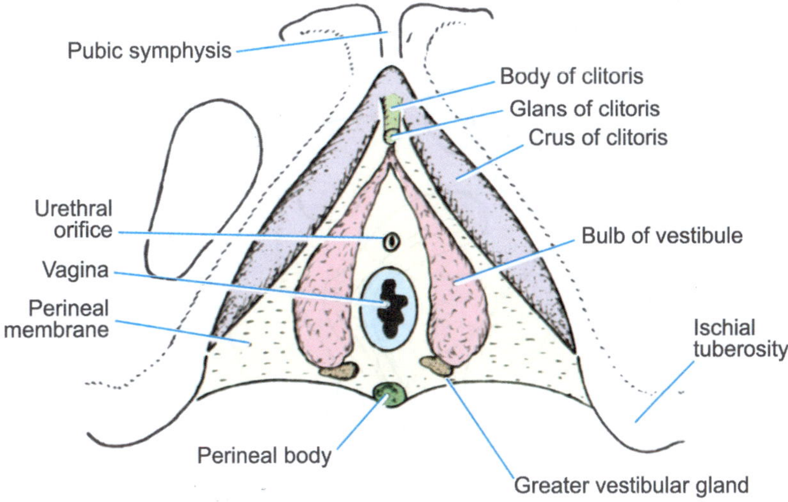

Fig. 21.3 Some deeper structures in the female perineum.

THE OVARIES

The right and left ovaries are the female gonads. Female gametes, called ***ova*** (singular = ovum), are produced in them. The ovary also produces female sex hormones (oestrogens). Each ovary is shaped like an almond: it is approximately 3 cm in length; 1.5 cm in width; and 1 cm in thickness. It is covered by a germinal epithelium that is continuous with the peritoneum. From Fig. 21.1 it will be seen that the uterus is attached, on either side, to a fold of peritoneum called the ***broad ligament***. The broad ligament stretches from the side of the uterus to the lateral wall and floor of the pelvis. The ovary is attached to the posterosuperior aspect of the broad ligament by a fold of peritoneum called the ***mesovarium***. The part of the broad ligament between the attachment of the mesovarium and the lateral wall of the pelvis is called the ***suspensory ligament of the ovary***. The ***lateral surface*** of the ovary lies in contact with the peritoneum covering the lateral wall of the pelvis. It lies in a depression called the ***ovarian fossa***. The ***lower pole*** gives attachment to the ***ligament of the ovary***: this ligament passes in the interval between the two layers of the broad ligament to reach the uterus (near the attachment of the uterine tube to the latter) (Fig. 21.1).

The free surface of the ovary is lined by a single layer of cuboidal cells (***germinal epithelium***). The substance of the ovary is divisible into a thick cortex and a much smaller medulla (Fig. 21.5).

Immediately deep to the germinal epithelium the ***cortex*** is covered by a condensation of connective tissue called the ***tunica albuginea***. The tunica albuginea of the ovary is much thinner, and less dense, than that of the testis.

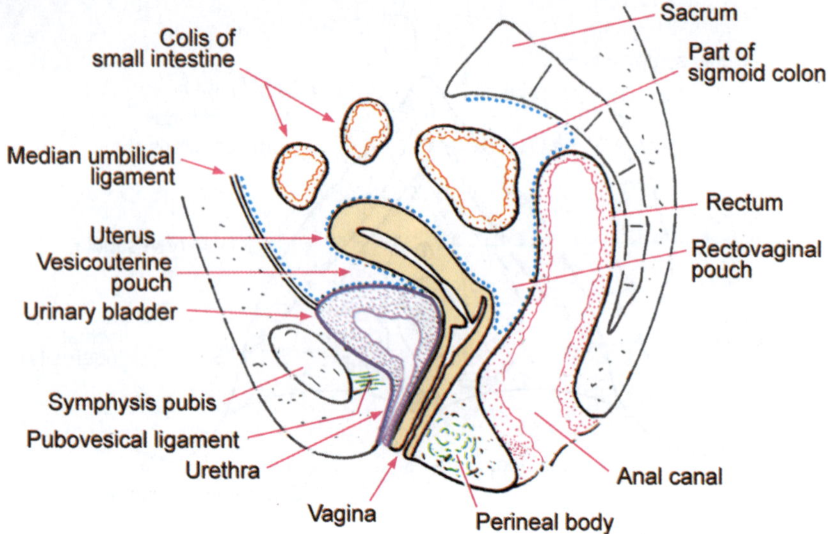

Fig. 21.4 Sagittal section through female pelvis.

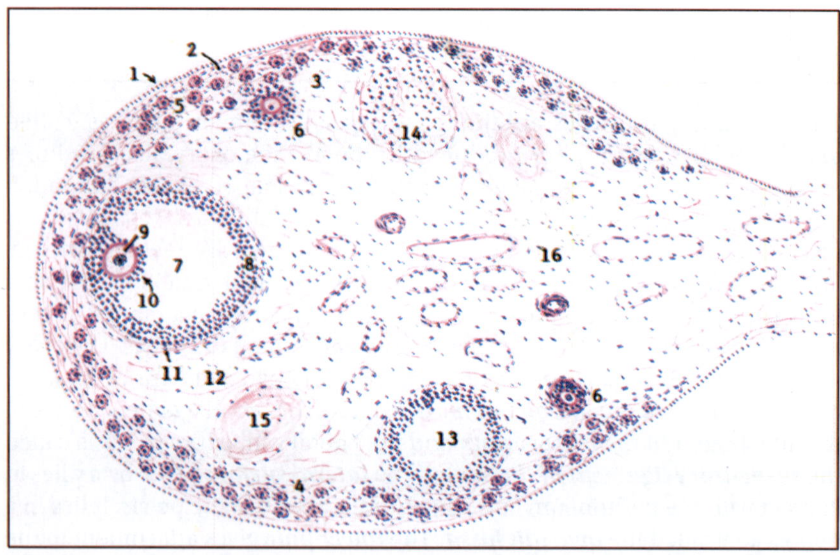

Fig. 21.5 Ovary, panoramic view. 1-Cuboidal epithelium over surface. 2-Tunica albuginea. 3, 4-Cortex. 5-Primordial follicle. 6-Secondary follicle. 7-Follicular cavity. 8-Granulosa cells. 9-Ovum. 10-Cumulus oophoricus. 11-Capsule of follicle. 12-Stroma. 14-Corpus luteum.

Deep to the tunica albuginea the cortex has a stroma made up of reticular fibres and numerous fusiform cells that resemble mesenchymal cells. Scattered in this stroma there are ***ovarian follicles*** at various stages of development. Each follicle contains a developing ovum (Fig. 21.9). The formation of ova, and the development and fate of ovarian follicles are described below.

The ***medulla*** consists of connective tissue in which numerous blood vessels (mostly veins) are seen.

OOGENESIS

The stem cells from which ova are derived are called ***oogonia***. These are large round cells present in the cortex of the ovary. Oogonia are derived (in fetal life) from ***primordial germ cells***.

An oogonium enlarges to form a ***primary oocyte*** (Fig. 21.6). The primary oocyte contains the diploid number of chromosomes i.e., 46. It undergoes the first meiotic division to form two daughter cells each of which has 23 chromosomes. However, the cytoplasm of the primary oocyte is not equally divided. Most of it goes to one daughter cell that is large and is called the ***secondary oocyte***. The second daughter cell has hardly any cytoplasm, and forms the ***first polar body***. The secondary oocyte now undergoes the second meiotic division, the daughter cells being again unequal in size. The larger daughter cell produced as a result of this division is the ***mature ovum***. The smaller daughter cell (which has hardly any cytoplasm) is the ***second polar body***. From the above it will be seen that one primary oocyte ultimately gives rise to only one ovum.

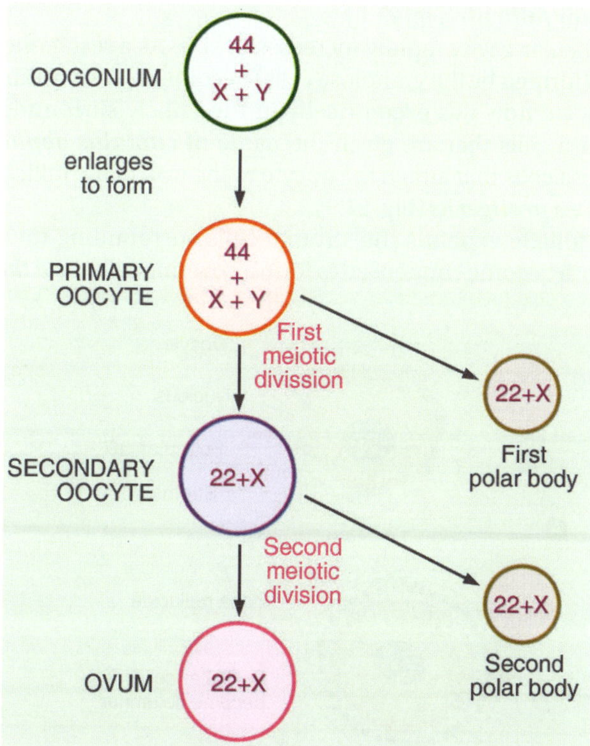

Fig. 21.6 Scheme to show the stages in oogenesis.

Formation of Ovarian Follicles

Ovarian follicles (or ***Graafian follicles***) are derived from stromal cells that surround developing ova as follows.

1. Some cells of the stroma become flattened and surround an oocyte (Fig. 21.7A). These stromal cells are now called ***follicular cells.***
   The ovum and the flat surrounding cells form a ***primordial follicle.*** Numerous primordial follicles are present in the ovary at birth. They undergo further development only at puberty.
2. The first indication that a primordial follicle is beginning to undergo further development is that the flattened follicular cells become columnar (Fig. 21.7B). Follicles at this stage of development are called ***primary follicles.***
3. A homogeneous membrane, the ***zona pellucida***, appears between the follicular cells and the oocyte (Fig.21.7B).
4. The follicular cells proliferate to form several layers of cells which constitute the ***membrana granulosa***. The cells are now called ***granulosa cells***. This is a ***secondary follicle.***
5. So far the granulosa cells are in the form of a compact mass. However, the cells of the granulosa to one side of the ovum soon partially separate from one another. In this way a ***follicular cavity*** (or ***antrum folliculi***) appears between them. The follicular cavity comes to be filled by a fluid, the ***liquor folliculi*** (Fig. 21.8).
6. The follicular cavity rapidly increases in size. As a result, the wall of the follicle (formed by the granulosa cells) becomes relatively thin (Fig. 21.8). The oocyte now lies eccentrically in the follicle surrounded by some granulosa cells that are given the name of ***cumulus oophoricus***. The granulosa cells that attach the oocyte to the wall of the follicle constitute the ***discus proligerus*** (Fig. 21.9).
7. As the follicle expands the stromal cells surrounding the membrana granulosa become condensed to form a covering called the ***theca interna***

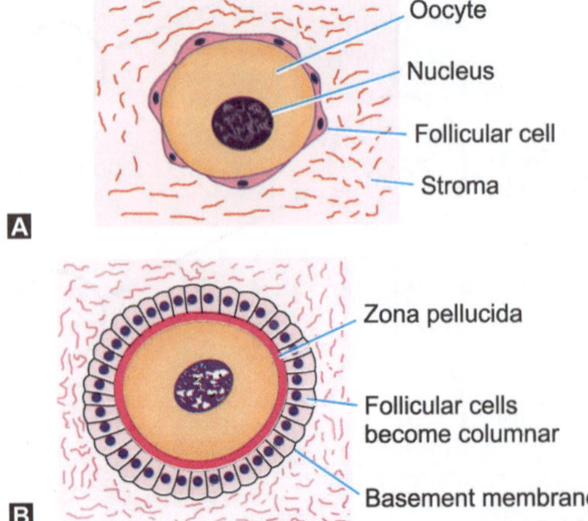

Fig. 21.7 Diagrammatic presentation of: A. Primordial follicle. B. Primary follicle.

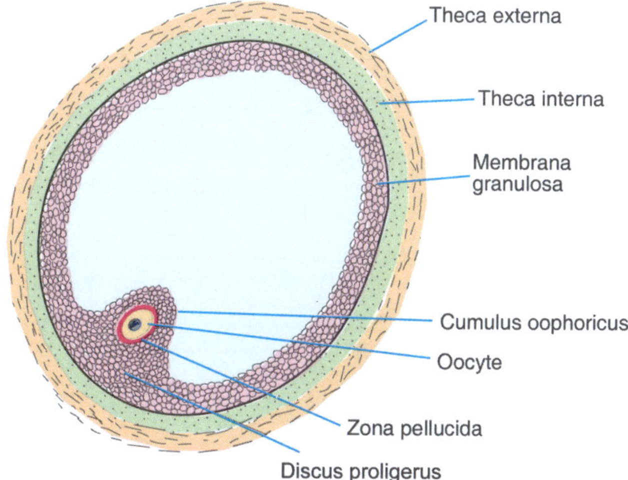

Fig. 21.8 Mature ovarian follicle.

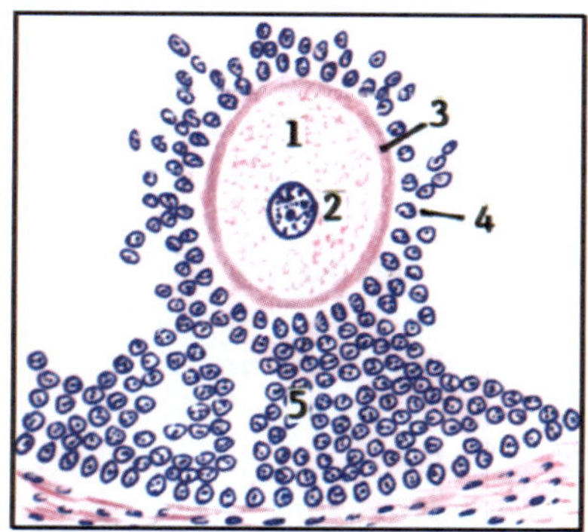

Fig. 21.9 Part of ovarian follicle seen at high magnification. 1-Ovum, 2-Nucleus of ovum, 3-Zona pellucida, 4-Cumulus oophoricus, 5-Discus proligerus.

(theca = cover). The cells of the theca interna later secrete a hormone called ***oestrogen***, and they are then called the cells of the ***thecal gland***.

8. Outside the theca interna some fibrous tissue becomes condensed to form another covering for the follicle. This is the ***theca externa***.
9. The ovarian follicle is at first very small. It gradually increases in size. Ultimately it ruptures and the ovum is shed from the ovary. The shedding of the ovum is called ***ovulation***.
10. After ovulation, the remaining part of the follicle undergoes changes that convert it into an important structure called the ***corpus luteum***.

Corpus Luteum

The corpus luteum is an important structure. It secretes a hormone, ***progesterone***. The corpus luteum is derived from the ovarian follicle, after the latter has ruptured to shed the ovum (Fig. 21.10).

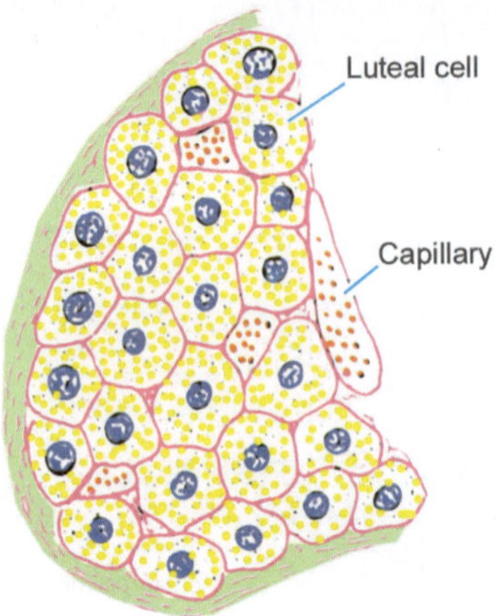

Fig. 21.10 Corpus luteum (diagrammatic). Note the large hexagonal cells filled with yellow granules.

At this stage, the follicular cells are small and rounded. They now enlarge rapidly. Their cytoplasm becomes filled with a yellow pigment called ***lutein***. They are now called ***luteal cells***. The presence of this yellow pigment gives the structure a yellow colour, and that is why it is called the corpus luteum (= yellow body).

a. If the ovum is not fertilized, the corpus luteum persists for about 14 days. During this period it secretes progesterone. It remains relatively small and is called the ***corpus luteum of menstruation***.
b. If the ovum is fertilized and pregnancy results, the corpus luteum persists and becomes large. It is called the ***corpus luteum of pregnancy***. The progesterone secreted by it is essential for the maintenance of pregnancy in the first few months. After the fourth month, the corpus luteum is no longer needed, as the placenta begins to secrete progesterone.

The series of changes that begin with the formation of an ovarian follicle, and end with the degeneration of the corpus luteum constitute what is called an ***ovarian cycle***.

The changes taking place during the ovarian cycle are greatly influenced by certain hormones produced by the hypophysis cerebri. The hormones produced by the theca interna and by the corpus luteum in turn influence other parts of the female reproductive system, notably the uterus, resulting in a cycle of changes referred to as the ***uterine cycle*** or ***menstrual cycle***. The menstrual cycle is described later in this chapter.

THE UTERINE TUBES

Each uterine tube (right or left) lies in the free margin of the corresponding broad ligament. It has medial and lateral ends (Fig. 21.1). The ***medial end*** is attached to the corresponding side of the uterus. Here its lumen communicates with the cavity of the uterus. The ***lateral end*** of the tube lies near the ovary. At this end it has an opening through which its lumen is in communication with the peritoneal cavity: this opening is called ***abdominal ostium*** (Fig. 21.1).

The uterine tube is about 10 cm long. About 1 cm of the tube, near the medial end, is embedded in the muscle wall of the uterus: this is the ***uterine part*** of the tube. The next 3 cm or so is thick-walled and has a narrow lumen so that it is cord like: this part is called the ***isthmus***. The next 5 cm or so is thin walled and has a much larger lumen than the rest of the tube. This dilated part is called the ***ampulla***. The lateral end of the uterine tube is funnel shaped and is called the ***infundibulum.*** The walls of the infundibulum are prolonged into a number of irregular processes called ***fimbria***.

Ova discharged from the ovary enter the uterine tube through the infundibulum and pass into the ampulla. They slowly travel towards the uterus. If sexual intercourse takes place at the appropriate time spermatozoa enter the uterine tube through the vagina and uterus and meet the ovum in the ampulla of the tube: fertilisation normally takes place here. The fertilised ovum travels through the uterine tube towards the uterus to enter its cavity. Here it gets implanted in the uterine wall. If fertilisation does not occur the unfertilised ovum degenerates.

The wall of the uterine tube is made up of mucous membrane, surrounded by a muscle coat (Fig. 21.11). It is covered externally by peritoneum.

The mucous membrane shows numerous branching folds which almost fill the lumen of the tube. These folds are most conspicuous in the ampulla. Each fold has a highly cellular core of connective tissue. It is lined by columnar epithelium that rests on a basement membrane. Some of the lining cells are ciliated: ciliary action helps to move ova towards the uterus. Other cells are secretory.

The muscle coat has an inner circular layer and an outer longitudinal layer of smooth muscle.

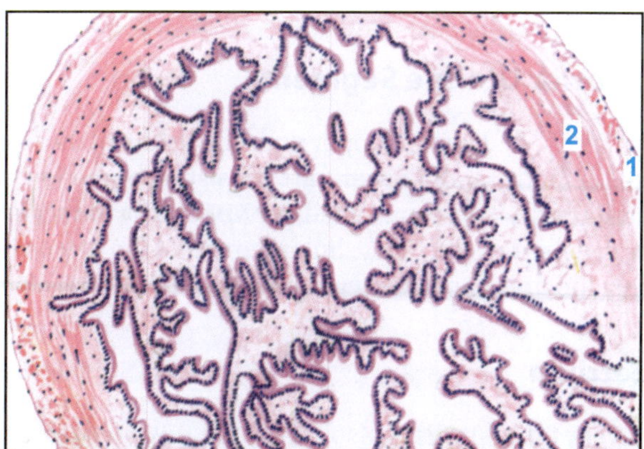

Fig. 21.11 Uterine tube. 1,2-Muscle layer (longitudinal and circular). Mucous membrane shows branching folds covered by ciliated columnar epithelium.

THE UTERUS

A general idea of the form of the uterus is presented in Fig. 21.1. It is seen that the organ is piriform. It is broader above and narrows down below. The uterus is about 7.5 cm (3 inches) in length. Its maximum width (near its upper end) is about 5 cm (2 inches). Its thickness (anteroposterior) is about 2.5 cm (1 inch). The exterior of the uterus shows a constriction at the junction of its upper two thirds with the lower one third. The part above the constriction is called the ***body***: it is broad above and narrow below. The part below the constriction is called the ***cervix***: this part is more or less cylindrical.

Sections across the uterus show that it has a thick wall, and a relatively narrow lumen. The wall is made up of a thick layer of muscle (called the ***myometrium***) and of an inner lining of mucosa (called the ***endometrium***). In a sagittal section (Fig. 21.1) the lumen is seen to be only a narrow slit, the anterior and posterior walls being close to each other. In the coronal plane the lumen of the body of the uterus is triangular (Fig. 21.1). The lumen of each uterine tube joins the lateral angle of this triangle. The part of the body of the uterus that lies above the level of the openings of the uterine tubes is called the ***fundus***. The cavity of the cervix (or ***canal of the cervix***) is roughly cylindrical. However, its upper and lower ends are somewhat narrower than the central part. The upper narrow end of the canal is called the ***internal os*** and the narrow lower end is called the ***external os***.

The uterus lies in the true pelvis. Its orientation is best appreciated in a sagittal section through the pelvis (Fig. 21.4). The long axis of the uterus is more or less at right angles to the long axis of the vagina. The forward bending of the uterus relative to the vagina is referred to as ***anteversion*** of the uterus. The uterus is also slightly bent forwards on itself: this is referred to as ***anteflexion***. The caudal part of the cervix projects into the upper part of vagina through the anterior wall of the latter: it is separated from the vaginal wall by recesses called the anterior, lateral, and posterior ***fornices*** (singular = fornix) of the vagina. The posterior fornix is deepest.

Upper and Lower Uterine Segments

The uterus can be divided into an upper part, consisting of the fundus and the greater part of the body; and a lower part consisting of the lower part of the body, and of the cervix. These are called the ***upper uterine segment***, and the ***lower uterine segment*** respectively. Enlargement of the uterus in pregnancy involves mainly the upper uterine segment.

The Myometrium

The muscle layer of the uterus is also called the ***myometrium***. It consists of bundles of smooth muscle amongst which there is connective tissue. Numerous blood vessels, nerves and lymphatics are also present in it.

The muscle cells of the uterus are capable of undergoing great elongation in association with the great enlargement of the organ in pregnancy. New muscle fibres are also formed. Contractions of the myometrium are responsible for expulsion of the fetus at the time of child birth.

The Endometrium

The mucous membrane of the uterus is called the ***endometrium***. The endometrium consists of a lining epithelium that rests on a stroma. Numerous uterine glands are present in the stroma.

The lining epithelium is columnar. The epithelium rests on a stroma which contains numerous blood vessels. It also contains numerous simple tubular uterine glands. The glands are lined by columnar epithelium (Fig. 21.14).

The endometrium undergoes marked cyclical changes that constitute the ***menstrual cycle.*** These are described below.

THE VAGINA

The vagina is a tubular structure with a muscular wall. Its lower end opens to the exterior through the vestibule (Fig. 21.1). At its upper end it is attached to the cervix of the uterus. We have seen that the cervix projects into the upper part of the vagina through the uppermost part of its anterior wall (Fig. 21.4); and that the space between the cervix and the adjoining part of the vaginal wall is divided (for descriptive purposes) into the anterior, posterior, and lateral fornices.

The wall of the vagina consists of a mucous membrane, a muscle coat, and an outer fibrous coat or adventitia (Fig. 21.12).

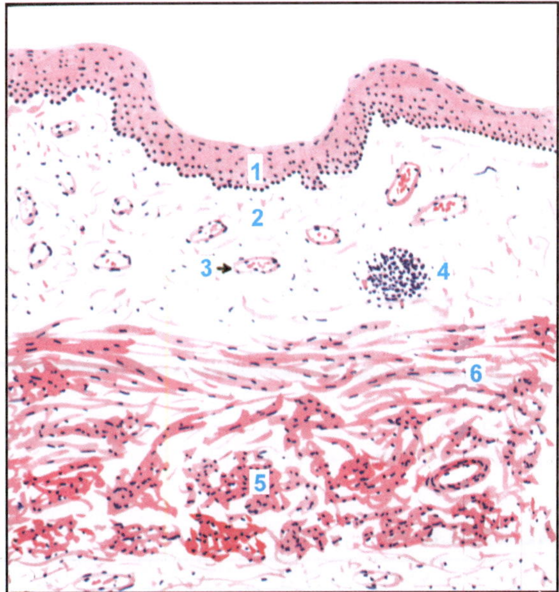

Fig. 21.12 Vagina. 1-Lining of stratified squamous epithelium. 2-Connective tissue. 3-Blood vessels. 4-Lymphoid follicle. 5,6-Muscle coat (longitudinal and circular).

The mucous membrane shows numerous longitudinal folds. It is lined by stratified squamous epithelium. No glands are seen in the mucosa, the vaginal surface being kept moist by secretions of glands in the cervix of the uterus.

Striated muscle fibres surrounding the lower end of the vagina form a sphincter for it.

THE MAMMARY GLANDS

Although the mammary glands are present in both sexes they remain rudimentary in the male. In the female, they are well developed after puberty. Each breast is a soft rounded elevation present over the pectoral region. The skin over the centre of the elevation shows a darkly pigmented circular area called the ***areola***. Overlying the central part of the areola there is a projection called the ***nipple***.

Each mammary gland has an outer covering of skin deep to which there are several discrete masses of glandular tissue. These masses are separated (and covered) by considerable quantities of connective tissue and of adipose tissue. The fascia covering the gland is connected to overlying skin by fibrous processes called the ***suspensory ligaments*** (of Cooper). (In cancer of the breast these processes contract causing pitting of the overlying skin).

The glandular tissue (or mammary gland proper) is made up of 15 to 20 lobes. Each lobe consists of a number of lobules. Each lobe drains into a ***lactiferous duct*** that opens at the summit of the nipple. Some distance from its termination each lactiferous duct shows a dilation called the ***lactiferous sinus***. The smaller ducts are lined by columnar epithelium. In the larger ducts the epithelium has two or three layers of cells. Near their openings on the nipple the lining becomes stratified squamous.

The structure of the glandular elements of the mammary gland varies considerably at different periods of life as follows:

a. Before the onset of puberty the glandular tissue consists entirely of ducts. The bulk of the breast consists of connective tissue and fat that widely separate the glandular elements (Fig. 21.13).
b. During pregnancy the ducts undergo marked proliferation and branching. Their terminal parts develop into proper alveoli. Each lobe is now a compound tubulo-alveolar gland. Towards the end of pregnancy the cells of the alveoli start secreting milk and the alveoli become distended.

Circular smooth muscle is present in the dermis of the areola. Contraction of this muscle causes erection of the nipple. Many sebaceous glands and apocrine sweat glands are also present in the areola. At the periphery of the areola there are large sebaceous glands that are responsible for the formation of surface elevations called the ***tubercles of Montgomery***.

MENSTRUAL CYCLE

The endometrium undergoes marked cyclical changes that constitute the ***menstrual cycle***. The most prominent feature of this cycle is the monthly flow of blood from the uterus. This is called ***menstruation***. The menstrual cycle is

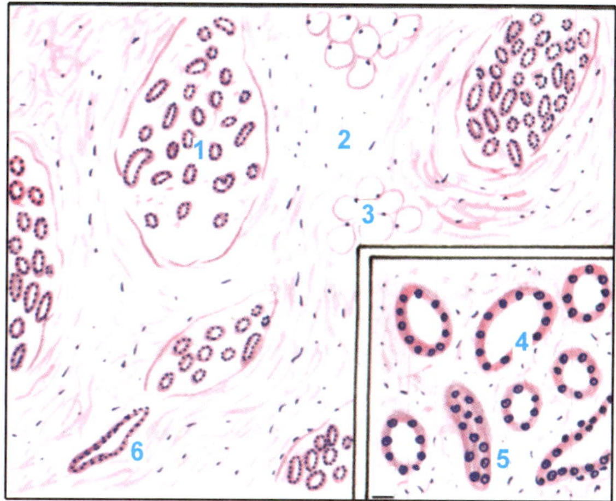

Fig. 21.13 Mammary gland (resting phase). 1, 4-Glandular tissue lined by cuboidal epithelium.2-Connective tissue. 3-Fat. 5-Duct.

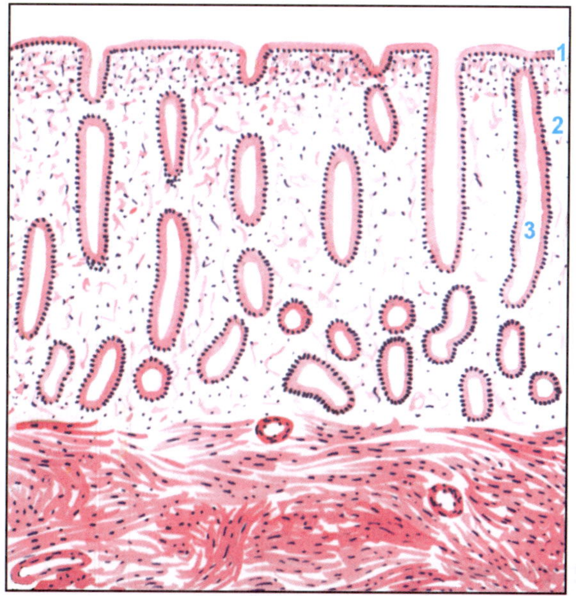

Fig. 21.14 Uterus (Proliferative phase). 1-Lining of columnar epithelium. 2-Stroma. 3-Uterine gland. Also observe the muscular coat.

divided into the following phases: ***postmenstrual***, ***proliferative***, ***secretory*** and ***menstrual***. The cyclical changes in the endometrium take place under the influence of hormones (oestrogen, progesterone) produced by the ovary.

1. In the postmenstrual phase the endometrium is thin. It progressively increases in thickness being thickest at the end of the secretory phase. At the time of the next menstruation the greater part of its thickness is shed off and flows out along with the menstrual blood. The part that remains is called the ***pars basalis***.

2. The uterine glands are straight in the postmenstrual phase. As the endometrium increases in thickness the glands elongate, increase in diameter, and become twisted (Fig. 21.15). Because of this twisting, they acquire a saw-toothed appearance in sections (Figs. 21.15, 21.16). At the time of menstruation the greater parts of the uterine glands are lost (along with the entire lining epithelium) leaving behind only their most basal parts. The lining epithelium is reformed (just after the cessation of menstruation) by proliferation of epithelial cells in the basal parts of the glands.

The thickening of endometrium during the secretory phase is a preparation for reception of a fertilized ovum. The thick soft endometrium provides a suitable environment for the fertilized ovum to get implanted in the uterine wall and grow. The shedding of the superficial layers of endometrium takes place if pregnancy does not occur. Now you will understand why a missed period is a sign of pregnancy.

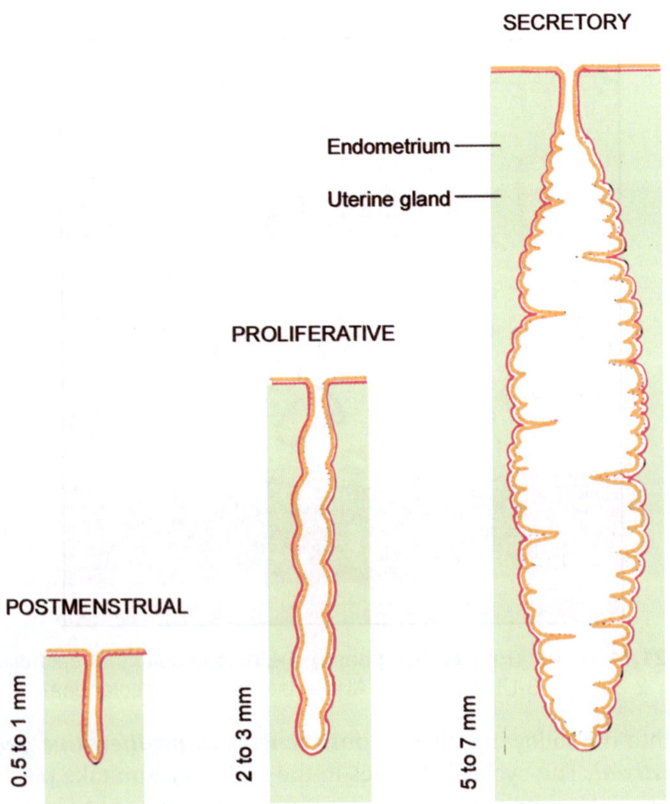

Fig. 21.15 Uterine glands at various stages of the menstrual cycle. The thickness of the endometrium is also indicated.

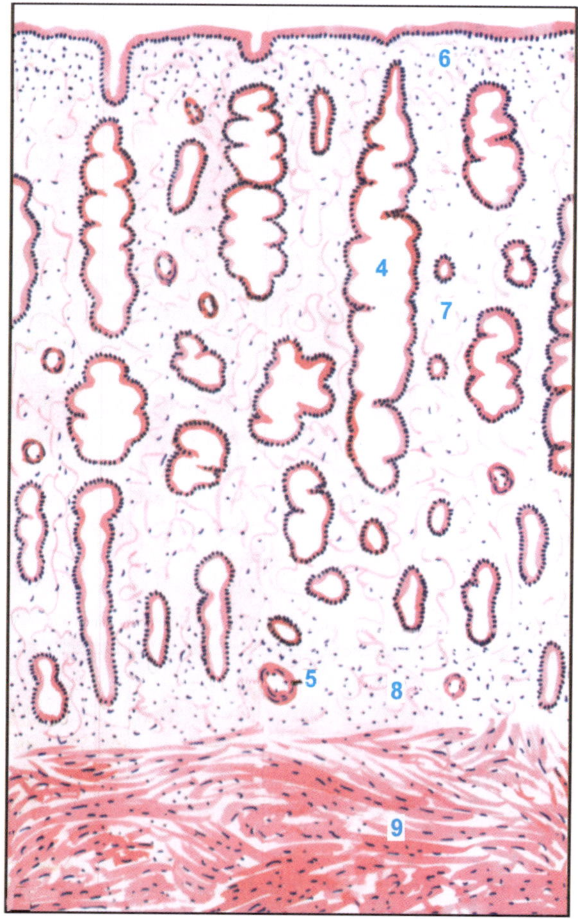

Fig. 21.16 Uterus (secretory phase). 4-Enlarged uterine gland. 5-Artery. 6-Stratum compactum. 7-Stratum spongiosum. 8-Stratum basale. 9-Muscle layer.

HORMONES INFLUENCING OVULATION AND MENSTRUATION

These cycles are under the control of various hormones, which can be briefly summarized as follows:

The hypothalamus acts as a major center for the control of reproduction. It secretes the ***Gonadotropin-releasing hormones*** (***GnRH),*** which in turn controls the secretion of ***gonadotrophic hormones*** from the adenohypophysis (anterior pituitary gland).

There are two gonadotrophic hormones. They are the ***follicle stimulating hormone (FSH)*** and the ***luteinizing hormone (LH).***

In the first half of the menstrual cycle the GnRH acts on the anterior pituitary to release FSH. The FSH acts on the ovary and stimulates the formation and maturation of ovarian follicles.

The maturing ovarian follicles now start secreting oestrogens. The repair and proliferation of endometrium takes place under the influence of oestrogens. The endometrial stroma progressively thickens, the glands in it elongate and the spiral arteries begin to grow towards the surface epithelium.

The level of oestrogen rises to a peak about two days before ovulation.

This leads to sudden increase in the level of LH secreted by the anterior pituitary (LH surge) about 24 to 36 hours before ovulation. The LH surge leads to ovulation; and the Graafian follicle is transformed to the corpus luteum.

The LH stimulates the secretion of projesterone by the corpus luteum. Though the secretion of projesterone predominates, some oestrogen is also produced.

If fertilization does not occur the granulosa cells produce the protein ***inhibin,*** which acts on the anterior pituitary and inhibits the secretion of gonadotrophins. This leads to regression of the corpus luteum.

Due to the regression of the corpus luteum there is a fall in the blood level of oestrogen and projesterone. The withdrawal of these hormones causes the endometrium to regress and triggers the onset of menstruation.

If fertilization occurs the corpus luteum does not regress. It continues to secrete progesterone and oestrogen. The secretory phase of endometrium continues and menstruation does not occur.

OESTROGENS

There are three oestrogens. These are (a) oestradiol, (b) oestrone and (c) oestriol. Oestradiol is the chief oestrogen. It is produced in the ovary. Oestrone is also produced in the ovary. Oestriol is formed by degradation of oestradiol and oestrone. The production of oestrogens varies in different phases of the menstrual cycle and in pregnancy. During pregnancy oestrogens are produced by the placenta.

The actions produced by oestrogens are as follows.

1. Oestrogens stimulate ***growth of all female reproductive organs*** including the female breast.
   a. ***Uterus***: Endometrium increases in thickness. Uterine glands become longer. Spiral arteries grow in length. The myometrium grows in thickness. Cervical secretion is watery. When dried on a glass slide the secretion forms a characteristic fern-like pattern.
   b. ***Uterine tubes***: Secretory activity, ciliary movements and contractility of smooth muscle increase.
   c. ***Vagina***: There is thickening of mucosa and cornification of epithelium. Glycogen accumulates in the cells.
   d. ***Mammary glands***: Enlargement of the breast at puberty is caused by growth of ducts, proliferation of stroma, and deposition of fat.
2. Oestrogens are responsible for development of ***secondary sex characters*** that distinguish the female from the male. Deposition of fat in subcutaneous tissues, specially in some regions (breast, buttocks) gives the body smoother and more rounded contours. Shoulders remain narrow, but the hips become broader. Growth of hair occurs in the pattern characteristic of the female.
3. Oestrogens cause the ***spurt in growth*** seen in girls at puberty. There is relatively early fusion of bony epiphyses, leading to shorter stature.
4. Oestogens lower cholesterol level. They cause salt and water retention.

PROGESTERONE

In the ovary, progesterone is secreted by the corpus luteum (which is formed after ovulation). If pregnancy occurs, secretion of progesterone by the corpus luteum continues for three months. Thereafter, progesterone is formed by the placenta.

The actions of progesterone are as follows.

1. ***Uterus***
   Progesterone is responsible for changes in uterine endometrium that are seen in the secretory phase of the menstrual cycle. However, these changes can be produced only after oestrogens have acted on the endometrium.
   Under the influence of progesterone there is further thickening of endometrium. The stroma becomes oedematous. Uterine glands enlarge and become tortuous. Cervical secretion becomes thick. Dried secretion does not form the fern-like pattern seen in the follicular phase.
2. ***Mammary gland***
   We have seen that under the influence of oestrogens there is proliferation of ducts. Subsequent influence of progesterone leads to proliferation of alveoli.
3. Progesterone tends to increase body temperature and rate of respiration.

PHYSIOLOGY OF PREGNANCY

FERTILIZATION

Transport of Ova and Spermatozoa

Pregnancy can be said to begin at the moment when an ovum is fertilized by a spermatozoon. Fertilization normally occurs in the ampulla of the uterine tube.

Transport of the ovum to this site is facilitated by ciliary movements in the uterine tube, and by the follicular fluid discharged by the ovarian follicle.

The transport of spermatozoa is aided by the following.

a. Motility of the spermatozoa.
b. Propulsive movements of the uterus and uterine tubes caused by oxytoccin (secreted by the pars posterior of the hypophysis cerebri).
c. Production of a thin watery secretion by cervical glands (under the influence of oestrogens).

Viability of Ova and Spermatozoa

After ovulation, the ovum is viable (i.e. it can be fertilized) for not more than two days. Spermatozoa introduced into the vagina die within four days. Therefore, fertilization can occur only if intercourse takes place during a period between four days before ovulation to two days after ovulation.

Some Facts about Fertilization

1. Only one spermatozoon can enter the ovum. After the entry of a single spermatozoon chemical alterations in the zona pellucida prevent entry of any other spermatozoon.
2. Proteolytic enzymes released from the acrosomal cap of the spermatozoon facilitate entry of the sperm into the ovum.
3. At the time of ovulation the second meiotic division of the ovum is in progress. The division is completed as soon as a sperm enters the ovum.
4. The nucleus of the ovum becomes the female pronucleus. The head of the spermatozoon becomes the male pronucleus. These pronuclei lose their nuclear membranes. The 23 chromosomes of the female pronucleus and the 23 chromosomes of the male pronucleus combine to form 23 pairs. A mitotic division starts immediately and results in an embryo having two cells.

Effects of Fertilization

a. The diploid number of chromosomes is restored.
b. Determination of sex of the child takes place.
c. Division of the fertilized ovum begins.

Test Tube Babies

The so-called test tube babies are produced by the technique of ***in vitro fertilization***. (***In vitro*** = outside the body, as against ***in vivo*** = within the body). This technique is being increasingly used in couples who are not able to achieve fertilization in the normal way.

Gonadotropins are administered to the woman to stimulate growth of follicles in the ovary. Just before ovulation, the ovum is removed (using an aspirator) and is placed in a suitable medium. Spermatozoa are added to the medium. Fertilization and early development of the embryo take place in this medium. The process is carefully monitored, and when the embryo is at the 8-cell stage it is put inside the uterus. Successful implantation takes place in about 20 per cent of such trials.

Sex Determination

We know that all ova contain 22 + **X** chromosomes. However, spermatozoa are of two types. Half of them have 22 + **X** chromosomes and the other half of them have 22 + **Y** chromosomes. We speak of these as '**X**-bearing', or '**Y**-bearing', spermatozoa. An ovum can be fertilized by either type of spermatozoon. If the sperm is **X**-bearing, the zygote has 44 + **X** + **X** chromosomes and the offspring is a girl. If the sperm is **Y**-bearing the zygote has 44 + **X** + **Y** chromosomes and the offspring is a boy.

Thus the sex of a child is 'determined' at the time of fertilization. It will now be clear that one chromosome of each of the 23 pairs is derived from the mother and the other from the father.

PLACENTA

Functions of Placenta

1. The placenta enables the transport of oxygen, water, electrolytes and nutrition (in the form of carbohydrates, lipids, polypeptides, amino acids and vitamins) from maternal to fetal blood. A full term fetus takes up about 25 ml of oxygen per minute from maternal blood. Even a short interruption of oxygen supply is fatal for the fetus.
2. It also provides for excretion of carbon dioxide, urea and other waste products produced by the fetus into the maternal blood.
3. Maternal antibodies (IgG gamma globulins) reaching the fetus through the placenta give the fetus immunity against some infections (e.g. diphtheria and measles).
4. The placenta acts as a barrier and prevents many bacteria and other harmful substances from reaching the fetus. However, most viruses (including poliomyelitis, measles and rubella) and some bacteria can pass across it. Drugs taken by the mother may also enter the fetal circulation and can produce congenital malformations.

   As a rule, maternal hormones do not reach the fetus. However, synthetic progestins and synthetic oestrogens (e.g., diethylstilbestrol) easily cross the placenta and can have adverse effects on the fetus (including carcinoma in later life).
5. While permitting the exchange of several substances between the maternal and fetal blood, it keeps these blood streams separate, thereby, preventing antigenic reactions between them.
6. The placenta synthesizes several hormones.
   Progesterone secreted by the placenta is essential for maintenance of pregnancy after the fourth month (when the corpus luteum degenerates).
   Oestrogens (mainly estriol) produced by the placenta reach maternal blood and promote uterine growth and development of the mammary gland.
   Human chorionic gonadotropin (hCG) produced by the placenta is similar in its actions to luteinizing hormone of the hypophysis cerebri. Gonadotropins are excreted through maternal urine where their presence is used as a test to detect a pregnancy in its early stages.
   Somatomammotropin (hCS) has an anti-insulin effect on the mother leading to increased plasma levels of glucose and amino acids in the maternal circulation. In this way it increases availability of these materials for the fetus. It also enhances glucose utilization by the fetus.

PHYSIOLOGICAL CHANGES IN THE MOTHER DURING PREGNANCY

1. The uterus undergoes marked enlargement. It becomes large enough to accommodate a full term fetus.
2. The corpus luteum enlarges. It continues to secrete progesterone during the first three months of pregnancy.

3. There is considerable growth of the breast. Both the ducts and alveoli proliferate. The nipples become larger and also become pigmented.
4. The mother gains weight. The factors responsible are as follows.
   a. Weight of the fetus.
   b. Weight of the placenta.
   c. Weight of amniotic fluid.
   d. Weight of enlarged uterus.
   e. Deposition of fat all over the body.
   f. Increased blood volume.
   g. Increased retention of sodium chloride and water by the body.
5. ***Changes in blood***
   a. Blood volume is increased, mainly to meet the needs of the placental circulation.
   b. Plasma volume is increased.
   c. Absolute number of red blood cells increases.
   d. Total leucocyte count increases up to 16000 to 20000/mm^3.
   e. Because of dilution of blood plasma protein concentration decreases slightly. The proportion of various proteins is also altered.
6. ***Changes in cardiovascular system***
   a. Cardiac output increases progressively during pregnancy, mainly to ensure adequate flow through the uterus and kidneys.
   b. In spite of increased blood volume and cardiac output blood pressure remains normal.
   c. Pressure of the enlarged uterus on the inferior vena cava increases venous pressure in the area drained through it. This leads to oedema of feet. There is increased tendency for development of piles, varicose veins, and venous thrombosis.
   d. Pressure of the enlarged uterus on the diaphragm makes the heart more horizontal, and displaces the apex beat.
7. ***Changes in the respiratory system***
   Tidal volume and pulmonary ventilation increase because of increased sensitivity of the respiratory centre to carbon dioxide.
8. ***Changes in gastrointestinal tract***
   In the first three months of pregnancy the mother frequently complains of nausea and vomitting, specially in the morning (morning sickness). This is because of decreased motility of the stomach and intestines caused by progesterone.
   Absorption of glucose is acclerated. This can cause disturbances of glucose metabolism. Glycosuria may occur.
9. ***Effect on kidneys***
   There is considerable increase in glomerular filtration rate. There may be some excretion of calcium, of glucose and of amino acids in urine.
10. ***Effects on metabolism***
    a. There is considerable increase in consumption of oxygen, mainly to meet needs of the fetus.
    b. There is positive nitrogen balance.
    c. Fat is stored in adipose tissue. The quantity of cholesterol, phospholipids and triglycerides in plasma increases.
    d. The quantity of calcium and phosphorus stored in the body increases. This is necessary for deposition of calcium and phosphorus in fetal bones. In addition there is increased need of these during lactation.

e. The requirement of iron is greatly increased during pregnancy and lactation. Iron is needed for the following.
   1. Production of red blood cells both in the mother and in the fetus.
   2. Production of myoglobin for uterine musculature.
   3. Loss of blood during parturition.

11. ***Changes in activity of endocrine glands and hormones.***
   a. The placenta secretes oestrogen, progesterone, human chorionic gonadotropin, and human chorionic somatomammotropin.
   b. There is increased production of prolactin by the hypophysis cerebri.
   c. Production of cortisol by the adrenal cortex is increased. This plays a role in deposition of fat in adipose tissue.

      There is marked increase in secretion of aldosterone, because of increased renin and angiotensin levels. The concentration of deoxycorticosterone is also greatly increased. These hormones serve to maintain positive sodium balance and high plasma volume.
   d. The secretion of parathormone by the parathyroid glands is greatly increased. This increases absorption of calcium from the gut to meet requirements of the fetus. Plasma levels of vitamin D are increased.
   e. Islets of the pancreas increase in size. Plasma insulin levels increase.
   f. Increased activity of the thyroid gland raises BMR, pulse rate and iodine uptake.

LACTATION

Growth of breasts begins at puberty under the influence of oestrogens. Glandular elements (alveoli) develop only at the time of the first pregnancy under the combined influence of oestrogens and progestrone produced by the placenta. Other hormones responsible for this growth are prolactin, chorionic somatomammotropin, growth hormone, cortisol and thyroxine.

The secretion of milk is stimulated by the hormone prolactin produced by the pars anterior of the hypophysis cerebri (anterior pituitary). However, during pregnancy this action of prolactin is inhibited by the high levels of oestrogen and progesterone secreted by the placenta. After birth of the child, and expulsion of the placenta, the levels of oestrogen and progesterone fall sharply. The uninhibited action of prolactin now induces secretion of milk.

Feeding the baby acts as a strong stimulus for secretion of milk. Sensory impulses arising from the nipples reach the hypothalamus. They stimulate secretion of prolactin and flow of milk.

Between feeds milk gets stored in alveoli. Ejection of stored milk takes place under the effect of oxytoccin, produced by the pars posterior of the hypophysis cerebri (posterior pituitary).

The quantity of milk produced by the breasts every day can be as much as 1.5 litres.

Milk secreted in the first few days is called colostrum. It is rich in antibodies that provide immunity against some diseases to the baby.

Breast-feeding inhibits secretion of gonadotropins by the hypophysis cerebri. Hence the ovarian and menstrual cycles do not occur, and recurrence of pregnancy does not normally take place for about three months.

CONTRACEPTIVES

These are measures that can be used to prevent unwanted pregnancy.

1. Mechanical methods

a. A condom is a baloon-like sheath that can be worn over the penis. Spermatozoa remain within it and do not reach the vagina. This is the simplest method of contraception.
b. A diaphragm can be fitted over the cervix of the uterus. It prevents entry of spermatozoa into the uterus.
c. Insertion of some foreign substance into the uterus can prevent implantation of an ovum. Two devices that are commonly used are (i) loop, and (ii) copper T.
d. A jelly containing some spermicidal chemical can be inserted into the vagina. This is often used in combination with a diaphragm.

2. Operation

a. ***Vasectomy***: Bilateral cutting and ligation of the ductus deferens (vas deferens) prevents spermatozoa from being ejaculated. This is a permanent method of avoiding pregnancy.
b. ***Tubectomy***: The uterine tubes are cut and ligated. This is also a permanent method, but the procedure carries more risk than vasectomy.

3. Hormonal Methods

a. ***Contraceptive pills:***

Ovulation in a woman (and by corollary, pregnancy) can be prevented by administration of contraceptive pills. The most important ingredients of such pills are progestins (in the form of synthetic compounds). Better results are obtained when a small amount of oestrogen is also given.

In the most common variety of pill (distributed by government agencies in India) the progestin is ***norethisterone acetate*** (1 mg); and the oestrogen is in the form of ***oestradiol*** (50μg). The pills are distributed in packets, each packet containing 28 pills out of which 21 pills contain these hormones, and 7 pills do not (for use in the last 7 days). The use of pills is started 5 days after onset of menstruation. They are taken continuously without any break as long as contraception is desired. Normal menstruation occurs during the 7 days in which pills without hormones are being taken. If the pills are taken regularly there is a regular menstrual cycle of 28 days duration.

Presence of progesterone in the pre-ovulatory phase prevents occurrence of ovulation. This is because the progesterone in the pill prevents the secretion of FSH and LH by the pituitary. This inhibits the maturation of follicles, and ovulation.

Stoppage of pills reduces levels of these hormones in blood. It is this withdrawal that leads to menstrual bleeding. Such pills have almost 100 per cent success in suppressing maturation of follicles and ovulation.

b. ***Safe period:***
Conception can be avoided if there is no sexual intercourse for 4 days before ovulation and 3 days after ovulation. However, the so-called ***rhythm method*** has not proved to be successful as the exact day of ovulation cannot be reliably predicted.

SOME DISEASES OF FEMALE REPRODUCTIVE ORGANS

Diseases that can be transmitted to a woman through sexual intercourse have been considered in Chapter 20. Some other conditions are given below.

1. ***Infections*** in the vulva and vagina readily spread to the cervix, the body of the uterus and the uterine tubes. Infection in the uterus is called ***endometritis.*** Inflammation of uterine tubes is called ***salpingitis***. Inflammation can reach the peritoneum through uterine tubes. This leads to peritonitis and pelvic inflammation. Pelvic inflammation can lead to infertility and pelvic pain.
2. The cervix is a common site of ***carcinoma***. Various kinds of growths can occur in the uterus. ***Fibroids*** are growths of uterine muscle. They are often multiple. Various tumours can arise in the ovaries.
3. Endometrial cells can reach tissues outside the uterus and can start growing there forming growths. The condition is called ***endometriosis***. It can be seen in the ovaries and in other pelvic organs.

CHAPTER

22

The Endocrine System

Endocrine tissue is made up essentially of cells that produce secretions that are poured directly into blood. The secretions of endocrine cells are called ***hormones***. Hormones travel through blood to target cells whose functioning they may influence profoundly. A hormone acts on cells that bear specific receptors for it. Some hormones act only on one organ or on one type of cell, while other hormones may have widespread effects. Acting along with the autonomic nervous system, the endocrine organs co-ordinate and control the metabolic activities and the internal environment of the body.

Endocrine cells are distributed in three different ways.

Some organs are entirely endocrine in function. They are referred to as ***endocrine glands*** (or ***ductless glands***). Those traditionally included under this heading are the hypophysis cerebri (or pituitary), the pineal gland, the thyroid gland, the parathyroid glands, and the suprarenal (or adrenal) glands.

Groups of endocrine cells may be present in organs that have other functions. Several examples of such tissue have been described in previous chapters. They include the islets of the pancreas, the interstitial cells of the testes, the kidneys, and the follicles and corpora lutea of ovaries.

HYPOTHALAMUS

The hypothalamus is a part of the brain that controls visceral functions. Some cells in it produce hormones that are also called releasing factors. These factors have a profound influence on activity of the hypophysis cerebri and of other endocrine organs. The production of these factors is influenced by emotional and other impulses reaching the brain. In this way mental stress or other emotions can influence the functions of various systems through the endocrine glands (and through the autonomic nervous system). The releasing factors produced by the hypothalamus are listed below.

Releasing and inhibiting factors produced by the hypothalamus

Abbreviations	*Full name*
GRH or GHRH	Growth hormone releasing hormone
GIH or GHRIH	Growth hormone inhibitory hormone or somatostatin
CRH	Corticotropin releasing hormone
TRH	Thyrotropin releasing hormone
LHRH or GnRH	Luteinizing hormone releasing hormone
PRH	Prolactin releasing hormone
PIH	Prolactin inhibiting hormone

THE HYPOPHYSIS CEREBRI (PITUITARY GLAND)

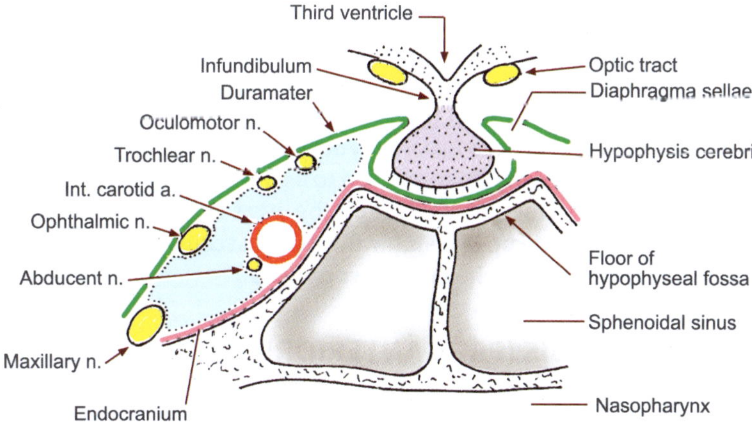

Fig. 22.1 Coronal section through hypophysis cerebri to show some of its relations.

The hypophysis cerebri is also called the ***pituitary gland***. It is suspended from the floor of the third ventricle (of the brain) by a narrow funnel shaped stalk called the ***infundibulum***, and lies in a depression on the upper surface of the sphenoid bone (Fig. 22.1).

The hypophysis cerebri is one of the most important endocrine glands. It produces several hormones some of which profoundly influence the activities of other endocrine tissues. Its own activity is influenced by the hypothalamus, and by the pineal body.

Subdivisions of the Hypophysis Cerebri

The hypophysis cerebri has, in the past, been divided into an anterior part, the ***pars anterior***; an intermediate part, the ***pars intermedia***; and a posterior part

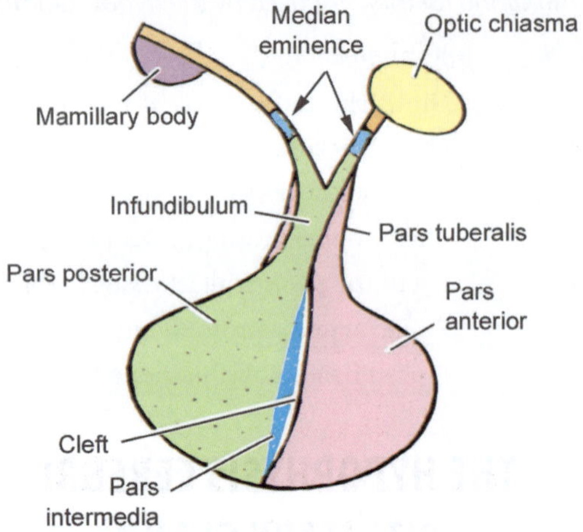

Fig. 22.2 Subdivisions of the hypophysis cerebri.

the ***pars posterior*** (or ***pars nervosa***) (Fig. 22.2). The pars posterior contains numerous nerve fibres. It is directly continuous with the central core of the infundibular stalk that is made up of nervous tissue. The pars posterior and the infundibular stalk are together referred to as the ***neurohypophysis***.

The pars anterior (which is also called the ***pars distalis***), and the pars intermedia, are both made up of cells having a direct secretory function. They are collectively referred to as the ***adenohypophysis***.

ADENOHYPOPHYSIS (PARS ANTERIOR)

The pars anterior is made up of cords of cells separated by fenestrated sinusoids. Several types of cells, responsible for the production of different hormones, are present (Fig. 22.3).

Using routine staining procedures the cells of the pars anterior can be divided into ***chromophil cells*** that have brightly staining granules in their cytoplasm; and ***chromophobe cells*** in which granules are not prominent. Chromophil cells are further classified as ***acidophil*** when their granules stain with acid dyes (like eosin or orange G); or ***basophil*** when the granules stain with basic dyes (like haematoxylin). Basophil granules are also PAS positive. The acidophil cells are often called ***alpha cells***, and the basophils are called ***beta cells***.

Types of Acidophil Cells

1. ***Somatotrophs*** produce the ***somatropic hormone*** (also called ***somatotropin [STH]***, or ***growth hormone [GH]***). This hormone controls body growth, particularly before puberty.

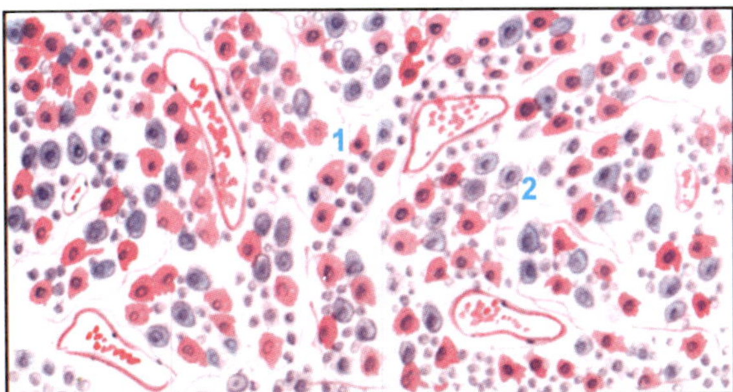

Fig. 22.3 Hypophysis cerebri. Pars anterior. 1-Acidophil. 2-Basophil. Cells in which cytoplasm is not conspicuous are chromophobes.

2. ***Mammotrophs*** (or ***lactotrophs***) produce the ***mammotropic hormone*** (also called ***mammotropin, prolactin (PRL), lactogenic hormone***, or LTH) which stimulates the growth and activity of the female mammary gland during pregnancy and lactation.

Types of Basophil Cells

1. The ***corticotrophs*** (or ***corticotropes***) produce the ***corticotropic hormone*** (also called ***adreno-corticotropin*** or ACTH). This hormone stimulates the secretion of some hormones of the adrenal cortex.
2. ***Thyrotrophs*** (or ***thyrotropes***) produce the ***thyrotropic hormone*** (***thyrotropin*** or TSH) which stimulates the activity of the thyroid gland.
3. ***Gonadotrophs*** (***gonadotropes***, or ***delta basophils***) produce two types of hormones each type having a different action in the male and female.
   a. In the female, the first of these hormones stimulates the growth of ovarian follicles. It is, therefore, called the ***follicle stimulating hormone*** (FSH). It also stimulates the secretion of oestrogens by the ovaries. In the male the same hormone stimulates spermatogenesis.
   b. In the female, the second hormone stimulates the maturation of the corpus luteum, and the secretion by it of progesterone. It is called the ***luteinizing hormone*** (LH). In the male the same hormone stimulates the production of androgens by the interstitial cells of the testes, and is called the ***interstitial cell stimulating hormone*** (ICSH).

Pars Tuberalis

The pars tuberalis consists mainly of undifferentiated cells. Some acidophil and basophil cells are also present.

Pars Intermedia

This is poorly developed in the human hypophysis. In ordinary preparations the most conspicuous feature is the presence of colloid filled vesicles. These vesicles are remnants of the pouch of Rathke. Beta cells, other secretory cells, and chromophobe cells are present. Some cells of the pars intermedia produce the ***melanocyte stimulating hormone*** (MSH) which causes increased pigmentation of the skin. Other cells produce ACTH. The secretion of hormones from the adenohypophysis is under control of the hypothalamus.

Functions of Adenohypophysis

1. The growth hormone, or somatotropic hormone is responsible for physical growth including that of bones and soft tissues. Deficiency leads to dwarfism and excess leads to gigantism.
2. Growth hormone influences protein metabolism by increasing protein synthesis and reducing protein breakdown.
3. Growth hormone increases utilisation of free fatty acids for production of energy.
4. Utilisation of glucose for production of energy is decreased. Growth hormone has an anti-insulin effect.
5. Growth hormone has an anabolic effect. A positive nitrogen balance is produced. Absorption of calcium is increased. Urinary excretion of calcium, sodium and phosphorus is decreased.
6. Prolactin stimulates growth of the breasts during pregnancy. After childbirth it stimulates lactation.
7. Thyroid stimulating hormone (TSH) increases secretion of hormones by the thyroid gland.
8. The adrenocorticotropic hormone (ACTH) stimulates secretion of hormones by the adrenal cortex.
9. The follicle stimulating hormone (FSH) and the luteinizing hormone (LH) control the ovarian and uterine cycles. See chapter 21 for details.
10. The melanocyte stimulating hormone stimulates melanin production by melanocytes.

NEUROHYPOPHYSIS (PARS POSTERIOR)

The pars posterior of the hypophysis is associated with the release into the blood of two hormones. One of these is ***vasopressin*** (also called the ***antidiuretic hormone*** or ADH). This hormone controls reabsorption of water by kidney tubules. The second hormone is oxytocin. It controls the contraction of smooth muscle of the uterus and also of the mammary gland.

It is now known that these two hormones are not produced in the hypophysis cerebri at all. They are synthesized in neurons located in the hypothalamus (Fig. 22.4). They reach the pars posterior of the hypophysis cerebri through axons. (This is called neurosecretion).

Functions of the Neurohypophysis

1. The antidiuretic hormone (ADH) acts on the collecting tubules of the kidneys and increases their permeability to water. It facilitates reabsorption of water and controls the water content of urine. (For details see chapter 19). Deficiency of this hormone leads to diabetes insipidus.
2. ADH causes vasoconstriction. Hence it is also called vasopressin.

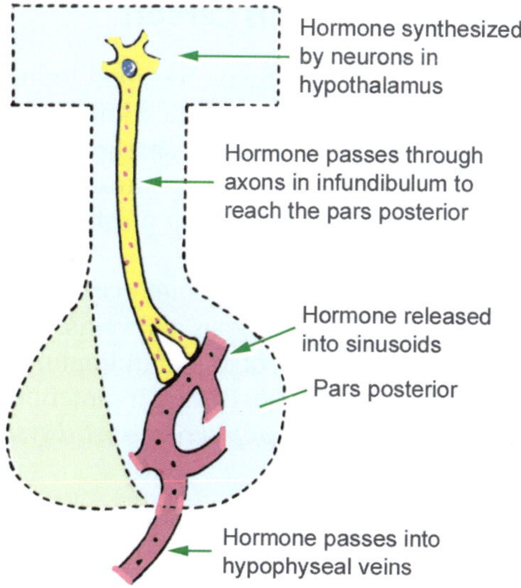

Fig. 22.4 Scheme to show the relationship of the hypothalamus and the pars posterior of the hypophysis cerebri.

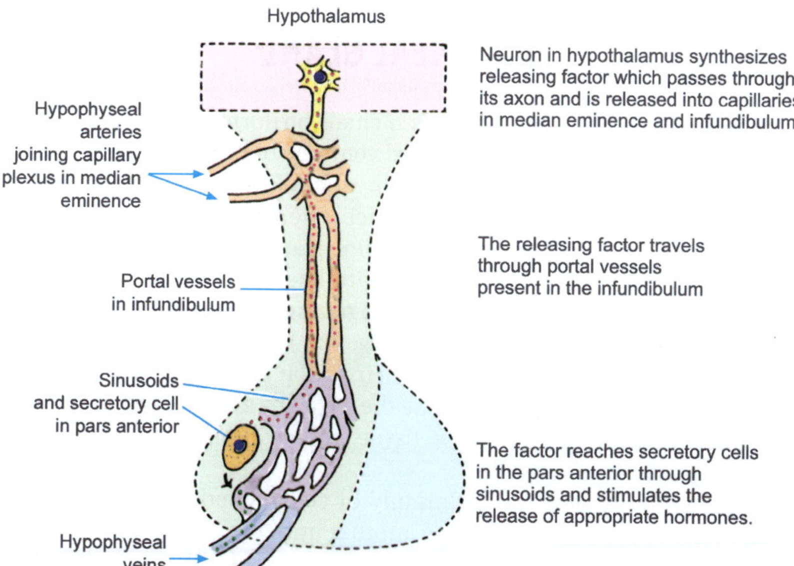

Fig. 22.5 Scheme to show the hypothalamo-hypophyseal portal circulation.

3. Oxytoccin triggers milk ejection from the breast (in a lactating mother) by causing contraction of myoepithelial cells.
4. Oxytoccin produces powerful contractions of uterine muscle at the time of childbirth.

Blood Supply of the Hypophysis Cerebri

The hypophysis cerebri is supplied by many small branches arising from the internal carotid arteries and their ramifications. The branches end in capillary plexuses from which portal vessels arise. These portal vessels descend through the infundibular stalk and end in the sinusoids of the pars anterior. The sinusoids are drained by veins that end in neighbouring venous sinuses (Fig. 22.5).

It will be noticed that the above arrangement is unusual in that two sets of capillaries intervene between the arteries and veins. One of these is in the median eminence and the upper part of the infundibulum. The second set of capillaries is represented by the sinusoids of the pars anterior. This arrangement is referred to as the ***hypothalamo-hypophyseal portal system***.

Control of Secretion of Hormones of the Adenohypophysis

The secretion of hormones by the adenohypophysis takes place under higher control of neurons in the hypothalamus. Different neurons produce specific ***releasing factors.*** These factors are released into the capillaries mentioned above. Portal vessels arising from the capillaries carry these factors to the pars anterior of the hypophysis. Here they stimulate the release of appropriate hormones.

THE PINEAL GLAND

The pineal gland (or pineal body) is a small piriform structure present in relation to the posterior wall of the third ventricle of the brain (Fig. 22.6). It is also called the ***epiphysis cerebri***. The pineal has for long been regarded as a vestigial organ of no functional importance. (Hence the name pineal body). However, it is now known to be an endocrine gland of great importance.

Sections of the pineal gland stained with haematoxylin and eosin reveal very little detail. The organ appears to be a mass of cells amongst which there are blood capillaries and nerve fibres (Fig. 22.7). A distinctive feature of the pineal in such sections is the presence of irregular masses made up mainly of calcium salts. These masses constitute the ***corpora arenacea*** or ***brain sand***. The organ is covered by connective tissue (representing the piamater) from which septa pass into its interior.

The pineal body is made up mainly of cells called ***pinealocytes***. The pinealocytes are separated from one another by neuroglial cells.

The nerve fibres present in the pineal are sympathetic (adrenergic, unmyelinated). Release of pineal secretions appears to require sympathetic stimulation.

The pinealocytes produce a number of hormones. These hormones have an important regulating influence on many other endocrine organs. The organs influenced include the adenohypophysis, the neurohypophysis, the thyroid, the parathyroids, the adrenal cortex and medulla, the gonads, and the pancreatic islets.

The best known hormone of the pineal gland is the amino acid ***melatonin***.

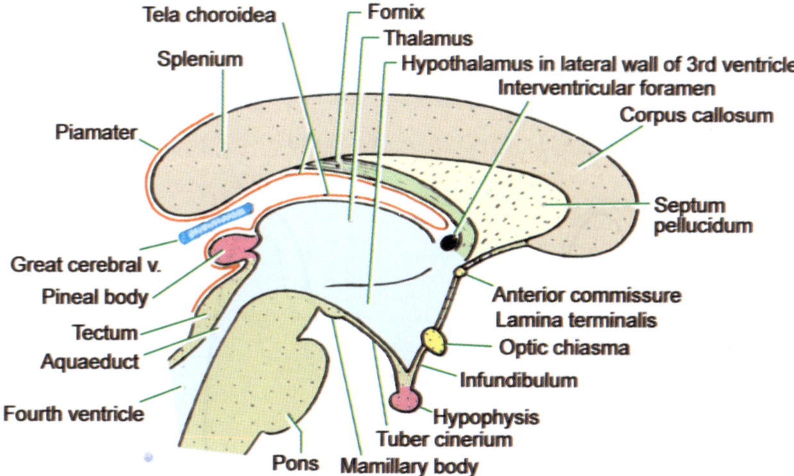

Fig. 22.6 Diagram to show the position of the hypophysis cerebri and of the pineal body relative to the third ventricle of the brain.

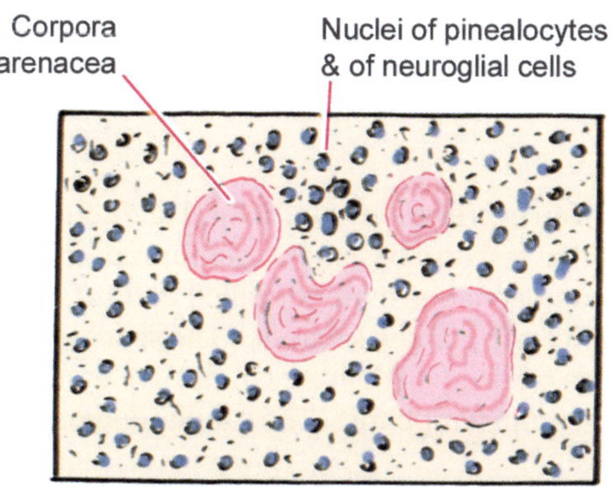

Fig. 22.7 Drawing of a section of the pineal body as seen with a light microscope.

THE THYROID GLAND

The thyroid gland is a very important endocrine organ. It is placed in the front of the neck, anterior to the larynx and trachea (Fig. 22.8).

Elementary Histology

The thyroid gland is covered by a fibrous capsule. Septa extending into the gland from the capsule divide it into lobules. On microscopic examination each

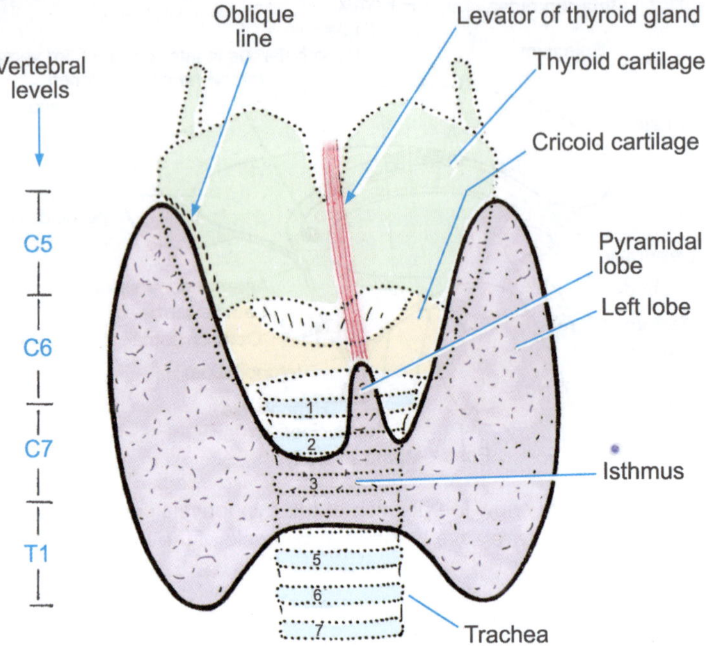

Fig. 22.8 Outline of the thyroid gland as seen from the front, and its relationship to the larynx and trachea.

lobule is made up of an aggregation of ***follicles*** (Fig. 22.9). Each follicle is lined by ***follicular cells***, that rest on a basement membrane. The follicle has a cavity that is filled by a homogeneous material called ***colloid*** (which appears pink in haematoxylin and eosin stained sections). The spaces between the follicles are filled by a stroma made up of delicate connective tissue in which there are numerous capillaries and lymphatics. The capillaries lie in close contact with the walls of follicles.

Apart from follicular cells the thyroid gland contains C-cells (or ***parafollicular cells***) which intervene (here and there) between the follicular cells and the basement membrane. They may also lie in the intervals between the follicles. Connective tissue stroma surrounding the follicles contains a dense capillary plexus, lymphatic capillaries and sympathetic nerves.

The Follicular Cells

1. The follicular cells vary in shape depending on the level of their activity (Fig. 22.10). Normally (at an average level of activity) the cells are cuboidal, and the colloid in the follicles is moderate in amount. When inactive (or resting) the cells are flat (squamous) and the follicles are distended with abundant colloid. Lastly, when the cells are highly active they become columnar and colloid is scanty.

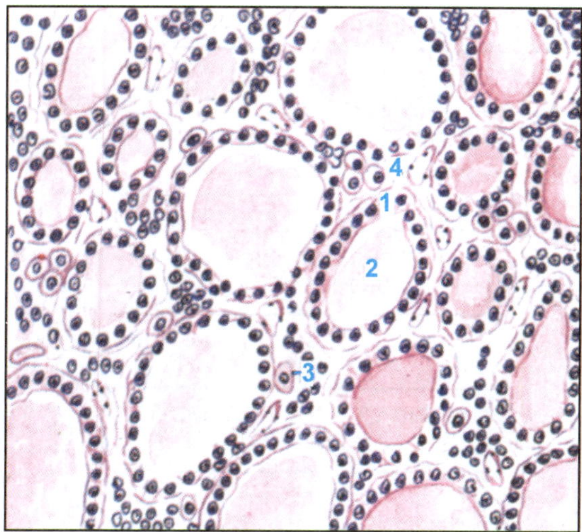

Fig. 22.9 Thyroid gland. 1-Follicle lined by cuboidal epithelium. 2-Colloid. 3-Parafollicular cells. 4-Connective tissue.

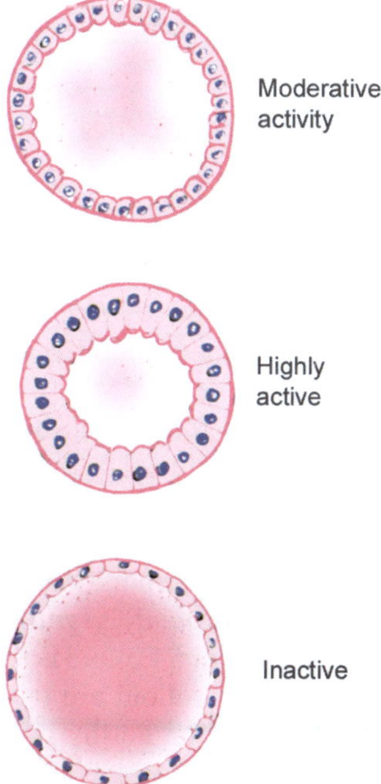

Fig. 22.10 Variations in appearance of thyroid follicles at different levels of activity.

2. The follicular cells secrete two hormones that influence the rate of metabolism. Iodine is an essential constituent of these hormones. One hormone containing three atoms of iodine in each molecule is called

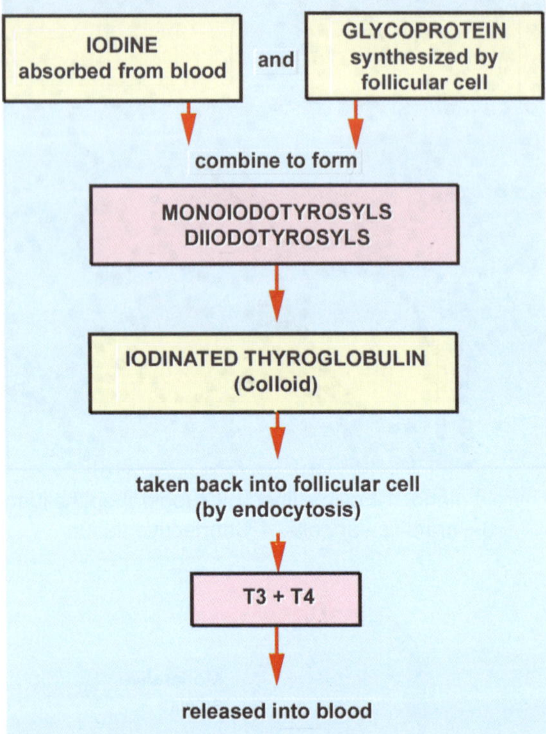

Fig. 22.11 Some steps in the formation of hormones by the thyroid gland.

triiodothyronine or T_3. The second hormone containing four atoms of iodine in each molecule is called tetraiodothyronine, T_4, or thyroxine. T_3 is much more active than T_4 (Fig. 22.11).

3. The activity of follicular cells is influenced by the thyroid stimulating hormone (TSH or thyrotropin) produced by the hypophysis cerebri. There is some evidence to indicate that their activity may also be increased by sympathetic stimulation.
4. The synthesis and release of thyroid hormone takes place in two phases. In the first phase thyroglobulin (a glycoprotein) is synthesized. The thyroglobulin combines with iodine to form colloid. Colloid is iodinated thyroglobulin.

In the second phase particles of colloid are taken back into the cell by endocytosis. Within the cell the iodinated thyroglobulin is acted upon by enzymes releasing hormones T_3 and T_4 which are released into blood.

The C-Cells (Parafollicular Cells)

They are also called ***clear cells***, or ***light cells***. C-cells secrete the hormone ***thyrocalcitonin***. This hormone has an action opposite to that of the parathyroid hormone on calcium metabolism. This hormone comes into play when serum calcium level is high. It tends to lower the calcium level by suppressing release of calcium ions from bone. This is achieved by suppressing bone resorption by osteoclasts.

Functions of the Thyroid Gland

Thyroid hormones have widespread effects all over the body.

1. There is increase in BMR, in heat production, and in oxygen consumption.
2. Thyroid hormones are necessary for normal growth of the body. In the absence of these hormones, fusion of bony epiphyses is delayed. Growth of the skull and eruption of teeth are affected.
   Congenital hypothyroidism leads to cretinism, in which there is mental retardation.
3. The thyroid hormones are necessary for normal functioning of the nervous system. In hypothyroidism memory is impaired, there is increased somnolence, and speech becomes slow. In hyperthyroidism the person becomes hyper-excitable and restless. There is insomnia.
4. Excess of thyroid hormone causes tacchycardia, increased cardiac output and vasodilatation.
5. Carbohydrate metabolism as activated. There is increased absorption of carbohydrates. Intake of glucose by cells is accelerated, there is increased glucolysis, increased gluconeogenesis, and insulin secretion.
6. Fat metabolism is stimulated. Free fatty acid concentration and utilisation are accelerated (for energy production).
7. Thyroid hormone has an anabolic effect, and protein synthesis is increased. However, in hyperthyroidism there is increased catabolism and negative nitrogen balance. There is muscle weakness.
8. Thyroid hormone leads to increased secretion of intestinal juice, and absorption of food. In hyperthyroidism there is diarrhoea. In hypothyroidism there is constipation.
9. Thyroid hormones are necessary for normal ovarian cycles and lactation.

Features of hyperthyroidism and hypothyroidism

Hyperthyroidism	**Hypothyroidism**
Increased BMR	Low BMR
Tacchycardia	Slow heart rate
Excessive sweating	
Loss of weight	Obesity
Increased appetite	Decreased appetite
Muscular weakness	Muscular weakness
Insomnia	Somnolence
Hyper-excitability	Mental sluggishness

Hypothyroidism in adults leads to ***Myxoedema***. In congenital thyroid deficiency there is ***cretinism***.

Goitre

Adequate intake of iodine is required for normal thyroid function. In iodine deficiency there is enlargement of the thyroid gland. This is called ***goitre***.

THE PARATHYROID GLANDS

The parathyroid glands are so called because they lie in close relationship to the thyroid gland (Fig. 22.12). Normally, there are two parathyroid glands, one superior and one inferior, on either side; there being four glands in all.

Each gland has a connective tissue capsule from which some septa extend into the gland substance. Within the gland a network of reticular fibres supports the cells. Many fat cells (adipocytes) are present in the stroma.

The parenchyma of the gland is made up of cells that are arranged in cords. Numerous sinusoids lie in close relationship to the cells.

The cells of the parathyroid glands are of two main types: ***chief cells*** (or ***principal cells***), and ***oxyphil cells*** (or ***eosinophil cells***) (Fig. 22.13). The chief cells are much more numerous than the oxyphil cells. The latter are absent in the young and appear a little before the age of puberty.

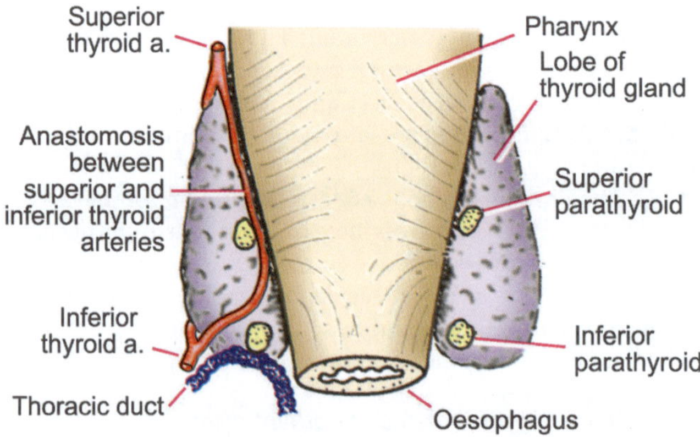

Fig. 22.12 Thyroid and parathyroid glands seen from behind.

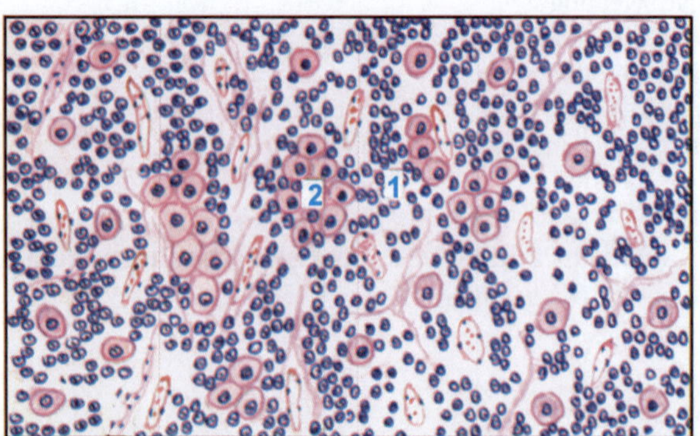

Fig. 22.13 Parathyroid gland. 1-Chief cells (only nuclei seen). 2-Oxyphil cells with pink cytoplasm. Note numerous capillaries.

The chief cells produce the parathyroid hormone (or parathormone). This hormone tends to increase the level of serum calcium by:

a. increasing bone resorption through stimulation of osteoclastic activity;
b. increasing calcium resorption from renal tubules (and inhibiting phosphate resorption);
c. enhancing calcium absorption from the gut.

HORMONES CONTROLLING CALCIUM METABOLISM

Calcium Metabolism

The human body contains about 1kg of calcium. Of this 99% is deposited in the skeleton and one per cent is in tissues. In plasma calcium is in the form of free ions, in combination with proteins, or in combination with bicarbonate and citrate. Calcium is obtained chiefly from milk. It is absorbed mainly in the duodenum.

Calcium in bones and in tissue fluid is readily exchangeable. Plasma calcium level is controlled within narrow limits. The level plays an important role in the following.

a. proper bone mineralisation.
b. maintaining cell membrane integrity.
c. control of neuromuscular excitability.
d. control of cardiac excitability.
e. blood coagulation.

Plasma calcium level is controlled by three hormones. These are:

1. Parathyroid hormone (PTH).
2. Calcitonin (produced by parafollicular cells of the thyroid gland).
3. Cholecalciferol (vitamin D).

Role of Vitamin D

Vitamin is obtained from diet. It is also produced by the action of sunlight on skin. Ultraviolet rays act on 7-dehydrocholesterol and convert it into vitamin D. In the liver vitamin D_3 is converted to 25-OH-cholecalciferol. Enzymes in the kidney convert this to 1,25(OH_2)-cholecalciferol (also written as 1,25(OH_2)-D_3. This is the active metabolite of vitamin D_3. This active form is often regarded as a hormone.

The effects of 1,25(OH_2)-D_3 are as follows.

1. It increases absorption of calcium from diet by increasing available calcium binding protein.
2. It increases reabsorption of calcium from distal convoluted tubules.
3. It helps parathormone to remove calcium from bone.

Role of Parathyroid Hormone (Parathormone)

1. Parathormone maintains the level of plasma calcium. When necessary it increases plasma calcium level by removing calcium from bone.
2. Existing osteoclasts are activated, and new ones are formed.
3. Reabsorption of calcium from distal convoluted tubules is increased.
4. Reabsorption of phosphorus by proximal convoluted tubules is decreased..

Role of Calcitonin

Calcitonin promotes deposition of calcium in bones. In other words it has an action opposite to that of parathormone. Secretion of calcitonin is stimulated by increased plasma calcium level. However, the main control of plasma calcium level is through parathormone which can maintain correct levels even in the absence of calcitonin.

THE SUPRARENAL (ADRENAL) GLANDS

As implied by their name the right and left suprarenal glands lie in the abdomen, close to the upper poles of the corresponding kidneys. In many animals they do not occupy a 'supra' renal position, but lie near the kidneys (Fig. 22.14). They are, therefore, commonly called the ***adrenal glands***.

The suprarenal gland is covered by a connective tissue capsule. Septa extend into the gland substance from the capsule. The gland is made up of two functionally distinct parts: a superficial part called the ***cortex***, and a deeper part called the ***medulla***. The volume of the cortex is about ten times that of the medulla (Fig. 22.15).

The Suprarenal Cortex

Layers of the Cortex

The suprarenal cortex is made up of cells arranged in cords. Sinusoids intervene between the cords. On the basis of the arrangement of its cells the cortex can be divided into three layers as follows.

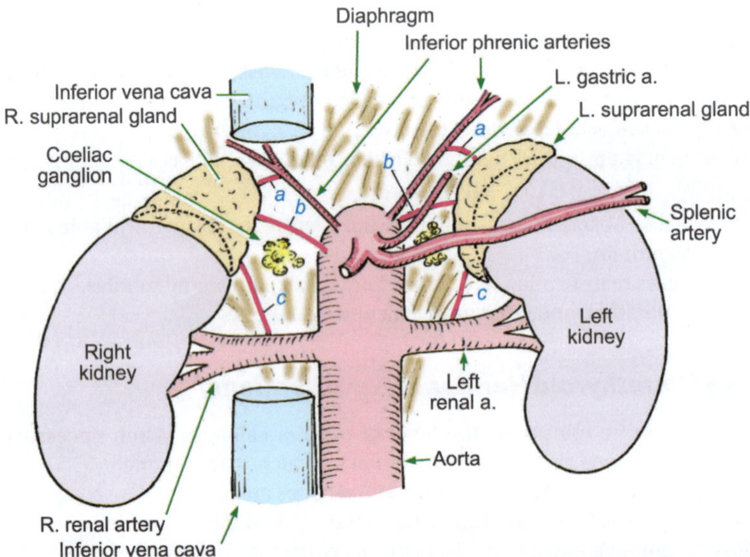

Fig. 22.14 Suprarenal glands and some related structures as seen from the front. a, b and c = superior, middle and inferior arteries to the suprarenal glands.

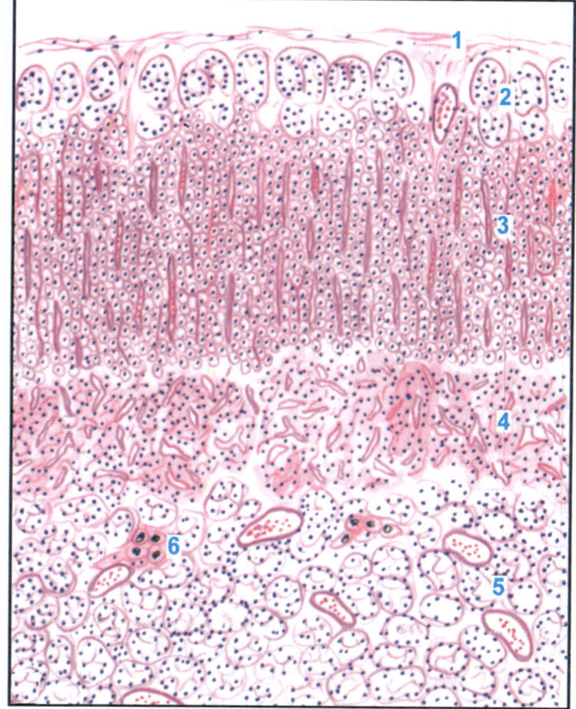

Fig. 22.15 Suprarenal gland. Upper 2/3 is cortex, lower 1/3 is medulla. 1-Capsule. 2-Zona glomerulosa. 3-Zona fasciculata. 4-Zona reticularis. 5-Medulla. 6-Sympathetic neurons.

a. The outermost layer is called the ***zona glomerulosa***. Here the cells are arranged as inverted U-shaped formations, or acinus-like groups. The zona glomerulosa constitutes the outer one-fifth of the cortex.
b. The next zone is called the ***zona fasciculata***. Here the cells are arranged in straight columns, two cell thick. Sinusoids intervene between the columns. This layer forms the middle three fifths of the cortex.
c. The innermost layer of the cortex (inner one fifth) is called the ***zona reticularis***. It is so called because it is made up of cords that branch and anastomose with each other to form a kind of reticulum.

Hormones Produced by the Suprarenal Cortex

All the hormones produced in the suprarenal cortex are corticosteroids. These are of three types.

Glucocorticoids:	Cortisol (Dihydrocortisone), Corticosterone (Cortisone).
Mineralo-corticoids:	Aldosterone, Deoxycorticosterone.
Sex hormones:	Dehydroepiandrosterone.

a. The cells of the zona glomerulosa produce the mineralocorticoid hormones ***aldosterone*** and ***deoxycorticosterone***. These hormones influence the electrolyte and water balance of the body. The secretion of aldosterone is influenced by renin secreted by juxta-glomerular cells of the kidney. The secretion of hormones by the zona glomerulosa appears to be largely independent of the hypophysis cerebri.
b. The cells of the zona fasciculata produce the glucocorticoids ***cortisone*** and ***cortisol*** (***dihydrocortisone***). Secretion of glucocorticoids is increased by the action of ACTH. These hormones have widespread effects including those on carbohydrate metabolism and protein metabolism. They appear to decrease antibody responses and have an anti-inflammatory effect.
c. The cells of the zona reticularis also produce some glucocorticoids; and sex hormones, both oestrogens and androgens.

The suprarenal cortex is essential for life. Removal or destruction leads to death unless the hormones produced by it are supplied artificially. Increase in secretion of corticosteroids causes dramatic reduction in number of lymphocytes.

Functions of Glucocorticoids

1. Gluconeogenesis is stimulated.
2. Utilisation of glucose is decreased. This is an anti-insulin or diabetogenic effect.
3. Protein synthesis is inhibited, and breakdown is increased.
4. Utilisation of fats for energy production is increased.
5. They help in dealing with stress. In stressful states ACTH is released and causes increased secretion of cortisol.
6. They cause vasoconstriction and maintain blood pressure.
7. Glucocorticoids are required for maintaining normal glomerular filtration rate.
8. Circulating oesinophils and basophils decrease. The production of lymphocytes is inhibited.
9. Glucocorticoids have an anti-inflammatory and anti-allergic effect. They prevent release of histamine.

Function of Mineralocorticoids (Aldosterone)

1. Renal tubular reabsorption of sodium ions and secretion of potassium ions is increased.
2. They also have similar action on salivary glands, sweat glands and gastric glands.
3. They control serum potassium levels.

Functions of Dehydroepiandrosterone

It is a weak androgen. In fetal life it is needed as a precursor for progesterone production. In the adult female it increases muscle mass, and growth of axillary and pubic hair. It produces libido (sex urge) in the female.

THE SUPRARENAL MEDULLA

Functionally the medulla of the suprarenal (or adrenal) gland is distinct from the cortex. The medulla is made up of groups or columns of cells. The cell groups or columns are separated by wide sinusoids. Functionally, the cells of the suprarenal medulla are regarded as modified postganglionic sympathetic neurons. Like typical postganglionic sympathetic neurons they secrete noradrenalin (norepinephrine) and adrenalin (epinephrine) into the blood. This secretion takes place mainly at times of stress (fear, anger) and results in widespread effects similar to those of stimulation of the sympathetic nervous system (e.g., increase in heart rate and blood pressure).

The secretions of the adrenal medulla are chemically catecholamines. In addition to norepinephrine and epinephrine the medulla secretes dopamine.

Functions of Epinephrine and Norepinephrine

1. The hormones are secreted whenever there is stimulation of sympathetic nerves. They add to the effect of sympathetic stimulation. There is increase in blood pressure, and increased blood flow through muscles.
2. Blood glucose level is increased through (a) secretion of glucagon, (b) glycogenolysis in the liver and in skeletal muscle.
3. They cause lipolysis (breakdown of fats) and free fatty acids are released.
4. Along with thyroxine and glucocorticoids catecholamines have a calorigenic effect (i.e., they cause heat production).
5. There is increased mental alertness (by action on the reticular activating system of the brain).

PANCREATIC ISLETS

The pancreas has been described in Chapter 17. The endocrine part of the pancreas is in the form of numerous rounded collections of cells that are embedded within the exocrine part of the gland. These collections of cells are called the ***pancreatic islets***, or the ***islets of Langerhans*** (Fig. 17.18). The human pancreas has about one million islets. They are most numerous in the tail of the pancreas.

a. The ***alpha cells*** (or ***A-cells***) secrete the hormone ***glucagon***. They form about 20% of the islet cells.
b. The ***beta cells*** (or ***B-cells***) secrete the hormone ***insulin***. About 70% of the cells are of this type.
c. The ***delta cells*** (or ***D-cells***) probably produce the hormones ***gastrin*** and ***somatostatin***. Somatostatin inhibits the secretion of glucagon by alpha cells, and (to a lesser extent) that of insulin by beta cells. It also inhibits actions of secretin and gastrin.

Actions of Insulin

1. Insulin reduces plasma glucose level by (a) increasing glucose uptake by tissues and (b) by reducing production of glucose and its release into the circulation.
2. In the liver, there is increased storage of glycogen, and reduced glucose release into blood.
3. In skeletal muscle insulin promotes greater use of glucose for energy production, and increases storage as glycogen.

4. Insulin reduces release of free fatty acids from adipose tissue. At the same time conversion of fatty acids into triglycerides, and their storage in adipose tissue is increased.
5. Insulin promotes storage of protein. Transport of amino acids into tissues is increased. Their utilisation for synthesis of proteins is also increased.
6. Breakdown of proteins by gluconeogenesis is reduced.
7. Insulin has an important anabolic action. It is essential for normal growth.

Actions of Glucagon

1. Glucagon increases blood sugar level. It causes glycogenolysis in the liver (but not in skeletal muscle). It also increases gluconeogenesis.
2. Glucagon promotes lipolysis.

Secretion of glucagon is stimulated when there is fall in blood glucose level. Hyperglycaemia has the opposite effect.

CLINICAL CORRELATIONS OF ENDOCRINE ORGANS

HYPOPHYSIS CEREBRI

Various types of tumours may arise in this organ. The effects of the tumour (adenoma) may be caused by pressure on surrounding structures, or by increased or decreased production of hormones.

An adenoma arising from chromophobe cells can become quite large and can produce pressure effects as follows.

a. Pressure on the walls of the hypophyseal fossa (sella turcica) leads to its enlargement, and this enlargement can be seen in a skiagram.
b. The enlarging tumour presses on and destroys other cells (acidophils, basophils) of the pars anterior, and gives rise to deficiency of the hormones produced by them. Pressure on the pars posterior can lead to diabetes insipidus.
c. Pressure on the optic chiasma can lead to loss of vision in the temporal halves of vision in both eyes (***bitemporal hemianopia***). Stretching of the optic nerves can lead to optic atrophy.
d. Pressure on the hypothalamus can interfere with various visceral functions. It can lead to ***Frohlich's syndrome*** which is characterized by obesity, poor development of sex organs including the gonads, and altered secondary sex characters.
e. Pressure on the third ventricle, can result in obstruction to flow of CSF, and raised intracranial tension.

In an ***eosinophil adenoma*** pressure effects are negligible. The main effects arise from excessive production of growth hormone. In a young individual (before the epiphyses have fused) the condition results in excessive growth (***gigantism***). If the adenoma is formed after the epiphyses have fused overgrowth mainly affects the head, the hands and the feet (***acromegaly***). The scalp, lips, tongue and face become thick because of increased amount of subcutaneous tissue, and the same happens to the hands and feet. The paranasal sinuses enlarge making the facial region prominent. There is overgrowth of hair, and the man's appearance tends to resemble that of an ape.

In a ***basophil adenoma*** there is excessive secretion of adrenotropic hormones. It leads to ***Cushings's syndrome*** which can also be caused by a tumour of the adrenal cortex. The syndrome is seen mostly in females. Abnormal deposition of fat takes place over the face, neck and trunk. The limbs remain thin and weak.

The posterior lobe of the hypophysis cerebri produces antidiuretic hormone (ADH) which is responsible for reabsorption of water from renal tubules. Destruction of the posterior lobe (e.g., by pressure from an adenoma) can result in ***diabetes insipidus***. In this condition large amounts of urine are passed (***polyuria***). The urine is of very low specific gravity and contains no sugar or albumin. The resultant dehydration leads to excessive thirst (***polydipsia***) and to dryness of skin.

THYROID GLAND

1. Thyroid tissue may develop at an abnormal site. Thyroid tissue present under the mucosa of the dorsum of the tongue is called a ***lingual thyroid***.
2. ***Ectopic thyroid tissue*** may be present in the larynx, the trachea, the oesophagus, the pleura or pericardium, and the ovaries.
3. Deficient intake of iodine (common in areas where drinking water does not contain iodine) can lead to benign enlargement of the thyroid gland. The enlarged thyroid is referred to as ***goitre***. The symptoms are those of hypothyroidism.
4. Hypothyroidism in infants leads to ***cretinism***. A child with cretinism has a puffed face with a protruding tongue, a bulky belly, and sometimes an umbilical hernia.
5. Hypothyroidism in adults is manifested by symptoms including a slow pulse, cold intolerance, mental and physical lethargy, and a hoarse voice. In advanced cases the condition is called ***myxoedema***. There is deposition of mucopolysaccharides in subcutaneous tissue at various sites resulting in a non-pitting oedema. The face is bloated, the lips are thick and protuberant and the expression is dull.
6. ***Hyperthyroidism*** is also referred to as ***thyrotoxicosis***, or ***toxic goitre***. The condition is much more common in women than in men. The condition is marked by nervousness, loss of weight, tachycardia and palpitation, excitability, tremors of the outstretched hands, and exophthalmos.
7. Tumours of the thyroid may be benign or malignant.
8. An operation for removal of the thyroid gland is called ***thyroidectomy***. This may be required in some cases of hyperthyroidism.
9. Inflammation of the thyroid gland is called ***thyroiditis***. It can be caused by infection or by various other causes. One variety of thyroiditis is caused by an autoimmune process (***autoimmune or lymphatic thyroiditis***). It is also called ***Hashimoto's disease***. The thyroid gland is enlarged and is infiltrated with lymphocytes.

PARATHYROID GLANDS

Hyperparathyroidism

Excessive amounts of circulating parathormone can be present in tumours of the parathyroid gland (parathyroid adenoma). As a result calcium is depleted from bones which become weak (and can fracture). Increased urinary excretion of calcium may lead to formation of urinary calculi.

Hypoparathyroidism

Calcium levels in blood fall leading to muscular irritability and convulsions. The condition may be spontaneous or may occur following accidental removal of parathyroid glands during thyroidectomy.

PANCREAS

1. The beta cells of pancreatic islets produce insulin, deficiency of which causes ***diabetes mellitus***.
2. Inflammation of the pancreas is called ***pancreatitis***.
3. ***Tumours***: Carcinoma of the pancreas is relatively common. It can lead to biliary obstruction and jaundice. It can also cause obstruction at the pylorus or duodenum, and ascites by pressure on the portal vein.

Tumours arising from beta cells of pancreatic islets (***beta cell tumours*** or ***insulinoma***) can produce features of hyperinsulinism.

A gastrin producing cell tumour can be responsible for repeated formation of peptic ulcers (***Zollinger Ellison syndrome***).

SUPRARENAL GLANDS

1. Adrenal cortical tissue may be present at various abnormal sites.
2. Congenital hyperplasia (over-development) of the cortex in the males leads to the ***adrenogenital syndrome*** marked by very early development of secondary sexual characters. In the female it may cause enlargement of the clitoris and the child may be mistaken for a male (***pseudo-hermaphroditism***).
3. After puberty hyperplasia of the adrenal cortex, or a cortical tumour, leads to ***Cushing's syndrome***. In this syndrome, seen mostly in females, there is abnormal deposit of fat in the face, neck and trunk but the limbs remain thin and weak.
4. Chronic deficiency of cortical hormones leads to ***Addison's disease***.
5. Tumours in the adrenal may arise from sympathetic nervous tissue (***neuroblastoma***) or from chromaffin cells (***phaeochromocytoma***).

CHAPTER

23

The Nervous System

A brief introduction to the nervous system has been given in Chapter 3. The nervous system is made up of nervous tissue, and this has been described in Chapter 10. These sections must be read before studying this chapter.

CRANIAL CAVITY AND VERTEBRAL CANAL

The skull is divisible into a large upper and posterior part, the ***cranial cavity***, and the ***facial skeleton*** forming the anterior and inferior part.

The cranial cavity is occupied by the brain, which is surrounded by three membranes (meninges) called the ***duramater*** (outermost), the ***arachnoidmater*** and the ***piamater*** (innermost). Between the arachnoidmater and the piamater there is the ***subarachnoid space,*** which is filled by ***cerebrospinal fluid*** (usually abbreviated to CSF). In addition to the brain, meninges, and CSF, the cranial cavity contains twelve pairs of cranial nerves that emerge from the brain and leave the cranial cavity through foramina in its walls. The cranial cavity also contains arteries that enter it from the neck to supply the brain and meninges. Venous blood drains into a series of ***intracranial venous sinuses***.

The roof and lateral walls of the cranial cavity are formed by the vault of the skull. The skin and other soft tissues that cover the vault of the skull constitute the ***scalp***. The floor of the cranial cavity is in the form of three large depressions. These are the ***anterior, middle and posterior cranial fossae*** (Fig. 23.1). Apart from the brain the cranial cavity contains two important endocrine glands. These are the hypophysis cerebri and the pineal gland.

Inferiorly, the cranial cavity has a large opening the ***foramen magnum***, through which it communicates with the ***vertebral canal***. The vertebral canal contains the spinal cord that is continuous with the lower end of the brain. Like the brain the spinal cord is surrounded by duramater, arachnoidmater and piamater. The subarachnoid space and CSF extend into it. The vertebral canal also contains blood vessels and roots of a series of spinal nerves that emerge from the spinal cord. The vertebral canal descends through the length of the

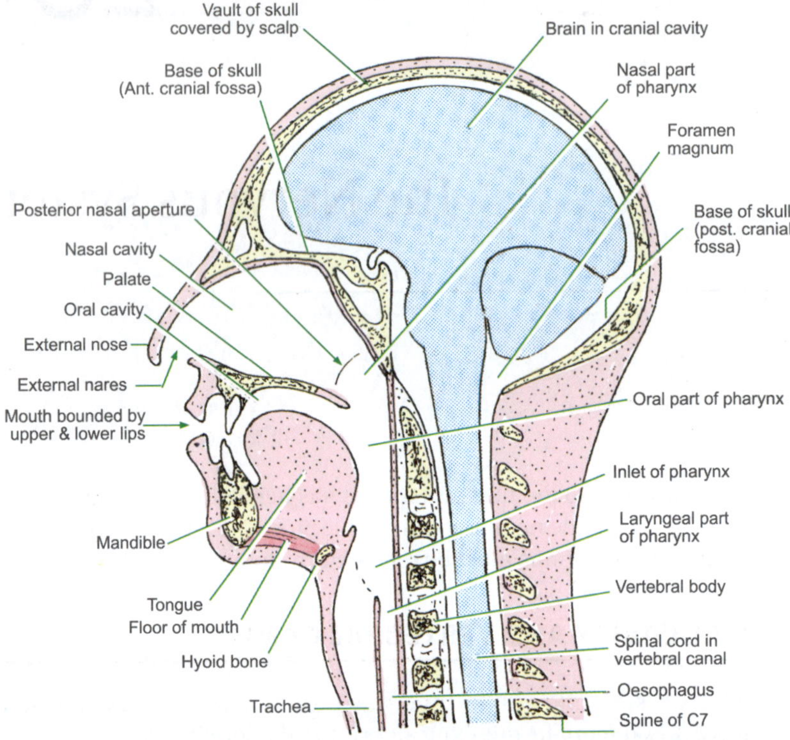

Fig. 23.1 Highly simplified presentation of some structures to be seen in a median section through the head and neck.

vertebral column and reaches up to the sacrum. However, the spinal cord extends only up to the lower border of the first lumbar vertebra.

THE SPINAL CORD

The spinal cord is the most important content of the vertebral canal. The upper end of the spinal cord becomes continuous with the medulla oblongata at the level of the upper border of the first cervical vertebra. (This means that it is the medulla oblongata that passes through the foramen magnum, not the spinal cord). The lower end of the spinal cord generally lies at the level of the lower border of the first lumbar vertebra (Fig. 23.2).

The lowest part of the spinal cord is conical and is called the ***conus medullaris***. The conus is continuous with a filamentous structure called the ***filum terminale***.

When seen in transverse section the grey matter of the spinal cord forms an H-shaped mass (Fig. 23.3). In each half of the cord the grey matter is divisible into a larger ventral mass, the ***anterior (or ventral) grey column***, and a narrow elongated ***posterior (or dorsal) grey column***. (The anterior and posterior grey columns are frequently miscalled the anterior and posterior ***horns***). In some parts of the spinal cord a small lateral projection of grey matter is seen between the ventral and dorsal grey columns. This is the ***lateral grey column***. The grey matter of the right and left halves of the spinal cord is connected across the middle line by the ***grey commissure***, that is traversed by the ***central canal***.

The white matter of the spinal cord is divided into right and left halves, in front by a deep ***anterior median fissure***, and behind by the ***posterior median septum***. In each half of the cord the white matter medial to the dorsal grey column forms the ***posterior funiculus*** (or ***posterior white column***). The white matter medial and ventral to the anterior grey column forms the ***anterior funiculus*** (or ***anterior white column***), while the white matter lateral to the anterior and posterior grey columns forms the ***lateral funiculus***.

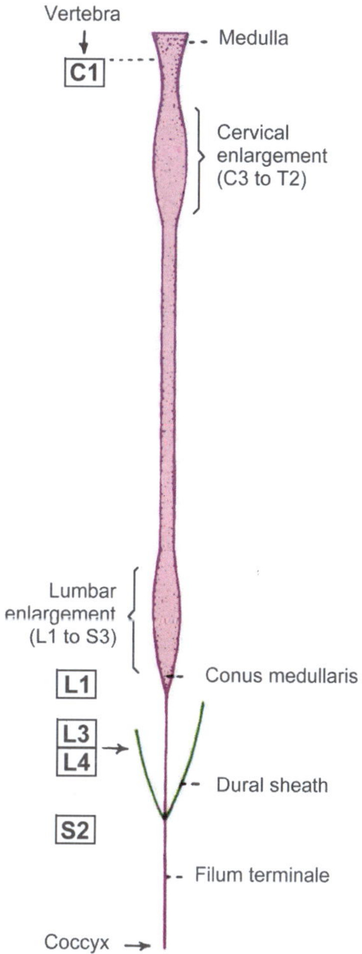

Fig. 23.2 Diagram showing some features of the spinal cord.

SPINAL NERVES AND SPINAL SEGMENTS

The spinal cord gives attachment, on either side, to a series of spinal nerves. Each spinal nerve arises by two roots, anterior (or ventral) and posterior (or dorsal) (Fig. 23.3). Each root is formed by aggregation of a number of rootlets that arise from the cord over a certain length (Fig. 23.4). The length of the spinal cord giving origin to the rootlets of one spinal nerve constitutes one ***spinal segment***. The spinal cord is made up of thirty one segments: 8 cervical, 12 thoracic, 5 lumbar, 5 sacral and one coccygeal. [Note that in the cervical and coccygeal regions the number of spinal segments, and of spinal nerves, does not correspond to the number of vertebrae].

The rootlets that make up the dorsal nerve roots are attached to the surface of the spinal cord along a vertical groove (called the posterolateral sulcus) opposite the tip of the posterior grey column (Fig. 23.3). The rootlets of the ventral nerve roots are attached to the anterolateral aspect of the cord opposite the anterior grey column. The ventral and dorsal nerve roots join each other to form a spinal nerve. Just proximal to its junction with the ventral root, the

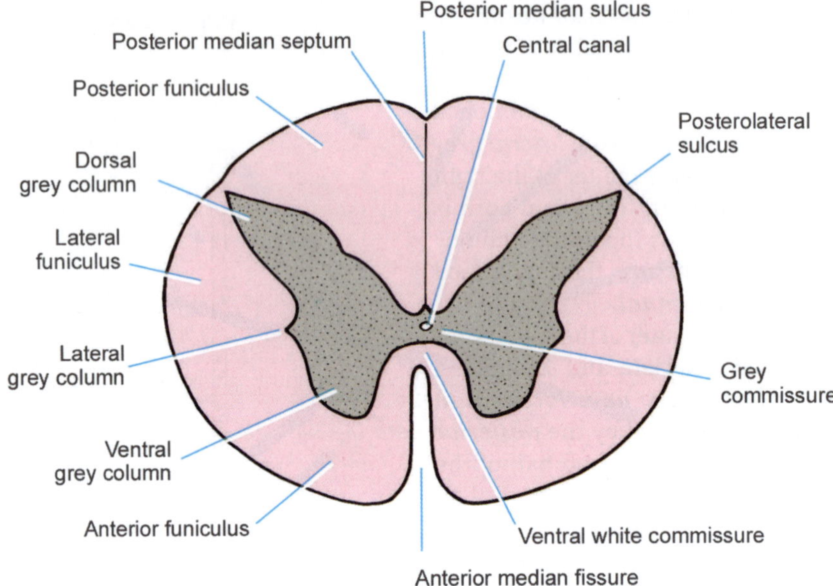

Fig. 23.3 Main features to be seen in a transverse section through the spinal cord.

dorsal root is marked by a swelling called the ***dorsal nerve root ganglion***, or ***spinal ganglion*** (Fig. 23.5).

The spinal cord is not of uniform thickness. The spinal segments that contribute to the nerves of the upper limbs are enlarged to form the ***cervical enlargement*** of the cord. Similarly, the segments innervating the lower limbs form the ***lumbar enlargement*** (Fig. 23.2).

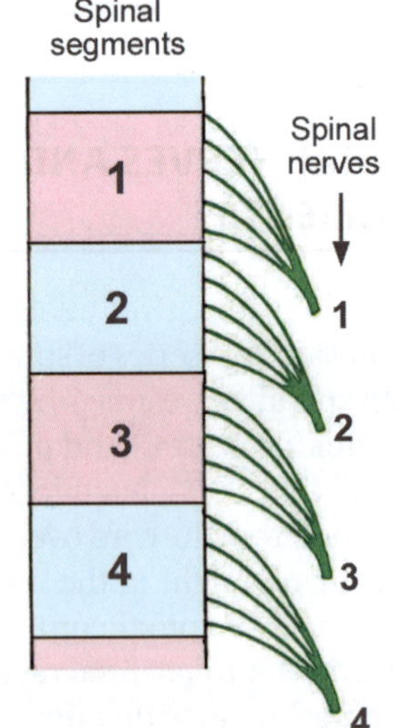

Fig. 23.4 Scheme to illustrate the concept of spinal segments.

Blood Supply of the Spinal Cord

The spinal cord receives its blood supply from three longitudinal arterial channels that extend along the length of the spinal cord (Fig. 23.6). The ***anterior spinal artery*** is present in relation to the anterior median fissure. Two ***posterior spinal arteries*** (one on each side) run along the posterolateral sulcus (i.e., along the line of attachment of the dorsal nerve roots). In addition to these channels the pia mater covering the spinal cord has an arterial plexus (called the ***arterial vasocorona***) which also sends branches into the substance of the cord.

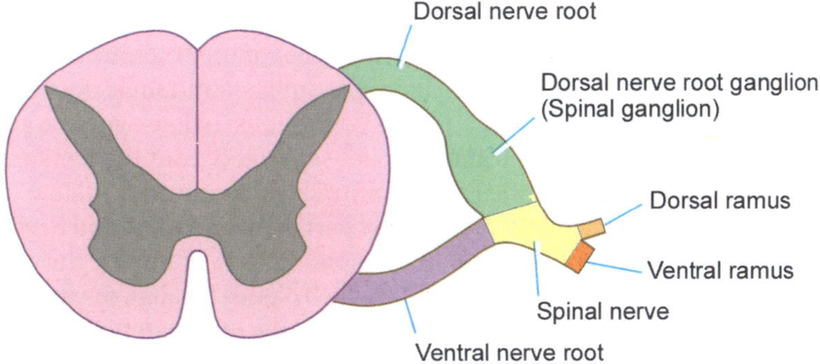

Fig. 23.5 Relationship of a spinal nerve to the spinal cord.

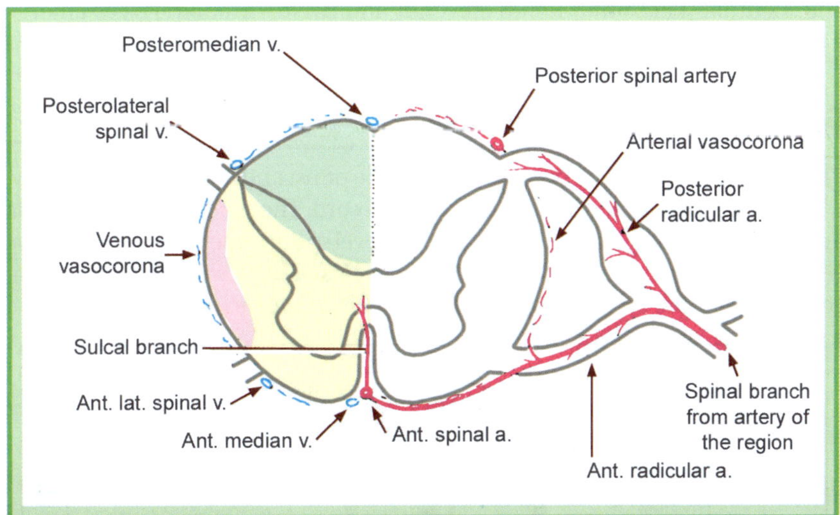

Fig. 23.6 Blood vessels supplying the spinal cord. In the left half of the figure, the area shaded green is supplied by the posterior spinal artery; the areas shaded pink is supplied by the arterial vasocorona; and the area shaded yellow is supplied by the anterior spinal artery.

The veins draining the spinal cord are arranged in the form of six longitudinal channels. These are ***anteromedian*** and ***posteromedian*** channels that lie in the midline; and ***anterolateral*** and ***posterolateral*** channels that are paired (Fig. 23.6). These channels are connected to one another by a plexus of veins that form a ***venous vasocorona.*** The blood from these veins is drained into radicular veins that open into a venous plexus lying between the dura mater and the bony vertebral canal (***epidural*** or ***internal vertebral venous plexus***) and through it into various segmental veins.

GROSS ANATOMY OF THE BRAINSTEM

The brainstem consists (from above downwards) of the midbrain, the pons and the medulla (Figs. 23.7, 23.8). The midbrain is continuous, above, with the cerebral hemispheres. The medulla is continuous, below, with the spinal cord. Posteriorly, the pons and medulla are separated from the cerebellum by the fourth ventricle (Fig. 23.9). The ventricle is continuous, below, with the central canal, which traverses the lower part of the medulla, and becomes continuous with the central canal of the spinal cord. Cranially, the fourth ventricle is continuous with the aqueduct, which passes through the midbrain. The midbrain, pons and medulla are connected to the cerebellum by the superior, middle and inferior cerebellar peduncles respectively.

A number of cranial nerves are attached to the brainstem. The third and fourth nerves emerge from the surface of the midbrain; and the fifth from the pons. The sixth, seventh and eighth nerves emerge at the junction of the pons and medulla. The ninth, tenth, eleventh and twelfth cranial nerves emerge from the surface of the medulla.

Gross Anatomy of the Medulla

The medulla is broad above, where it joins the pons; and narrows down below, where it becomes continuous with the spinal cord. The junction of the medulla and cord is usually described as lying at the level of the upper border of the atlas vertebra. The medulla is divided into a lower ***closed part***, which surrounds the central canal; and an upper ***open part***, which is related to the lower part of the

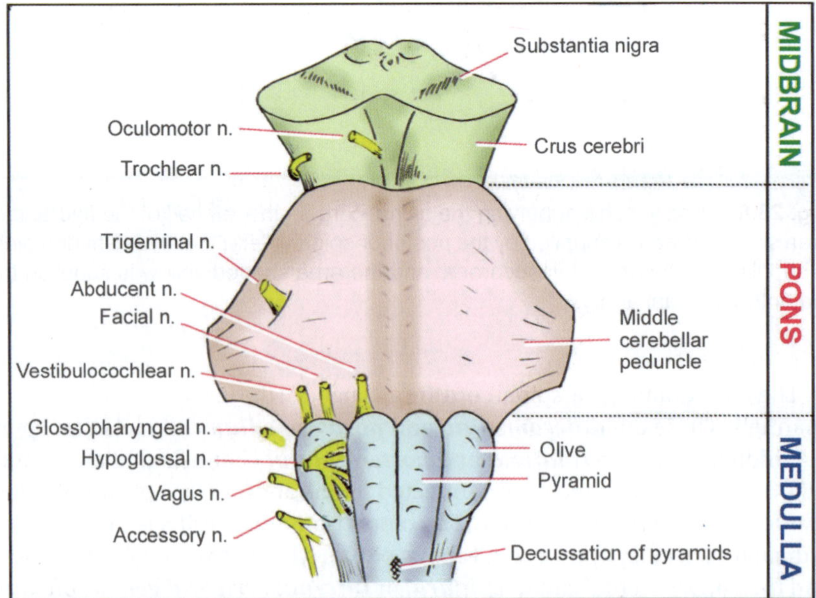

Fig. 23.7 Ventral aspect of the brainstem.

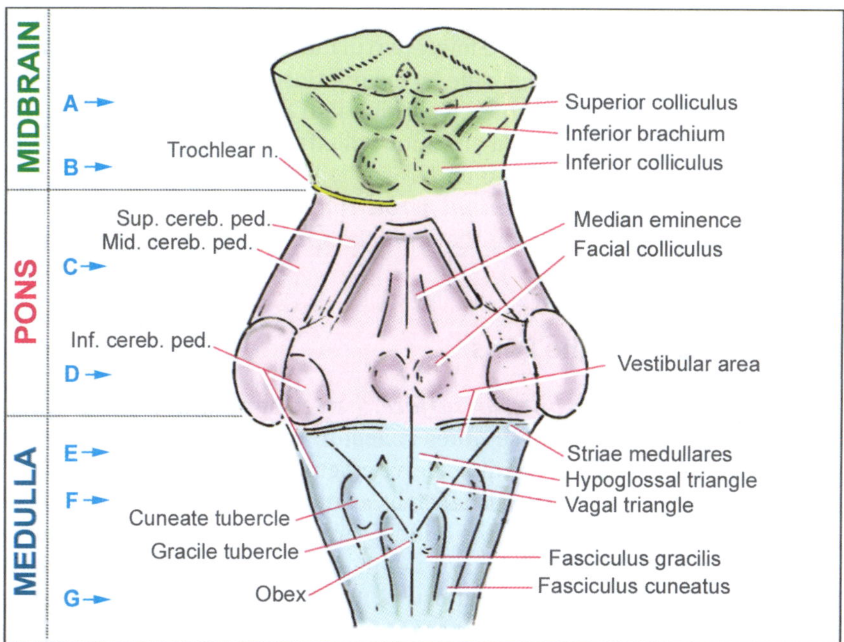

Fig. 23.8 Dorsal aspect of the brainstem. Letters G to A represent levels at which transverse sections are shown in Fig. 23.10 to 23.16.

fourth ventricle. The surface of the medulla is marked by a series of fissures or sulci that divide it into a number of regions. The ***anterior median fissure*** and the ***posterior median sulcus*** are upward continuations of the corresponding features seen on the spinal cord. On each side the ***anterolateral sulcus*** lies in line with the ventral roots of spinal nerves. The rootlets of the hypoglossal nerve emerge from this sulcus. The ***posterolateral sulcus*** lies in line with the dorsal nerve roots of spinal nerves, and gives attachment to rootlets of the glossopharyngeal, vagus and accessory nerves. The region between the anterior median sulcus and the anterolateral sulcus is occupied (on either side of the midline) by an elevation called the ***pyramid.*** The elevation is caused by a large bundle of fibres that descend from the cerebral cortex to the spinal cord. Some of these fibres cross from one side to the other in the lower part of the medulla, obliterating the anterior median fissure. These crossing fibres constitute the ***decussation of the pyramids***. In the upper part of the medulla, the region between the anterolateral and posterolateral sulci shows a prominent, elongated, oval swelling named the ***olive.*** It is produced by a large mass of grey matter called the ***inferior olivary nucleus.*** The posterior part of the medulla, between the posterior median sulcus and the posterolateral sulcus, contains tracts that enter the medulla from the posterior funiculus of the spinal cord. These are the ***fasciculus gracilis*** lying medially, next to the middle line, and the ***fasciculus cuneatus*** lying laterally. These fasciculi end in rounded elevations called the ***gracile*** and ***cuneate tubercles.*** These tubercles are produced by masses of grey matter called the ***nucleus gracilis*** and the ***nucleus cuneatus*** respectively.

Just above these tubercles the posterior aspect of the medulla is occupied by a triangular fossa which forms the lower part of the floor of the fourth ventricle. This fossa is bounded on either side by the inferior cerebellar peduncle. The lower part of the medulla, immediately lateral to the fasciculus cuneatus, is marked by another longitudinal elevation called the ***tuberculum cinereum.*** This elevation is produced by an underlying collection of grey matter called the ***spinal nucleus of the trigeminal nerve.*** The grey matter of this nucleus is covered by a layer of nerve fibres that form the ***spinal tract of the trigeminal nerve.***

Gross Anatomy of the Pons

The pons shows a convex ***anterior surface***, marked by prominent transversely running fibres. Laterally, these fibres collect to form a bundle, the ***middle cerebellar peduncle***. The trigeminal nerve emerges from the anterior surface, and the point of its emergence is taken as a landmark to define the plane of junction between the pons and the middle cerebellar peduncle. The anterior surface of the pons is marked, in the midline, by a shallow groove, the ***sulcus basilaris,*** which lodges the basilar artery. The line of junction between the pons and the medulla is marked by a groove through which a number of cranial nerves emerge. The abducent nerve emerges just above the pyramid and runs

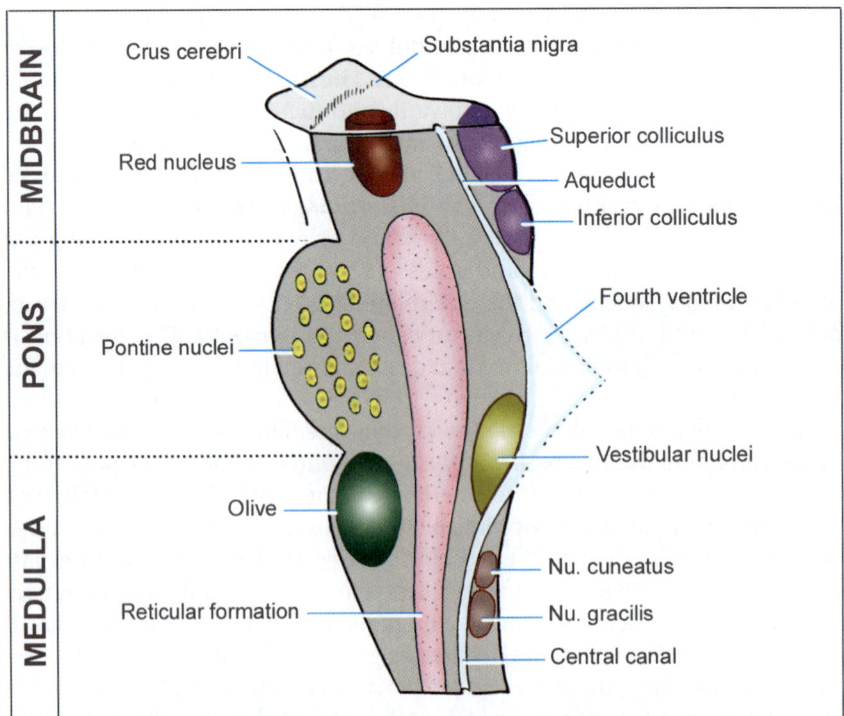

Fig. 23.9 Median section through the brainstem. Some important masses of grey matter are shown projected on to the median plane.

upwards in close relation to the anterior surface of the pons. The facial and vestibulo-cochlear nerves emerge in the interval between the olive and the pons. The posterior aspect of the pons forms the upper part of the floor of the fourth ventricle.

Gross Anatomy of the Midbrain

When the midbrain is viewed from the anterior aspect, we see two large bundles of fibres, one on each side of the middle line. These are the ***crura*** of the midbrain. The crura are separated by a deep fissure. Near the pons the fissure is narrow, but broadens as the crura diverge to enter the corresponding cerebral hemispheres. The oculomotor nerve emerges from the medial aspect of the crus (singular of crura) of the same side.

The posterior aspect of the midbrain is marked by four rounded swellings. These are the ***colliculi,*** one ***superior*** and one ***inferior*** on each side. Each colliculus is related laterally to a ridge called the ***brachium.*** The ***superior brachium*** connects the superior colliculus to the lateral geniculate body, while the ***inferior brachium*** connects the inferior colliculus to the medial geniculate body. Just below the colliculi, there is the uppermost part of a membrane, the ***superior medullary velum,*** which stretches between the two superior cerebellar peduncles, and helps to form the roof of the fourth ventricle. The trochlear nerve emerges from the velum, and then winds round the side of the midbrain to reach its ventral aspect.

INTERNAL STRUCTURE OF THE BRAINSTEM

The following description is confined to those features of internal structure that can be seen with the naked eye. The main features of the internal structure of the brainstem are most easily reviewed by examining transverse sections at various levels. These are illustrated in Figs. 23.10 to 23.14. The levels represented in these figures are indicated in Fig. 23.8.

Internal Structure of the Medulla

A section at the level of the pyramidal decussation (Fig. 23.10) shows some similarity to sections through the spinal cord. The central canal is surrounded by central grey matter. The ventral grey columns are present, but are separated from the central grey matter by decussating pyramidal fibres. The region behind the central grey matter is occupied by the fasciculus gracilis, medially; and by the fasciculus cuneatus laterally. Closely related to these fasciculi there are two tongue-shaped extensions of the central grey matter. The medial of these extensions is the ***nucleus gracilis***, and the lateral is the ***nucleus cuneatus***. More laterally, there is the ***spinal nucleus of the trigeminal nerve***. The spinal nucleus of the trigeminal nerve is related superficially to the ***spinal tract*** of the nerve. The ventral part of the medulla is occupied, on either side of the middle line, by a prominent bundle of fibres: these fibres form the ***pyramid***.

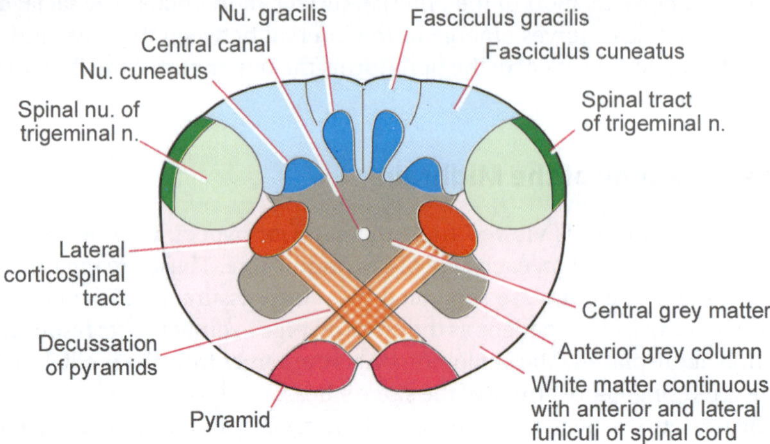

Fig. 23.10 Main features to be seen in a transverse section through the medulla at the level of the pyramidal decussation.

The fibres of the pyramids are ***corticospinal fibres*** on their way from the cerebral cortex to the spinal cord. At this level in the medulla many of these fibres run backwards and medially to cross in the middle line. These crossing fibres constitute the ***decussation of the pyramids***. Having crossed the middle line, the corticospinal fibres turn downwards to enter the lateral white column of the spinal cord. The anterolateral region of the medulla is continuous with the anterior and lateral funiculi of the spinal cord.

A section through the medulla at a somewhat higher level is shown in Fig. 23.11. The central canal surrounded by central grey matter, the nucleus gracilis, the nucleus cuneatus, the spinal nucleus of the trigeminal nerve, and the pyramids occupy the same positions as at lower levels. The nucleus gracilis and the nucleus cuneatus are, however, much larger and are no longer continuous with the central grey matter. The fasciculus gracilis and the fasciculus cuneatus are less prominent. The region just behind the pyramids is occupied by a prominent bundle of fibres, the ***medial lemniscus,*** on either side of the middle line. The medial lemniscus is formed by fibres arising in the nucleus gracilis and the nucleus cuneatus. These fibres cross the middle line and turn upwards in the lemniscus of the opposite side. Crossing fibres of the two sides constitute the ***sensory decussation.*** The region lateral to the medial lemniscus contains scattered neurons mixed with nerve fibres. This region is the ***reticular formation***. More laterally there is a mass of white matter containing various tracts.

A section through the medulla at the level of the olive is shown in Fig. 23.12. The pyramids, the medial lemniscus, the spinal nucleus and tract of the trigeminal nerve, and the reticular formation are present in the same relative position as at lower levels. The medial lemniscus is, however, much more prominent and is somewhat expanded anteriorly. Lateral to the spinal nucleus (and tract) of the trigeminal nerve we see a large compact bundle of fibres. This is the ***inferior cerebellar peduncle*** that connects the medulla to the cerebellum. Posteriorly, the medulla forms the floor of the fourth ventricle. Here it is lined by a layer of grey matter in which are located several important

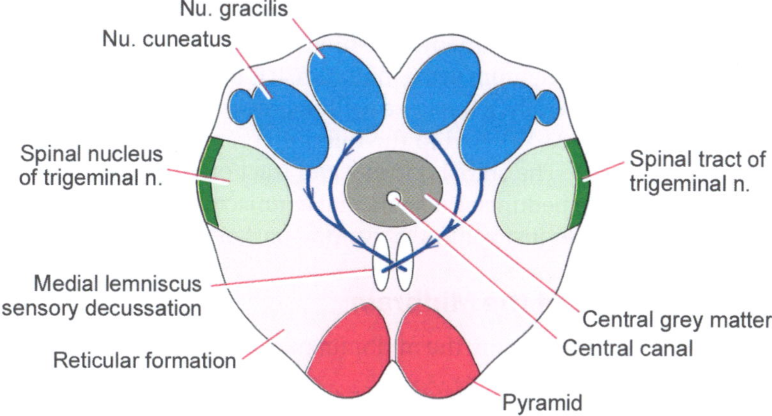

Fig. 23.11 Transverse section through the medulla to show the main features seen at the level of the sensory decussation.

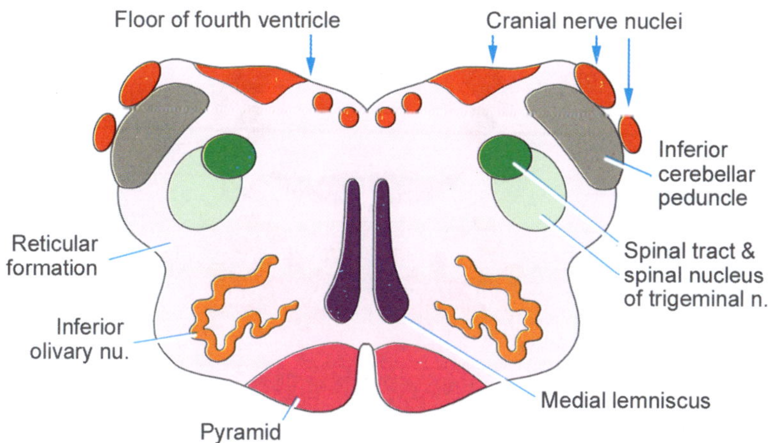

Fig. 23.12 Main features to be seen in a transverse section through the medulla at the level of the olive.

cranial nerve nuclei. The ***inferior olivary nucleus*** forms a prominent feature in the anterolateral part of the medulla at this level. It is made up of a thin lamina of grey matter that is folded on itself like a crumpled purse. The nucleus has a hilum that is directed medially.

Internal Structure of the Pons

The pons is divisible into a ventral part and a dorsal part (Fig. 23.13).

The ***ventral (or basilar) part*** consists of transverse and vertical fibres. Amongst the fibres are groups of cells that constitute the ***pontine nuclei***. When traced laterally the transverse fibres form the ***middle cerebellar peduncle***. The vertical fibres are of two types. Some of them descend from the cerebral cortex to end in the pontine nuclei. Others are corticospinal fibres that descend through the pons into the medulla where they form the pyramids.

The ***dorsal part (or tegmentum)*** of the pons may be regarded as an upward continuation of the part of the medulla behind the pyramids. Superiorly, it is continuous with the tegmentum of the midbrain. It is bounded, posteriorly, by the fourth ventricle. Laterally, it is related to the ***superior cerebellar peduncles*** in its upper part (Fig. 23.13), and to the inferior cerebellar peduncles in its lower part (Fig. 23.14). The spinal nucleus and tract of the trigeminal nerve lie just medial to these peduncles. The medial lemniscus forms a transversely elongated band of fibres just behind the ventral part of the pons.

Internal Structure of the Midbrain

For convenience of description, the midbrain may be divided as follows (Fig. 23.15):

1. The part lying behind a transverse line drawn through the cerebral aqueduct is called the ***tectum.*** It consists of the superior and inferior colliculi of the two sides.

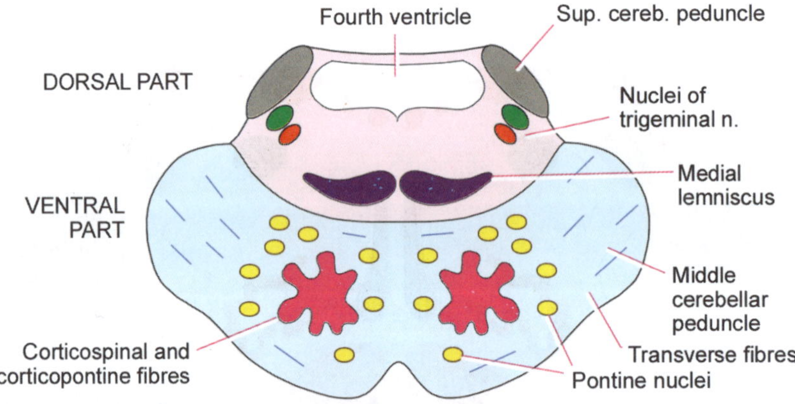

Fig. 23.13 Main features to be seen in a transverse section through the upper part of the pons.

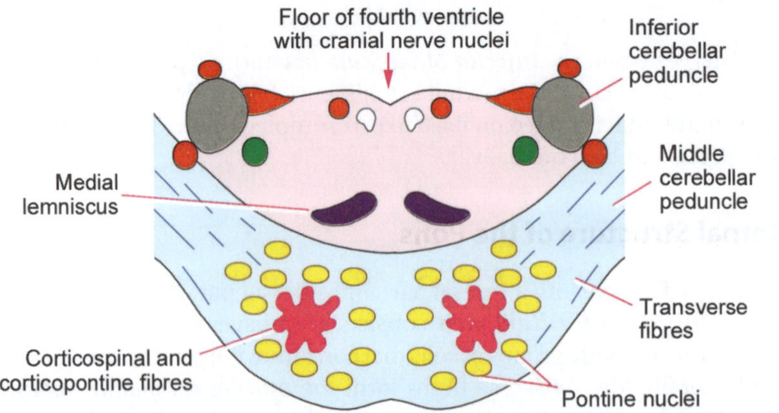

Fig. 23.14 Main features to be seen in a transverse section through the lower part of the pons.

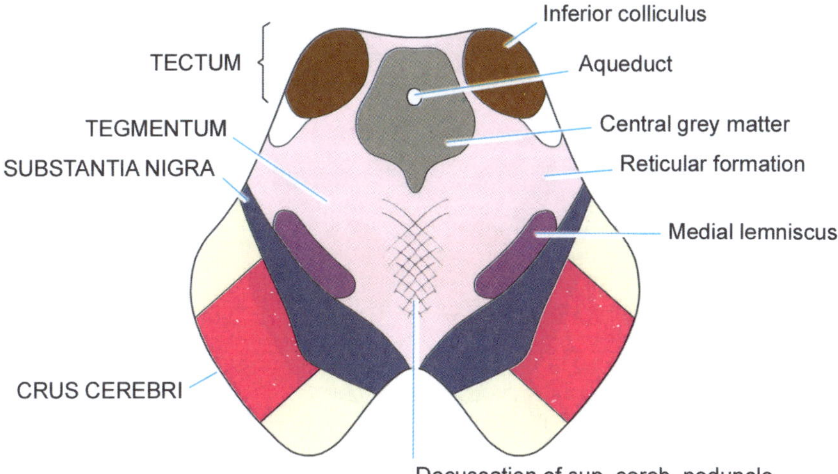

Fig. 23.15 Main features to be seen in a transverse section through the lower part of the midbrain.

2. The part lying in front of the transverse line is made up of right and left halves called the ***cerebral peduncles.*** Each peduncle consists of three parts. From anterior to posterior side these are the ***crus cerebri*** (or ***basis pedunculi),*** the ***substantia nigra*** and the ***tegmentum.***

The ***crus cerebri*** consists of a large mass of vertically running fibres. These fibres descend from the cerebral cortex. Some of these pass through the midbrain to reach the pons, while others reach the spinal cord. The two crura are separated by a notch seen on the anterior aspect of the midbrain.

The ***substantia nigra*** is made up of pigmented grey matter and, therefore, appears dark in colour.

The ***tegmentum*** of the two sides is continuous across the middle line. It contains important masses of grey matter as well as fibre bundles. The largest of the nuclei is the ***red nucleus*** (Fig. 23.16) present in the upper half of the midbrain. The tegmentum also contains the ***reticular formation*** which is continuous below with that of the pons and medulla. The fibre bundles of the tegmentum include the medial lemniscus which lies just behind the substantia nigra, lateral to the red nucleus. These are the fibres of the superior cerebellar peduncles that have their origin in the cerebellum and decussate before ending in the red nucleus (and in some other centres).

Functions of the Reticular Formation

Because of its diverse connections the reticular formation of the brainstem is believed to have a controlling or modifying influence on many functions. Some of them are as follows.

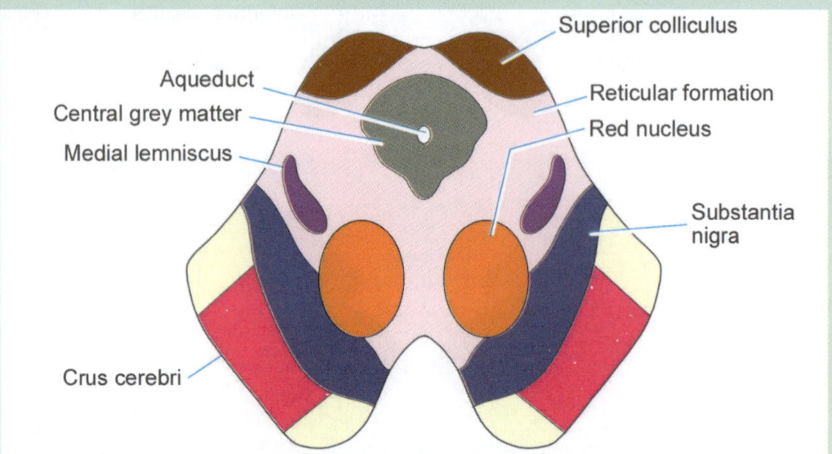

Fig. 23.16 Main features to be seen in a transverse section through the upper part of the midbrain.

A. Somatomotor control

Through its direct connections with the spinal cord; and indirectly through the corpus striatum, the cerebral cortex and the cerebellum, the reticular formation has an influence on fine control of movements including those involved in postural adjustments, locomotion, skilled use of the hands, speech etc.

B. Somatosensory control

The reticular formation influences conduction through somatosensory pathways. Similar effects may also be exerted on visual and auditory pathways.

C. Visceral control

Physiological studies have shown that stimulation of certain areas in the reticular formation of the medulla has great influence on respiratory and cardiovascular function. These effects are produced through connections between the reticular formation and autonomic centres in the brainstem and spinal cord.

D. Neuroendocrine control

Through its connections with the hypothalamus, the reticular formation influences activity of the adenohypophysis and of the neurohypophysis.

E. Some other functions

1. The reticular formation also influences other hypothalamic functions. These include a possible effect on circadian rhythms.
2. The reticular formation controls arousal and the state of consciousness of a person through the ascending reticular activating system.

F. Serotoninergic Raphe System

The reticular formation has a complex system made up of serotoninergic fibres. These fibres form a pain controlling pathway. Cranially, this pathway connects to some centres in the midbrain that constitute a pain control centre.

Some fibres descending into the spinal cord influence sympathetic control of the cardiovascular system.

PHYSIOLOGY OF PAIN

Every individual experiences at one time or another. Pain is basically a protective phenomenon, that warns us. When the cause of pain is obvious (e.g. touching a hot object) we instinctively move away from the cause. When a part of the body is hurt the pain causes us to give rest to the part.

Pain may arise in any part of the body. It can be caused by mechanical damage, by extreme heat or by extreme cold. Pain arises from viscera when their walls are stretched, or when there is strong contraction of muscle in the walls. Examples of the latter are intestinal colic, biliary colic, renal colic and pain during labour (childbirth).

Release of some chemicals causes pain. These are 5-hydroxytryptamine (5-HT), prostaglandins, potassium, AMP and ADP. Injured tissues release kinogen that is acted upon by enzymes to form kinins. The kinins (e.g. bradykinin, kallidin) cause pain.

Impulses of pain are picked up mainly by free nerve endings. They travel through spinal nerves to the spinal cord. From here they travel through the spinothalamic tracts and reach the thalamus. From the thalamus impulses pass to the somatosensory area of the cerebral cortex. Pain from the face travels through the trigeminal nerve.

Pain can be perceived by the thalamus and in the reticular formation of the brainstem. However the quality and localisation of pain are perceived by the cerebral cortex.

Pain from viscera travels along sympathetic and parasympathetic nerves. In the spinal cord the impulses travel through spinothalamic tracts to the thalamus and from there to the cerebral cortex.

GROSS ANATOMY OF THE CEREBELLUM

Subdivisions of the Cerebellum

The cerebellum lies in the posterior cranial fossa, behind the pons and the medulla. It is separated from the cerebrum by a fold of dura mater called the ***tentorium cerebelli.***

The cerebellum consists of a part lying near the middle line called the ***vermis,*** and of two lateral ***hemispheres.*** It has two surfaces, ***superior*** and ***inferior.*** On the superior aspect, there is no line of distinction between vermis and hemispheres. On the inferior aspect, the two hemispheres are separated by a deep depression called the ***vallecula.*** The vermis lies in the depth of this depression. Anteriorly and posteriorly the hemispheres extend beyond the vermis and are separated by anterior and posterior ***cerebellar notches.***

The surface of the cerebellum is marked by a series of fissures that run more or less parallel to one another. The fissures subdivide the surface of the cerebellum into narrow leaf like bands or ***folia***. The long axis of the majority of folia is more or less transverse. Sections of the cerebellum cut at right angles to this axis have a characteristic tree-like appearance to which the term ***arbor-vitae*** (tree of life) is applied.

Some of the fissures on the surface of the cerebellum are deeper than others. They divide the cerebellum into ***lobes*** within which smaller ***lobules*** may be recognised. To show the various subdivisions of the cerebellum in a single illustration it is usual to represent the organ as if it has been 'opened out' so that the superior and inferior aspects can both be seen. Such an illustration is shown in Fig. 23.17. This should be compared with Figs. 23.18 A, B which are more realistic drawings of the superior and inferior surfaces, and with Fig. 23.19 which is a middle line section showing the subdivisions of the vermis.

The deepest fissures in the cerebellum are (i) the ***primary fissure*** seen on the superior surface, and (ii) the ***posterolateral fissure*** seen on the inferior aspect. These fissures divide the cerebellum into three lobes. The part anterior to the primary fissure is the ***anterior lobe.*** The part between the two fissures is the ***middle lobe*** (sometimes called the ***posterior lobe***). The remaining part is the ***flocculonodular lobe.***

The central core of each cerebellar hemisphere is formed by white matter. The peduncles are continued into this white matter.

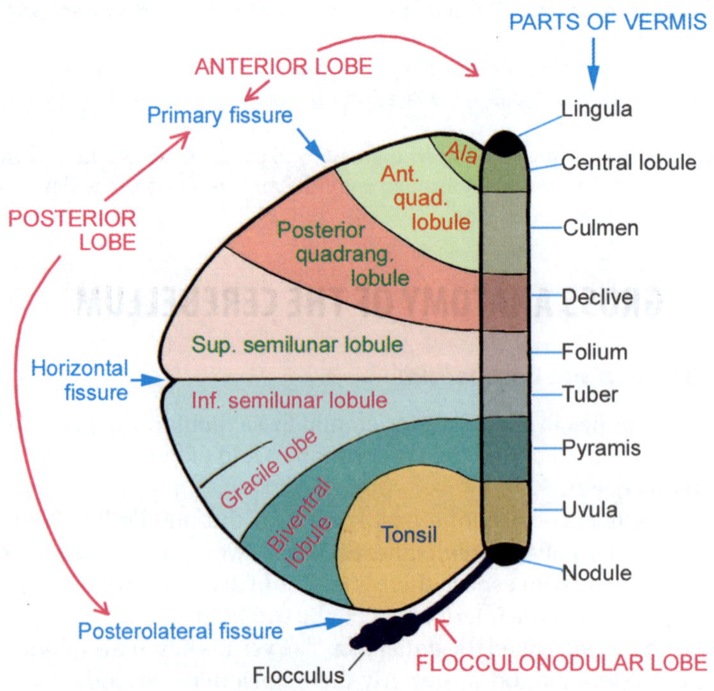

Fig. 23.17 Scheme to show the subdivisions of the cerebellum.

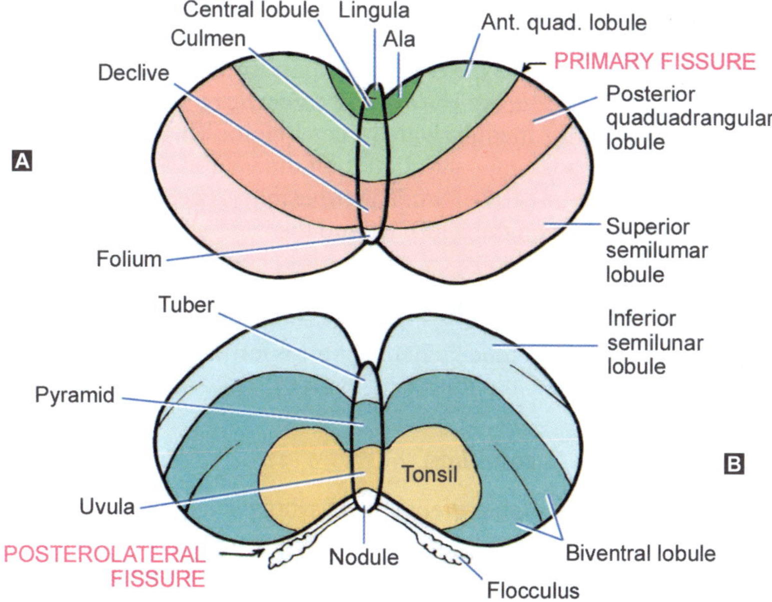

Fig. 23.18 Subdivisions of the cerebellum. A. As seen on the superior aspect. B. As seen on the inferior aspect.

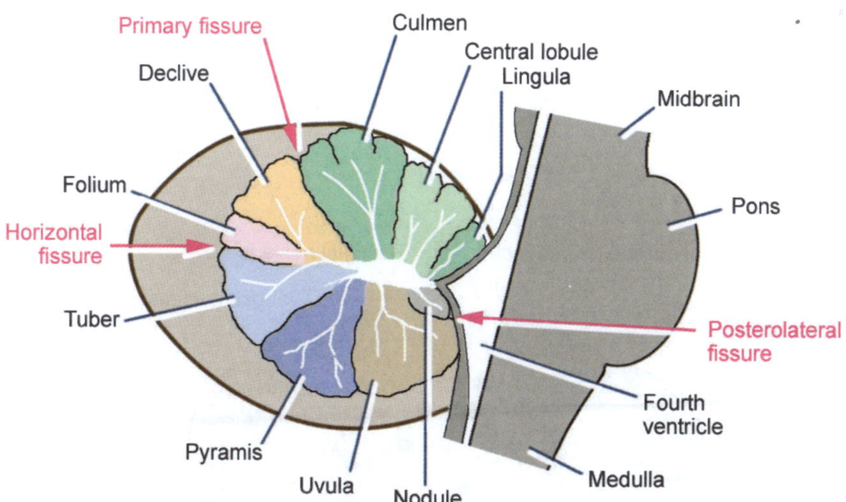

Fig. 23.19 Subdivisions of the vermis of the cerebellum as seen in a median section.

Cerebellar Peduncles

The fibres entering or leaving the cerebellum pass through three thick bundles called the cerebellar peduncles. The ***inferior cerebellar peduncle*** connects the posterolateral part of the medulla with the cerebellum. The ***middle cerebellar peduncle*** looks like a lateral continuation of the ventral part of the pons. It connects the pons to the cerebellum. The ***superior cerebellar peduncle*** is the main connection between the midbrain and the cerebellum.

White Matter of the Cerebellum

The central core of each cerebellar hemisphere is formed by white matter. The peduncles are continued into this white matter.

Grey Matter of the Cerebellum

Most of the grey matter of the cerebellum is arranged as a thin layer covering the central core of white matter. This layer is the ***cerebellar cortex***. The subdivisions of the cerebellar cortex correspond to the subdivisions of the cerebellum described above. Embedded within the central core of white matter there are masses of grey matter which constitute the ***cerebellar nuclei.*** These are as follows (Fig. 23.20):

1. The ***dentate nucleus*** lies in the centre of each cerebellar hemisphere. Cross sections through the nucleus have a striking resemblance to those through the inferior olivary nucleus. Like the latter it is made up of a thin lamina of grey matter that is folded upon itself so that it resembles a crumpled purse. Both the nuclei have a hilum directed medially.
2. The ***emboliform nucleus*** lies on the medial side of the dentate nucleus.
3. The ***globose nucleus*** lies medial to the emboliform nucleus.
4. The ***fastigial nucleus*** lies close to the middle line in the anterior part of the superior vermis.

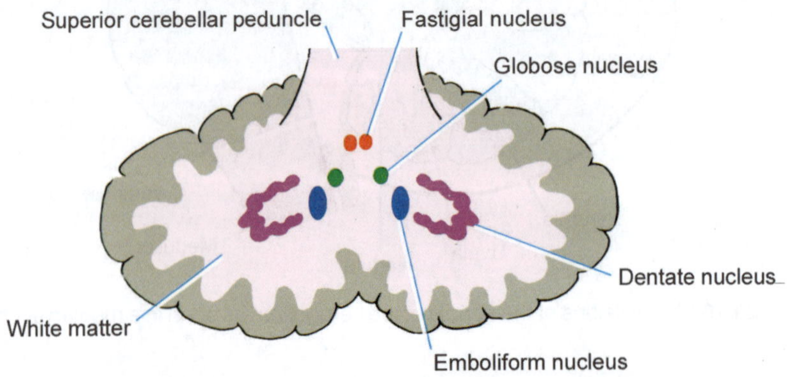

Fig. 23.20 Scheme to show the cerebellar nuclei.

Functions of the Cerebellum

1. The cerebellum plays an essential role in the control of movement. It is responsible for ensuring that movement takes place smoothly, in the right direction, and to the right extent. The cerebellar cortex is also important for learning of movements (e.g., in learning to write).
2. Through its vestibular and spinal connections the cerebellum is responsible for maintaining the equilibrium of the body.
3. These functions are possible because the cerebellum receives constant information regarding the state of contraction of muscles, and of the position of various joints. It also receives information from the eyes, the ears, the vestibular apparatus, the reticular formation and the cerebral cortex. All this information is integrated, and is used to influence movement through motor centres in the brainstem and spinal cord, and also through the cerebral cortex.

GROSS ANATOMY OF THE CEREBRAL HEMISPHERES

EXTERIOR OF THE CEREBRAL HEMISPHERES

Poles, Surfaces, and Borders

The cerebrum consists of two cerebral hemispheres that are partially connected with each other. When viewed from the lateral aspect each cerebral hemisphere has the appearance shown in Fig. 23.21. Three somewhat pointed ends or ***poles*** can be recognised. These are the ***frontal pole*** anteriorly, the ***occipital pole*** posteriorly, and the ***temporal pole*** that lies between the frontal and occipital poles, and points forwards and somewhat downwards. A coronal section through the cerebral hemispheres (Fig. 23.22) shows that each hemisphere has three borders, ***superomedial, inferolateral*** and ***inferomedial.*** These borders divide the surface of the hemisphere into three large surfaces, ***superolateral, medial*** and ***inferior.*** The inferior surface is further subdivided into an anterior ***orbital*** part and a posterior ***tentorial*** part (Fig. 23.23). The surfaces of the cerebral hemisphere are not smooth. They show a series of grooves or ***sulci*** which are separated by intervening areas that are called ***gyri.***

Lobes

For convenience of description each cerebral hemisphere is divided into four major subdivisions or ***lobes.*** To consider the boundaries of these lobes reference has to be made to some sulci and other features to be seen on each hemisphere (Fig. 23.21).

1. On the superolateral surface of the hemisphere there are two prominent sulci. One of these is the ***posterior ramus of the lateral sulcus*** which begins near the temporal pole and runs backwards and slightly upwards. Its posteriormost part curves sharply upwards. The second sulcus that is

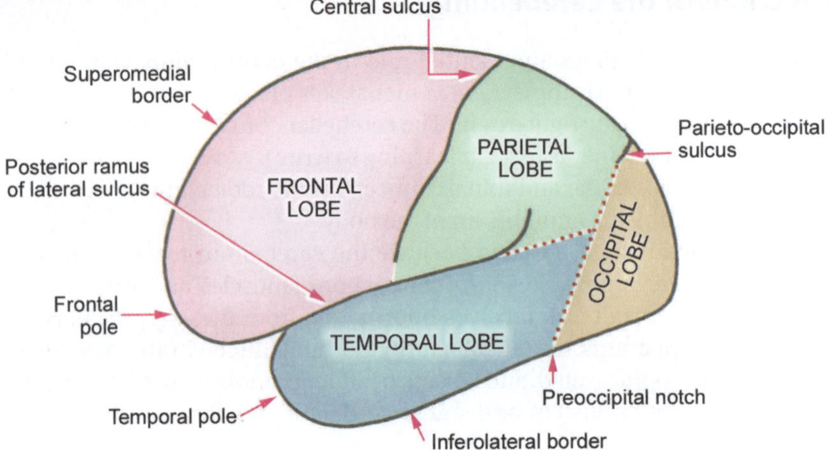

Fig. 23.21 Lateral aspect of the cerebral hemisphere to show borders, poles and lobes.

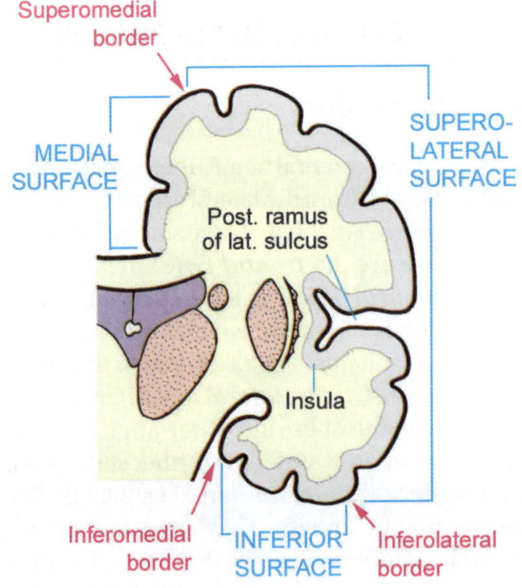

Fig. 23.22 Coronal section through a cerebral hemisphere to show its borders and surfaces.

used to delimit the lobes is the ***central sulcus.*** It begins on the superomedial margin a little behind the midpoint between the frontal and occipital poles, and runs downwards and forwards to end a little above the posterior ramus of the lateral sulcus.

2. On the medial surface of the hemisphere, near the occipital pole, there is a sulcus called the ***parieto-occipital sulcus*** (Fig. 23.25). The upper end of this sulcus reaches the superomedial border and a small part of it can be seen on the superolateral surface (Fig. 23.21).

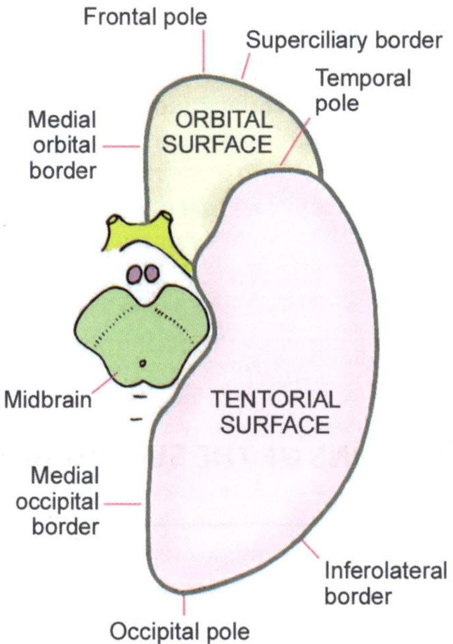

Fig. 23.23 Inferior aspect of a cerebral hemisphere to show its borders, poles and surfaces.

3. A little anterior to the occipital pole the inferolateral border shows a slight indentation called the ***preoccipital notch*** (or ***preoccipital incisure***).

To complete the subdivision of the hemisphere into lobes we now have to draw two imaginary lines. The first imaginary line connects the upper end of the parieto-occipital sulcus to the preoccipital notch. The second imaginary line is a backward continuation of the posterior ramus of the lateral sulcus (excluding the posterior upturned part) to meet the first line. We are now in a position to define the limits of the various lobes as follows:

a. The ***frontal lobe*** lies anterior to the central sulcus, and above the posterior ramus of the lateral sulcus.
b. The ***parietal lobe*** lies behind the central sulcus. It is bounded below by the posterior ramus of the lateral sulcus and by the second imaginary line; and behind by the upper part of the first imaginary line.
c. The ***occipital lobe*** is the area lying behind the first imaginary line.
d. The ***temporal lobe*** lies below the posterior ramus of the lateral sulcus and the second imaginary line. It is separated from the occipital lobe by the lower part of the first imaginary line.

Before going on to consider further subdivisions of each of the lobes named above, attention has to be directed to details of some structures already mentioned.

a. The upper end of the central sulcus winds round the superomedial border to reach the medial surface. Here its end is surrounded by a gyrus called the ***paracentral lobule*** (Fig. 23.25). The lower end of the central sulcus is always separated by a small interval from the posterior ramus of the lateral sulcus (Fig. 23.21).

b. The lateral sulcus begins on the inferior aspect of the cerebral hemisphere where it lies between the orbital surface and the anterior part of the temporal lobe (Fig. 23.27). It runs laterally to reach the superolateral surface. On reaching this surface it divides into three rami (branches). These rami are ***anterior*** (or ***anterior horizontal***), ***ascending*** (or ***anterior ascending***) and ***posterior*** (Fig. 23.24). The anterior and ascending rami are short and run into the frontal lobe in the directions indicated by their names. The posterior ramus has already been considered. Unlike most other sulci, the lateral sulcus is very deep. Its walls cover a fairly large area of the surface of the hemisphere called the ***insula*** (Fig. 23.23).

FURTHER SUBDIVISIONS OF THE SUPEROLATERAL SURFACE

Frontal Lobe

The frontal lobe is further subdivided as follows (Fig. 23.24). The ***precentral sulcus*** runs downwards and forwards parallel to and a little anterior to the central sulcus. The area between it and the central sulcus is the ***precentral gyrus.*** In the region anterior to the precentral gyrus there are two sulci that run in an anteroposterior direction. These are the ***superior*** and ***inferior frontal sulci.*** They divide this region into ***superior***, ***middle*** and ***inferior frontal gyri.*** The anterior and ascending rami of the lateral sulcus extend into the inferior frontal gyrus dividing it into three parts. The part below the anterior ramus is the ***pars orbitalis***; that between the anterior and ascending rami is the ***pars triangularis***; and the part posterior to the ascending ramus is the ***pars opercularis.***

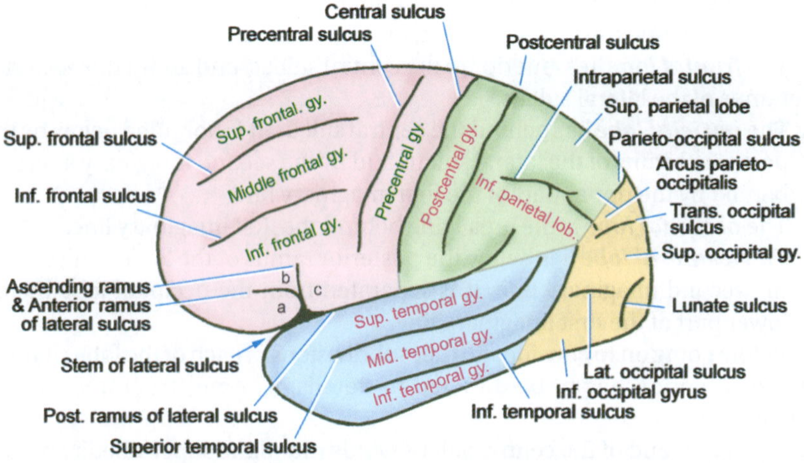

Fig. 23.24 Simplified presentation of sulci and gyri on the superolateral surface of the cerebral hemisphere. a = pars orbitalis. b = pars triangularis. c = pars opercularis.

Temporal Lobe

The temporal lobe has two sulci that run parallel to the posterior ramus of the lateral sulcus. They are termed the ***superior and inferior temporal sulci.*** They divide the superolateral surface of this lobe into ***superior, middle and inferior temporal gyri.***

Parietal Lobe

The parietal lobe shows the following subdivisions:

The ***postcentral sulcus*** runs downwards and forwards parallel to and a little behind the central sulcus. The area between these two sulci is the ***postcentral gyrus.*** The rest of the parietal lobe is divided into a ***superior parietal lobule*** and an ***inferior parietal lobule*** by the ***intraparietal sulcus.*** Some other sulci are shown in Fig. 23.24.

Occipital Lobe

The occipital lobe shows three rather short sulci. One of these, the ***lateral occipital sulcus*** lies horizontally and divides the lobe into ***superior and inferior occipital gyri.*** The ***lunate sulcus*** runs downwards and slightly forwards just in front of the occipital pole. The upper end of the parieto-occipital sulcus (which just reaches the superolateral surface from the medial surface) is surrounded by the ***arcus parieto-occipitalis.***

Insula

In the depth of the stem and posterior ramus of the lateral sulcus there is a part of the cerebral hemisphere called the insula (insula = insulated or hidden). During development of the cerebral hemisphere this area grows less than surrounding areas which, therefore, come to overlap it and occlude it from surface view. These surrounding areas are called ***opercula*** (= lids). The ***frontal operculum*** lies between the anterior and ascending rami of the lateral sulcus. The ***frontoparietal operculum*** lies above the posterior ramus of the lateral sulcus. The ***temporal operculum*** lies below this sulcus. The temporal operculum has a superior surface hidden in the depth of the lateral sulcus (Fig. 23.23). On this surface we see two gyri called the ***anterior and posterior transverse temporal gyri.***

Medial Surface of Cerebral Hemisphere

When the two cerebral hemispheres are separated from each other by a cut in the middle line the appearances seen are shown in Figs. 23.25 and 23.26. The structures seen are as follows:

The ***corpus callosum*** is a prominent arched structure consisting of commissural fibres passing from one hemisphere to the other (Fig. 23.26). It consists of a central part called the ***trunk,*** a posterior end or ***splenium,*** and an anterior end or ***genu.*** A little below the corpus callosum we see the third

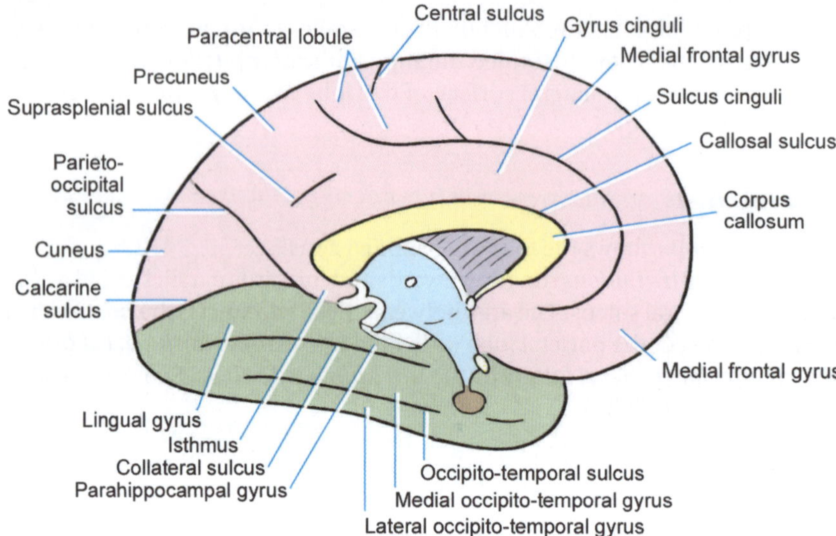

Fig. 23.25 Simplified presentation of sulci and gyri on the cerebral hemisphere as seen from the medial aspect. The medial surface and the tentorial surface (shaded green) are seen. The corpus callosum and some other median structures have been cut across.

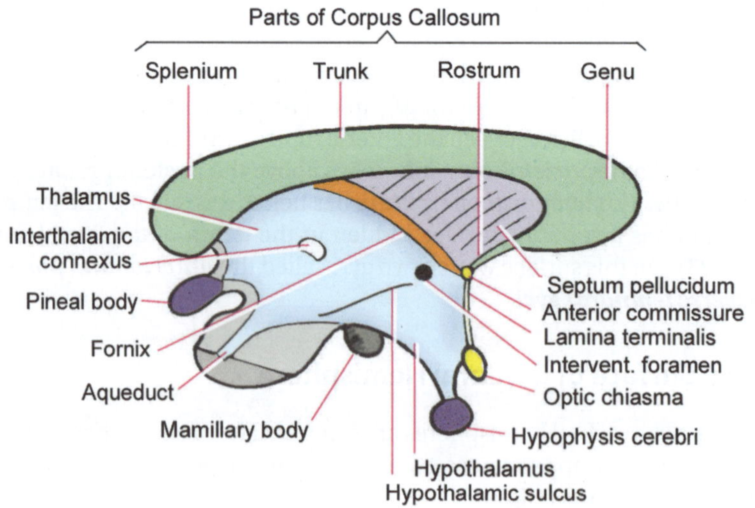

Fig. 23.26 Enlarged view of part of Fig. 23.25 to show some structures to be seen on the medial aspect of the cerebral hemisphere.

ventricle of the brain. A number of structures can be identified in relation to this ventricle. The ***interventricular foramen*** through which the third ventricle communicates with the lateral ventricle can be seen in the upper and anterior part. Posteroinferiorly, the ventricle is continuous with the ***cerebral aqueduct.*** The lateral wall of the ventricle is formed in greater part by a large mass of grey matter called the ***thalamus.*** The right and left thalami are usually interconnected (across the middle line) by a strip of grey matter called the ***interthalamic connexus.*** The anteroinferior part of the lateral wall of the third ventricle is formed by a collection of grey matter that constitutes the ***hypothalamus.***

Above the thalamus there is a bundle of fibres called the ***fornix.*** Posteriorly, the fornix is attached to the undersurface of the corpus callosum, but anteriorly it disappears from view just in front of the interventricular foramen. Extending between the fornix and the corpus callosum there is a thin lamina called the ***septum pellucidum*** (or ***septum lucidum***), which separates the right and left lateral ventricles from each other. Removal of the septum pellucidum brings the interior of the lateral ventricle into view.

In the anterior wall of the third ventricle there are the ***anterior commissure*** and the ***lamina terminalis.*** The anterior commissure is attached to the genu of the corpus callosum through a thin lamina of fibres that constitutes the ***rostrum*** of the corpus callosum. Below, the anterior commissure is continuous with the lamina terminalis which is a thin lamina of nervous tissue. The lower end of the lamina terminalis is attached to the optic chiasma. Posteriorly, the third ventricle is related to the ***pineal gland*** and inferiorly to the ***hypophysis cerebri.***

Above the corpus callosum (and also in front of and behind it) we see the sulci and gyri of the medial surface of the hemisphere (Fig. 23.25). The most prominent of the sulci is the ***cingulate sulcus*** which follows a curved course parallel to the upper convex margin of the corpus callosum. Anteriorly, it ends below the rostrum of the corpus callosum. Posteriorly, it turns upwards to reach the superomedial border a little behind the upper end of the central sulcus. The area between the cingulate sulcus and the corpus callosum is called the ***gyrus cinguli.*** It is separated from the corpus callosum by the ***callosal sulcus.*** The part of the medial surface of the hemisphere between the cingulate sulcus and the superomedial border consists of two parts. The smaller posterior part which is wound around the end of the central sulcus is called the ***paracentral lobule***. The large anterior part is called the ***medial frontal gyrus.*** These two parts are separated by a short sulcus continuous with the cingulate sulcus.

The part of the medial surface behind the paracentral lobule and the gyrus cinguli shows two major sulci that cut off a triangular area called the ***cuneus.*** The triangle is bounded anteriorly and above by the ***parieto-occipital sulcus***; inferiorly by the ***calcarine sulcus***; and posteriorly by the superomedial border of the hemisphere. The calcarine sulcus extends forwards beyond its junction with the parieto-occipital sulcus and ends a little below the splenium of the corpus callosum. The small area separating the splenium from the calcarine sulcus is called the ***isthmus.*** Between the parieto-occipital sulcus and the paracentral lobule there is a quadrilateral area called the ***precuneus.*** Anteroinferiorly the precuneus is separated from the posterior part of the gyrus cinguli by the ***suprasplenial (or subparietal) sulcus.***

The precuneus and the posterior part of the paracentral lobule form the medial surface of the parietal lobe.

Inferior Surface of Cerebrum

When the cerebrum is separated from the hindbrain by cutting across the midbrain, and is viewed from below, the appearances seen are shown in Fig. 23.27. Posterior to the midbrain we see the undersurface of the splenium of the corpus callosum. Anterior to the midbrain there is a depressed area called the ***interpeduncular fossa***. The fossa is bounded in front by the ***optic chiasma*** and on the sides by the right and left ***optic tracts***. The optic tracts wind round the sides of the midbrain to terminate on its posterolateral aspect. In this region two swellings, the ***medial and lateral geniculate bodies***, can be seen.

Certain structures are seen within the interpeduncular fossa. These are closely related to the floor of the third ventricle (see also Fig. 23.26). Anterior and medial to the crura of the midbrain there are two rounded swellings called the ***mamillary bodies.*** Anterior to these bodies there is a median elevation called the ***tuber cinereum,*** to which the infundibulum of the hypophysis cerebri is attached. The triangular interval between the mamillary bodies and the midbrain is pierced by numerous small blood vessels and is called the ***posterior perforated substance.*** A similar area lying on each side of the optic chiasma is called the ***anterior perforated substance***.

In addition to these structures we see the sulci and gyri on the orbital and tentorial parts of the inferior surface of the each cerebral hemisphere (described

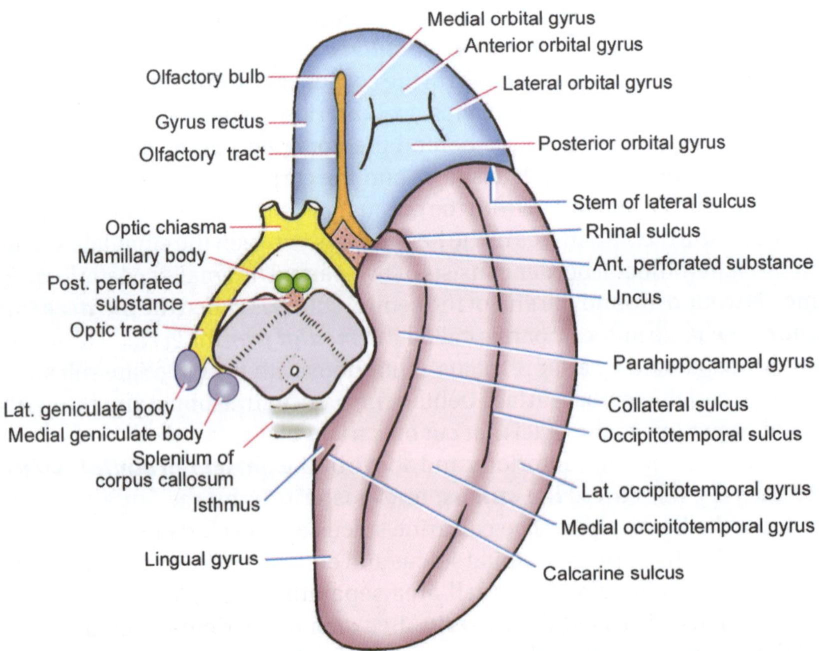

Fig. 23.27 Structures to be seen on the inferior aspect of the cerebral hemisphere.

below). The orbital and tentorial parts of the inferior surface are separated from each other by the stem of the lateral sulcus.

Orbital Surface

Close to the medial border of the orbital surface there is an anteroposterior sulcus: it is called the ***olfactory sulcus*** because the olfactory bulb and tract lie superficial to it. The area medial to this sulcus is called the ***gyrus rectus***. The rest of the orbital surface is divided by an H-shaped ***orbital sulcus*** into ***anterior***, ***posterior***, ***medial*** and ***lateral orbital gyri.***

Tentorial Surface

The tentorial surface is marked by two major sulci that run in an anteroposterior direction. These are the ***collateral sulcus*** medially, and the ***occipitotemporal sulcus*** laterally. The posterior part of the collateral sulcus runs parallel to the calcarine sulcus: the area between them is the ***lingual gyrus.*** Anteriorly, the lingual gyrus becomes continuous with the ***parahippocampal gyrus*** which is related medially to the midbrain and to the interpeduncular fossa. The anterior end of the parahippocampal gyrus is cut off from the curved temporal pole of the hemisphere by a curved ***rhinal sulcus.*** This part of the parahippocampal gyrus forms a hook-like structure called the ***uncus.*** Posteriorly, the parahippocampal gyrus becomes continuous with the gyrus cinguli through the isthmus (Fig. 23.25). The area between the collateral sulcus and the rhinal sulcus medially, and the occipitotemporal sulcus laterally, is the ***medial occipitotemporal gyrus.*** The area lateral to the occipitotemporal sulcus is called the ***lateral occipitotemporal gyrus.*** This gyrus is continuous (around the inferolateral margin of the cerebral hemisphere) with the inferior temporal gyrus.

SOME STRUCTURES WITHIN THE CEREBRAL HEMISPHERES

For a proper understanding of the structure of the cerebrum, brief reference to the development of the brain is necessary. At an early stage of development the brain is made up of three hollow vesicles. These are the ***prosencephalon,*** the ***mesencephalon*** and the ***rhombencephalon*** (in craniocaudal sequence) (Fig. 23.28). The mesencephalon gives rise to the midbrain, while the rhombencephalon forms the hindbrain (i.e., the pons, the medulla, and the cerebellum). The cerebrum develops from the prosencephalon which soon shows a subdivision into a median part, the ***diencephalon,*** and two lateral evaginations (the ***telencephalic vesicles***) which together constitute the ***telencephalon.*** In subsequent development, the telencephalic vesicles grow much faster than the diencephalon. As they enlarge they eventually overlap the diencephalon and fuse with its lateral aspect. One telencephalic vesicle, along with the corresponding half of the diencephalon constitutes one cerebral hemisphere. From what has been said above it will be clear that the diencephalic part of the hemisphere lies medially and inferiorly relative to the part derived from the telencephalon.

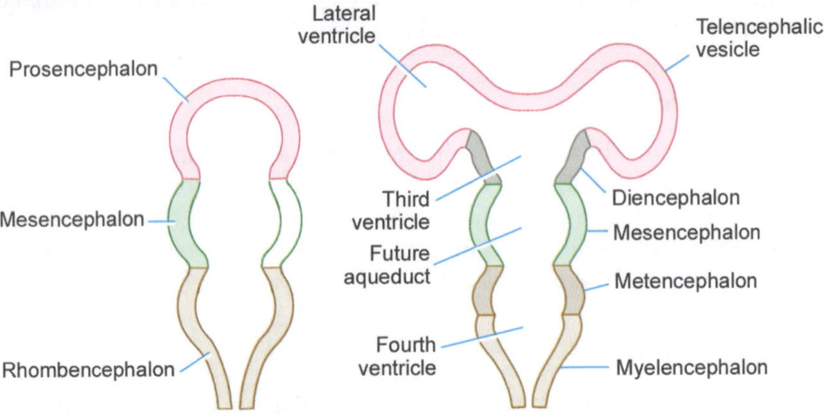

Fig. 23.28 Two stages in the development of the brain.

The developing brain has a series of cavities within it. The cavity of each telencephalic vesicle becomes one ***lateral ventricle.*** The ***third ventricle*** may be regarded as the cavity of the diencephalon. The interventricular foramina connecting the lateral ventricles to the third ventricle represent the sites of the original telencephalic evaginations.

Keeping these facts in mind we may now examine the basic structure of the cerebral hemispheres as seen in a coronal section (Fig. 23.29).

The surface of the cerebral hemisphere is covered by a thin layer of grey matter called the ***cerebral cortex***. The cortex follows the irregular contour of the sulci and gyri of the hemisphere and extends into the depths of the sulci. As a result of this folding of the cerebral surface, the cerebral cortex acquires a much larger surface area than the size of the hemispheres would otherwise allow.

The greater part of the cerebral hemisphere deep to the cortex is occupied by white matter within which are embedded certain important masses of grey matter. Immediately lateral to the third ventricle there are the ***thalamus*** and ***hypothalamus*** (and certain smaller masses) derived from the diencephalon. More laterally there is the ***corpus striatum*** which is derived from the telecephalon. It consists of two masses of grey matter, the ***caudate nucleus*** and the ***lentiform nucleus***. A little lateral to the lentiform nucleus we see the cerebral cortex in the region of the insula. Between the lentiform nucleus and the insula there is a thin layer of grey matter called the ***claustrum.*** The caudate nucleus, the lentiform nucleus, the claustrum and some other masses of grey matter (all of telencephalic origin) are referred to as ***basal ganglia.***

The white matter that occupies the interval between the thalamus and caudate nucleus medially, and the lentiform nucleus laterally, is called the ***internal capsule.*** It is a region of considerable importance as major ascending and descending tracts pass through it. The white matter that radiates from the upper end of the internal capsule to the cortex is called the ***corona radiata.***

The two cerebral hemispheres are interconnected by fibres passing from one to the other. These fibres constitute the ***commissures*** of the cerebrum.

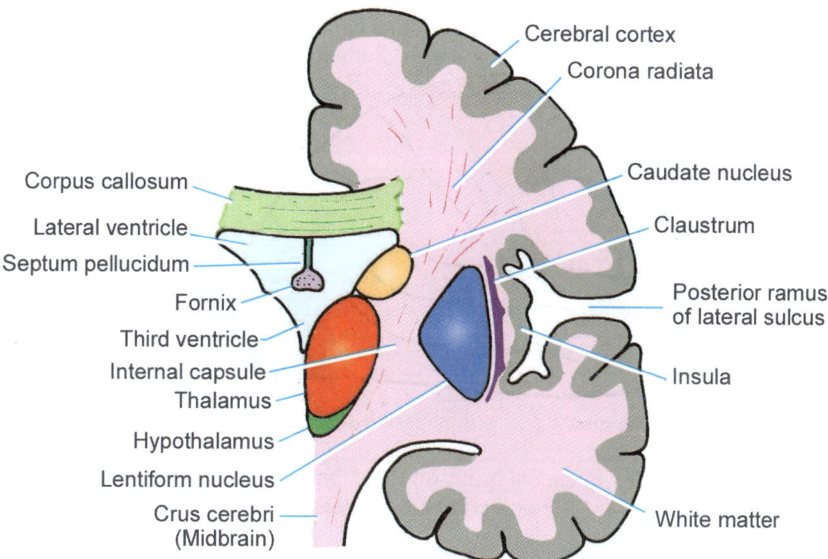

Fig. 23.29 Coronal section through a cerebral hemisphere to show some important masses of grey matter, and some other structures, within it.

The largest of these the ***corpus callosum*** which is seen just above the lateral ventricles in Fig. 23.29.

IMPORTANT FUNCTIONAL AREAS OF THE CEREBRAL CORTEX

Some areas of the cerebral cortex can be assigned specific functions. These areas can be defined in terms of sulci and gyri described in preceding pages.

Motor Area

The motor area is located in the precentral gyrus on the superolateral surface of the hemisphere (Fig. 23.30), and in the anterior part of the paracentral lobule on the medial surface.

Specific regions within the area are responsible for movements in specific parts of the body. Stimulation of the paracentral lobule produces movement in the lower limbs. The trunk and upper limb are represented in the upper part of the precentral gyrus, while the face and head are represented in the lower part of the gyrus.

Premotor Area

The premotor area is located just anterior to the motor area. It occupies the posterior parts of the superior, middle and inferior frontal gyri (Fig. 23.30).

Stimulation of the premotor area results in movements, but these are somewhat more intricate than those produced by stimulation of the motor area.

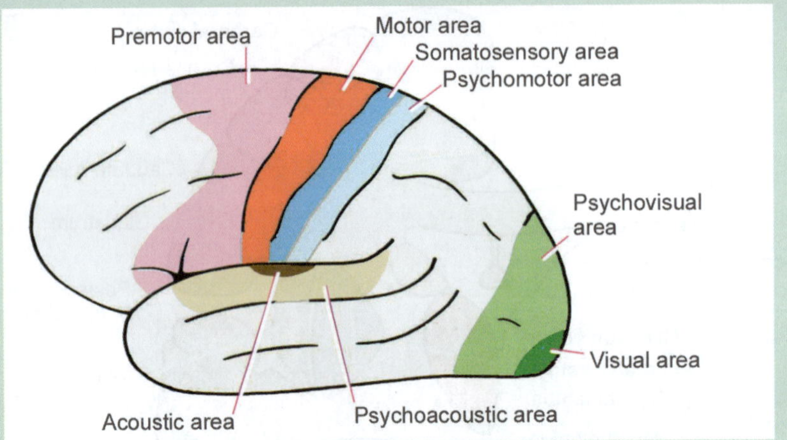

Fig. 23.30 Functional areas on the superolateral aspect of the cerebral hemisphere.

Motor Speech Area

The motor speech area of Broca lies in the inferior frontal gyrus). Injury to this region results in inability to speak (***aphasia***) even though the muscles concerned are not paralysed. These effects occur only if damage occurs in the left hemisphere in right handed persons; and in the right hemisphere in left handed persons. In other words motor control of speech is confined to one hemisphere: that which controls the dominant upper limb.

Sensory Area

The sensory area of classical description is located in the postcentral gyrus (Fig. 23.30). It also extends on to the medial surface of the hemisphere where it lies in the posterior part of the paracentral lobule. Responses can be recorded from the sensory area when individual parts of the body are stimulated. A definite representation of various parts of the body can be mapped out in the sensory area. It corresponds to that in the motor area in that the body is represented upside down.

Visual Areas

The areas concerned with vision are located in the occipital lobe, mainly on the medial surface, both above and below the calcarine sulcus.

Acoustic Area

The acoustic area, or the area for hearing, is situated in the temporal lobe. It lies in that part of the superior temporal gyrus which forms the inferior wall of the posterior ramus of the lateral sulcus.

WHITE MATTER OF CEREBRAL HEMISPHERES

Deep to the cerebral cortex the greater part of each cerebral hemisphere is occupied by nerve fibres that constitute the white matter. These fibres may be:

a. ***Association fibres*** that interconnect different regions of the cerebral cortex.
b. ***Projection fibres*** that connect the cerebral cortex with other masses of grey matter; and ***vice versa.***
c. ***Commissural fibres*** that interconnect identical areas in the two hemispheres.

Association Fibres

These may be short and may connect adjoining gyri. Alternatively, they may be long and may connect distant parts of the cerebral cortex. Some association fibres pass through commissures to connect ***dissimilar*** areas in the two cerebral hemispheres.

Projection Fibres

These fibres connect the cerebral cortex to centres in the brainstem and spinal cord, in both directions. Fibres to the cortex are often referred to as ***corticopetal fibres***, while those going away from the cortex are referred to as ***corticofugal fibres.*** Fibres connecting the cortex with the thalamus, the hypothalamus and the basal ganglia, are also projection fibres. Many of the major projection fibres pass through the internal capsule, which is considered below.

THE INTERNAL CAPSULE

We have seen that a large number of nerve fibres interconnect the cerebral cortex with centres in the brainstem and spinal cord, and with the thalamus. Most of these fibres pass through the interval between the thalamus and caudate nucleus medially, and the lentiform nucleus laterally. This region is called the ***internal capsule.*** Superiorly, the internal capsule is continuous with the corona radiata; and, below, with the crus cerebri (of the midbrain). The internal capsule may be divided into the following parts (Fig. 23.31).

a. The ***anterior limb*** lies between the caudate nucleus medially, and the anterior part of the lentiform nucleus laterally.
b. The ***posterior limb*** lies between the thalamus medially, and the posterior part of the lentiform nucleus on the lateral side.
c. In transverse sections through the cerebral hemisphere the anterior and posterior limbs of the internal capsule are seen to meet at an angle open outwards. This angle is called the ***genu*** (genu = bend).
d. Some fibres of the internal capsule lie behind the posterior end of the lentiform nucleus. They constitute its ***retrolentiform part.***
e. Some other fibres pass below the lentiform nucleus (and not medial to it). These fibres constitute the ***sublentiform part*** of the internal capsule.

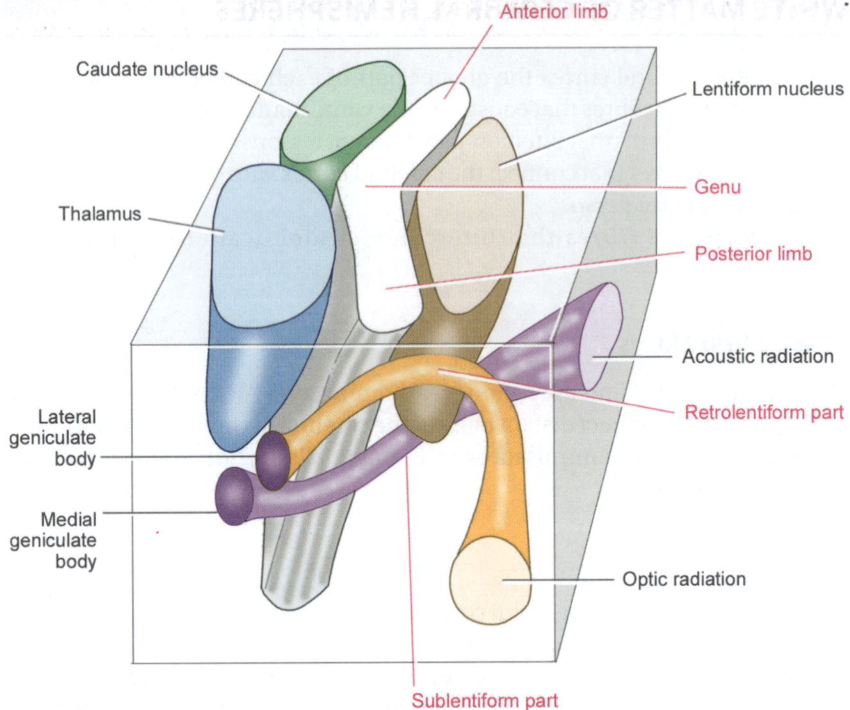

Fig. 23.31 Scheme to show the subdivisions of the internal capsule.

CORPUS CALLOSUM

The corpus callosum is made up of a large mass of nerve fibres that connect the two cerebral hemispheres (Fig. 23.26). It is subdivided into a central part or ***trunk,*** an anterior end that is bent on itself to form the ***genu***, and an enlarged posterior end called the ***splenium.*** A thin lamina of nerve fibres connects the genu to the upper end of the lamina terminalis. These fibres form the ***rostrum*** of the corpus callosum. The corpus callosum is intimately related to the lateral ventricles. Its undersurface gives attachment to the septum pellucidum (Figs. 23.26).

The fibres of the corpus callosum interconnect the corresponding regions of almost all parts of the cerebral cortex of the two hemispheres.

SOME IMPORTANT TRACTS

We have seen that a collection of nerve fibres within the central nervous system, that connects two masses of grey matter, is called a tract. Tracts may be ascending or descending. They are usually named after the masses of grey matter connected by them. Thus a tract beginning in the cerebral cortex and descending to the spinal cord is called the corticospinal tract, while a tract

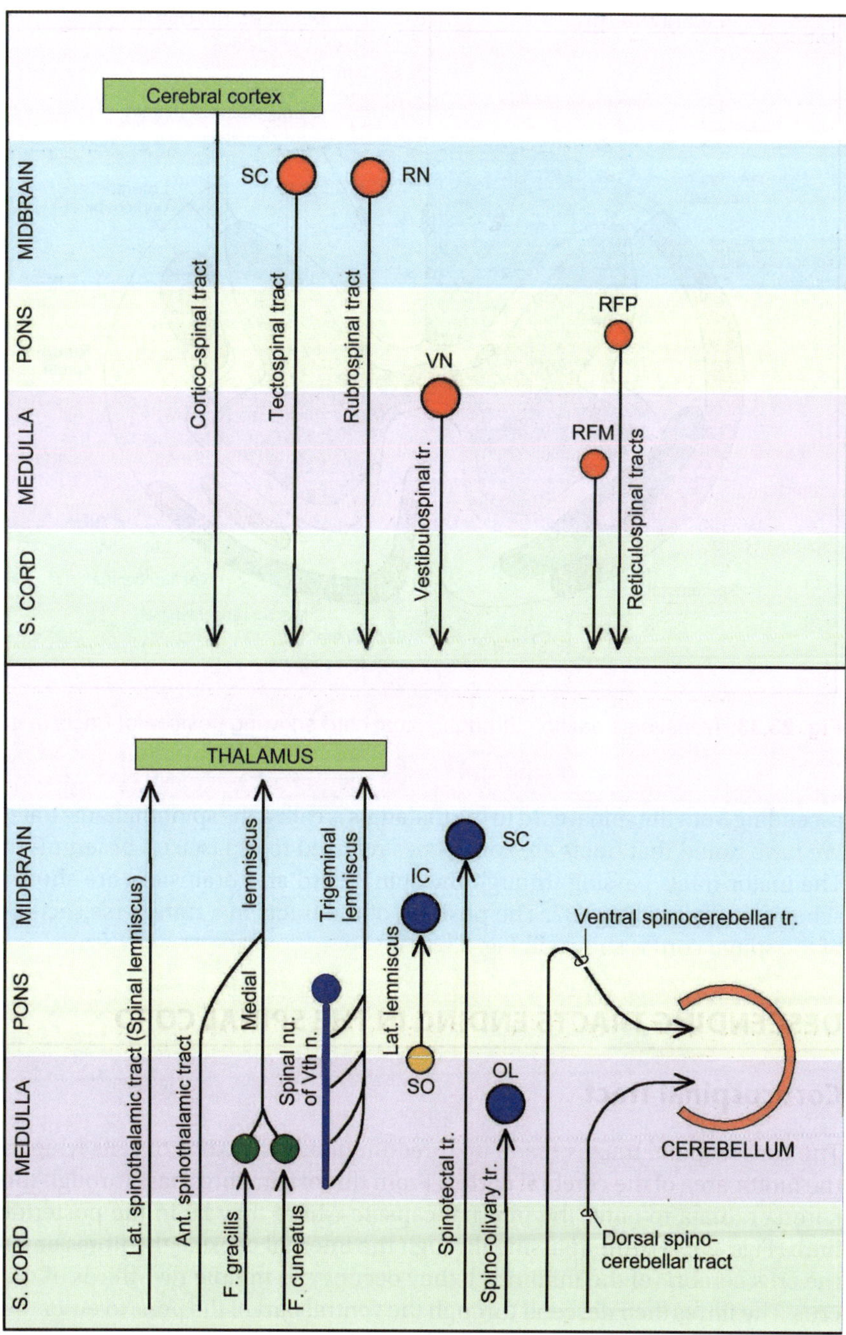

Fig. 23.32 1. Scheme to show the various tracts passing through the brainstem. SC = superior colliculus; RN = red nucleus; VN = vestibular nuclei; OL = inferior olivary nucleus. RFP = reticular formation of pons. RFM = reticular formation of medulla; IC = inferior collicus; SO = superior olivary nucleus.

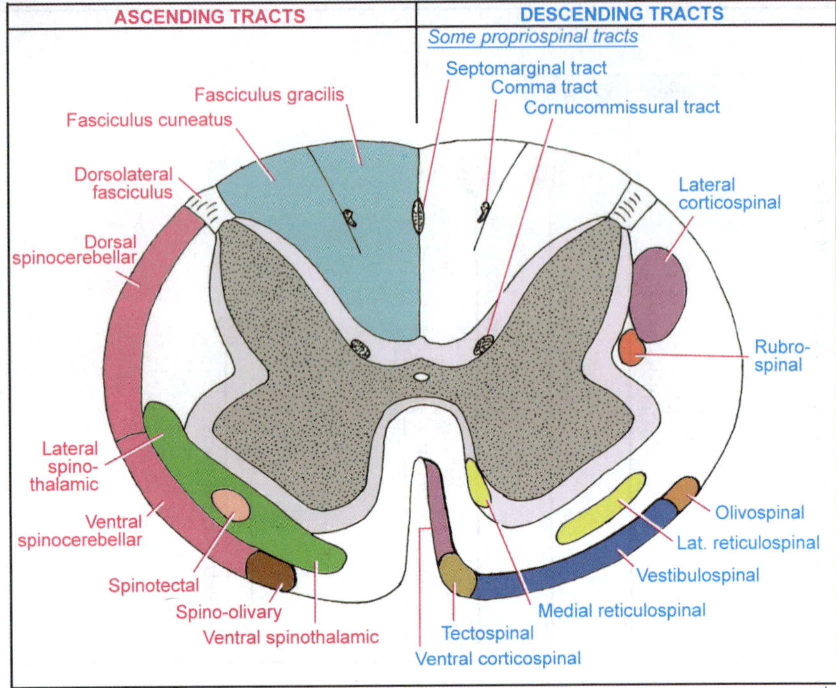

Fig. 23.33 Transverse section through spinal cord showing position of tracts in it.

ascending from the spinal cord to the thalamus is called the spinothalamic tract. We have noted that tracts are sometimes referred to as fasciculi or lemnisci. The major tracts passing through the spinal cord and brainstem are shown schematically in Fig. 23.32. The position of the tracts in a transverse section of the spinal cord is shown in Fig. 23.33A.

DESCENDING TRACTS ENDING IN THE SPINAL CORD

Corticospinal Tract

The corticospinal tract is made up, predominantly, of axons of cells lying in the motor area of the cerebral cortex. From this origin fibres pass through the corona radiata to enter the internal capsule where they lie in the posterior limb (Figs. 23.34). After passing through the internal capsule the fibres enter the crus cerebri (of the midbrain): they occupy the middle two-thirds of the crus. The fibres then descend through the ventral part of the pons to enter the pyramids in the upper part of the medulla. Near the lower end of the medulla about 80 per cent of the fibres cross to the opposite side. (The crossing fibres of the two sides constitute the ***decussation of the pyramids***.)

The fibres that have crossed in the medulla enter the lateral funiculus of the spinal cord and descend as the ***lateral corticospinal tract*** (Fig. 23.33). The fibres of this tract terminate in grey matter at various levels of the spinal cord.

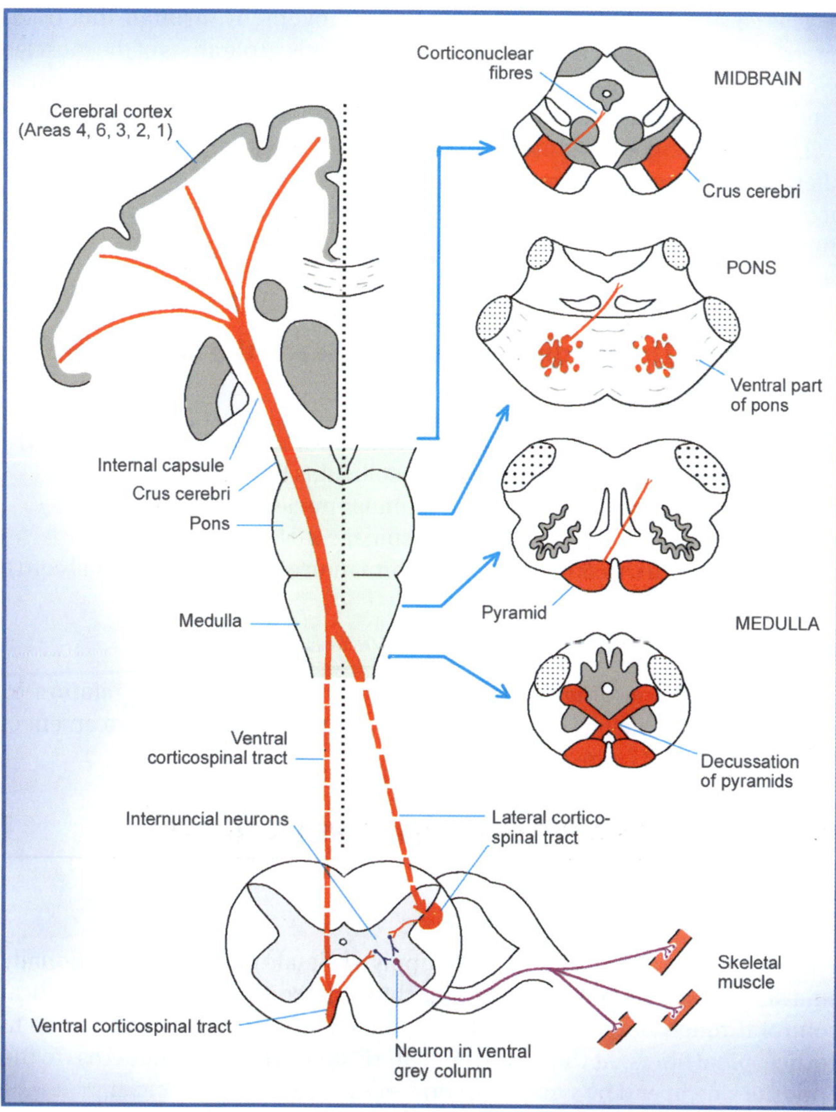

Fig. 23.34 Scheme to show the course of the corticospinal tracts. Note the position of the tracts at various levels of the brainstem.

The fibres end by synapsing with cells in the ventral grey column (directly or through intervening neurons).

The corticospinal fibres that do not cross in the pyramidal decussation enter the anterior funiculus of the spinal cord to form the ***anterior corticospinal tract.*** On reaching the appropriate level of the spinal cord the fibres of this tract cross the middle line to reach grey matter on the opposite side of the cord. Their manner of termination is similar to that of fibres of the lateral corticospinal tract. In this way the corticospinal fibres of both the lateral and anterior tracts ultimately connect the cerebral cortex of one side with ventral column neurons in the opposite half of the spinal cord.

The cerebral cortex controls voluntary movement through this tract. Interruption of the tract anywhere in its course leads to paralysis of the muscles concerned. As the fibres are closely packed in their course through the internal capsule and brainstem small lesions here can cause widespread paralysis.

The neurons that give origin to the fibres of the corticospinal tracts are often referred to as ***upper motor neurons*** in distinction to the ventral column neurons and their processes which constitute the ***lower motor neurons.*** Interruption of either of these neurons leads to paralysis, but the nature of the paralysis is distinctive in each case.

Some Other Descending Tracts That Reach the Spinal Cord

These are (Fig. 23.32):

1. The ***rubrospinal tract*** (from red nucleus in the midbrain to spinal cord).
2. The ***tectospinal tract*** (from superior colliculus to spinal cord).
3. The ***vestibulospinal tract*** (from vestibular nuclei to spinal cord).
4. The ***olivospinal tract*** (from olive to spinal cord).
5. ***Reticulospinal tracts*** (from reticular formation of brainstem to spinal cord).

Significance of Descending Tracts

The various descending tracts mentioned above, that end in relation to ventral column neurons, influence their activity, and thereby have an effect on contraction and tone of skeletal muscle.

DESCENDING TRACTS ENDING IN THE BRAINSTEM

Corticonuclear Tracts

The nuclei of cranial n⊠erves that supply skeletal muscle are functionally equivalent to ventral column neurons of the spinal cord. They are under cortical control through fibres that are closely related in their origin and course to corticospinal fibres. At various levels of the brainstem these fibres cross to the opposite side to end by synapsing with cells in cranial nerve nuclei.

Cortico-ponto-cerebellar Pathway

Fibres arising in the cerebral cortex of the frontal, temporal, parietal and occipital lobes descend through the corona radiata and internal capsule to reach the crus cerebri. These fibres enter the ventral part of the pons to end in pontine nuclei of the same side.

Axons of neurons in the pontine nuclei form the transverse fibres of the pons. These fibres cross the middle line and pass into the middle cerebellar peduncle of the opposite side. The fibres of this peduncle reach the cerebellar cortex.

The cortico-ponto-cerebellar pathway forms the anatomical basis for control of cerebellar activity by the cerebral cortex.

ASCENDING TRACTS

Introductory Remarks

The ascending tracts of the spinal cord and brainstem represent one stage of multineuron pathways by which afferent impulses arising in various parts of the body are conveyed to different parts of the brain. The ***first order neurons*** of these pathways are usually located in spinal (dorsal nerve root) ganglia. We have seen that the neurons in these ganglia are unipolar. Each neuron gives off a peripheral process and a central process. The peripheral processes of the neurons form the afferent fibres of peripheral nerves. They end in relation to sensory end organs (receptors) situated in various tissues. The central processes of these neurons enter the spinal cord through the dorsal nerve roots. Having entered the cord the central processes, as a rule, terminate by synapsing with cells in spinal grey matter. Some of them may run upwards in the white matter of the cord to form ascending tracts (Fig. 23.35). The majority of ascending tracts are, however, formed by axons of cells in spinal grey matter. These are ***second order*** sensory neurons (Fig. 23.37). In the case of pathways that convey sensory information to the cerebral cortex the second order neurons end by synapsing with neurons in the thalamus. ***Third order*** sensory neurons located in the thalamus carry the sensations to the cerebral cortex.

The Posterior Column — Medial Lemniscus Pathway

Fasciculus Gracilis and Fasciculus Cuneatus

These tracts occupy the posterior funiculus of the spinal cord and are, therefore, often referred to as the ***posterior column tracts*** (Fig. 23.33). They are formed predominantly by central processes of neurons located in dorsal nerve root ganglia i.e., by first order sensory neurons (Fig. 23.35). The fibres of these fasciculi extend upwards as far as the lower part of the medulla. Here the fibres of the gracile and cuneate fasciculi terminate by synapsing with neurons in the nucleus gracilis and nucleus cuneatus respectively.

Medial Lemniscus

The neurons of the gracile and cuneate nuclei are second order sensory neurons. Their axons run forwards and medially (as ***internal arcuate fibres***) to cross the middle line. The crossing fibres of the two sides constitute the ***sensory decussation.*** Having crossed the middle line, the fibres turn upwards to form a prominent bundle called the ***medial lemniscus*** (Fig. 23.35). The medial lemniscus runs upwards through the medulla, pons and midbrain to end in the thalamus (ventral posterolateral nucleus).

(c) Third order sensory neurons located in the thalamus give off axons that pass through the internal capsule and the corona radiata to reach the somatosensory areas of the cerebral cortex.

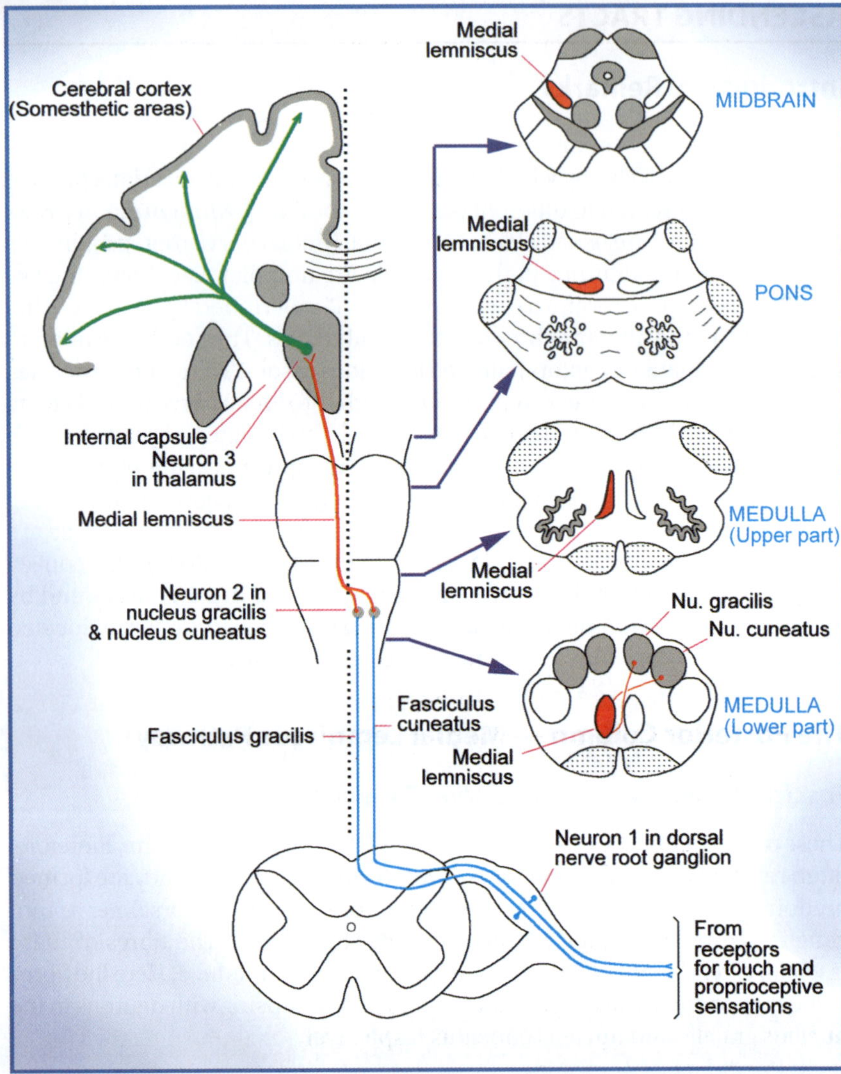

Fig. 23.35 Scheme to show the main features of the posterior column - medial lemniscus pathway. Note the position of the medial lemniscus at various levels of the brainstem.

The pathway described above carries:

1. Some components of the sense of touch. These include deep touch and pressure, the ability to localise exactly the part touched (tactile localisation), the ability to recognise as separate two points on the skin that are touched simultaneously (tactile discrimination), and the ability to recognise the shape of an object held in the hand (stereognosis).
2. Proprioceptive impulses that convey the sense of position and of movement of different parts of the body.
3. The sense of vibration.

Spinothalamic Pathway

a. The first order neurons of this pathway are located in spinal ganglia. The central processes of these neurons enter the spinal cord and terminate in relation to spinal grey matter (Fig. 23.36).
b. The second order neurons of this pathway are located in the spinal grey matter. The axons of these neurons constitute the anterior and lateral spinothalamic tracts. They ascend through the medulla, pons and midbrain to end in the thalamus.

Other Ascending Tracts

1. The ***spinotectal tract*** connects the spinal grey matter to the superior colliculus. It carries impulses that regulate reflex movements of the head and eyes in response to stimulation of some parts of the body.
2. The ***spino-olivary tract*** is carries proprioceptive impulses to olivary nuclei. The tract may also carry exteroceptive impulses.

SPINOCEREBELLAR PATHWAYS

These pathways carry proprioceptive impulses arising in muscles and tendons to the cerebellum.
a. The first order neurons of these pathways are located in dorsal nerve root ganglia. They end in spinal grey matter.
b. The second order neurons of the pathway begin in spinal grey matter. They run up the spinal cord as spinocerebellar tracts (ventral and dorsal).

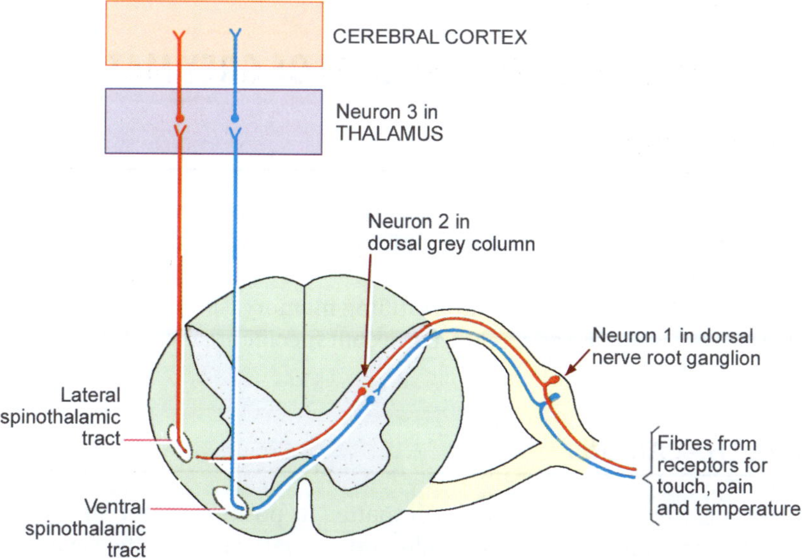

Fig. 23.36 Scheme to illustrate the main features of the spinothalamic tracts.

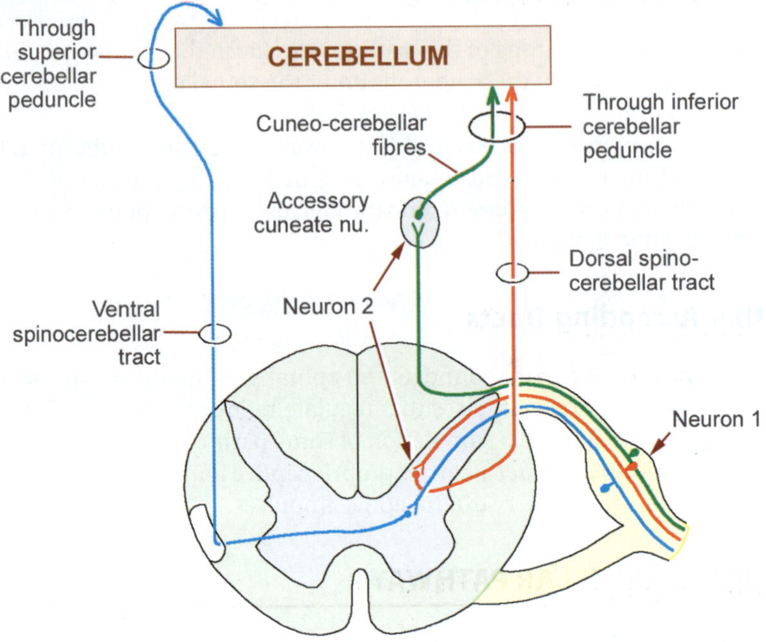

Fig. 23.37 Scheme to illustrate the main features of spinocerebellar pathways.

The ***dorsal spinocerebellar tract*** passes through the inferior cerebellar peduncle to reach the cerebellum (Fig. 23.37). The ***ventral (anterior) spinocerebellar tract*** ascends to the pons. Here it enters the superior cerebellar peduncle to reach the cerebellum.

SOME IMPORTANT MASSES OF GREY MATTER

THE CEREBRAL CORTEX

The most important grey matter in the brain is the *cerebral cortex* which has already been considered. The various functional area and their functions have been considered.

Higher functions of the brain including memory, speech and intelligence are also controlled by the cerebral cortex but specific areas cannot be assigned to these functions.

THE THALAMUS

The thalamus is a large mass of grey matter. Its position is seen in Fig. 23.38. The thalami of the right and left sides are separated only by the cavity of the third ventricle. The upper surface of the thalamus lies in the floor of the lateral ventricle. Lateral to the thalamus we see the internal capsule.

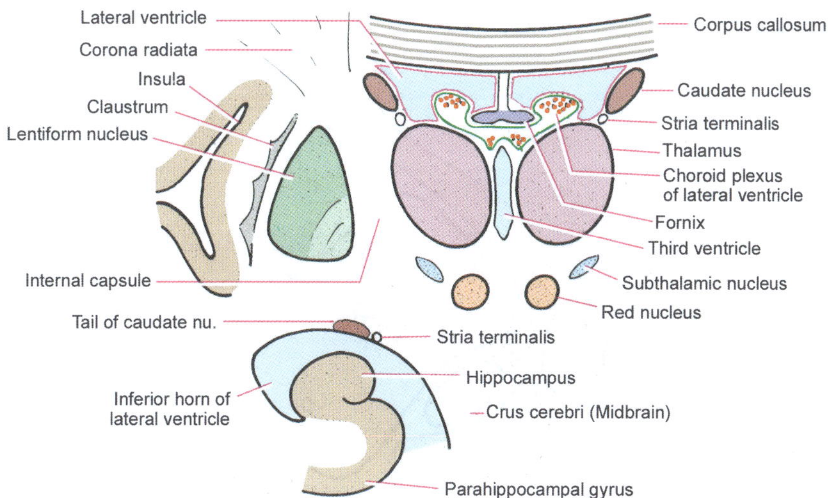

Fig. 23.38 Coronal section through the cerebrum to show structures related to the thalamus.

The thalamus receives the terminations of major sensory pathways ascending from the spinal cord and brainstem. These include the medial lemniscus, and the spinothalamic tracts. The sensations are relayed to the sensory areas of the cerebral cortex.

Medial and Lateral Geniculate Bodies

Lying below the posterior part of the thalamus there are the medial and lateral geniculate bodies. Earlier they were considered to be independent structures but they are now regarded as parts of the thalamus. The ***medial geniculate body*** is a relay station on the pathway of hearing. The ***lateral geniculate body*** is a relay station on the pathway of vision (Fig. 23.39).

Functions of the Thalamus

1. The thalamus receives somatic sensory inputs from various parts of the body. These include sensations of touch, pain and temperature, and proprioceptive sensations from muscles, joints and tendons. The thalamus also receives sensations from viscera, from special sense organs of vision hearing and of taste. It relays all these to the cerebral cortex.
2. Apart from being a great relay station the thalamus is believed to have some degree of ability to perceive some exteroceptive sensations, specially pain.

THE HYPOTHALAMUS

The hypothalamus lies immediately below the thalamus. It is one of the most important parts of the brain being responsible for control of numerous functions that are vital for the survival of an animal as described below.

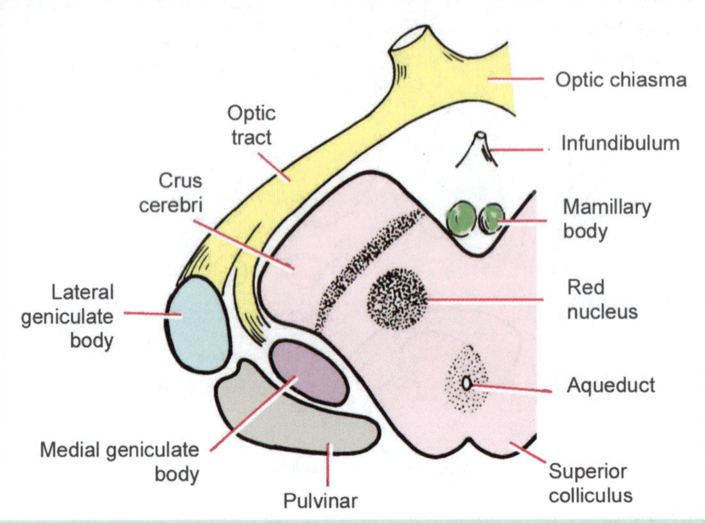

Fig. 23.39 Diagram to show the location of the medial and lateral geniculate bodies.

Functions of the Hypothalamus

The hypothalamus plays an important role in the control of many functions that are vital for the survival of an animal. In exercising such control the hypothalamus acts in close coordination with higher centres including the limbic system and the prefrontal cortex, and with autonomic centres in the brainstem and spinal cord. The main functions attributed to the hypothalamus are as follows.

Regulation of Eating and Drinking Behaviour

The hypothalamus is responsible for feelings of hunger and of satiety, and this determines whether the animal will accept or refuse food. It is also responsible for thirst and drinking. A ***feeding centre***, and a ***satiety centre*** have been described in it.

Correlate this with the fact that some neurons in the hypothalamus are sensitive to osmolarity (preoptic nucleus), glucose content and fatty acid content of blood.

Regulation of Sexual Activity and Reproduction

The hypothalamus controls sexual activity, both in the male and female. It also exerts an effect on gametogenesis, on ovarian and uterine cycles, and on the development of secondary sexual characters. These effects are produced by influencing the secretion of gonadotropic hormones by the hypophysis cerebri.

Control of Autonomic Activity

The hypothalamus exerts an important influence on the activity of the autonomic nervous system, and thus has considerable effect on cardiovascular, respiratory and alimentary functions.

Emotional Behaviour

The hypothalamus has an important influence on emotions like fear, anger and pleasure. Stimulation of some areas of the hypothalamus produces sensations of pleasure, while stimulation of other regions produces pain or other unpleasant effects.

Control of Endocrine Activity

The influence of the hypothalamus in the production of hormones by the pars anterior of the hypophysis cerebri, and the elaboration of oxytocin and the antidiuretic hormone by the hypothalamus itself, have been described above. Through control of the adenohypophysis, the hypothalamus indirectly influences the thyroid gland, the adrenal cortex, and the gonads.

Response to Stress

Through control over the autonomic nervous system, and hormones, the hypothalamus plays a complex role in the way a person responds to stress.

Temperature Regulation

Some neurons in the hypothalamus act as a thermostat to control body temperature. When body temperature rises or falls, appropriate mechanisms are brought into play to bring the temperature back to normal.

Biological Clock

Several functions of the body show a cyclic variation in activity, over the twentyfour hours of a day. The most conspicuous of these is the cycle of sleep and waking. Such cycles (called ***circadian rhythms***) are believed to be controlled by the hypothalamus, which is said to function as a biological clock.

CORPUS STRIATUM

The ***caudate nucleus*** and the ***lentiform nucleus*** are closely related to the internal capsule and the thalamus (Figs. 23.40, 23.41). They are also closely related to the lateral ventricle. The two nuclei together form the ***corpus striatum***. Dopamine is important in functioning of the corpus striatum.

The corpus striatum plays an important role in control of motor activity. It is important in maintaining muscle tone and body posture.

Degenerative changes in the corpus striatum lead to ***Parkinsonism***, in which the body becomes rigid and movements become very difficult. Characteristic involuntary movements of the hands are often present.

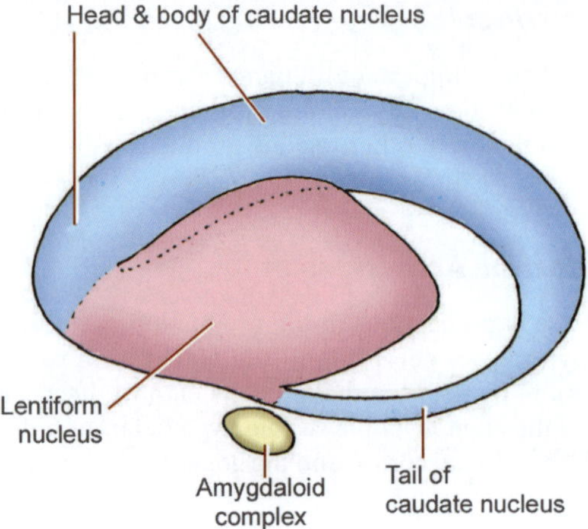

Fig. 23.40 The corpus striatum viewed from the lateral aspect.

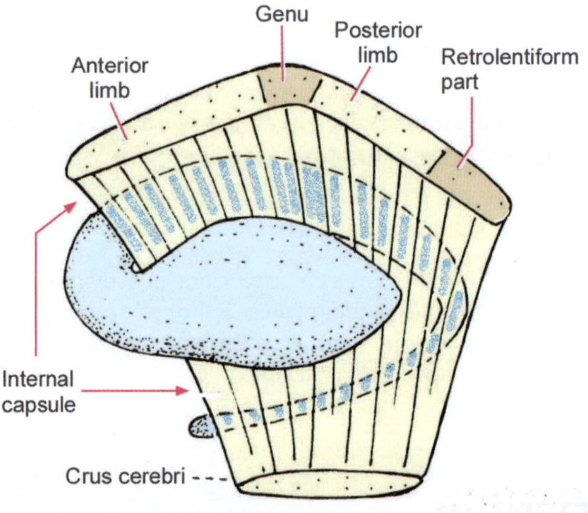

Fig. 23.41 Relationship of the corpus striatum to the internal capsule (viewed from the lateral side).

THE VENTRICLES OF THE BRAIN

The interior of the brain contains a series of cavities (Fig. 23.42). The cerebrum contains a median cavity, the ***third ventricle***, and two ***lateral ventricles***, one in each cerebral hemisphere (right or left) (Fig. 23.43). The lateral ventricle has a complex shape. It has a central part, and three horns: anterior, posterior and inferior. Each lateral ventricle opens into the thirds ventricle through an interventricular foramen. The third ventricle is continuous caudally with the cerebral aqueduct (Fig. 23.44), which passes through the midbrain, and opens into the fourth ventricle. The fourth ventricle is situated dorsal to the pons and medulla, and ventral to the cerebellum (Fig. 23.45). It communicates, inferiorly, with the central canal, which passes through the lower part of the medulla and the spinal cord. The ventricular system is filled with cerebrospinal fluid (CSF). Some additional details about the ventricles can be seen in Figs. 23.43, 23.44 and 23.45.

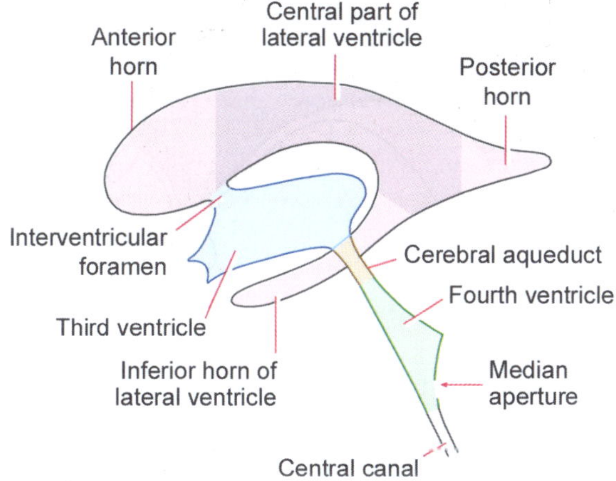

Fig. 23.42 The ventricular system of the brain. Lateral view.

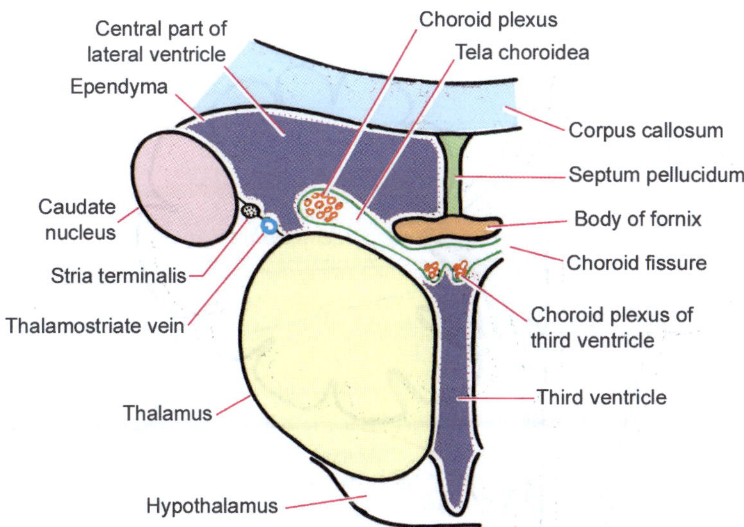

Fig. 23.43 Central part of the lateral ventricle and the third ventricle. Note the structures forming the walls of the ventricles. Note also the relationship of the tela choroidea and choroid plexuses to these ventricles.

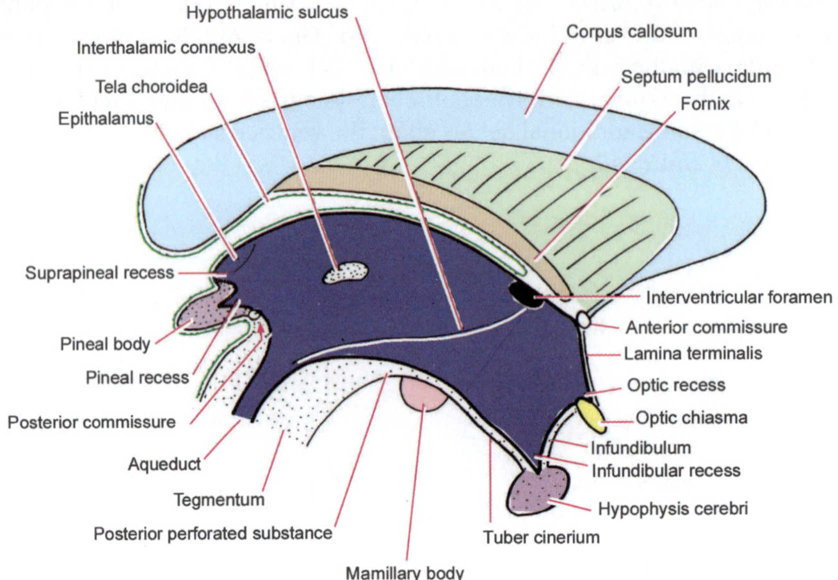

Fig. 23.44 Boundaries and recesses of the third ventricle. Note the mode of formation of the tela choroidea that lies in the roof of the ventricle.

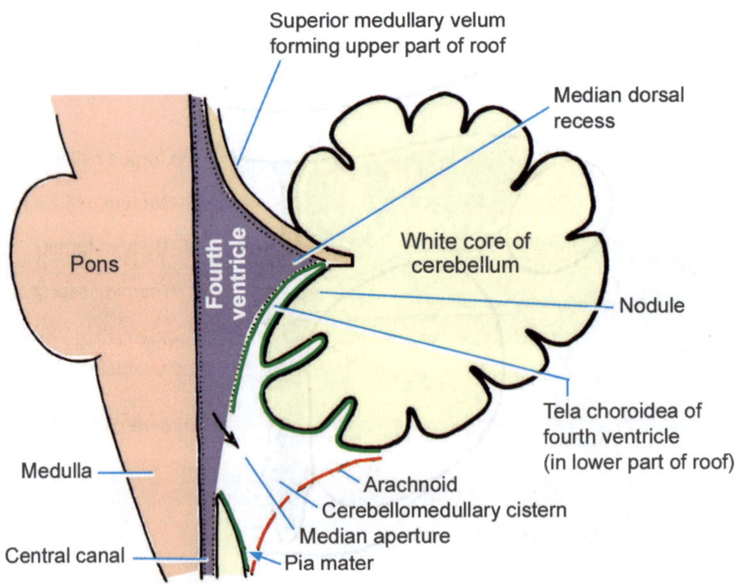

Fig. 23.45 Mid-sagittal section through the fourth ventricle and related structures. The piamater is shown in green.

CEREBROSPINAL FLUID

In addition to the ventricular system, cerebrospinal fluid fills the subarachnoid space which surrounds the brain. The CSF provides a fluid cushion which protects the brain from injury. It also helps to carry nutrition and remove waste products.

CSF is formed in ***choroids plexuses*** present in the ventricles. These are bunches of capillaries. The fluid formed in each lateral ventricle flows into the third ventricle through the interventricular foramen. From the third ventricle it passes through the aqueduct into the fourth ventricle. Here it passes through apertures in the roof of the fourth ventricle to enter the subarachnoid space. CSF is reabsorbed into the circulation through ***arachnoid villi*** present in intracranial venous sinuses.

CSF can be obtained for examination by introducing a needle into the subarachnoid space in the lumbar region. This procedure is called ***lumbar puncture.***

SOME CLINICAL CONSIDERATIONS

Damage to nervous tissue can occur in various ways. Any part of the brain or spinal cord may be damaged by direct injury (***trauma***). Apart from other obvious causes such injury may occur during child birth. We have seen that if nervous tissue is deprived of blood even for a short period irreversible damage may result. Localised damage of this kind may occur if one of the arteries supplying the brain is blocked. This may occur by clotting of blood within the vessel (***thrombosis***). Such an event is more likely in older individuals in whom the arteries have undergone a degenerative change known as ***arteriosclerosis.*** A vessel can also be blocked by some extraneous material (e.g., clot, fat, air) reaching it from some other part of the body through the circulation. Such matter is called an ***embolus.*** Sometimes an artery may rupture, the blood leaking into brain tissue (***haemorrhage***) causing considerable damage. A haemorrhage in the brain is often fatal. Bleeding may be caused by rupture of small abnormal dilatations of arteries (***aneurysms***). Aneurysms may be congenital, or may be produced due to weakening of the arterial wall in the region.

Another cause of brain damage is the presence of any abnormal mass within the cranial cavity. As the cranial cavity cannot expand such a mass inevitably presses on brain tissue. Such a ***space occupying lesion*** may be a tumour, a collection of pus, a collection of blood (in the epidural space) etc. Apart from producing general signs of increased intracranial tension, local effects are produced depending on the area involved.

Increased intracranial tension, specially when it is rapid in progression, can lead to further brain damage in a number of ways. Swelling of the brain (***cerebral oedema***) following trauma, or infection, can itself act like a space occupying lesion. Such oedema can be a result of the breakdown of the blood brain barrier, or because of increased vascular permeability. Initially, space for the expanding contents of the cranial cavity is obtained at the expense of the ventricular system, the CSF being pushed out of the ventricles, and the subarachnoid space. Thereafter, brain tissue is pressed against the wall of the cranial cavity leading to flattening of sulci and gyri. Unequal pressure in different regions can cause brain tissue to herniate in various directions.

Part of the brain may herniate through a wound in the skull. Basal parts of the cerebral hemisphere may herniate into the posterior cranial fossa, and the brainstem can be pushed down into the foramen magnum.

As pressure on a region of brain tissue increases it can lead to occlusion of blood vessels and infarctions. When intracranial pressure increases to the level of arterial pressure, blood flow ceases and brain death ensues.

Nervous tissue may be affected by infections, both acute and chronic. An infection in the brain is referred to as ***encephalitis***; and that in the spinal cord is called ***myelitis.*** Defects in neural tissue may also be caused by ***maldevelopment*** (congenital anomalies), by ***degeneration*** in old age, and by various ***metabolic disorders.*** Finally, alterations in nervous function may occur in the absence of recognisable structural changes. These are called ***functional disorders.***

From the above it will be obvious that in some cases a neurological disorder will be of acute onset (as in trauma, vascular accidents, or acute infections). In such cases the patient may at first show signs indicative of widespread functional deficit quite out of proportion to the actual area involved. Deep unconsciousness (***coma***) is often present. In course of time, however, considerable recovery may take place, leaving residual defects dependent upon the area involved. In slowly developing diseases on the other hand, considerable structural damage may occur before symptoms become obvious. In the descriptions that follow we will deal only with signs and symptoms referable to the actual area of lesion.

DISORDERS OF MOTOR FUNCTION

Inability to move a part of the body is referred to as ***paralysis.*** This can be produced by interruption of motor pathways anywhere between the motor area of the cerebral cortex and the muscles themselves. We have seen that the pathway from cortex to muscle involves at least two neurons. The first of these is located in the cerebral cortex. Its axon terminates in the spinal cord or in motor cranial nerve nuclei in the brainstem. From a physiological and clinical point of view this neuron is referred to as the ***upper motor neuron***. The second neuron is located in the anterior grey column of the spinal cord (or in motor nuclei of the brainstem) and sends out an axon that travels through a peripheral nerve to innervate muscle. This neuron is referred to as the ***lower motor neuron.*** (For the present purpose we may ignore interneurons present in the pathway). When lower motor neurons are destroyed, or their continuity interrupted, the muscles supplied by them lose their tone (i.e., they become flaccid); and in course of time the muscles undergo atrophy. Changes in electrical responses of the muscles also take place. These alterations constitute the ***reaction of degeneration.*** In addition, because of interruption of the efferent part of reflex pathways tendon reflexes are abolished.

Destruction or interruption of the upper motor neuron is not followed by any of these changes. On the other hand it is usually accompanied by an increase in muscle tone, and exaggeration of tendon reflexes. It is, therefore, possible to distinguish between an upper motor neuron paralysis (often called ***spastic paralysis***) and a lower motor neuron (or ***flaccid***) paralysis. Paralysis may be confined to one limb (***monoplegia***) or to both limbs on one side of the body (***hemiplegia***). Paralysis of both lower limbs is called ***paraplegia,*** and that of all four limbs is called ***quadriplegia.*** Paralysis of muscles supplied by one or more cranial nerves may occur in isolation, or in combination with hemiplegia. Destruction of a particular region often destroys lower motor neurons situated at that level resulting in a localised flaccid paralysis of muscles supplied from that level. This lesion may at the same time interrupt descending tracts (representing upper motor neurons), resulting in a spastic paralysis below the level of the lesion. The presence of a localised flaccid paralysis can thus serve as a pointer to the level of lesion.

It is also important to remember that the fibres of upper motor neurons meant for the limbs cross the midline in the lower part of the medulla (in the decussation of the pyramids); and those for the cranial nerves cross just above the level of their termination. A lesion above the level of crossing produces a paralysis in the opposite half of the body, and a lesion below this level produces paralysis on the same side.

Keeping the considerations discussed above in mind we may now consider the effects of lesions of the motor pathways at various levels.

1. Because of the large extent of the ***motor areas of the cerebral cortex*** lesions here produce a relatively localised paralysis e.g., a monoplegia.
2. A lesion in the ***internal capsule*** is capable of producing widespread paralysis on the opposite half of the body (hemiplegia) which may also involve the lower part of the face and the tongue. (The cranial nerves having a bilateral corticonuclear supply are spared). A lesion in the internal capsule is most likely to result from thrombosis or rupture of one of the arteries supplying the capsule. The artery most often involved is Charcot's artery of cerebral haemorrhage.
3. Lesions of corticospinal fibres at various levels in the ***brainstem***, above the level of the pyramidal decussation, can produce contralateral hemiplegia. Involvement of motor cranial nerve nuclei (or of fibres arising from them) may result in various combinations. For example a lesion in the upper part of the midbrain can produce a paralysis of muscles supplied by the oculomotor nerve on the side of lesion, along with a hemiplegia on the opposite side (***Weber's syndrome***). A similar lesion in the pons, results in a paralysis of the lateral rectus muscle (abducent nerve) on the side of lesion with hemiplegia on the opposite side (***Raymond's syndrome***). Alternatively, facial paralysis of one side can be combined with contralateral hemiplegia (***Millard Gubler syndrome***). Various such combinations may result depending on the level of lesion. (Also see medial and lateral medullary syndromes).
4. Lesions affecting the lateral corticospinal tract in the spinal cord produce an upper motor neuron paralysis of muscles on the same side of the body. Lesions above the fifth cervical segment result in paralysis of both upper and lower extremities; while lesions below the first thoracic segment affect only the lower limbs. As in the brainstem, lesions in the spinal cord may be bilateral. Involvement of lower motor neurons at the level of lesion produces a flaccid paralysis of muscles supplied from that level, along with spastic paralysis below the level of injury.

   In some diseases (e.g., ***poliomyelitis***) damage may be confined to lower motor neurons, and the resulting paralysis may be purely flaccid.

DISORDERS OF EQUILIBRIUM

We have seen that the maintenance of equilibrium, and of correct posture, is dependent on reflex arcs involving various centres including the spinal cord, the cerebellum, and the vestibular nuclei. Afferent impulses for these reflexes are carried by the posterior column tracts (fasciculus gracilis and fasciculus cuneatus), the spinocerebellar tracts, and others. Efferents reach neurons of the ventral grey column (anterior horn cells) through rubrospinal, vestibulospinal, and other 'extrapyramidal' tracts. Interruption of any of these pathways; or lesions in the cerebellum, the vestibular nuclei and other centres concerned; can result in various abnormalities involving maintenance of posture and coordination of movements.

Inability to maintain the equilibrium of the body, while standing, or while walking, is referred to as ***ataxia.*** This may occur as a result of the interruption of afferent proprioceptive pathways (***sensory ataxia***). Disease of the cerebellum itself, or of efferent pathways, results in more severe disability. Coordination of the activity of different groups of muscles is interfered with, leading to various defects. The person is unable to stand with his feet close together: the body sways from side to side and the person may fall. While walking, the patient staggers and is unable to maintain progression in the desired direction. Lack of proprioceptive information can be compensated to a considerable extent by information received through the eyes. The defects mentioned are, therefore, much more pronounced with the eyes closed (***Romberg's sign***). Lack of coordination of muscles also interferes with purposeful movements (***asynergia***). Movements are jerky and lack precision. For example, the patient finds it difficult to touch his nose with a finger, or to move a finger along a line. There is difficulty in performing movements involving rapid alternating action of opposing groups of muscles (e.g., tapping one hand with the other; repeated pronation and supination of the forearm). This phenomenon is called ***dysdiadokokinesis.*** Incoordination of the muscles responsible for the articulation of words leads to characteristic speech defects (***dysarthria***). For the same reason, the eyes are unable to fix the gaze on an object for any length of time. Attempts to bring the gaze back to the same point result in repeated jerky movements of the eyes. This is called ***nystagmus.***

Apart from incoordination, cerebellar disease is characterised by diminished muscle tone (***hypotonia***). The muscles are soft, and tire easily (***asthenia***). Joints may lack stability (***flail joints***). Tendon reflexes may be diminished. Alternatively, tapping a tendon may result in oscillating movements of the part concerned, like a pendulum.

ABNORMAL MOVEMENTS

Various kinds of abnormal movements are seen in neurological disorders involving the basal nuclei (basal ganglia), the subthalamic nucleus and the cerebellum. These may take the form of involuntary shaking (***tremor***) of the hands, head or other parts of the body, because of rapid alternating contraction of opposing groups of muscles. In some instances the tremor comes on when the patient tries to perform voluntary movement (***intention tremor***). Intention tremor is seen in disorders of the cerebellum.

In many cases, abnormal movements are accompanied by rigidity of muscles, because of increased muscle tone. The increased tone is also a release phenomenon. One common syndrome marked by rigidity and abnormal movements is called ***Parkinsonism*** or ***paralysis agitans*** (shaking palsy). It is characterised by marked rigidity that leads to a stooped posture, a slow shuffling gait, difficulty in speech, and a mask-like face. Characteristic involuntary 'pill-rolling' movements of the hands are seen. The condition is believed to be due to degenerative changes in the striatum and the substantia nigra.

SENSORY DISORDERS

Interruption of ascending pathways carrying various sensations results in loss of sensory perception (***anaesthesia***) over parts of the body concerned. In case of peripheral nerves the area of anaesthesia following injury is often much less than the area of distribution of the nerve. This is so because of considerable overlap in the areas supplied by different nerves. The area of skin supplied from one spinal segment is called a ***dermatome.*** Dermatomes for adjoining segments overlap, a given area of skin being innervated by two or more segments.

In the case of spinal cord lesions, the level of disease can be inferred from the level of sensory loss. In this connection it must be remembered that the finer modalities of touch are carried by the posterior column tracts which are uncrossed. Crude touch, pain and temperature are carried by the spinothalamic tracts which are crossed. Thus a unilateral lesion in the spinal cord can result in loss of the power of tactile localisation, tactile discrimination and of stereognosis on the side of lesion; with loss of crude touch, pain and temperature on the opposite side.

In a disease called ***syringomyelia***, the region of the spinal cord near the central canal undergoes degeneration with formation of cavities. Fibres of spinothalamic tracts crossing in this region are interrupted. Sensations of pain and temperature are lost over the part of the skin from which fibres are interrupted, but touch is retained as there is an additional pathway for it through the posterior column tracts. This phenomenon is called ***dissociated anaesthesia.***

Sensory disturbances can also result from lesions in the brainstem because of damage to the medial lemniscus or to the spinal and trigeminal lemnisci. Lesions of the thalamus can produce bizarre sensory disturbances. Lesions in the internal capsule can cause sensory loss in the entire opposite half of the body as thalamocortical fibres pass through this region. Pressure on sensory areas of the cerebral cortex can result in various abnormal sensations, or in anaesthesia over certain regions. Damage to pathways carrying special sensations of smell, vision and hearing can result in various defects.

REFERRED PAIN

It sometimes happens that when one of the viscera is diseased pain is not felt in the region of the organ itself, but is felt in some part of the skin and body wall. This phenomenon is called ***referred pain.*** This pain is usually (but not always) referred to areas of skin supplied by the same spinal segments which innervate the viscus. Some classical examples of referred pain are as follows.

1. Pain arising in the diaphragm, or diaphragmatic pleura, is referred to the shoulder (C4).
2. Pain arising in the heart is referred to the lower cervical and upper thoracic segments. It is felt in the chest wall and along the medial side of the left arm. It may also be referred to the neck or jaw.
3. Referred pain from the stomach is felt in the epigastrium (T6 to T9); and that from the intestines is felt in the epigastrium and around the umbilicus (T7 to T10). Pain from the ileocaecal region is felt in the right iliac region. Pain from the appendix is felt in the umbilical region.
4. Pain from the gall bladder is referred to the epigastrium. It may also be referred to the back just below the inferior angle of the right scapula.

5. Pain arising in the area of distribution of one division of the trigeminal nerve may be referred along other branches of the same division, or even along branches of other divisions.

SPINAL REFLEXES

We have seen that the nervous system is involved in various types of reflex activity. Many of these reflexes can be demonstrated clinically, and constitute a valuable aid in establishing the integrity of various levels of the nervous system. Some of the reflexes that are used for this purpose are described below.

Myotatic or Stretch Reflexes

Sudden stretching of a muscle (by tapping its tendon) produces reflex contraction of the muscle. The pathway for this reflex involves two neurons only. Stretching of the muscle stimulates proprioceptive nerve endings located in muscle spindles and other receptors. These impulses are carried to the spinal cord by neurons that synapse with motor neurons in the ventral grey columns (Fig. 3.5). Fibres arising from these motor neurons reach the muscle and produce contraction. Stretch reflexes are abolished if any part of the pathway for it (i.e., the reflex arc) is interrupted. Under certain conditions these reflexes may be exaggerated. From a clinical point of view it is important to know the level of the spinal cord at which each reflex is mediated. Some of the important stretch reflexes are described below. The spinal segments concerned are given in brackets.

1. The ***knee jerk*** or ***patellar tendon reflex*** consists of extension of the leg by contraction of the quadriceps when the ligamentum patellae is tapped (L2, L3, L4).
2. The ***ankle jerk*** or ***Achilles tendon reflex*** consists of plantar flexion of the foot on tapping the tendo calcaneus (L5, S1, S2).
3. The ***biceps tendon reflex*** consists of flexion of the forearm on tapping the biceps tendon (C5, C6).
4. The ***triceps tendon reflex*** consists of extension of the forearm on tapping the triceps tendon (C6, C7, C8).
5. The ***supinator jerk*** (or ***radial periosteal reflex***) consists of flexion of the forearm when the distal end of the radius is tapped (C7, C8). Note that the muscle responsible for this reflex is the brachioradialis, not the supinator. It is called the supinator jerk because the brachioradialis was at one time called the supinator longus.
6. The ***wrist tendon reflex*** consists of flexion of the fingers on percussion on wrist tendons (C8, T1).
7. The ***jaw*** or ***masseter reflex*** is a myotatic reflex mediated through the trigeminal nerve (and not through the spinal cord). To elicit this reflex the patient is asked to open the mouth slightly. The examiner places his index finger over the middle of the patient's chin and taps it. This results in bilateral contraction of the masseter and temporalis muscles. Both afferent and efferent components of the reflex arc pass through the mandibular division of the trigeminal nerve, the nuclei concerned being located in the pons.

Superficial Reflexes

Stimulation of skin in certain regions of the body causes contraction of underlying muscles. This occurs reflexly, the reflex being mediated through the spinal cord. Some of these superficial reflexes are described below.

1. The ***abdominal reflexes*** consist of contraction of underlying muscles on stroking the skin of the abdomen in its upper (T6,7), middle (T8,9) and lower (T10 to T12) parts.
2. The ***cremasteric reflex*** consists of elevation of the scrotum on stroking the skin of the medial side of the thigh (T12 to L2).
3. The ***gluteal reflex*** consists of contraction of the glutei on stroking the overlying skin (L4 to S1).
4. The normal ***plantar reflex*** consists of plantar flexion of the toes on stroking the skin of the sole (L5 to S2). When there is an injury to the corticospinal system an abnormal response is obtained. There is extension (dorsiflexion) of the great toe and fanning out of other toes. This response is referred to as ***Babinski's sign.*** Such a response may also be seen in new born infants, and sometimes in sleeping or intoxicated adults.
5. The ***anal reflex*** consists of contraction of the external anal sphincter on stroking the perianal region (S4,5, coccygeal).

THE AUTONOMIC NERVOUS SYSTEM

The autonomic nervous system is responsible for the nerve supply of viscera and blood vessels. It is subdivided into two main parts. These are the ***sympathetic*** and ***parasympathetic*** nervous systems. Both these divisions contain efferent as well as afferent fibres.

The efferent fibres supply smooth muscle throughout the body. The influence of these nerves may be either to cause contraction or relaxation. In a given situation the sympathetic and parasympathetic nerves generally produce opposite effects. For example, sympathetic stimulation causes dilatation of the pupil, whereas parasympathetic stimulation causes constriction. In addition to the supply of smooth muscle, autonomic nerves supply glands: such nerves are described as ***secretomotor***. The secretomotor nerves to almost all glands are parasympathetic. The only exception are the sweat glands which have a sympathetic supply.

The sympathetic nervous system is represented by the right and left sympathetic trunks and their branches. Most parasympathetic fibres travel through the vagus nerves. Some fibres to pelvic viscera arise from sacral segments of the spinal cord. Autonomic fibres pass through a number of plexuses. These include cardiac and oesophageal plexuses present in the thorax, and numerous plexuses present in the abdomen and pelvis.

THE SYMPATHETIC TRUNK

There are two sympathetic trunks, right and left. Each trunk is a long nerve cord placed on either side of the vertebral column and extending from the base of the skull above, to the coccyx below. The trunk bears a number of sympathetic ganglia along its length. The ganglia contain sympathetic neurons.

Basically there is one ganglion corresponding to each spinal nerve, but in many situations the ganglia of adjoining segments fuse so that they appear to be fewer in number than the spinal nerves. The ventral primary ramus of each spinal nerve receives fibres from a sympathetic ganglion through a delicate communication called the ***grey ramus communicans***. In the case of spinal nerves T1 to L2 (or L3) there is, in addition to the grey ramus, a ***white ramus communicans*** through which fibres pass from the spinal nerve to the ganglion. Some sympathetic neurons are also present in autonomic plexuses.

Sympathetic neurons supply:

1. Sweat glands and some smooth muscle present in the skin.
2. Blood vessels.
3. Viscera.

CHAPTER

24

The Eye and Ear

THE EYE

THE EYELIDS AND CONJUNCTIVA

The part of the eye seen on the face consists of a part that is white, and a circular area in front that looks dark. The 'white of the eye' is formed by the outermost coat of the eyeball which is called the ***sclera***. The sclera is lined on the outside by a thin transparent membrane the ***ocular conjunctiva***. The circular dark part in the centre is the ***iris*** that we see through a transparent disc like structure the ***cornea*** which covers it. At the centre of the iris there is an aperture called the ***pupil***. The pupil appears black because the interior of the eye (which we see through the pupil) is dark. When we view the 'eyes' we see only a small part of the eyeball in the interval between the upper and lower eyelids. This interval is called the ***palpebral fissure*** (Fig. 24.1).

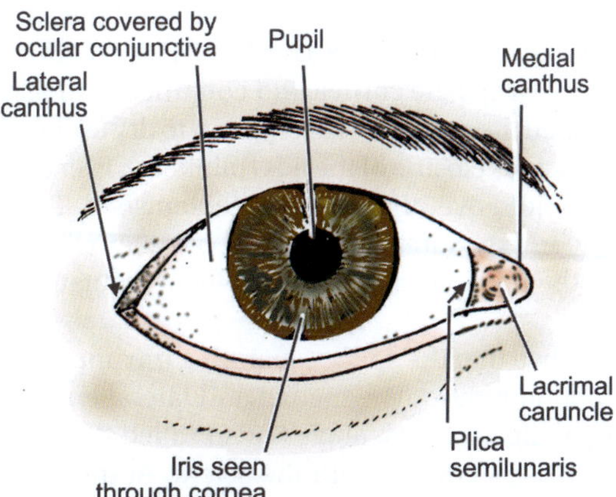

Fig. 24.1 Some features of the eye as seen on the face. The eyelashes are omitted. The interval between the two eyelids is the palpebral fissure.

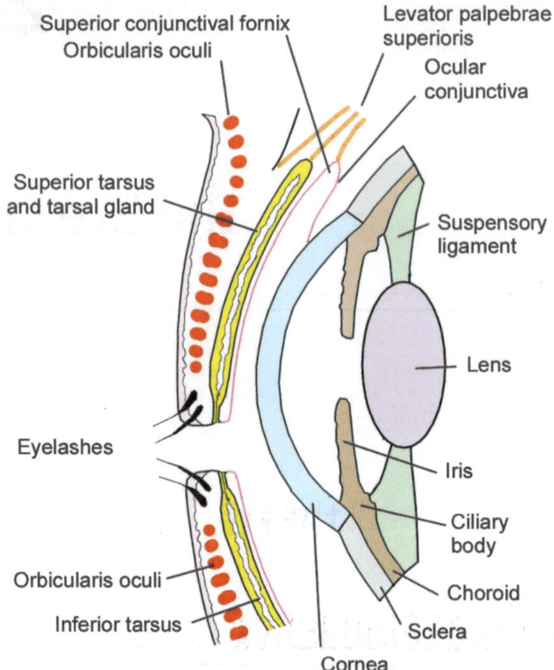

Fig. 24.2 Schematic sagittal section through the eyelids and anterior part of the eyeball.

The upper and lower eyelids (or palpebrae) protect the eyeball, specially the cornea, from injury in several ways.

Firstly, they provide protection against mechanical injury by reflex closure when any object suddenly approaches the eye. The same happens when the cornea is touched (***corneal reflex***).

Secondly, they help to keep the cornea moist as follows: When the eyelids are closed (i.e., when the upper and lower eyelids meet) a capillary space separates the posterior surfaces of the lids from the cornea and the anterior part of the sclera. This space is the ***conjunctival sac*** (Fig. 24.2). It contains a thin film of lacrimal fluid, which keeps the cornea and conjunctiva moist.

With the 'eyes' open the cornea has a tendency to dry up, but this is prevented by periodic, unconscious closure of the lids (blinking). Every time this happens the film of lacrimal fluid over the cornea is replenished. Thirdly, lids protect the eyes from sudden exposure to bright light by reflex closure. In bright light partial closure of the lids may assist the pupils in regulating the light falling on the retina.

We have seen above that the space separating the upper and lower eyelids is called the palpebral fissure. The medial and lateral ends of the fissure are called the ***angles*** of the eye. Each angle is also called the ***canthus*** (Fig. 24.1). The lateral canthus is in contact with the sclera. At the medial canthus the upper and lower lids are separated by a triangular interval called the ***lacus lacrimalis***. In the floor of this area there is a rounded pink elevation called the ***lacrimal caruncle***. Just lateral to the caruncle there is a fold of conjunctiva called the ***plica semilunaris***. Each eyelid has a free edge to which eyelashes are attached. Just lateral to the lacrimal caruncle each lid margin has a slight elevation called the ***lacrimal papilla***. On the summit of the papilla there is a small aperture called the ***lacrimal punctum***. It is important to note that the punctum is normally in direct contact with the ocular conjunctiva.

Each lacrimal punctum opens into a narrow canal that drains, away excessive lacrimal fluid into the ***lacrimal sac***. From here the fluid passes into a duct that opens into the nose (Fig. 24.3).

THE EYEBALL

It is common knowledge that the right and left eyes are the peripheral organs of vision. Each eyeball is like a camera. It has a ***lens*** that produces images of objects that we see. The images fall on a membrane called the ***retina***. Cells in the retina convert the light images into nervous impulses which pass through the optic nerves and other parts of the visual pathway to reach visual areas of the cerebral cortex. It is in the cortex that vision is actually perceived.

The greater part of the eyeball (posterior five sixths) is shaped like a sphere and has a diameter of about 24 mm. The anterior one sixth is much more convex than the posterior part. It represents part of a sphere having a diameter of about 15 mm. In its posterior five sixths the outer wall of the eyeball is formed by a thick white opaque membrane called the ***sclera***. The wall of the anterior one sixth is transparent and is called the ***cornea***.

A horizontal section across an eyeball is shown in Fig. 24.4. Note the following features:

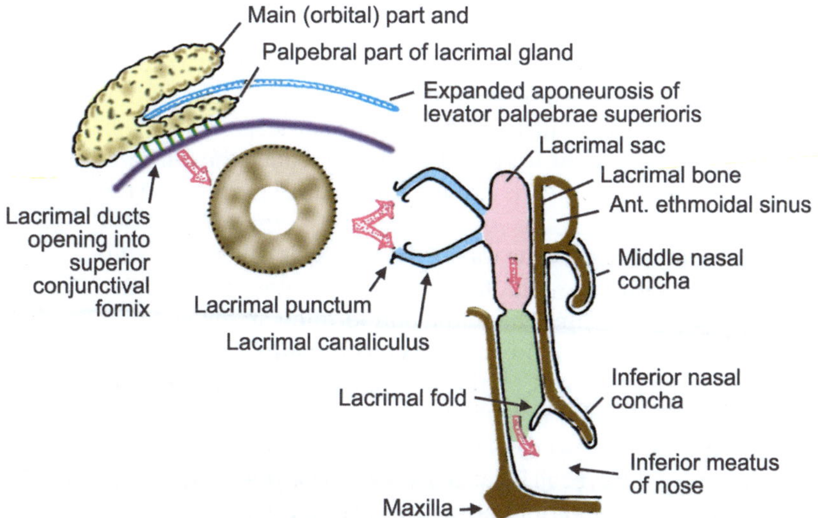

Fig. 24.3 Scheme to show the parts of the lacrimal apparatus. The pink arrows indicate the direction of flow of lacrimal fluid.

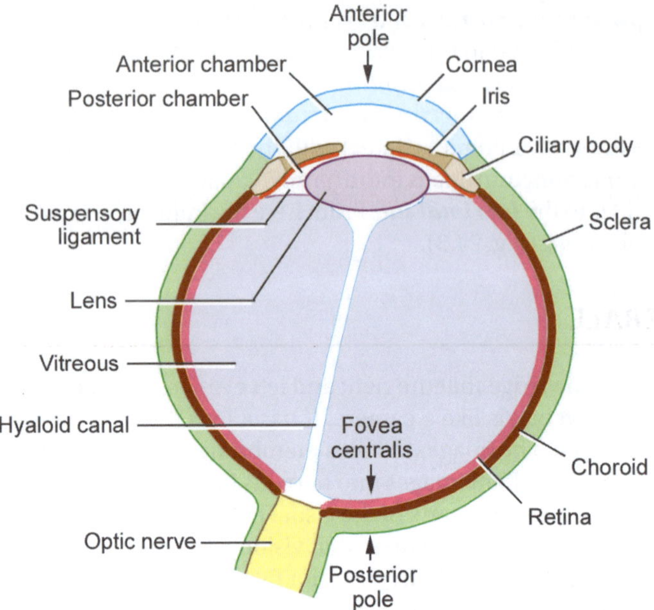

Fig. 24.4 Horizontal section across the eyeball to show the main features of its structure.

The wall of the eyeball is made up of three main layers.

1. The outermost layer is called the ***fibrous coat***. It is formed posteriorly by the sclera; and anteriorly by the cornea.
2. The next layer is the ***vascular coat***. It has the following subdivisions. The part lining the inner surface of most of the sclera is thin and is called the ***choroid***. Near the junction of the sclera with the cornea the vascular coat is thick and forms the ***ciliary body***. The ciliary body is continuous with the ***iris*** which lies a short distance behind the cornea.
   The space between the iris and the cornea is called the ***anterior chamber***. The space between the iris and the front of the lens is called the ***posterior chamber***.
3. The innermost layer of the wall of the eyeball is called the ***retina.***
   Light falling on the retina has to pass through a number of ***refracting media*** before reaching the retina and forming an image on it. These are (a) the cornea; (b) a fluid, the ***aqueous humour***, which fills the anterior and posterior chambers; (c) the lens; and (d) a jelly like ***vitreous body*** that fills the eyeball posterior to the lens.

The centre of the cornea is called the ***anterior pole*** of the eyeball. The opposite end of the eyeball is called the ***posterior pole***. The ***visual axis*** of the eye passes from the anterior pole to the posterior pole.

The Sclera

The sclera is made up mainly of fibrous tissue. Its external surface gives attachment to the extrinsic muscles of the eyeball. Posteriorly, in the region of the attachment of the optic nerve the sclera is perforated like a sieve. This area is called the ***lamina cribrosa***. Bundles of nerve fibres arising in the retina pass through these perforations to form the optic nerve.

Anteriorly, the sclera becomes continuous with the cornea at the ***sclerocorneal junction***. A circular channel called the ***sinus venosus sclerae*** (or ***canal of Schlemm***) is located in the sclera just behind the sclerocorneal junction.

The external surface of the sclera is covered, in its anterior part, by the ocular conjunctiva. The rest of the sclera is in contact with a ***fascial sheath*** that surrounds the eyeball.

The sclera provides a smooth external surface that facilitates movements of the eyeball. This surface also provides attachment to the extrinsic muscles of the eyeball.

The Cornea

The cornea is more convex than the sclera. The junction of the two is marked, on the exterior of the eyeball, by a groove called the ***sulcus sclerae***.

The cornea is made up of five layers that are shown in Fig. 24.5.

Because of its convexity the cornea adds greatly to the refractive power of the eye.

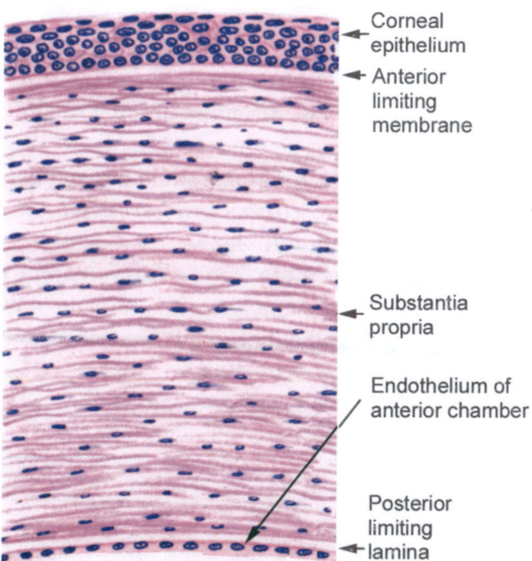

Fig. 24.5 Layers of the cornea.

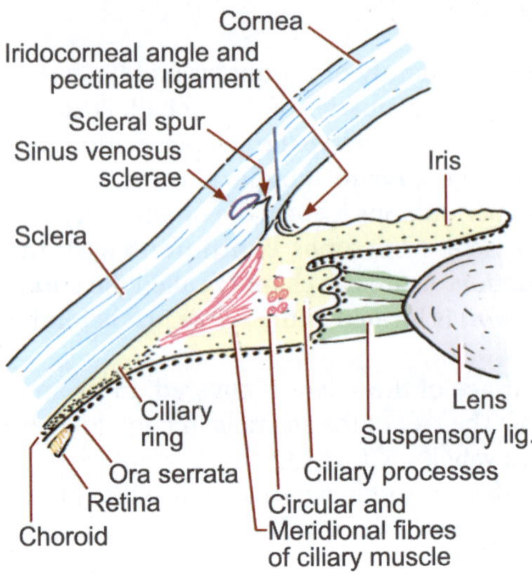

Fig. 24.6 Section through ciliary body and iris.

The Choroid

The choroid consists of a network of blood vessels supported by connective tissue containing many pigmented cells that give it a dark brown colour. It is the dark colour of the choroid that darkens the interior of the eyeball. It also prevents reflection of light within the eyeball. Both these factors are necessary for formation of sharp images on the retina.

The Ciliary Body

The ciliary body represents an anterior continuation of the choroid. Anteriorly, it becomes continuous with the iris. It is made up of vascular tissue, muscle and connective tissue.

The ciliary body can be divided into a posterior part called the ***ciliary ring***, and an anterior part made of the ***ciliary processes*** (Fig. 24.6). The ciliary processes secrete the aqueous humour.

Lateral to the ciliary processes there is the ***ciliary muscle***. Contraction of this muscle relaxes the fibres of the suspensory ligament. Release of tension on the lens makes it more convex and enables it to focus images of near objects on the retina. This is called ***accommodation***.

The ciliary muscle (or ciliaris) is supplied by parasympathetic nerve fibres. The fibres travel to it via the oculomotor nerve and the ciliary ganglion.

The Iris

The iris is the most anterior part of the vascular coat of the eyeball. It forms a diaphragm placed immediately in front of the lens. At its periphery it is continuous with the ciliary body. In its centre there is an aperture, the ***pupil***.

The pupil regulates the amount of light passing into the eye. In bright light the pupil contracts, and in dim light it dilates. In this way the optimum amount of light required for proper vision reaches the retina, within a considerable range in intensity of illumination. Changes in the size of the pupil are produced by the smooth muscle of the iris that consists of two parts.

a. The ***sphincter pupillae*** is a ring of circularly arranged muscle situated just around the pupil. Its contraction narrows the pupil.
b. The ***dilator pupillae*** is in the form of muscle fibres that are arranged radially in the iris. It dilates the pupil.

The sphincter pupillae has a parasympathetic nerve supply (similar to that of the ciliary muscle). The dilator pupillae is innervated by sympathetic nerves.

The Iridocorneal Angle

The angle between the peripheral margins of the iris and of the cornea is a region of importance. In it there are ***spaces of the iridocorneal angle***. These spaces communicate with the anterior chamber, and laterally with the sinus venosus sclerae. Aqueous humour secreted by the ciliary processes passes into the posterior chamber of the eye (i.e., the space between the posterior surface of the iris and the lens). It passes through the pupil into the anterior chamber. From here it filters through the spaces of the iridocorneal angle to enter the sinus venosus sclerae through which it is drained into the veins of the region. With advancing age these spaces may get blocked resulting in increased tension within the eyeball. This disease, called ***glaucoma,*** may have serious consequences.

THE RETINA

The retina has two layers. The outer layer is the ***pigment cell layer*** that is only one cell thick. The second layer is the ***nervous layer***. It is made up of several layers of cells.

The essential features of the structure of the retina are shown in Fig. 24.7. It contains photoreceptors that convert the stimulus of light into nervous impulses. These receptors are of two kinds, ***rods*** and ***cones***. There are about seven million cones in each retina. The rods are far more numerous: they number more than 100 million. The cones respond best to bright light. They are responsible for sharp vision and for discrimination of colour.

Opposite the posterior pole of the eyeball the retina shows a ***central region*** about 6 mm in diameter. This region is responsible for sharp vision. In the centre of this region an area about 2 mm in diameter has a yellow colour and is called the ***macula lutea.***

Each rod or cone consists of a cell body, a peripheral process and a central process. The basic neuronal arrangement within the retina is shown in Fig. 24.7. The central processes of rods and cones synapse with the peripheral processes of ***bipolar cells***. The central processes of bipolar cells synapse with dendrites of ***ganglion cells***. Axons arising from ganglion cells form the ***fibres of the optic nerve.***

We have seen that the optic nerve is attached to the eyeball a short distance medial to the posterior pole. The nerve fibres arising from the ganglion cells all over the retina converge to this region, where they pass through the lamina cribrosa to form the optic nerve. When viewed from the retinal side this region is seen as a circular area called the ***optic disc***. There are no photoreceptors here. The optic disc is, therefore, insensitive to light and is called the ***blind spot***.

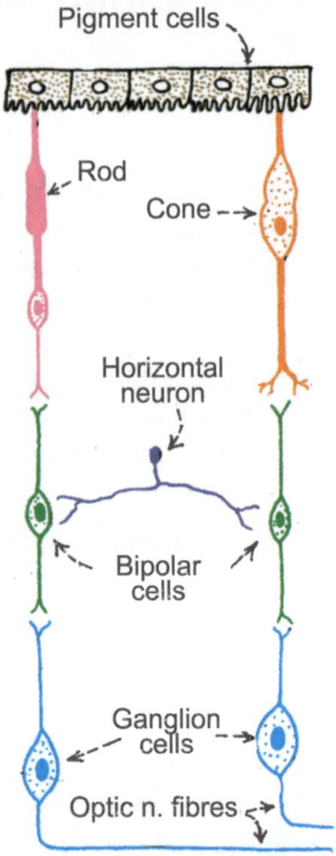

Fig. 24.7 Simplified scheme to show the main elements of the retina.

The Lens

The lens lies in front of the vitreous body and behind the iris. It is surrounded by a capsule. It has convex anterior and posterior surfaces, and a peripheral margin (or equator) to which the suspensory ligament is attached.

The Suspensory Ligament

The suspensory ligament of the lens is made up of fibres passing from the equator of the lens to the ciliary processes.

Changes in the tension on the suspensory ligament, produced by contraction of the ciliary muscle, produce alterations in the convexity of the lens and enable the eye to focus objects at varying distances from the eye.

MUSCLES OF THE ORBIT

The muscles of the orbit include the ***extraocular muscles*** which are the four recti (superior, inferior, medial and lateral), two oblique muscles (superior and inferior), and the levator palpebrae superioris (Fig. 24.8). They are responsible for movements of the eyeball. Two muscles (made up of smooth muscle), the ***sphincter pupillae*** and the ***dilator pupillae*** change the size of the pupil and control the amount of light entering the eye.

Movements of the Eyeball

As a convention movements of the eyeball are described with reference to its anterior end (or more simply, the cornea).

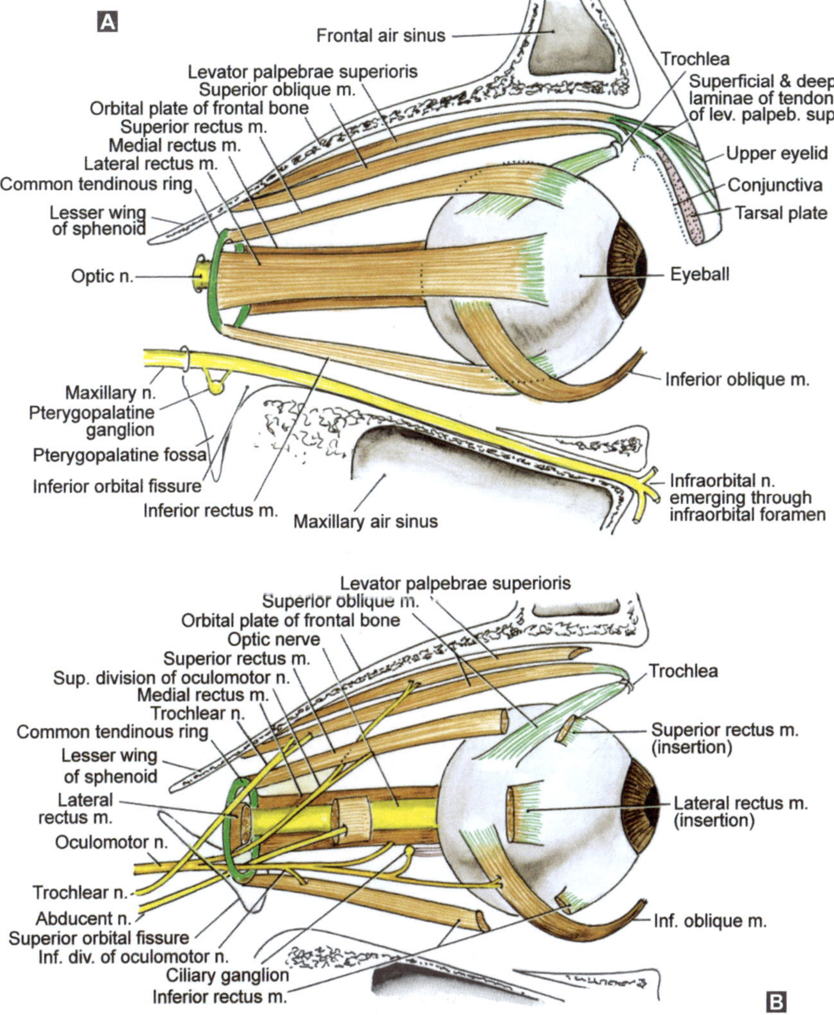

Fig. 24.8 Scheme to show extraocular muscles as seen from the lateral side.

A. The cornea can move upwards or downwards, the movement occurring on an imaginary axis passing transversely through the equator of the eyeball. Upward movement can be produced (a) by pulling the anterior part of the eyeball upwards (superior rectus), or (b) by pulling the posterior part downwards (inferior oblique) (Fig. 24.9). Similarly, downward movement can be produced by (a) pulling the anterior part downwards (inferior rectus) or (b) pulling the posterior part upwards (superior oblique).

B. The cornea can move medially or laterally on an axis passing vertically through the equator of the eyeball. Medial movement of the cornea can be produced by pulling the anterior part of the eyeball medially. This action is

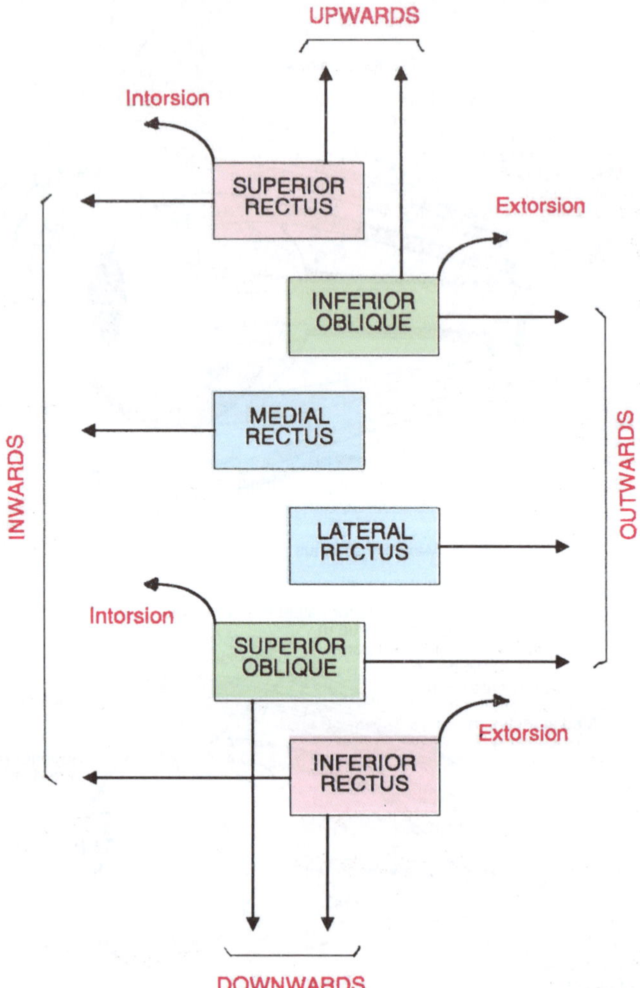

Fig. 24.9 Scheme showing the movements of the eyeball produced by individual extraocular muscles, and the muscles responsible for each movement.

performed by the medial rectus. The superior and inferior recti can also move the cornea medially as they pass forwards and laterally from origin to insertion. Lateral movement can be produced (a) by pulling the anterior part of the eyeball laterally (lateral rectus) or (b) by pulling the posterior part medially (superior and inferior oblique).

Nerve Supply of Muscles of the Eyeball

The lateral rectus is supplied by the abducent nerve. The superior oblique muscle is supplied by the trochlear nerve. All other muscles are supplied by the oculomotor nerve. Injury or disease of any of these nerves can interfere with eye movements.

The sphincter pupillae is supplied by parasympathetic nerves, and the dilator pupillae by sympathetic nerves.

THE VISUAL PATHWAY

The peripheral receptors for light are situated in the retina. These are called rods and cones (Fig. 24.7). Impulses received by them pass through other cells present in the retina. Nerve fibres arising in the retina constitute the optic nerves. The two optic nerves join to form the optic chiasma in which many of their fibres cross to the opposite side. The uncrossed fibres of the optic nerve, along with the fibres that have crossed over from the opposite side form the ***optic tract*** (Fig. 24.10). The optic tract terminates predominantly in the ***lateral geniculate body***. Fresh fibres arising in the lateral geniculate body form the ***geniculocalcarine tract*** (or optic radiation) that ends in the ***visual areas*** of the cerebral cortex. Vision is actually perceived in the cerebral cortex.

MECHANISM OF VISION

When we look at an object its image is formed on the retina of each eye. The layers of the eye through which light has to pass to reach the retina are the following.

1. Cornea.
2. Aqueous humour.
3. Lens of eye.
4. Vitreous.

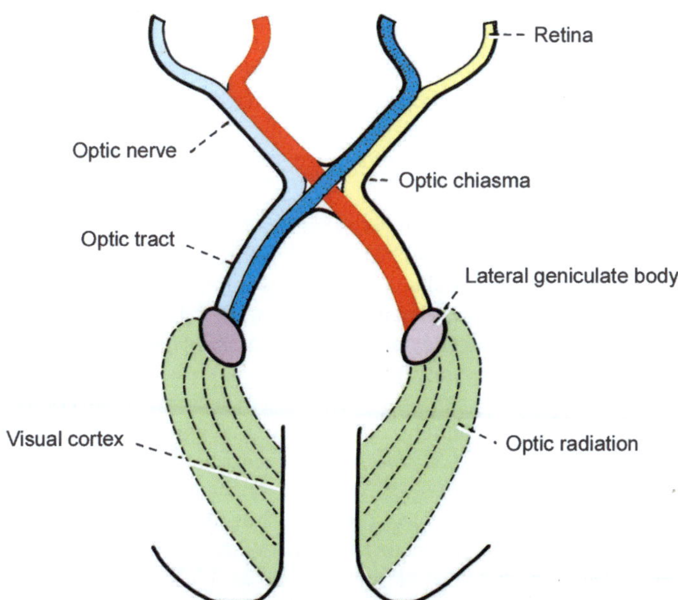

Fig. 24.10 The optic pathway. Note that the fibres from the medial (or nasal) half of each retina cross to the optic tract of the opposite side.

To understand how the image is formed you must understand some elementary principles of optics.

a. When an object is placed in front of a convex lens an image of the object is formed behind the lens. (The image can be seen if a sheet of paper is placed where the image is being formed.)
b. The image formed in inverted (upside down).
c. The lens is able to form an image because it has the power to 'bend' the ray of light. This is called refraction.
d. When two or more parallel rays fall on the lens, they are bent and meet at a point. The distance between the lens and this point is the focal length of the lens. A powerful lens has a shorter focal length than a less powerful one.
e. The power of a lens is measured in ***dioptres***. It is calculated as follows.

$$\text{Dioptre} = \frac{1}{\text{Focal length in metres.}}$$

It follows that if the focal length of a lens is one metre its power is one dioptre. If the focal length is 0.5 meter the power is two dioptres.

These principles also apply to a combination of lenses.

Diopteric Strength of the Eye

Calculation of the diopteric strength of the eye is more complex. This is because refraction takes place at two surfaces.

a. Because of its convexity the cornea acts as a lens.
b. Refraction is caused by the lens of the eye.

Some refraction is also done by the aqueous humour. The effective focal length of the combined system is 17 mm. The refractive power is 59 dioptres.

Accommodation

A very important feature of the lens of the eye is that the curvature (and power) of the lens can be adjusted. This makes it possible for images of objects at varying distances from the eye to be correctly focussed on the retina. This property is called accommodation.

The mechanism for accommodation is as follows.

1. The substance of the lens of the eye is made of elastic material. The lens is tightly enclosed by its capsule. The shape of the lens is maintained by tension produced by the capsule. The peripheral margin (or equator) of the lens gives attachment, all round, to the suspensory ligament. The other ends of the fibres of this ligament are attached to the ciliary body. Within this body there is the ciliary muscle. This muscle is attached to the suspensory ligament in such a way that contraction of the muscle relaxes the ligament. Relaxation of the ligament reduces its pull on the equator of the lens. This allows the lens to become more convex (because of its own elasticity).
2. When we look at a distant object the ciliary muscles are relaxed and the lens focusses the image of the object on the retina. When we look at a near object the image can be properly focussed only if the power of the lens increases. This is achieved by contraction of the ciliary muscle that makes the lens more convex. That is how accommodation is produced.

3. Accommodation is a reflex phenomenon. Whenever the eyes see a blurred image the parasympathetic nerves supplying the ciliary muscles are reflexly stimulated. The muscles contract and the image becomes sharp.
4. Simultaneously, there is (a) constriction of the pupil and (b) convergence of the two eyes. These factors help in near vision.

Photopic and Scotopic Vision

Vision in bright light is called photopic vision. Objects are seen clearly and colours can be appreciated. Photopic vision is the function of cones.

Vision in dim light is called scotopic vision. It is the function of rods. Colours are not seen and details of objects cannot be made out.

Rhodopsin

The substance in rods that is sensitive to light is called ***rhodopsin***. It is made up of a protein ***opsin***, and ***retinine*** (or ***retinal***) which is a derived from vitamin A. Exposure to light splits rhodopsin into opsin and retinine. This results in a change in sodium permeability and the rod is activated. When light is removed opsin and retinine recombine to form rhodopsin. Vitamin A that is present in rods is essential for vision in dim light. If Vitamin A is deficient the person cannot see in dim light. This is called ***night blindness***.

Iodopsin

The light sensitive chemical in cones is called iodopsin. It consists of retinine plus photopsin. There are three types of iodopsin: blue sensitive, green sensitive and red sensitive. There are three corresponding types of cones. All colours are made up of blue, green and red mixed in different proportions. When we look at a colour, the intensity of stimulation of cones responding to the three colours corresponds to the proportion of these in the colour itself. This is the basis of ***colour vision***.

Colour Blindness

Some persons cannot appreciate colours correctly. This is called colour blindness. It is an inherited abnormality. In its most severe form no colour can be seen. In other forms abnormal colours are seen.

Binocular Vision and Stereoscopic Vision

In those animals in which the eyes are directed laterally (as in a cow) the visual field of each eye is different. In the course of evolution the eyes have gradually moved to the front of the head. As a result some part of the field of vision can be seen by both eyes. This is called ***binocular vision***.

The biggest advantage of binocular vision is that perception of depth becomes possible. Distances can be judged accurately. The ability to perceive depth is called ***stereoscopic vision***.

REFLEXES RELATED TO THE EYEBALL

Pupillary Reflexes

Light thrown on an eye causes the pupil of that eye to contract. This is called the ***direct pupillary light reflex.*** At the same time the pupil of the other eye also contracts. This is called the ***consensual light reflex.*** The pathway for the light reflex is shown in Fig. 24.11. Impulses from the retina (of the eye on which light is thrown) travel through the optic nerve, chiasma and optic tracts. Near the lateral geniculate body the fibres concerned pass into the midbrain and end in the pretectal nucleus. Axons arising from this nucleus reach the Edinger Westphal nuclei of both sides. Fibres arising in these nuclei pass through the oculomotor nerve and supply the sphincter pupillae after relay in the ciliary ganglion.

Constriction of the pupil also takes place when we look at a near object i.e., during accommodation. This the ***accommodation reflex.*** The pathway is different from that for the light reflex. In certain diseases (notably syphlitic infection) of the nervous system the pupillary light reflex may be abolished, but pupillary constriction in response to accommodation remains. This condition is called ***Argyll-Robertson-pupil.***

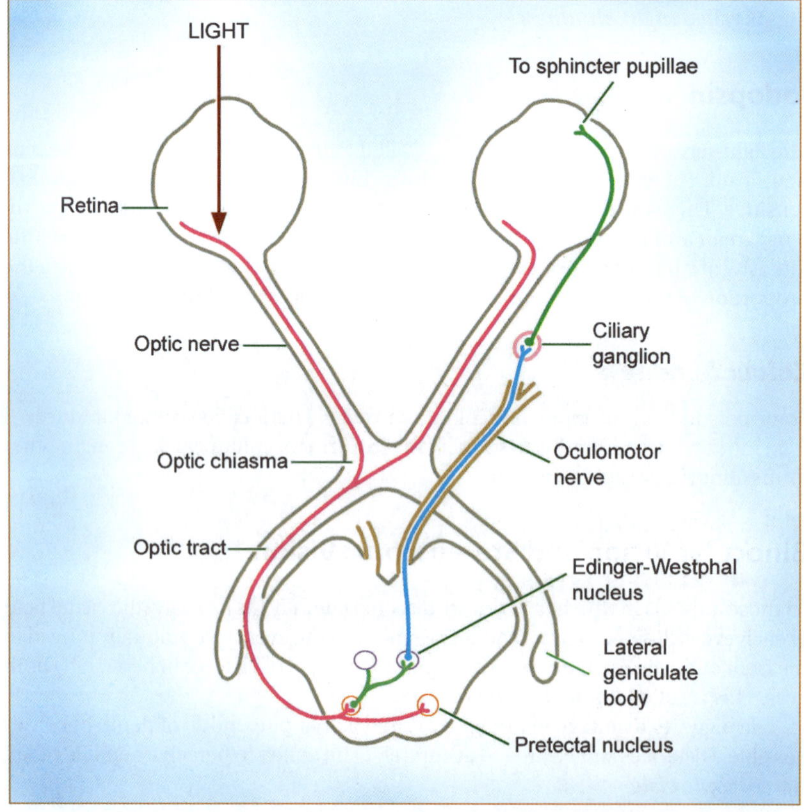

Fig. 24.11 Pathway for the light reflex.

Corneal Reflex

If the cornea is touched with a small wisp of cotton this results in closing of both eyes. This is called the ***corneal reflex***. Impulses from the cornea travel along branches of the ophthalmic division of the trigeminal nerve to the sensory nuclei of this nerve. Secondary fibres establish connections with the motor nuclei of the facial nerve of both sides. Fibres arising in the facial nuclei, and reaching the muscles closing the palpebral aperture, complete the reflex arc. In the case of injury to the ophthalmic division of the trigeminal nerve, the corneal reflex cannot be elicited from that side, but a bilateral response is obtained by stimulating the cornea of the normal side. In facial paralysis the response is seen only on the normal side.

SOME DISEASES OF THE EYE

1. A painful swelling appearing near the eyelid margin is called a ***stye***. This is caused by infection in tarsal glands present in the lid.
2. Chronic inflammation of the margin of an eyelid is called ***blepharitis***. It can be due to infection or to allergy.
3. Inflammation of the conjunctiva is ***conjunctivitis***. It can be caused by infection (bacterial or viral) or by allergy.
4. ***Trachoma*** is a common infection of the conjunctiva and cornea. It causes deformity and can lead to blindness.
5. Infection of the cornea is ***keratitis***.
6. Inflammation of the iris, ciliary body and choroid is called ***anterior uveitis*** or ***iridocyclitis***.
7. Inflammation of the retina and choroid is called ***posterior uveitis***.

Refractive Errors

A refractive error is one in which images are not properly focussed on the retina.

1. A normal eye is emetropic.
2. Sometimes there is difficulty in seeing near objects clearly (for example reading becomes difficult), but objects at a distance can be seen normally. This is called hypermetropia (or far sightedness). It can be corrected by using convex (+) lenses.
3. The opposite condition is called myopia (near sightedness). Reading a book is easy but something written on a blackboard in a class is not seen clearly. The condition is corrected by using concave (-) lenses.
4. In astigmatism there is distortion of vision because of abnormality in the cornea, or lens. In mild astigmatism vision may appear to be normal but the person gets headache after using the eyes for some time. It is corrected by using special (cylindrical) lenses. Astigmatism can occur along with myopia or hypermetropia.
5. In most persons vision is normal in young age, but after the age of 40 there is difficulty in reading, or in other work requiring close vision. This is regarded as a normal effect of age and is called presbyopia.

Other Disorders

1. In many old persons the lens gradually becomes opaque. This condition is called cataract. Vision can be restored by surgical removal of the opaque lens, and by

replacing it either with spectacles or with an intraocular lens (lens put into the eye).

2. Many people become blind because of infections or injuries that make the cornea opaque. Vision can be restored in such persons by replacing the cornea with that from another person (corneal transplantation).
3. Movements of eyes require coordinated action of many muscles. If one or more muscles do not work normally, the two eyes may appear to be looking in different directions. This is called strabismus or squint.
4. The eye maintains its shape because it is filled by aqueous and vitreous which exert pressure on the wall. Aqueous is constantly secreted and excess is removed. If there is obstruction to the circulation of aqueous, the pressure within the eye (intraocular pressure) increases. This condition is called glaucoma. It produces symptoms including pain, and ultimately it can cause blindness.
5. Diseases of the retina are called retinopathies. They can lead to blindness. They can be caused by interference with blood supply, because of diabetes, or can be congenital. A portion of the retina can get detached from the choroid. This causes abnormalities of vision.

THE EAR AND SOME RELATED STRUCTURES

INTRODUCTION

Anatomically speaking, the ear is made up of three main parts called the ***external ear***, the ***middle ear*** and the ***internal ear***. The external ear and the middle ear are concerned exclusively with hearing. The internal ear has a ***cochlear part*** concerned with hearing; and a ***vestibular part*** which provides information to the brain regarding the position and movements of the head.

The main parts of the ear are shown in Fig. 24.12. The part of the ear that is seen on the surface of the body (i.e., the part that the lay person calls the ear) is

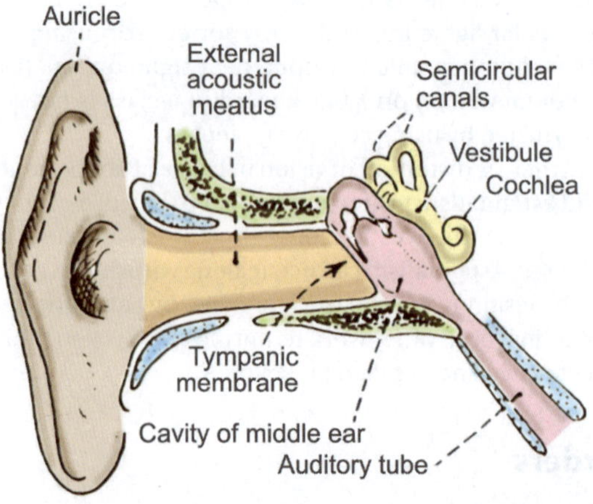

Fig. 24.12 Scheme to show the main parts of the ear. 1. Malleus; 2. Incus; 3. Stapes.

anatomically speaking the ***auricle*** or ***pinna***. Leading inwards from the auricle there is a tube called the ***external acoustic meatus***. The auricle and external acoustic meatus together form the external ear. The inner end of the external acoustic meatus is closed by a thin membranous diaphragm which is called the ***tympanic membrane***. This membrane separates the external acoustic meatus from the middle ear.

The middle ear is a small space placed deep within the temporal bone. It is also called the ***tympanum*** (from which we get the adjective tympanic applied to structures connected with the middle ear). Medially the middle ear is closely related to parts of the internal ear. The cavity of the middle ear is continuous with that of the nasopharynx through a passage called the ***auditory tube***. Within the cavity of the middle ear there are three small bones that are collectively called the ***ossicles*** of the ear. The ossicles are called ***malleus*** (= like a hammer); the ***incus*** (= like an anvil, used by blacksmiths); and the ***stapes*** (= like a stirrup in which the foot of a horse rider fits). The three ossicles form a chain that is attached on one side to the tympanic membrane and at the other to a part of the internal ear.

The internal ear is in the form of a cavity within the petrous temporal bone having a very complex shape. This bony cavity (or ***bony labyrinth***) has a central part called the ***vestibule***. Continuous with the front of the vestibule there is a spiral shaped cavity, the bony ***cochlea***. Posteriorly, the vestibule is continuous with three ***semicircular canals***.

Sound waves travelling through air reach the ears. In many lower animals in which the auricle is large and mobile it may help in directing the sound waves into the external acoustic meatus. The auricle is of doubtful functional significance in man. Waves striking the tympanic membrane produce vibrations in it. These vibrations are transmitted through the chain of ossicles present in the middle ear to reach the internal ear. Specialised end organs in the cochlea act as transducers that convert the mechanical vibrations into nervous impulses. These impulses travel through the cochlear part of the vestibulocochlear nerve to reach the brain. Actual perception of sound takes place in the auditory (or acoustic) areas in the cerebral cortex.

THE AURICLE

The auricle is made up of a skeleton of elastic cartilage and fibrous tissue, which is covered on both sides by a layer of thin skin. The cartilage of the auricle is continuous with that of the external acoustic meatus. The auricle has an external surface facing laterally, and an inner or cranial surface that lies against the side of the head.

The cartilage of the auricle is curved on it self in a complicated manner so that a number of elevations and depressions are produced. These elevations and depressions are given names that are shown in Fig. 24.13. In particular note that the lowest part of the auricle is soft. It does not contain cartilage and is composed only of a fold of skin with enclosed connective tissue. This part is called the ***lobule***. (It is through this part that perforations are made for wearing ear-rings). At the centre of the external surface of the auricle there is

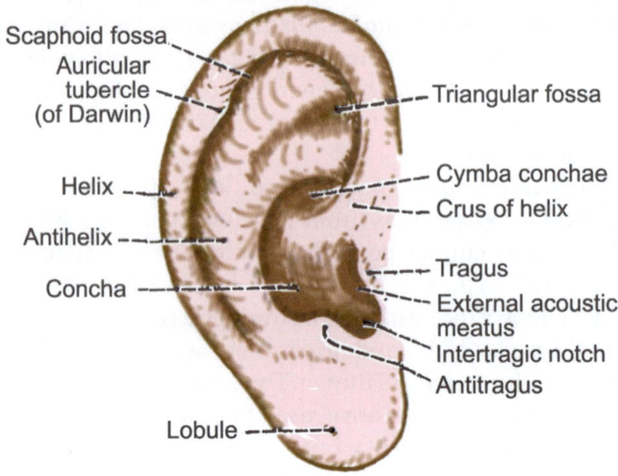

Fig. 24.13 Named features to be seen on the external aspect of the auricle.

a large depression called the ***concha***. Its anterior part is continued into the external acoustic meatus.

EXTERNAL ACOUSTIC MEATUS

The external acoustic meatus is a tube passing medially from the bottom of the concha of the auricle. It is closed medially by the tympanic membrane. The total length of the tube is approximately 24 mm. Of this the wall of the outer 8 mm is cartilaginous, while that of the inner 16 mm is bony (Fig. 24.12).

The medial end of the meatus is closed by the tympanic membrane.

The external acoustic meatus is not straight, but follows an S-shaped course. In clinical examination of the meatus, and through it of the tympanic membrane, the auricle is pulled upwards, backwards and somewhat laterally. This renders the meatus straight. It then has a uniform medial, forward and downward direction.

The meatus shows a narrowing at the junction of the cartilaginous and bony parts. It shows another narrowing called the ***isthmus*** about 4 mm from the tympanic membrane (i.e., 20 mm from the floor of the concha). The floor of the meatus shows a depression immediately lateral to the tympanic membrane. Foreign bodies entering the meatus can get stuck here.

The skin lining the external acoustic meatus contains numerous ***ceruminous glands***. These are modified sweat glands that produce the wax of the ear, or ***cerumen***.

THE MIDDLE EAR

The middle ear is also called the ***tympanic cavity*** or ***tympanum*** (Fig. 24.12). It is a space lying in the petrous temporal bone. The middle ear is separated from

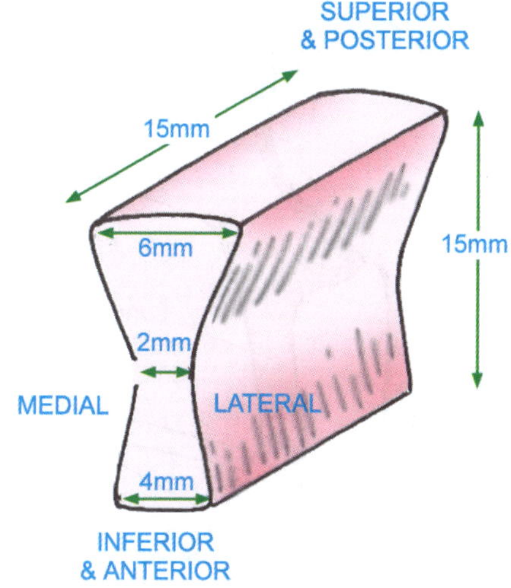

Fig. 24.14 Dimensions of the tympanic cavity.

the external acoustic meatus by the tympanic membrane. From Fig. 24.12 it will be seen that part of the tympanic cavity lies above the level of the tympanic membrane: this part is called the ***epitympanic recess.*** We have also seen that three ossicles, the malleus, the incus and the stapes lie within the middle ear. The tympanic cavity communicates with the cavity of the nasopharynx through the ***auditory tube***. It also communicates with a large space in the petrous part of the temporal bone, called the ***mastoid antrum;*** and with smaller spaces within the mastoid process called the ***mastoid air cells***. These spaces, the tympanic cavity itself, and the auditory tube are all lined by mucous membrane. Because of their communication with the nasopharynx these spaces are filled with air.

The tympanic cavity is shaped like a box (Fig. 24.14). It has six sides: a roof, a floor, and anterior, posterior, medial and lateral walls.

Ossicles of the Middle Ear

The ***malleus*** is so called because it resembles a hammer (mallet = hammer) (Fig. 24.15). It has an upper rounded part called the ***head*** to which is attached a relatively long ***handle*** (or ***manubrium***).

The ***incus*** (= anvil) has a main part or ***body*** and two ***processes, long and short***.

The ***stapes*** is shaped like a stirrup. It has a ***head***, two ***limbs*** or ***crura*** (anterior and posterior) and a ***base***. The constricted part adjoining the head is called the ***neck***.

The handle of the malleus is intimately attached to the tympanic membrane. The head of the malleus, articulates with the body of the incus. The lower end of the long process of the incus articulates with the head of the stapes. The base of the stapes is attached to the margins of an oval aperture (the fenestra vestibuli) in the medial wall of the middle ear.

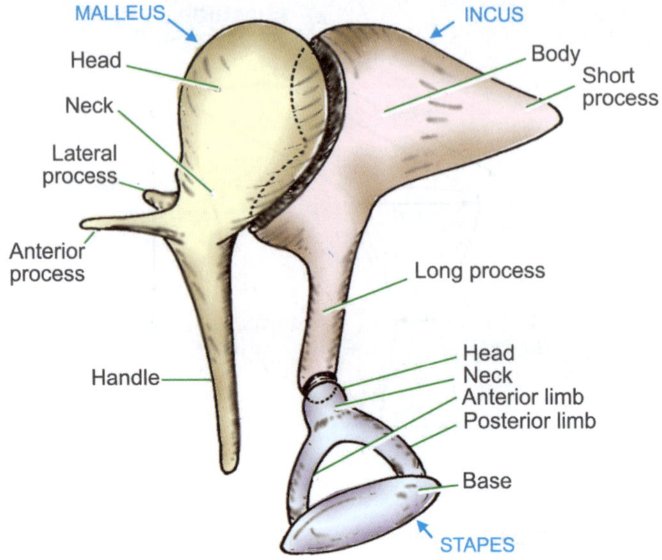

Fig. 24.15 Ossicles of the ear.

Walls of Middle Ear

The roof of the middle ear is formed of a plate of bone. This plate separates the middle ear from the cranial cavity. The floor of the middle ear is formed by a thin plate of bone that separates the middle ear from the bulb of the internal jugular vein.

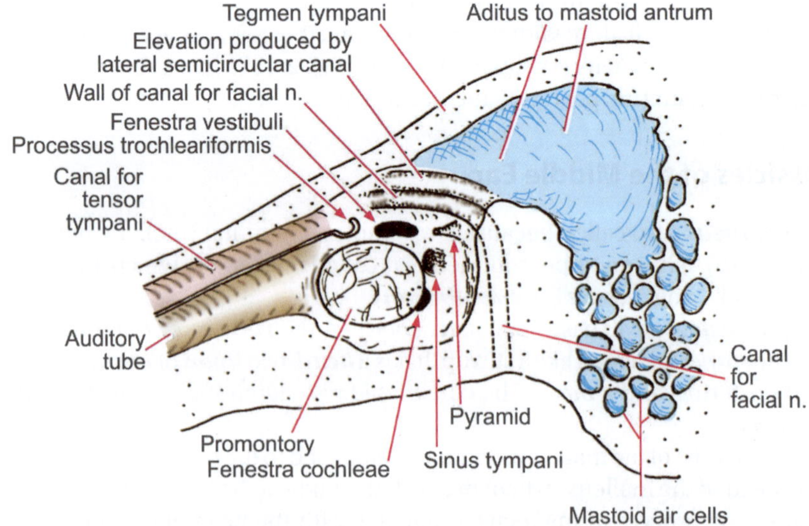

Fig. 24.16 Medial wall of middle ear. Parts of the anterior and posterior walls are also shown.

The greater part of the lateral wall of the middle ear is formed by the tympanic membrane. The part of the middle ear cavity lying above the level of the tympanic membrane is the ***epitympanic recess***.

The posterior wall of the middle ear shows a large round aperture through which the middle ear communicates with the mastoid antrum. This aperture is called the ***aditus to the mastoid antrum***. The posterior wall of the middle ear also bears a conical elevation called the ***pyramid***. The tip of the pyramid projects forwards, and has an opening that leads into a canal in which the stapedius muscle is lodged. The tendon of the stapedius emerges from the opening at the tip of the pyramid and runs forwards to be inserted into the neck of the stapes.

Medial Wall of Middle Ear

The medial wall of the middle ear is also the lateral wall of the internal ear (Fig. 24.16). The most prominent feature to be seen on the medial wall is the ***promontory***. Posterosuperior to the promontory we see the ***fenestra vestibuli*** that is also called the ***oval window***. The base of the stapes fits into this opening and is attached to its margins by the annular ligament. Posteroinferior to the promontory there is a round aperture called the ***fenestra cochleae*** (also called the ***round window***). This opening is continuous with part of the cavity of the cochlea. It is closed by the ***secondary tympanic membrane***.

The facial nere is closely related to the medial wall of the middle ear.

The middle ear contains two small muscles. These are the tensor tympani and the stapedius. They protect the ear against very loud sounds by restricting the vibrations of the tympanic membrane and the ossicles.

The Mastoid Antrum and Air Cells

The mastoid antrum (Fig. 24.16) is of considerable importance as it is a frequent site of infection, which may be difficult to eradicate. Furthermore, infection may spread from it to neighbouring structures with serious consequences. The antrum opens into the epitympanic recess.

The mastoid air cells are a series of intercommunicating spaces of variable size present within the mastoid process. They communicate above with the mastoid antrum. Their number varies considerably. Infection can reach the mastoid air cells though the tympanic cavity and the mastoid antrum, and can spread to any of the structures related to them.

The Auditory Tube

The auditory tube is also called the ***pharyngotympanic tube***, or the ***Eustachian tube***. It provides a communication between the nasopharynx and the middle ear (Fig. 24.12). Air therefore passes into the tympanic cavity (and into the mastoid antrum and air cells). As a result, air pressure on both sides of the tympanic membrane is the same: this is important for proper vibration of the tympanic membrane. However, the auditory tube is not patent all the time.

It opens during deglutition, or even during the swallowing of saliva. When we suddenly ascend to a higher altitude (as in going up a hill in a car) the air pressure on the outside of the tympanic membrane falls, but that on its inner side remains the same as before. This inequality in pressure gives rise to a change in the quality of sound perceived. However, on swallowing of saliva, and the consequent equalisation of pressure, the sound suddenly returns to normal.

The communication between the pharynx and the middle ear is also a path along which infection frequently reaches the middle ear. This occurs more commonly in children, in whom the auditory tube is shorter and wider than in the adult. In the presence of infection the tube is easily blocked. When this happens air within the tympanic cavity is gradually absorbed and pressure on the outside of the tympanic membrane becomes greater than on the inside. This can give rise to discomfort which can be relieved by introducing air into the auditory tube through a catheter. If obstruction to the auditory tube is prolonged pus can accumulate in middle ear resulting in severe pain. The pus may burst through the tympanic membrane leading to discharge from the ear, and to the formation of a perforation in the membrane. It is for these reasons that the anatomy of the auditory tube is of much practical importance.

THE INTERNAL EAR

The internal ear is made up of a complex system of cavities within the petrous temporal bone. Because of the complex shape of these intercommunicating cavities they are referred to as the ***bony labyrinth***. Within the bony labyrinth there are membrane lined intercommunicating cavities that constitute the ***membranous labyrinth***.

The basic arrangement of the labyrinth is best understood by looking at a transverse section through a relatively simple part of it like a semicircular canal (Fig. 24.17). The wall of the bony labyrinth is made up of dense bone. Its inner surface is lined by periosteum. Lying within the bony labyrinth there is the membranous labyrinth. The space within the membranous labyrinth is filled in by a fluid called the ***endolymph.*** The space between the membranous labyrinth and the bony labyrinth is filled by another fluid called the ***perilymph.***

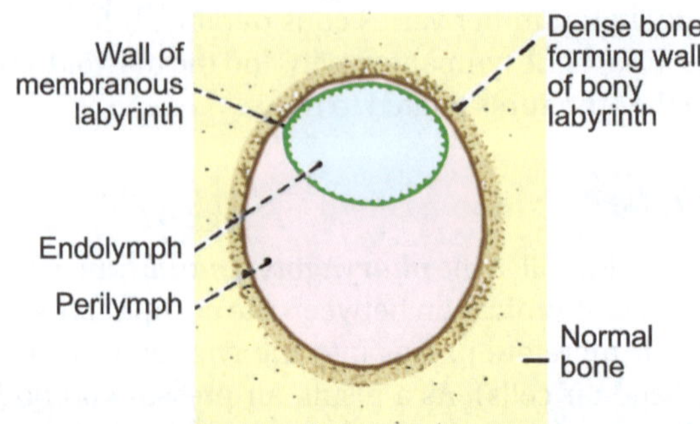

Fig. 24.17 Basic structure of the internal ear as seen in a section through a semicircular canal.

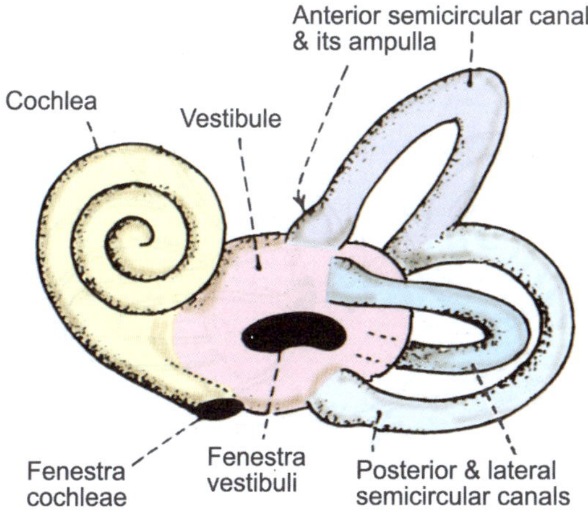

Fig. 24.18 Bony labyrinth seen from the lateral side.

The Bony Labyrinth

The parts of the bony labyrinth are shown in Fig. 24.18. These are as follows.

a. In the central part of the bony labyrinth there is a cavity called the ***vestibule***.
b. Anterior to the vestibule we see the ***bony cochlea***.
c. Posteriorly, the cavity of the vestibule is continuous with the three ***semicircular canals***.

The Bony Cochlea

The cochlea is continuous with the anterior part of the vestibule. From Fig. 24.18 it is seen that the cochlea is basically a tube that is coiled on itself for two and three quarter turns. The diameter of the tube is greatest at its junction with the vestibule, and this part is called the ***basal turn*** of the cochlea. The tube becomes progressively narrower towards the centre or ***apex*** of the cochlea. The basal turn of the cochlea produces an elevation, the promontory, on the medial wall of the middle ear.

If we examine the basal turn of the cochlea shown in Fig. 24.19 we find that it is made up of an upper channel the scala vestibuli which is continuous with the vestibule; and of a lower channel, the scala tympani, which opens into the middle ear through the fenestra cochleae. The fenestra cochleae is closed by the ***secondary tympanic membrane.***

The scala vestibuli and the scala tympani are partially separated from each other by a shelf of bone. The shelf follows the coiling of the cochlea and is, therefore, called the ***spiral lamina***. Further details of the cochlea can be appreciated if we study a transverse section through one turn of the cochlea (Fig. 24.20). In this figure we see that the spiral lamina extends only partially into the canal of the cochlea. The ***basilar membrane*** stretches from the 'free' edge of the spiral lamina to the outer wall of the cochlear canal. The ***vestibular***

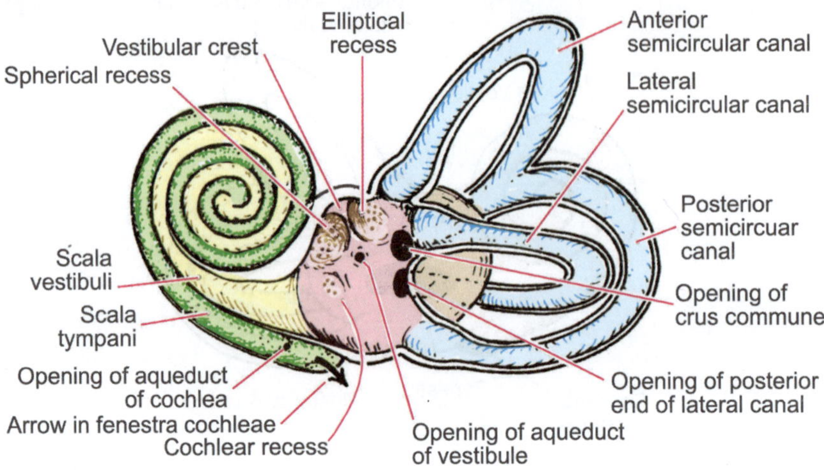

Fig. 24.19 Interior of the bony labyrinth as seen from the lateral side.

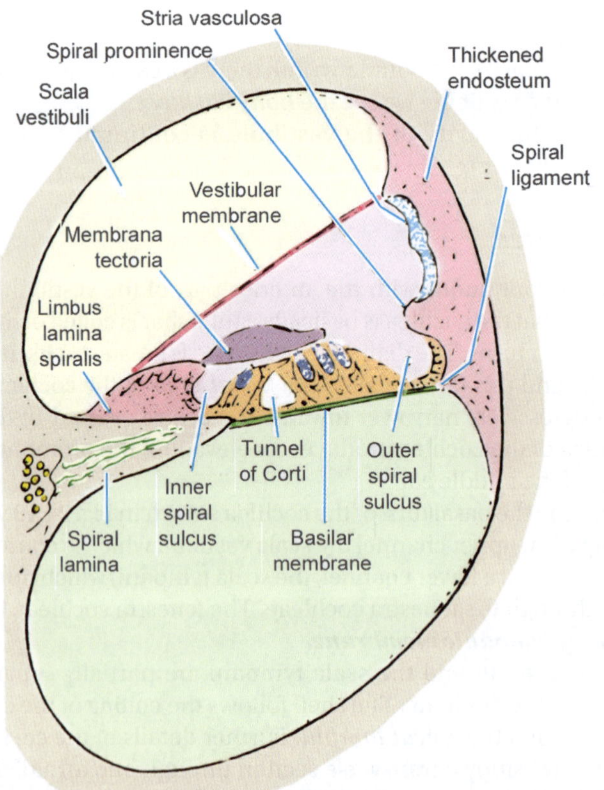

Fig. 24.20 Transverse section through one turn of the cochlea.

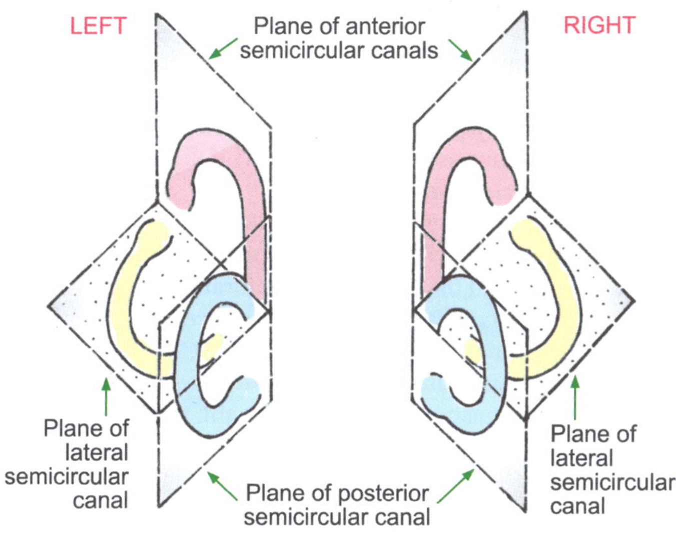

Fig. 24.21 Diagram to show how the semicircular canals are placed (as seen from behind).

membrane is also attached to the free end of the spiral lamina. Between the two membranes there is a triangular interval.

At the apex of the cochlea the scala vestibuli becomes continuous with the scala tympani (Fig. 24.19). This communication is called the ***helicotrema***.

The membranous labyrinth in the cochlea is called the ***duct of the cochlea***. This duct lies just above the basilar membrane. It is separated from the scala vestibuli by a thin ***vestibular membrane.***

Near the attached margin of the spiral lamina there is a canal. This canal is also shaped like a spiral and is called the ***spiral canal***. This canal contains a collection of neurons that constitute the ***spiral ganglion***. Fibres arising from the ganglion pass through the spiral lamina to supply the spiral organ (See below).

The Semicircular Canals

There are three semicircular canals, ***anterior*** (or superior), ***posterior,*** and ***lateral*** (Fig. 24.18). One end of each canal is dilated, and the dilatation is called an ***ampulla***. The non-ampullated ends of the anterior and posterior canals join to form a common channel, the ***crus commune***. As a result the semicircular canals open into the vestibule through five (not six) openings.

The most important facts about the semicircular canals concern their orientation. The three canals lie in planes at right angles to one another (Fig. 24.21). The anterior and posterior canals are both vertical, and are placed at right angles to each other. The lateral canal is horizontal. All the canals are therefore at right angles to one another. From Fig. 24.21 it will be clear that the right and left lateral semicircular canals lie in the same plane. The anterior canal of one side lies in the same plane as the posterior canal of the opposite side.

Membranous Labyrinth

The parts of the membranous labyrinth are shown in Figs. 24.22 and 24.23. They are as follows.

1. Within the vestibule there are two rounded sacs. The anterior sac is the ***saccule***. The posterior sac is the ***utricle***. The utricle is connected to the saccule by the ***utriculo-saccular duct***.
2. The part of the membranous labyrinth lying in the bony cochlea is called the ***duct of the cochlea***. It occupies the triangular interval between the basilar membrane and the vestibular membrane. Within this duct there is the organ of Corti, which is the end organ for reception of sound. It rests on the basilar membrane.
3. Lying within each semicircular canal there is a ***semicircular duct.*** (It is important to distinguish carefully between the terms semicircular canal, and semicircular duct). The semicircular ducts open into the utricle.
4. The ***saccus endolymphaticus*** is a blind pouch-like extension of the membranous labyrinth. It communicates with the saccule and also with the utricle.

ORGAN OF CORTI AND MECHANISM OF HEARING

The end organ for hearing is the ***spiral organ (of Corti).*** It lies in the duct of the cochlea, just above the basilar membrane (Fig. 24.20).

The organ has a complex structure and contains many types of cells. The most important of these are ***hair cells***. The hair cells are innervated by fibres of the cochlear nerve. These cells respond to vibrations produced by sound and convert them into nerve impulses that travel to the brain.

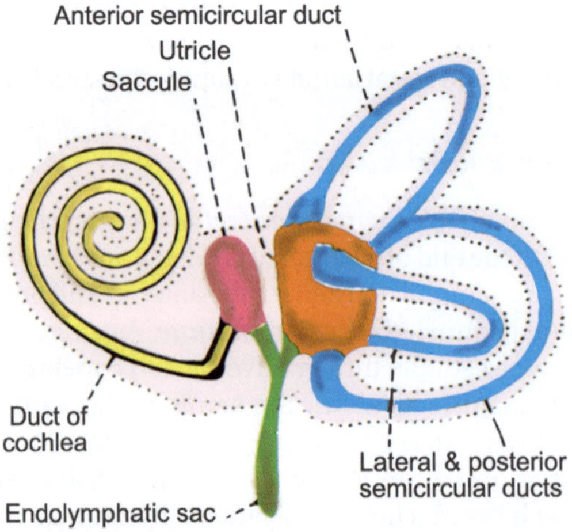

Fig. 24.22 Scheme to show the parts of the membranous labyrinth. Note the ampullated ends of the semicircular ducts.

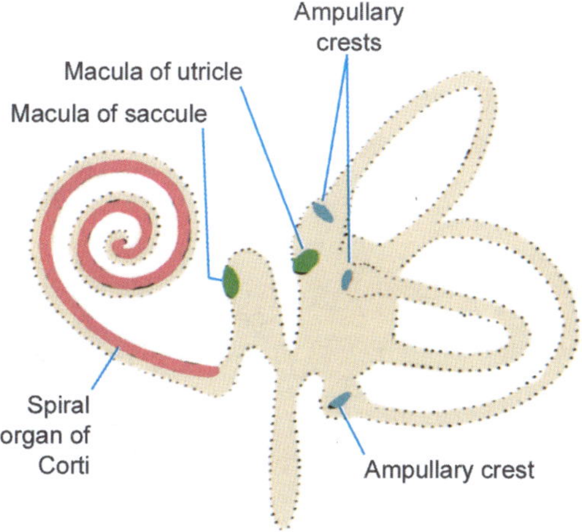

Fig. 24.23 End organs in the membranous labyrinth.

We have seen that sound waves travelling through air produce vibrations in the tympanic membrane. These are transmitted through the malleus and incus to the stapes. The base of the stapes (which fits into the fenestra vestibuli) transmits these vibrations to the perilymph of the vestibule. From there the vibrations pass into the scala vestibuli. Each time the base of the stapes moves inwards into the vestibule it creates a pressure wave which extends along the perilymph filling the entire length of the scala vestibuli. Reaching the helicotrema the pressure wave passes into the perilymph filling the scala tympani. Traversing the entire length of the scala tympani it reaches the secondary tympanic membrane (which closes the fenestra cochleae) causing it to bulge into the middle ear. The process is reversed when the base of the stapes moves outwards. These changes take place almost instantaneously. In this way vibrations are set up in the perilymph. These in turn produce vibrations of the basilar membrane and of the spiral organ. Distortions produced in the hair cells of the organ of Corti as a result of vibrations generate nervous impulses. These impulses travel along nerve fibres that are peripheral processes of neurons located in the spiral ganglia. These processes reach the hair cells through canals in the spiral lamina.

Central processes arising from neurons of the spiral ganglion constitute the cochlear nerve.

Pathway of Hearing

The first neurons of the pathway of hearing are located in the spiral ganglion which lies within a bony tunnel running along the cochlea. These neurons are bipolar. Peripheral processes of neurons lying in this ganglion innervate the hair cells of the ***spiral organ*** (organ of Corti) (Fig. 24.24). The central processes of the neurons form the cochlear nerve. The fibres of the cochlear nerve terminate in the ***cochlear nuclei*** present in the pons.

Fibres arising from the cochlear nuclei terminate in various masses of grey matter. These include the ***inferior colliculus*** and the ***medial geniculate body***. Fibres arising in the medial geniculate body form the ***acoustic radiation*** that ends in the acoustic area of the cerebral cortex.

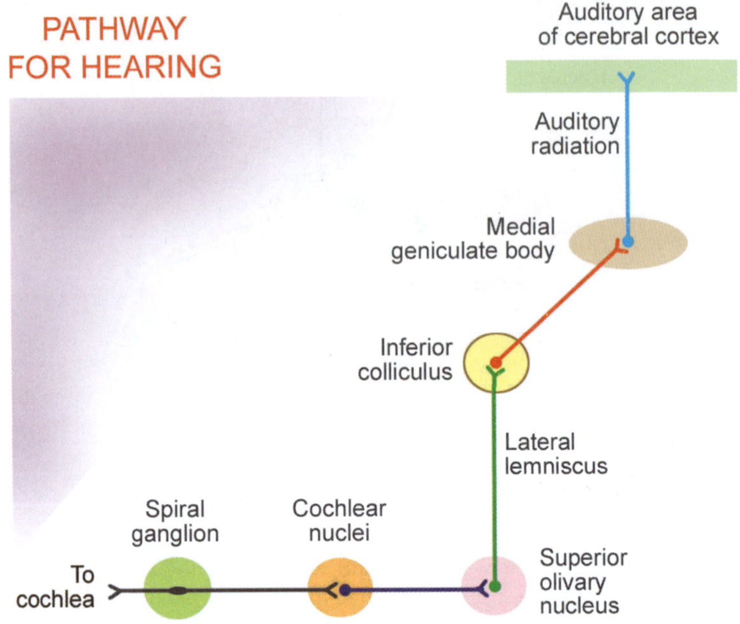

Fig. 24.24 Simplified scheme to show the pathway for hearing.

Other End Organs in the Membranous Labyrinth

Information about changes in the position of the head is provided by end organs called ***maculae*** (singular = macula) present in the utricle and the saccule.

Each macula consists essentially of hair cells, surrounded by supporting cells. The 'hair' of the hair cells are covered by a membrane which contains crystals of calcium carbonate (***otoliths***). With changes in the position of the head the otoliths are displaced leading to distortion of hair cells. Nervous impulses are generated as a result of this distortion.

Information about angular movements (acceleration) of the head is provided by end organs called the ***ampullary crests*** (or ***cristae ampullae***) one of which is present in the ampulla of each semicircular duct. Each crista consists of hair cells (and supporting cells) that are surmounted by a gelatinous covering that forms a partition (***cupola***) within the ampulla. Movements of the head produce currents in the endolymph within the semicircular ducts. These cause the cupolae to move resulting in deformation of hair cells and production of nerve impulses.

The nerve fibres innervating the cristae of the semicircular ducts and the maculae of the utricle and saccule are peripheral processes of neurons located in the vestibular ganglion. This ganglion lies in the internal acoustic meatus. The central processes of cells of the ganglion form the vestibular nerve.

SOME DISEASES OF THE EAR

1. The adjective for ear is ***otic***. Hence inflammation of the ear is called ***otitis***. Inflammation in the middle ear is called ***otitis media***. This may be acute or chronic. Infection from the throat can spread to the middle ear through the auditory tube. Pus accumulating in the middle ear can lead to perforation of the tympanic membrane. This pus flows to the outside through the external acoustic meatus. Inflammation from the middle ear can also spread to spaces within the mastoid temporal bone (mastoid antrum and mastoid air cells), and to the internal ear.
2. The internal ear is also called the labyrinth, and inflammation here is called ***labyrinthitis***. In labyrinthitis movement of the head creates giddiness and surrounding objects appear to move in circles. When the condition is severe the patient cannot stand up or walk because of giddiness. The condition can take several weeks to recover.
3. When traveling in a bus or train, many persons complain of nausea and vomiting. This is called ***motion sickness***. It is produced by excessive stimulation of the vestibular apparatus.
4. ***Deafness:*** There are many causes of deafness.
   a. Chronic infection in the middle ear can lead to destruction of ossicles or loss of movement in them. This interferes with conduction of sound waves and leads to conductive deafness.
      Some degree of temporary deafness can be caused by accumulation of wax in the external acoustic meatus, or by suddenly climbing to a higher altitude (as in an airplane).
   b. Deafness can be caused by pathology in the internal ear (cochlea). The defect can be present from birth (congenital). It can follow some viral infections, including labyrinthitis. Deafness can also be caused by degenerative changes in old age.

PART FOUR

Further Learning Through Pictures

In the various chapters of this book the main facts of human anatomy, that nursing students need to know, have been presented as simply as possible. In the pages that follow, the student will find many illustrations a study of which will enable them to know many details that have not been presented earlier. Each figure should be studied carefully and all labeled features identified. Once this has been done, the illustrations will be useful for reference whenever required

CHAPTER

25

Some Important Regions

In this Chapter a number of figures illustrating some important regions of the body are shown. The list given below should help you to locate any illustration easily.

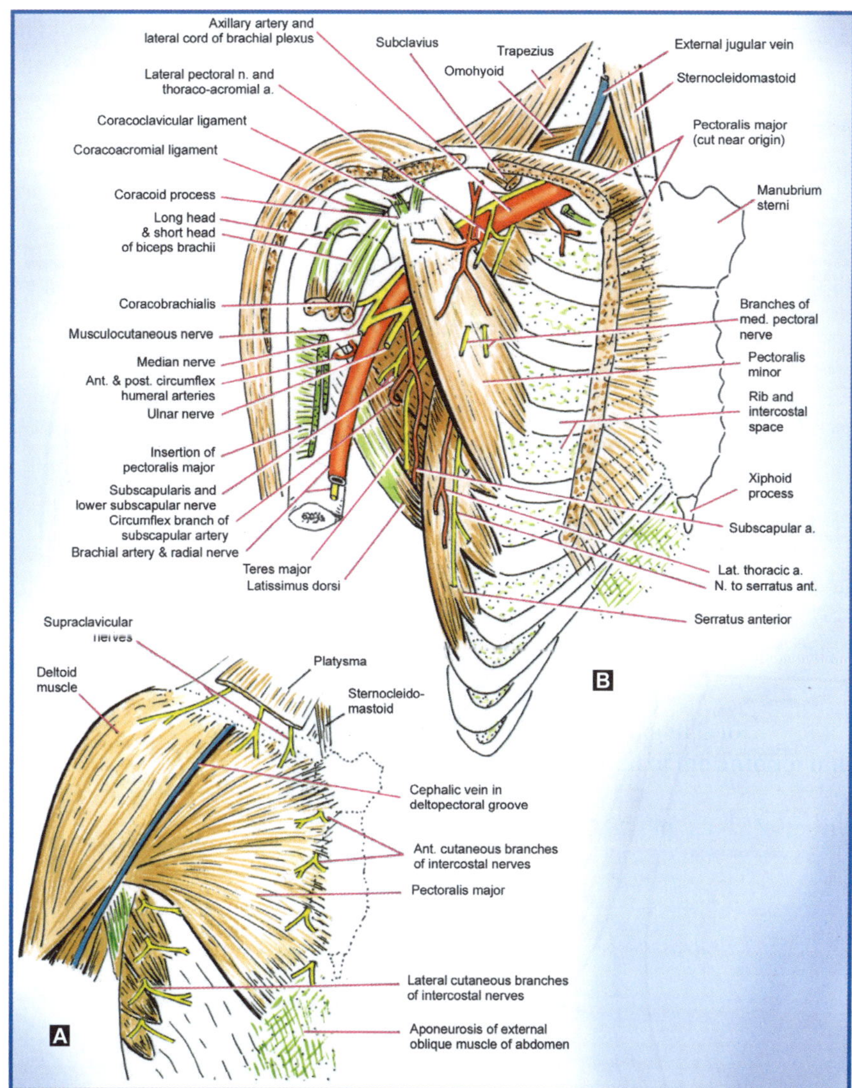

Figs 25.1A and B A. Pectoral region seen after removal of skin and fascia. Observe the pectoralis major. At the medial end it is attached to the chest wall. Its lateral end gains attachment to the upper end of the humerus. It causes powerful movements of the arm; B. Pectoral region seen after removal of greater parts of pectoralis major and anterior part of deltoid.

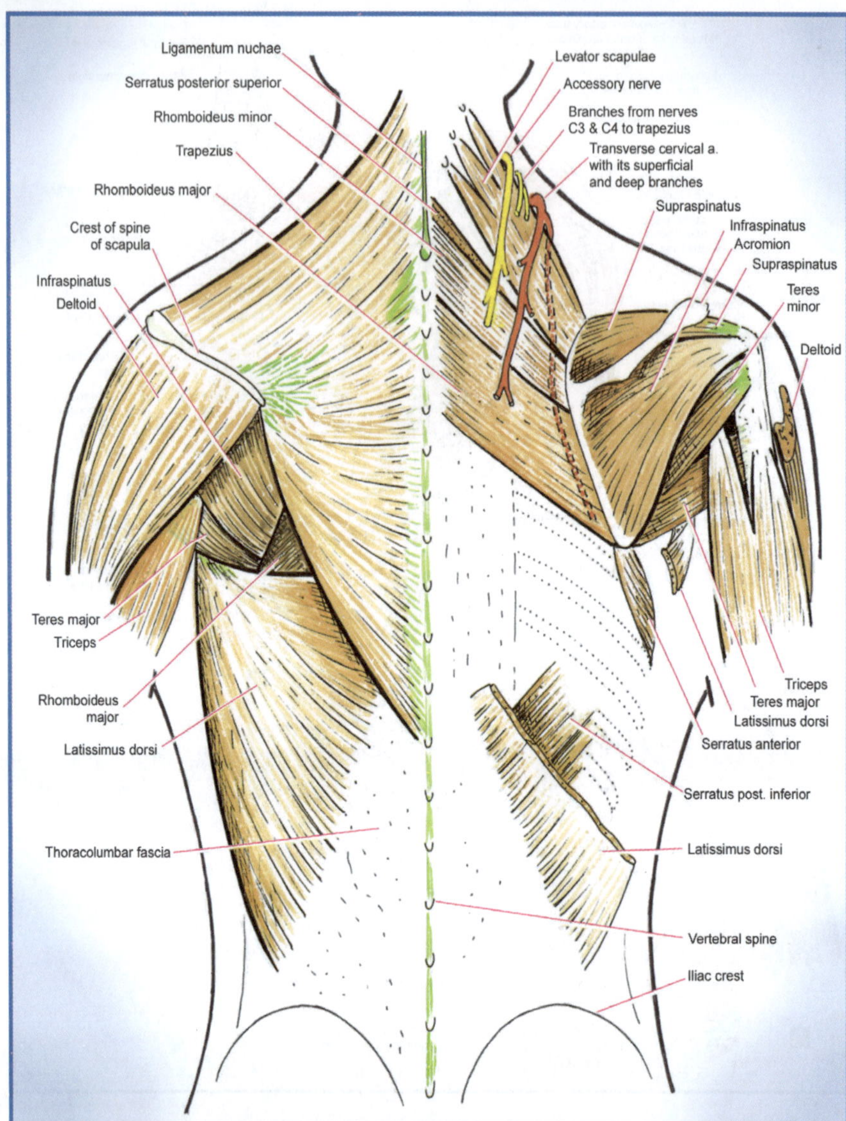

Fig. 25.2 Dissection showing some structures on the back of the trunk. Note the trapezius which is a large triangular muscle. Medially it is attached to the vertebral column. Above it reaches the skull. Laterally it gains attachment to the scapula and the clavicle. Also observe that the latissimus dorsi is another large muscle the fibres of which converge to reach the upper end of the humerus. Both muscles are responsible for powerful movements of the arm.

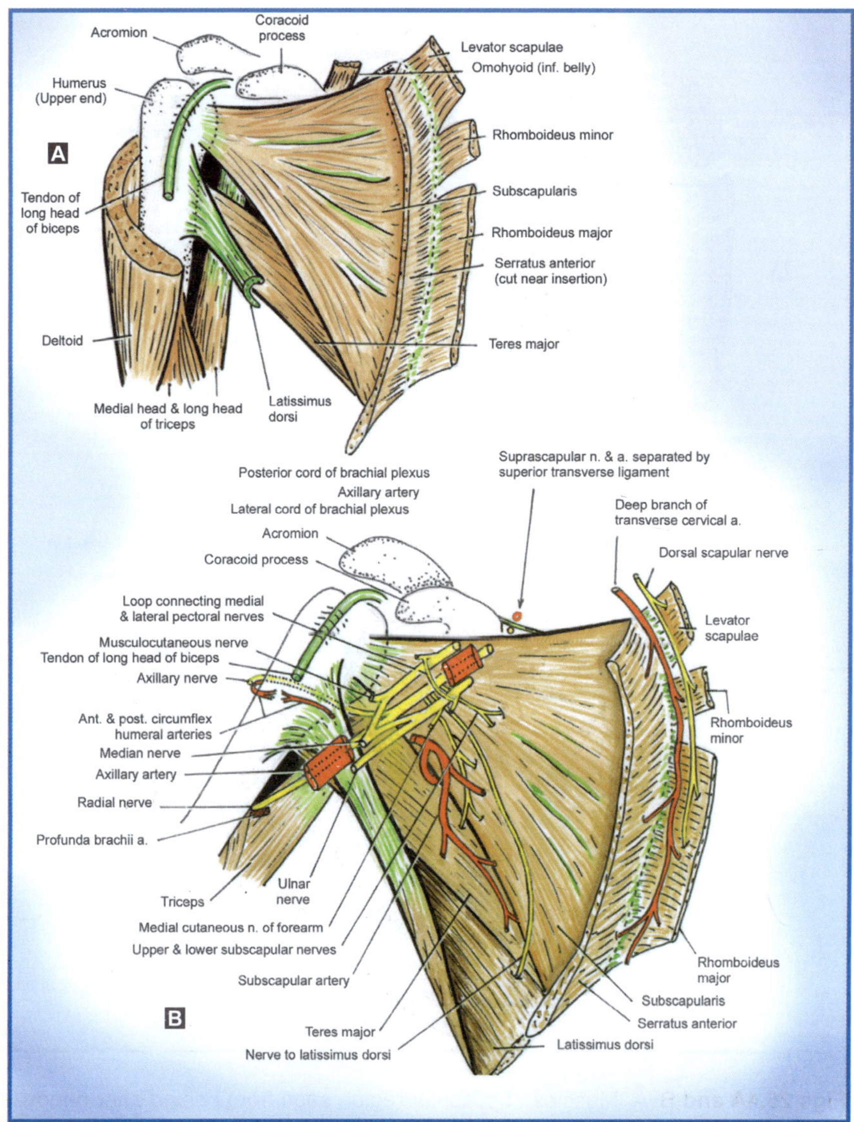

Figs 25.3A and B A. Scapular region seen from the front. The upper part of the deltoid has been removed. The muscles of this region help in movements at the shoulder joint; B. Scapular region seen from the front and showing the arteries and nerves of the region. Segments of the axillary artery have been removed to show deeper structures. Veins and lymph nodes are not drawn.

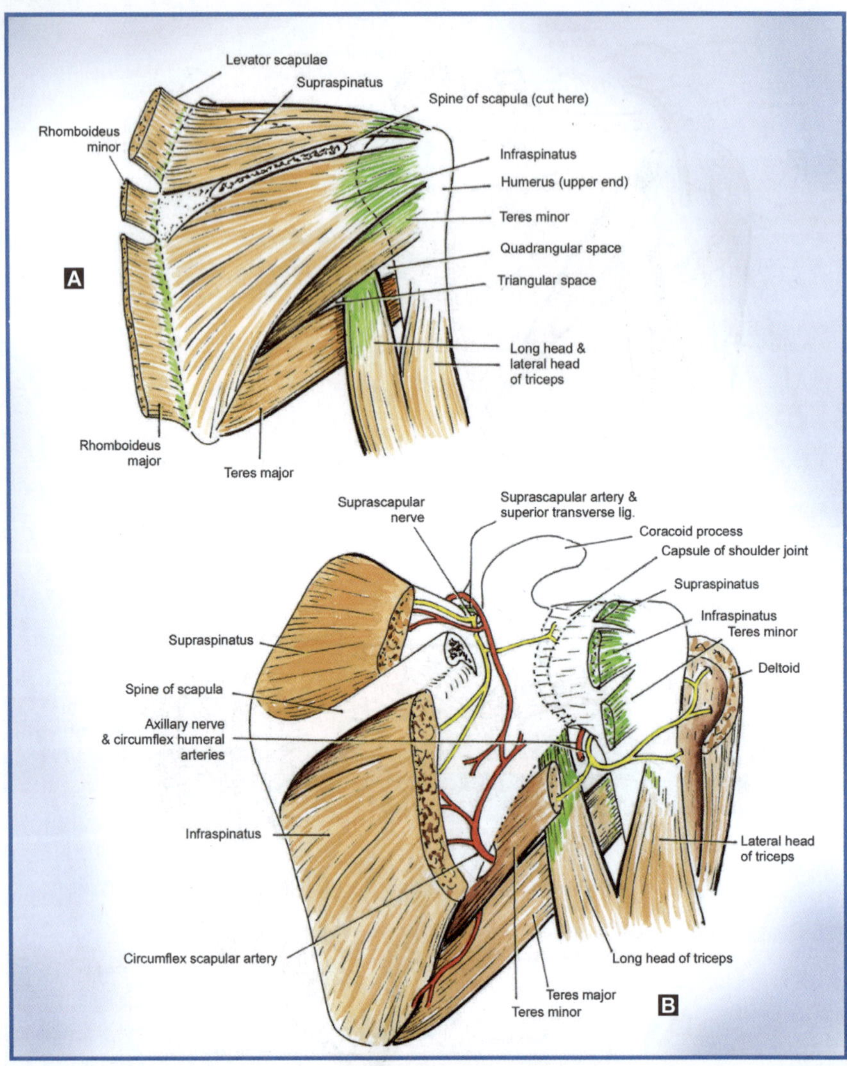

Figs 25.4A and B A. Muscles of scapular region seen from behind after removal of the deltoid; B. Scapular region seen from behind to show nerves and arteries of the region.

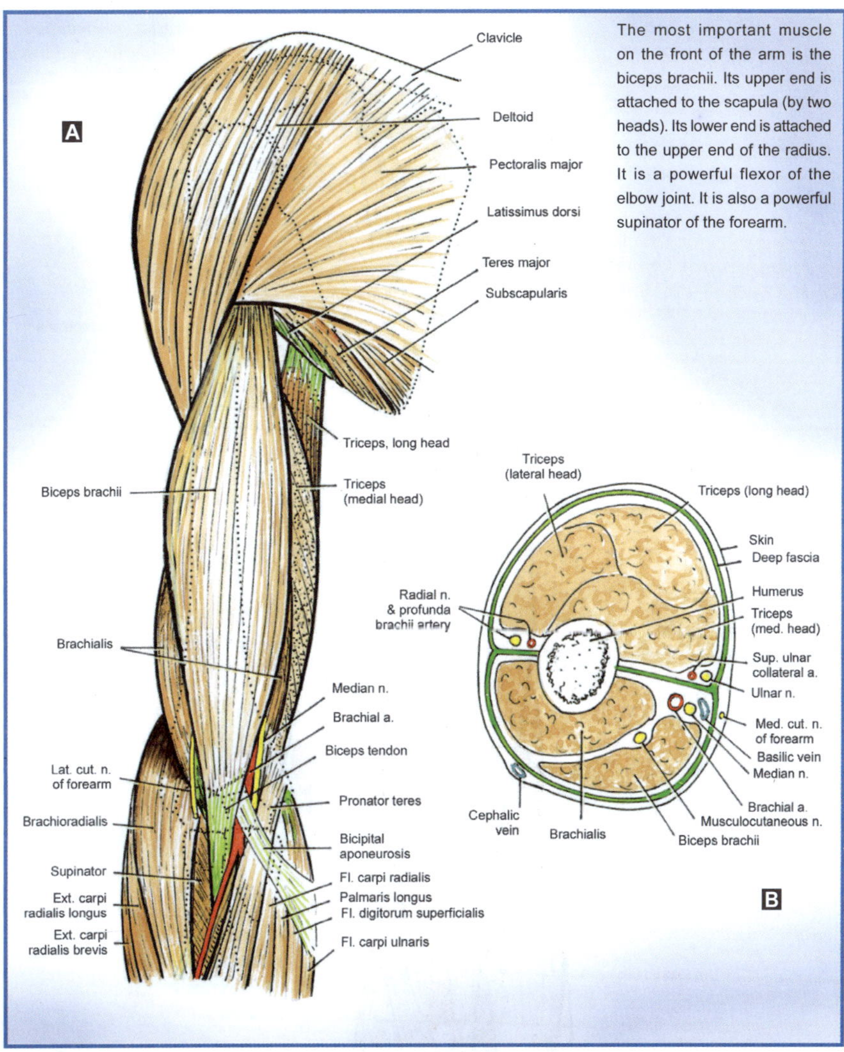

Figs 25.5A and B A. Front of arm. Note the large biceps brachii muscle. Also note the brachial artery lying just medial to the biceps tendon. In the upper part of the figure identify the deltoid and pectoralis major muscles; B. Transverse section through middle of arm.

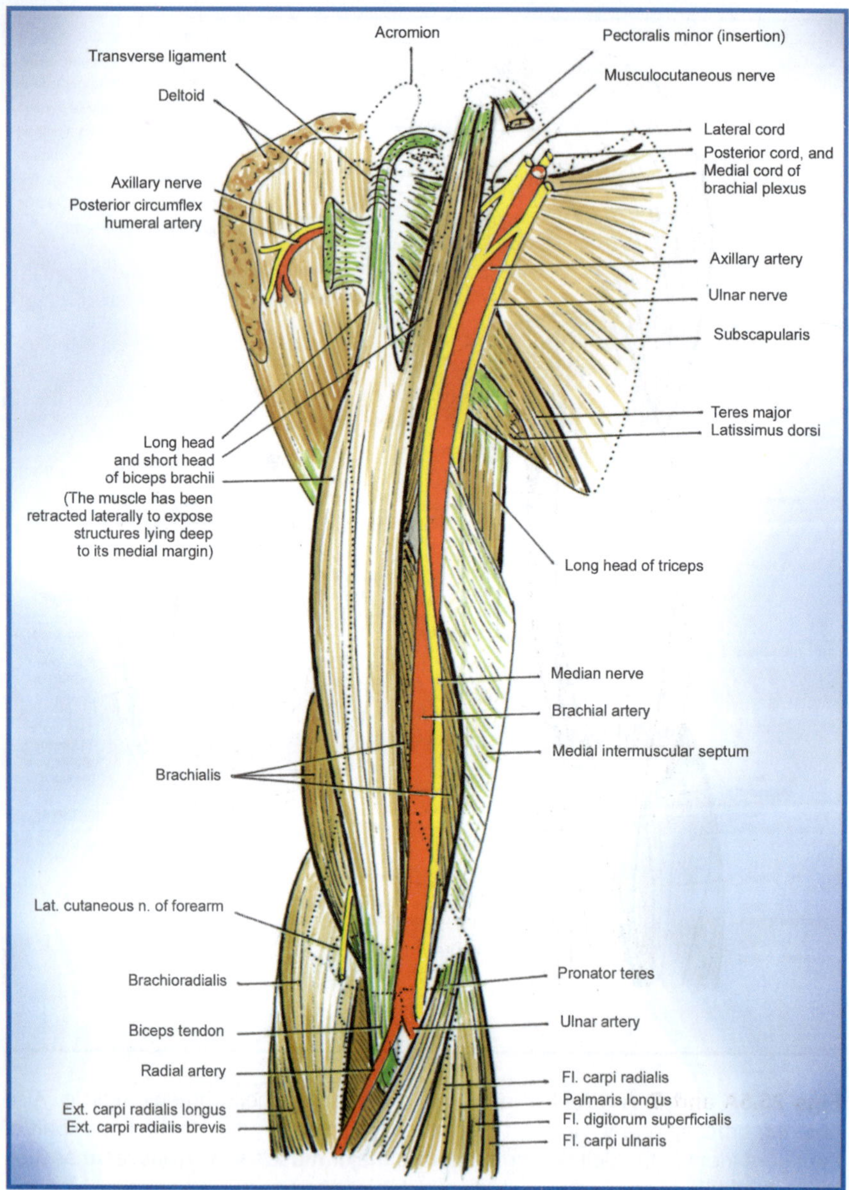

Fig. 25.6 Front of arm seen after removing the pectoralis major and part of the deltoid. Some structures of the axilla and scapular region are also seen. The brachial artery is the main artery of the arm. It is a continuation of the axillary artery. In front of the elbow it divides into radial and ulnar arteries.

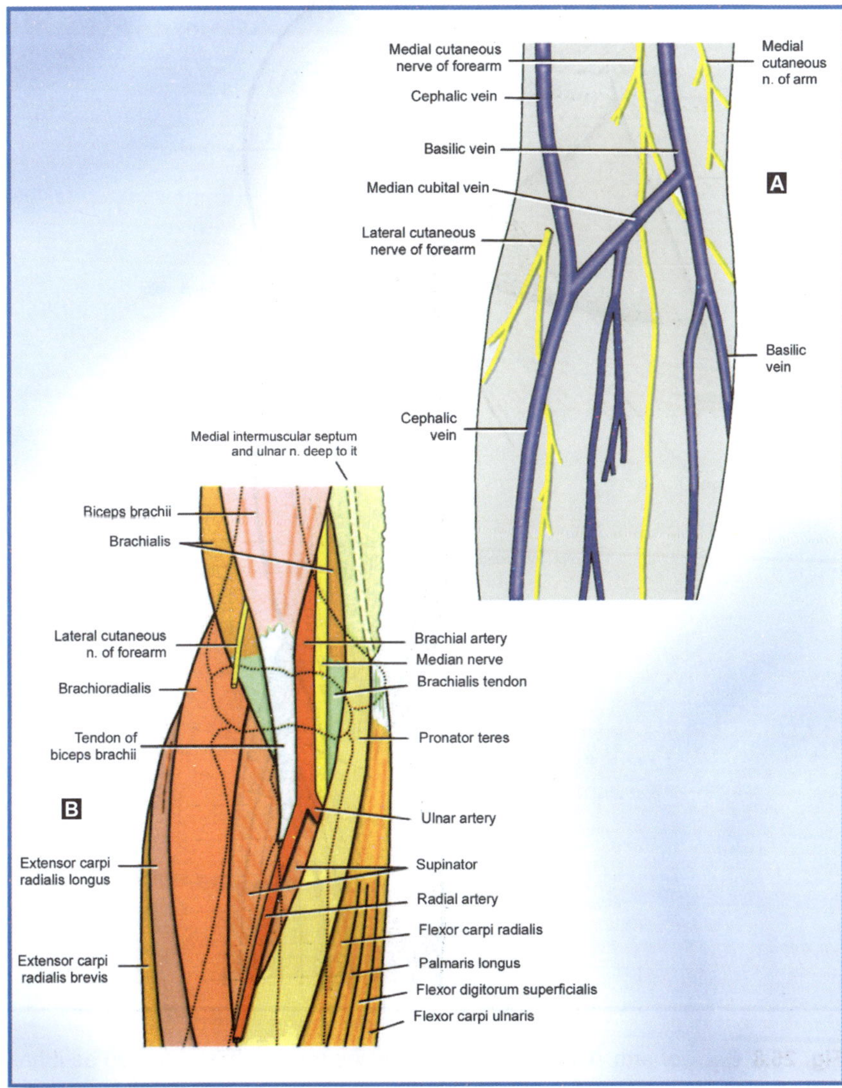

Figs 25.7A and B A. Superficial nerves and veins on the front of the elbow. The hollow in front of the elbow is called the cubital fossa. The arrangement of veins here is important as they are frequently used for intravenous injections. Identify the various structures present in the region; B. Cubital fossa seen after removal of superficial structures.

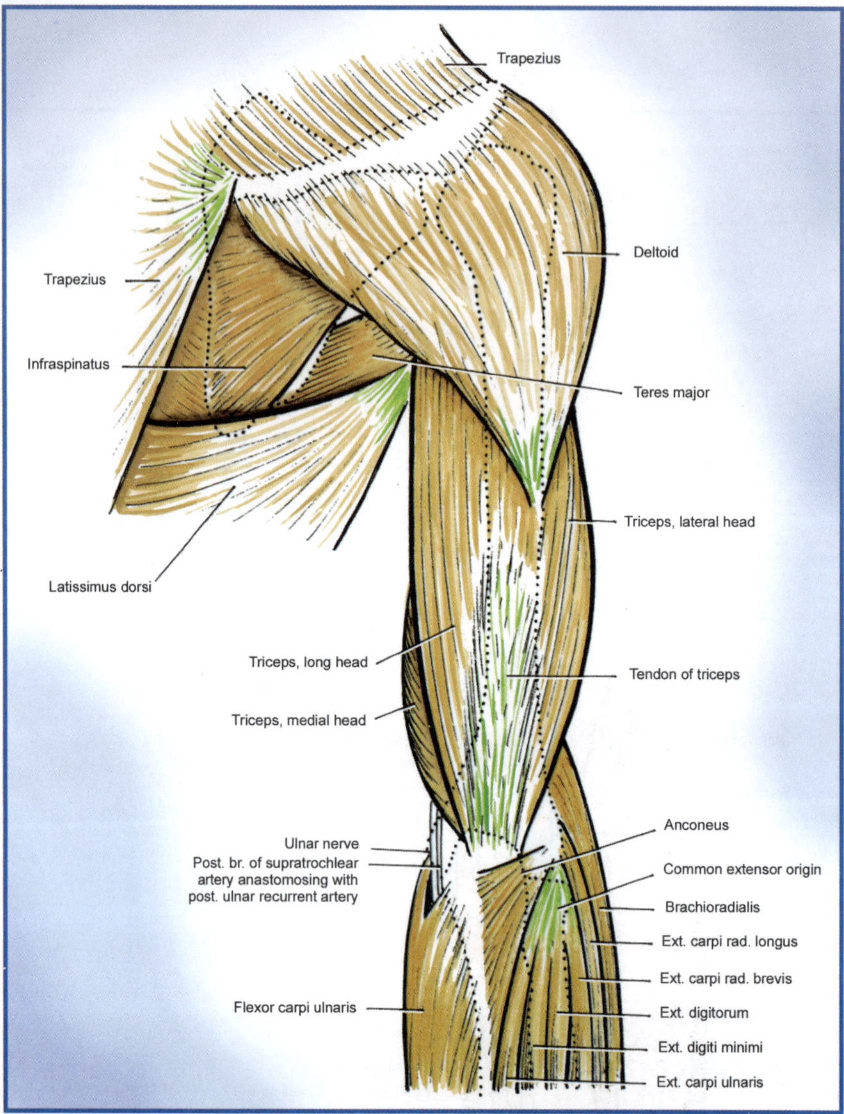

Fig. 25.8 Back of arm. The largest muscle is the triceps. It is so called as it has three heads. Its lower end is attached to the upper end of the ulna. It is powerful extensor of the forearm, at the elbow joint. Note that the upper part of the triceps is overlapped by the deltoid.

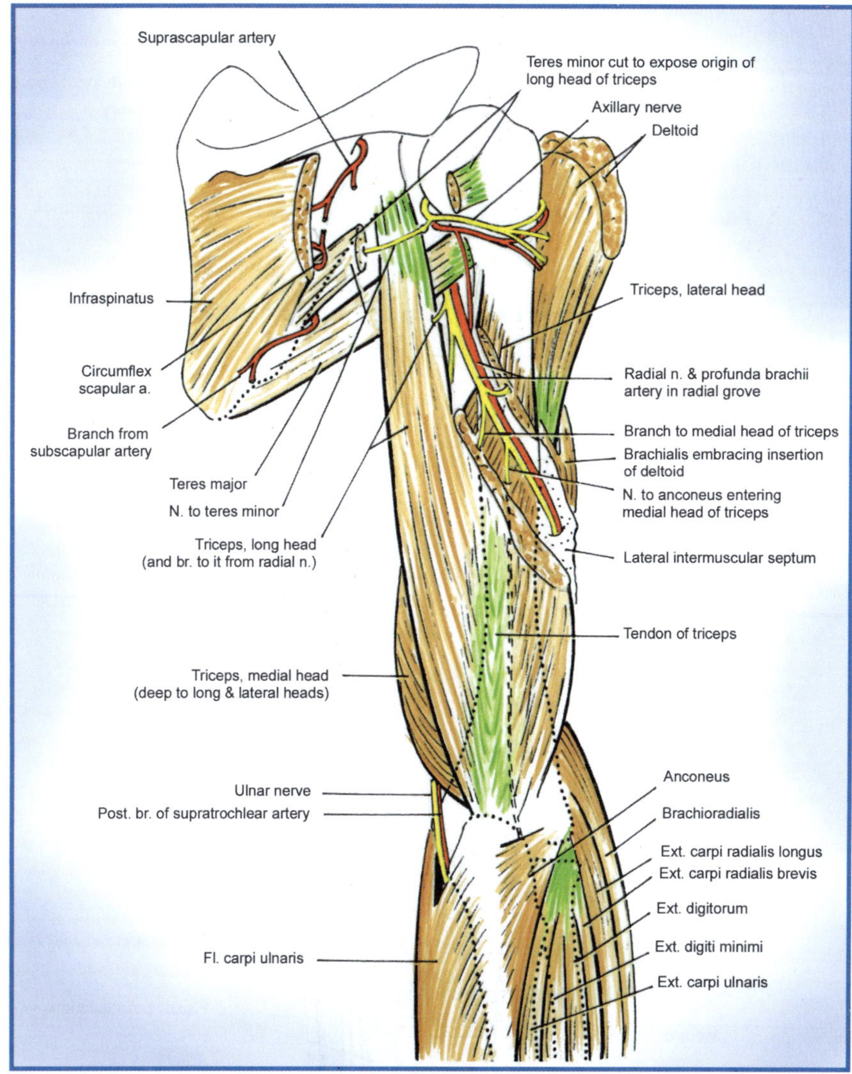

Fig. 25.9 Back of arm. Deep structures seen after removing the deltoid and a segment of the lateral head of triceps. Observe the radial nerve running obliquely behind the humerus. It is accompanied by the profunda brachii artery. The origin of the triceps is better seen in this figure.

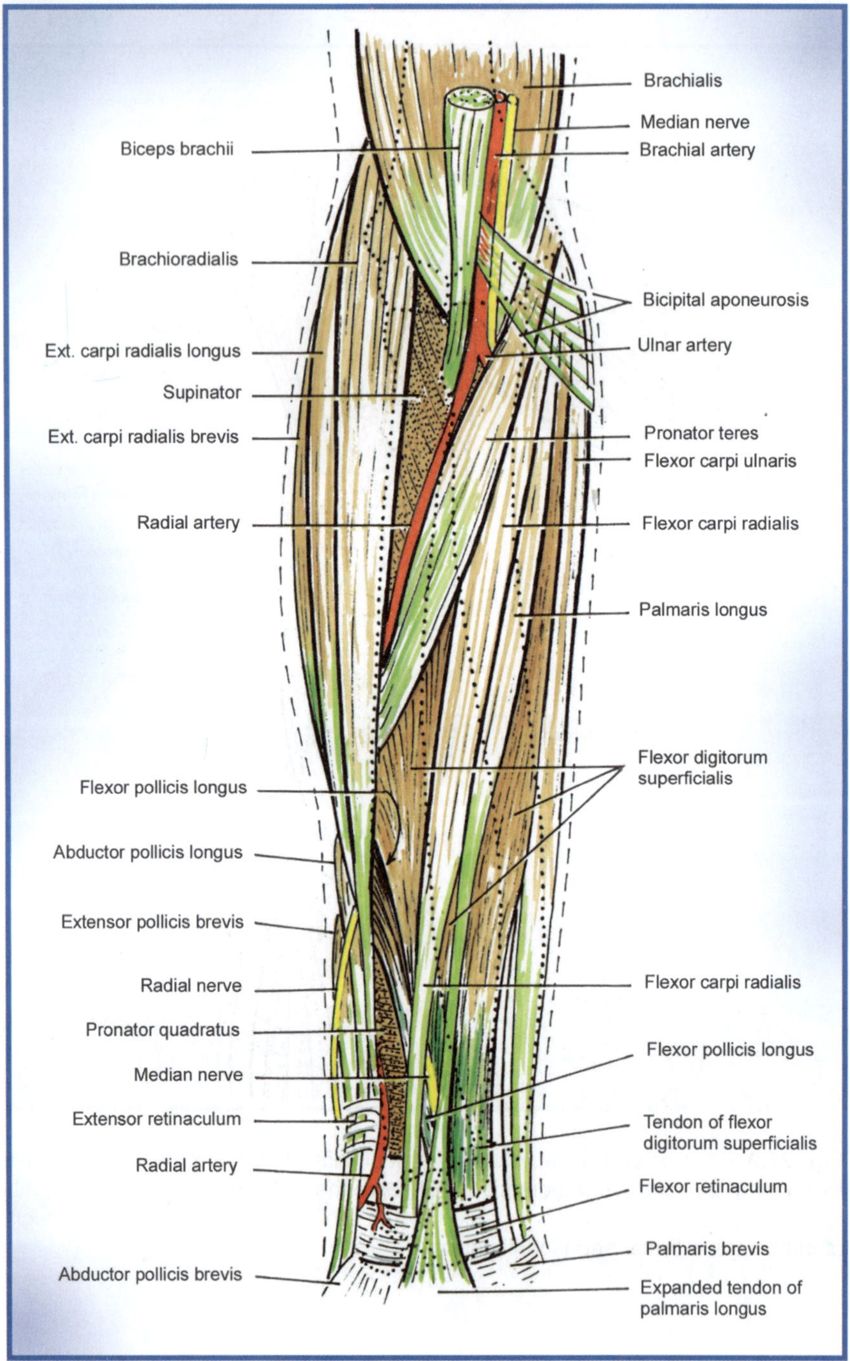

Fig. 25.10 Front of forearm. Observe that many muscles are present. Some of them produce movements at the wrist joint. Others send long tendons into the palm and fingers and produce movements of the fingers. Just above the wrist identify the radial artery. It is used for feeling the pulse.

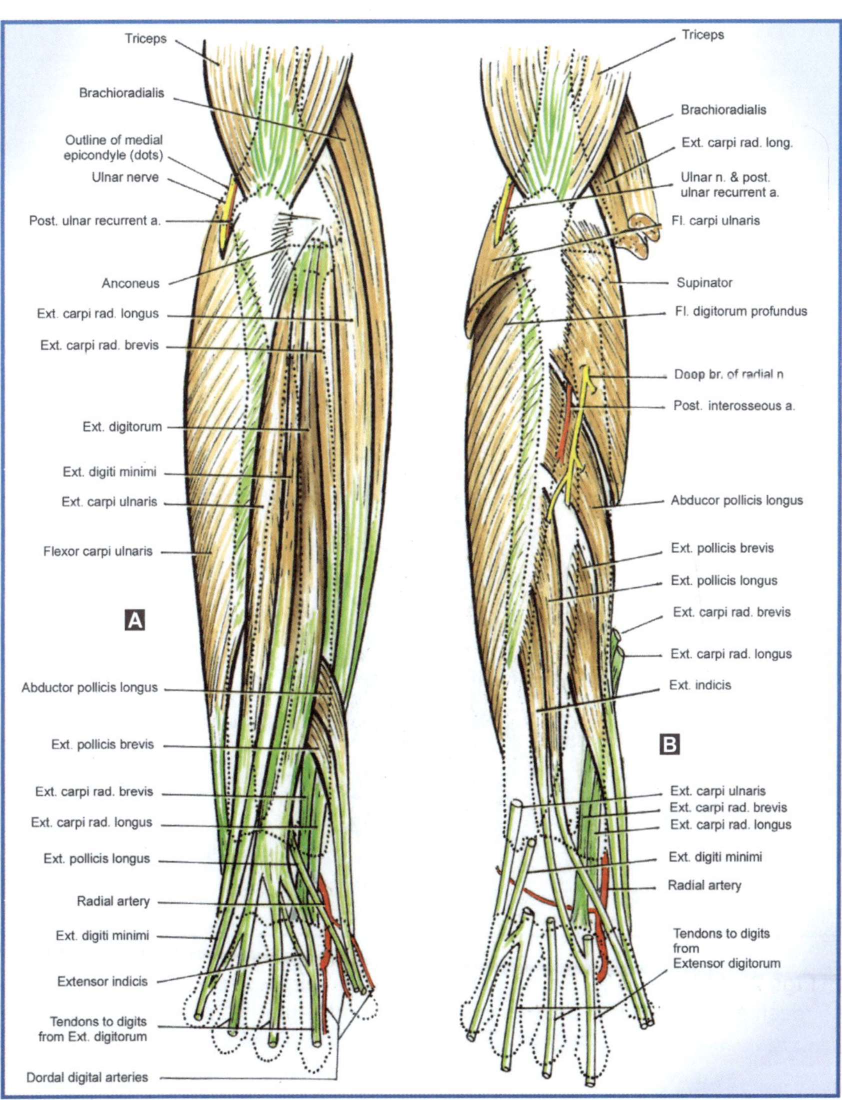

Figs 25.11A and B A. Back of forearm. Muscles seen after removal of superficial structures; B. Back of forearm. Deep structures seen after removal of parts of some muscles.

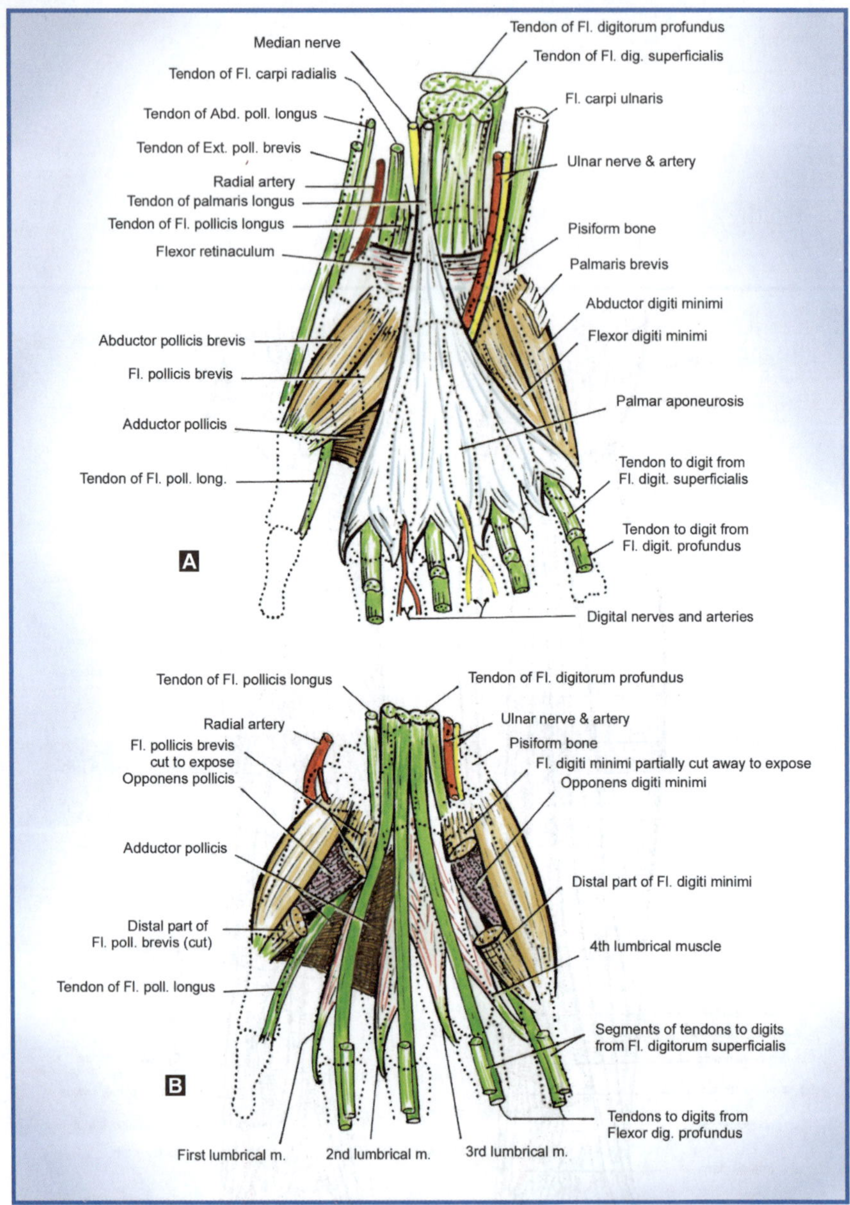

Figs 25.12A and B A. Palm. Superficial structures; B. Palm. Deep structures seen after removal of palmar aponeurosis and segments of some muscles.

There are many muscles on the front of the thigh. The sartorius runs diagonally from above downwards.Lateral to the sartorius observe the rectus femoris, the vastus lateralis and the vastus medialis. These are parts of a large muscle called the quadriceps femoris. The muscle ends in a tendon attached to the upper border of the patella. The lower end of the patella is connected to the tibia by the ligamentum patellae. Through this ligament the quadriceps acts as an extensor of the knee joint. This movement is very important in standing and walking.

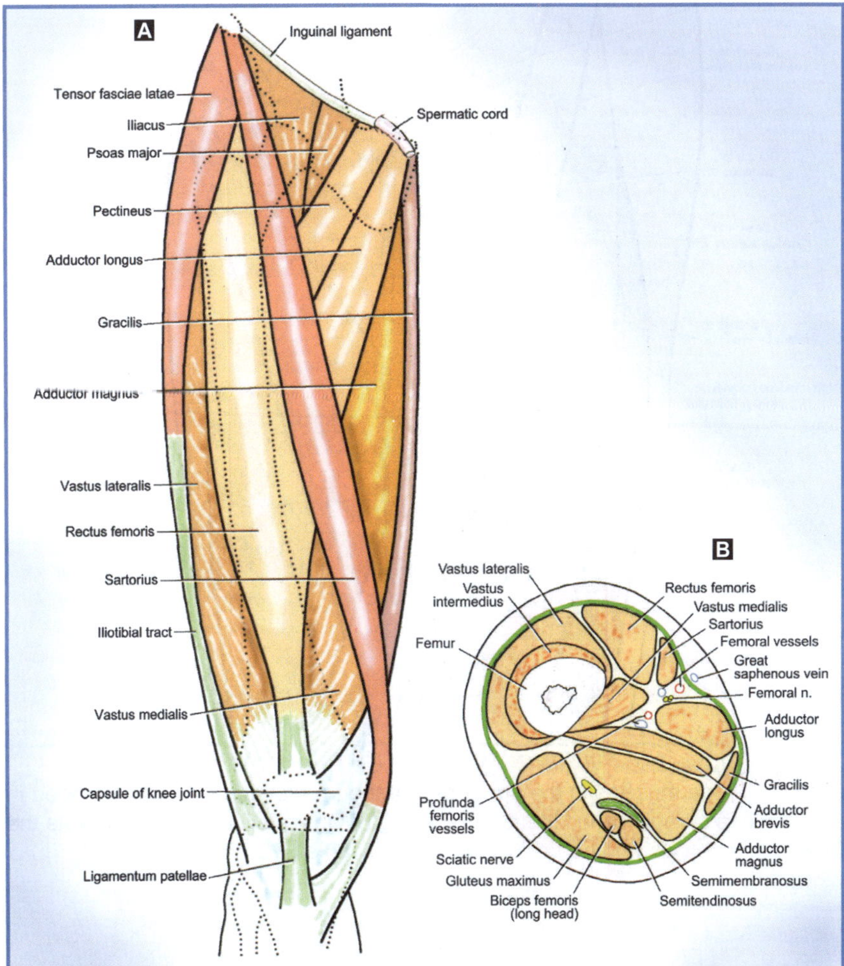

Figs 25.13A and B A. Front and medial side of thigh after removal of superficial structures; B. Transverse section across the thigh at the level of the apex of the femoral triangle.

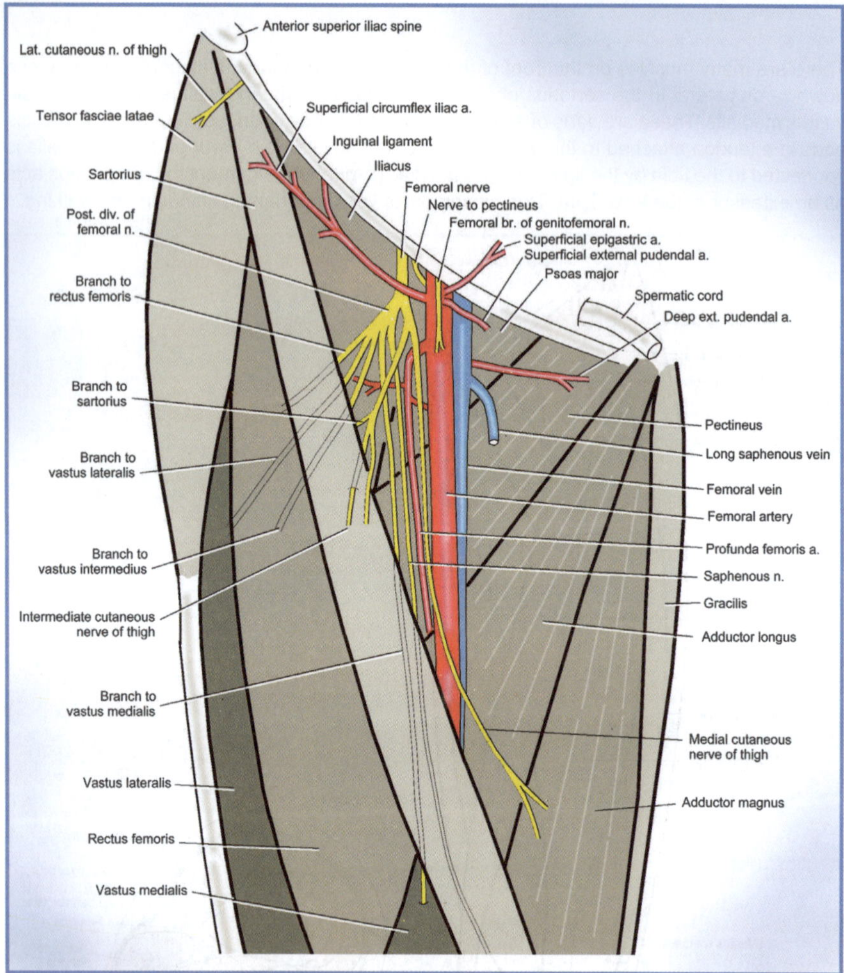

Fig. 25.14 The muscles in the upper part of the front of the thigh are arranged in the form of a triangle called the femoral triangle. Observe its boundaries. Note the femoral artery, vein and nerve present in the triangle.

In the upper part of this figure you see the gluteal region. The most important muscle here is the gluteus maximus. As it is a large and thick muscle it is used for giving intramuscular injections. The gluteal muscles play an important role in maintaining the erect posture of the body.

In the back of the thigh identify the biceps femoris, the semitendinosus, and the semimembranosus muscles. They are collectively referred to as the hamstring muscles. At the upper end they are attached to the ischial tuberosity. The lower end of the biceps femoris is attached to the upper end of the fibula. The lower ends of the other two hamstrings are attached to the upper end of the tibia.

The region behind the knee is called the popliteal fossa. In it identify the popliteal artery and vein, and the tibial and common peroneal nerves.

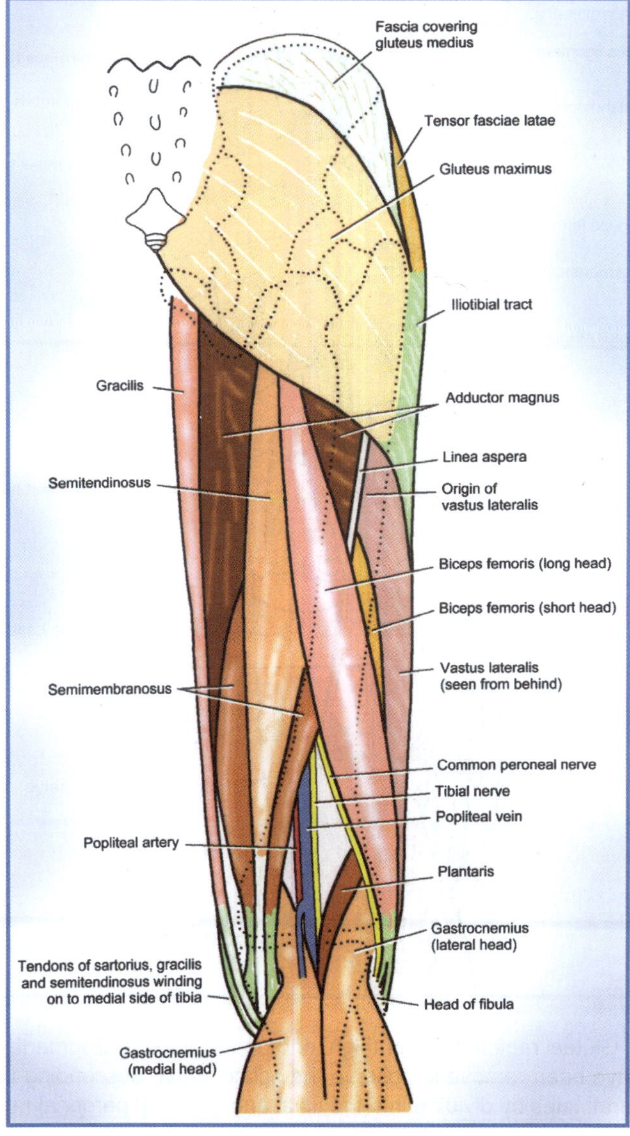

Fig. 25.15 Back of thigh and popliteal fossa seen after removal of superficial structures.

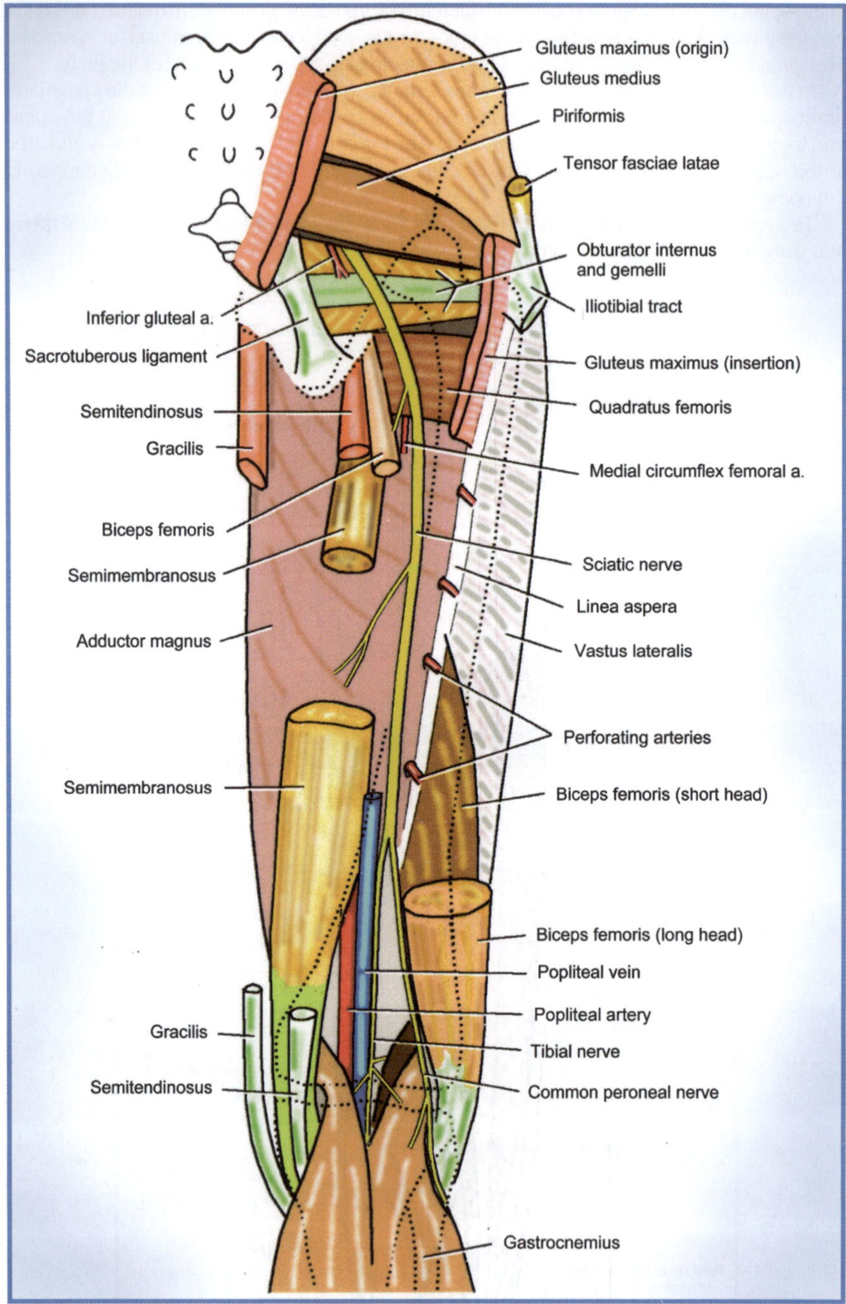

Fig. 25.16 Gluteal region, back of thigh, and popliteal fossa. Segments of several muscles have been removed. Observe the sciatic nerve descending through the region. It terminates by dividing into the tibial and common peroneal nerves.

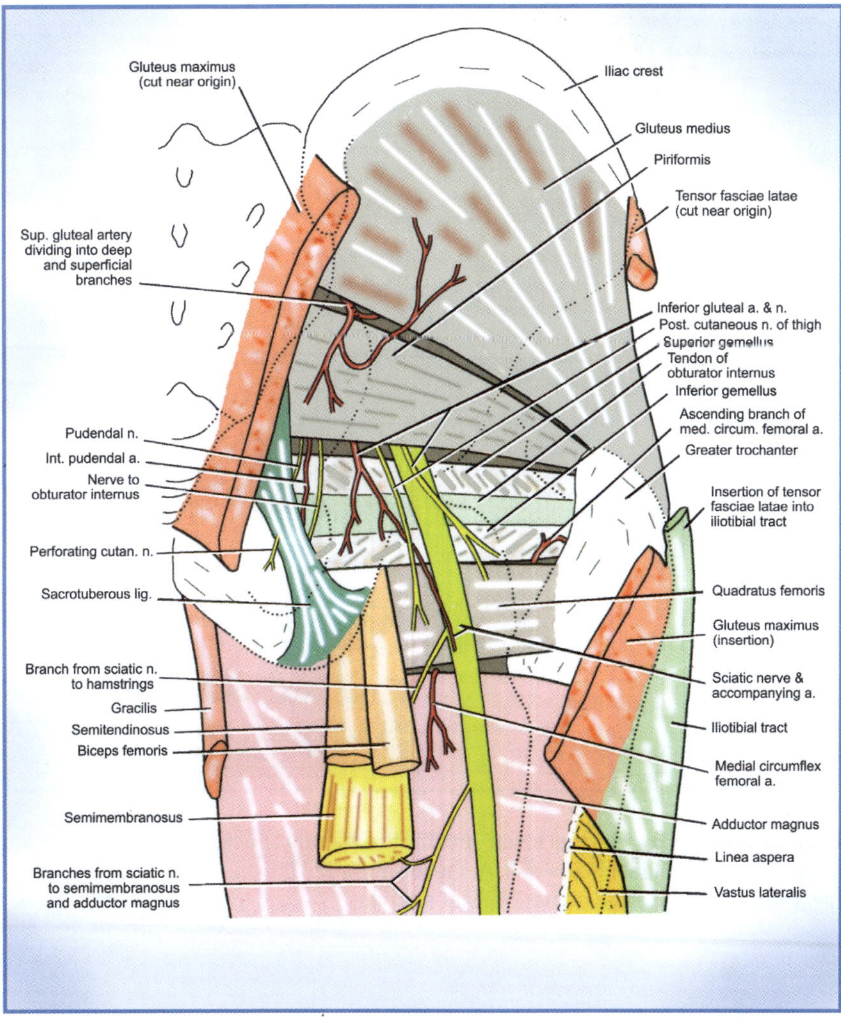

Fig. 25.17 Gluteal region seen after removal of the greater part of the gluteus maximus, and segments of some other muscles.

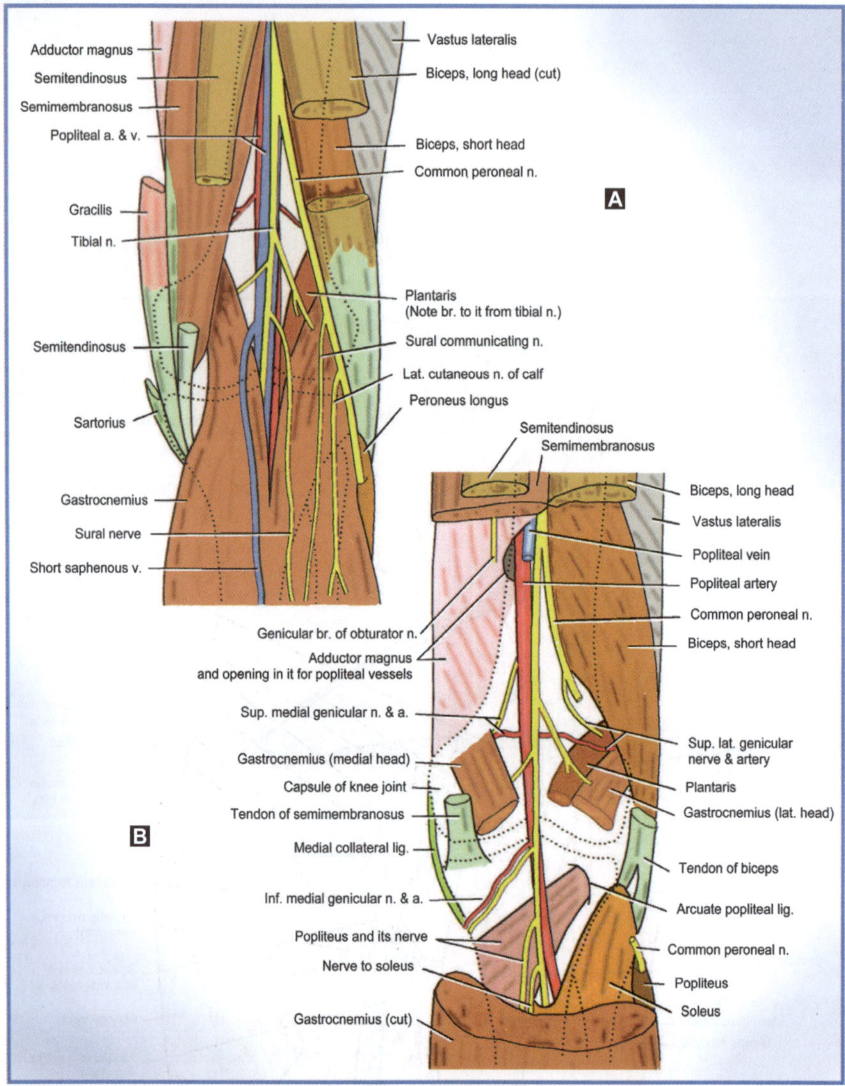

Figs 25.18A and B Popliteal fossa. Identify the various structures shown. B. Shows deeper level than that shown in A. At the lower end of the fossa the popliteal artery divides into anterior and posterior tibial arteries.

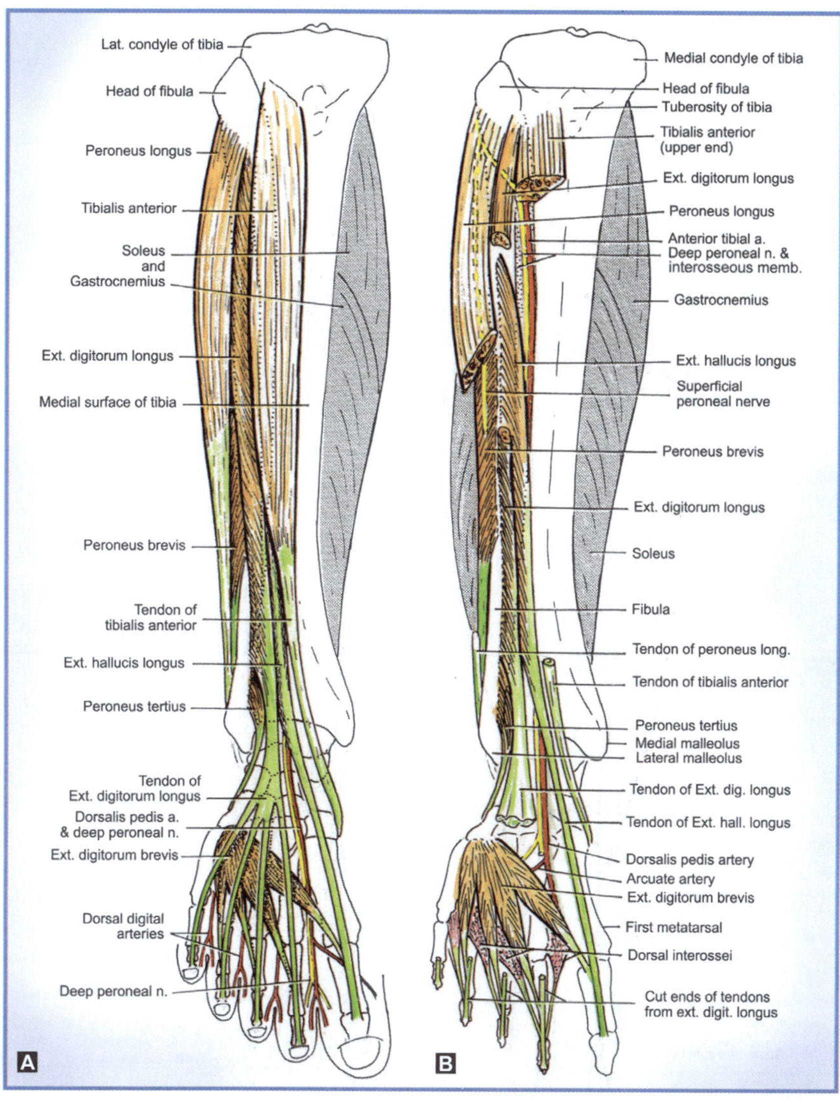

Fig. 25.19 Front and lateral side of leg. A. Superficial view of muscles. B. Deep structures in the region. The muscles are responsible for movements of the ankle and toes.

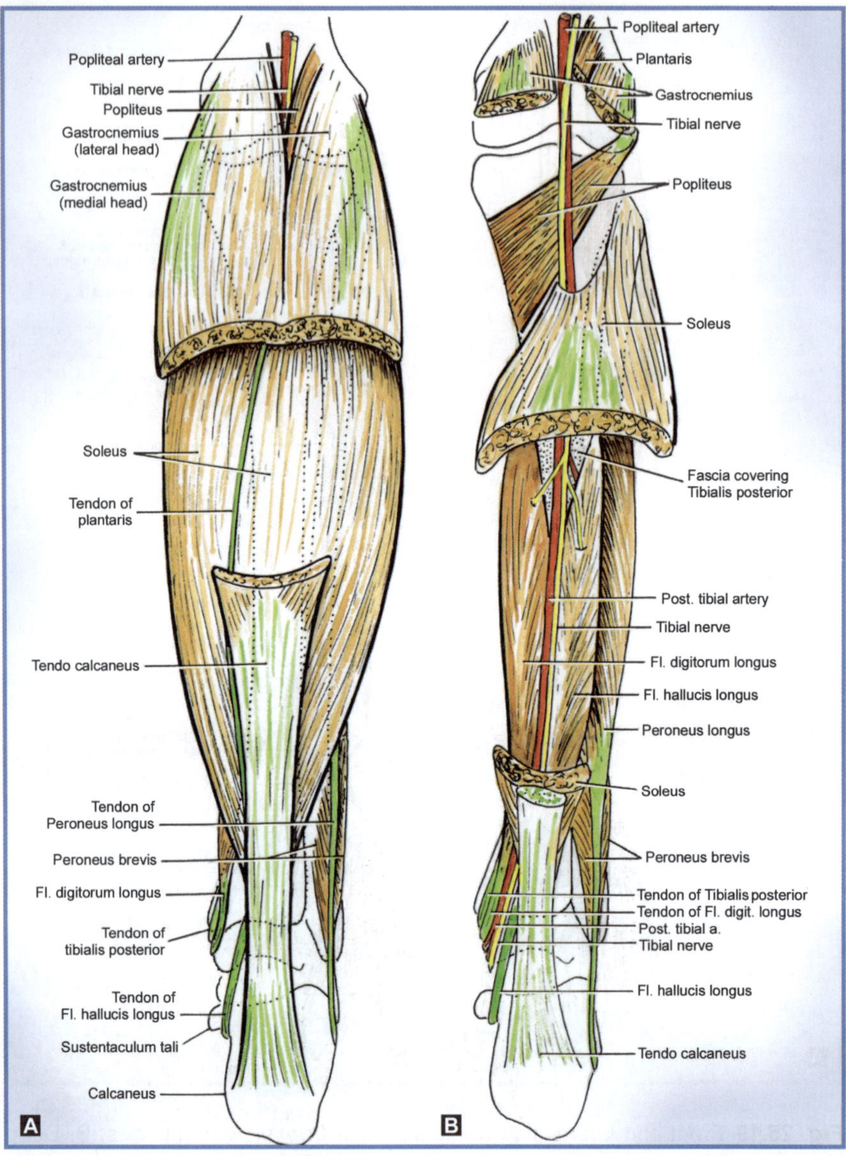

Fig. 25.20 Back of leg. The muscles here are called the calf muscles. One of these is the gastrocnemius and the other is the soleus. They end in a common tendon that is attached to the calcaneus. The muscles are very important for walking. In figure 'A' a segment of the gastrocnemius has been removed to expose deeper structures; B. The gastrocnemius has been completely removed and a segment of the soleus has been cut away.

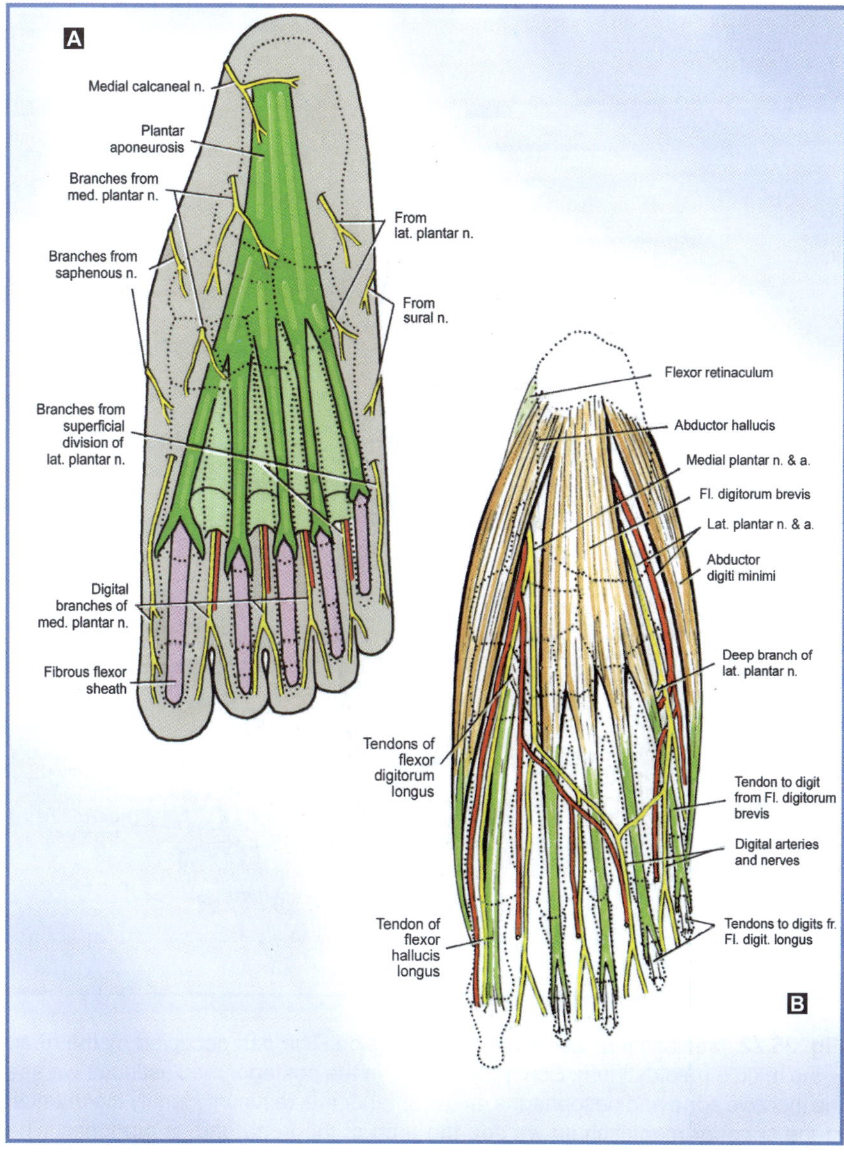

Figs 25.21A and B Sole of foot. A. Superficial structures; B. Structures seen after removal of the plantar aponeurosis.

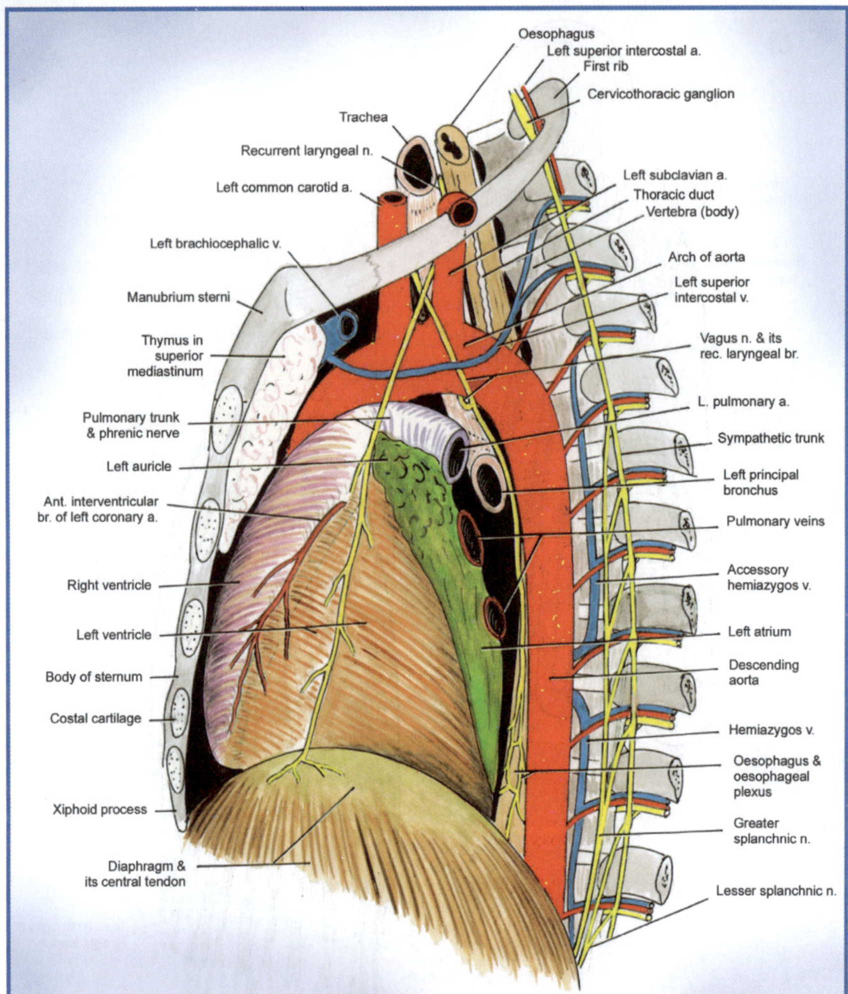

Fig. 25.22 Mediastinum viewed from the left side. The part occupied by the heart is the middle mediastinum. Behind the heart, in the posterior mediastinum, we see the thoracic aorta and oesophagus. In the anterior mediastinum identify the thymus. In the superior mediastinum we see the arch of the aorta and its branches. The trachea and the upper part of the oesophagus are also seen.

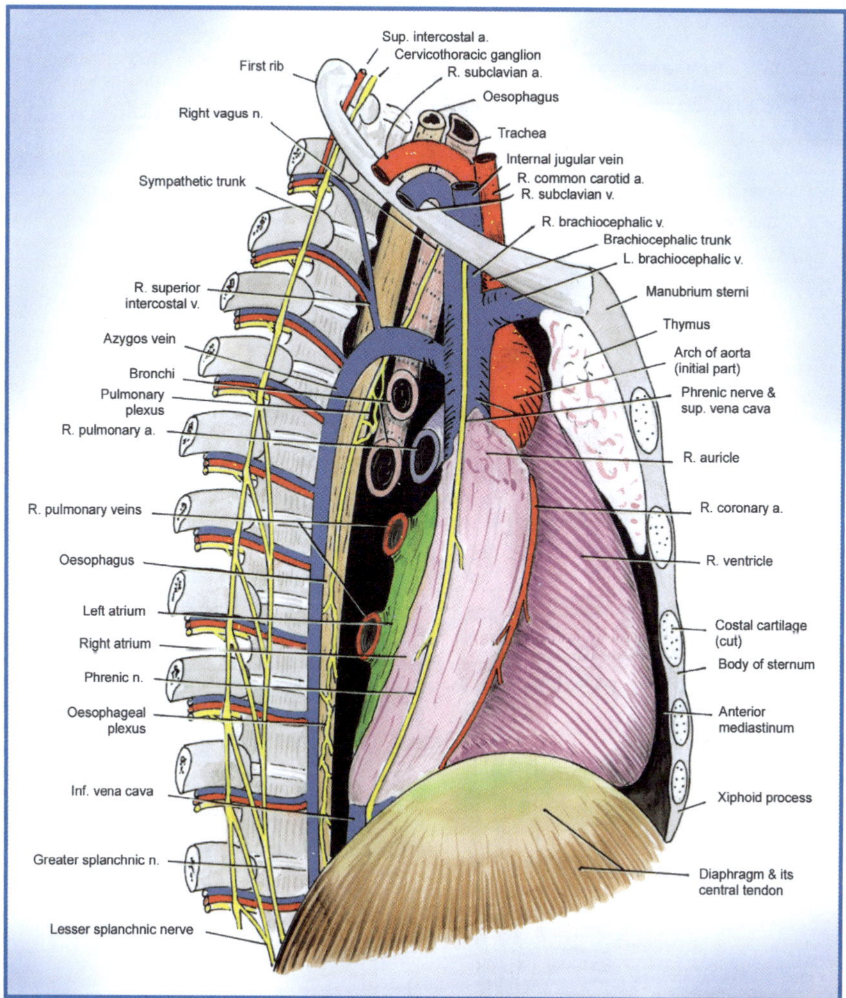

Fig. 25.23 Mediastinum viewed from the right side. In the middle mediastinum we see the right side of the heart. Identify the superior vena cava, the azygos vein, the trachea, and oesophagus. Between the heart and the sternum (anterior mediastinum) locate the thymus.

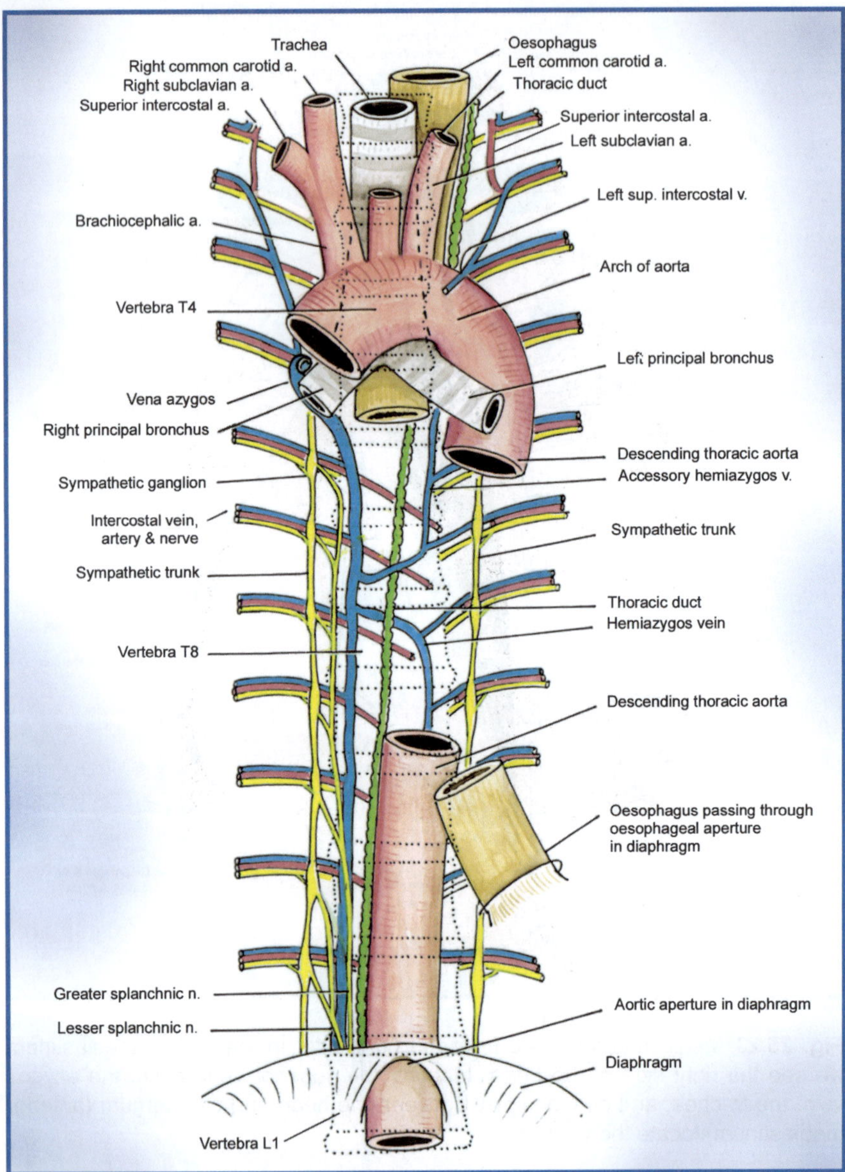

Fig. 25.24 Posterior wall of the thorax seen after removing the heart. Part of the aorta has also been removed. Observe the lower end of the aorta passing through the diaphragm. Note the relationship of the arch of the aorta to the trachea and principal bronchi. Identify the thoracic duct, the sympathetic trunk, and intercostal veins draining into the azygos and hemiazygos veins.

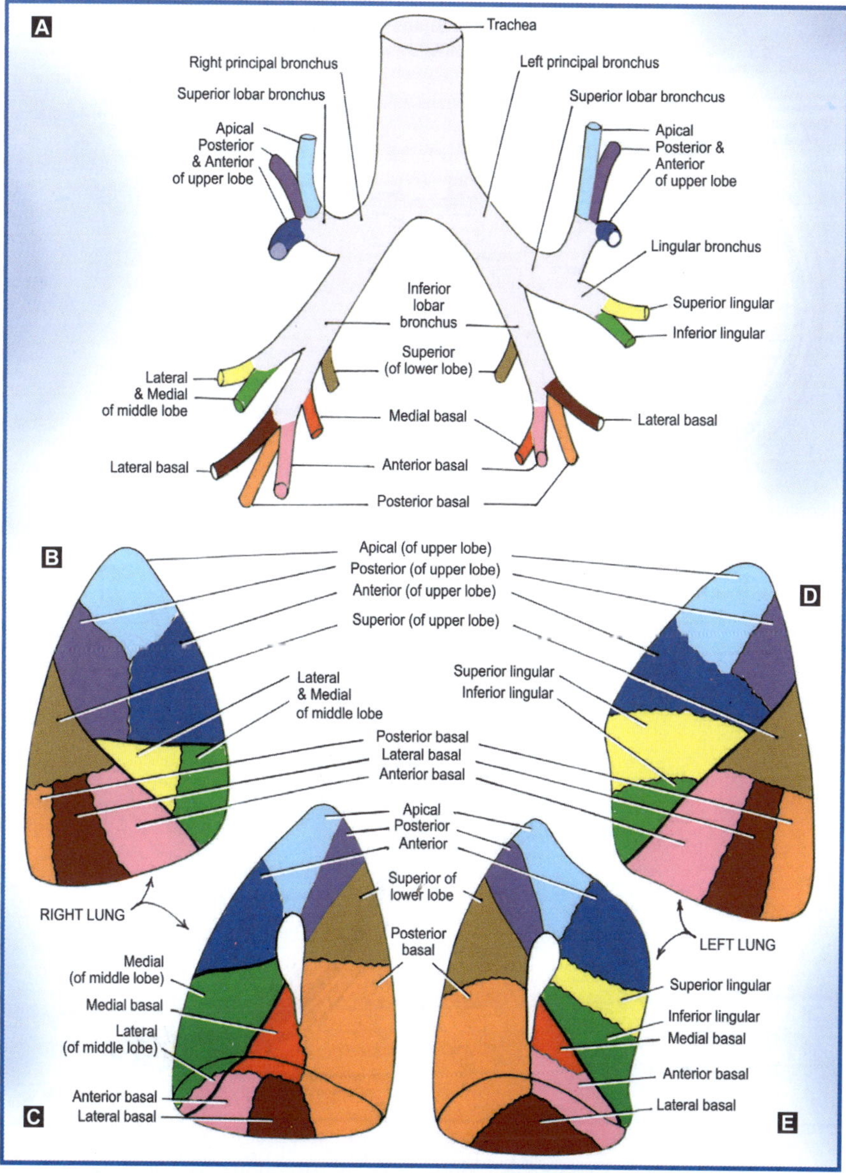

Figs 25.25A to E Scheme to show the bronchial tree as seen from the front. **B to E** Bronchopulmonary segments of the right and left lungs.

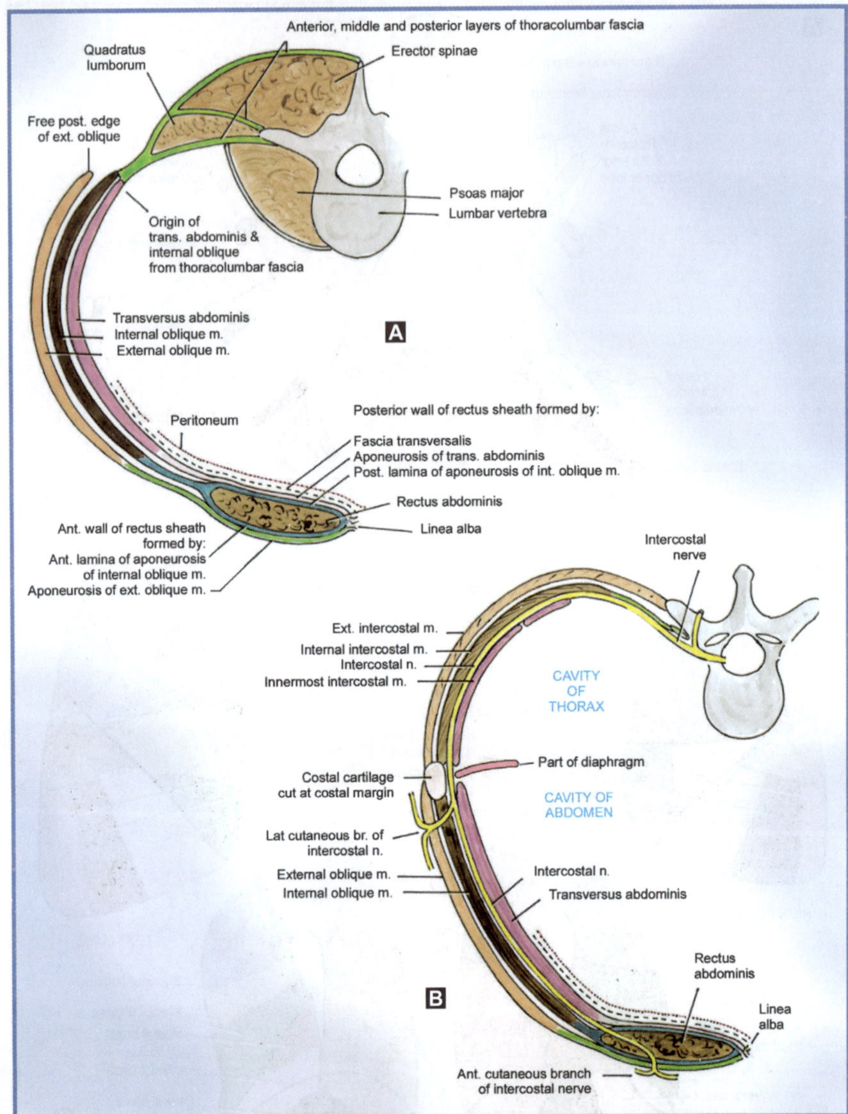

Figs 25.26A and B A. Schematic transverse section through abdominal wall to show its layers. Identify the external oblique, internal oblique and transversus muscles. Also identify the rectus abdominis; B. Schematic transverse section through thoracic and abdominal walls along the course of an intercostal nerve. Both in the thorax and abdomen the nerve lies between the second and third layers of the wall.

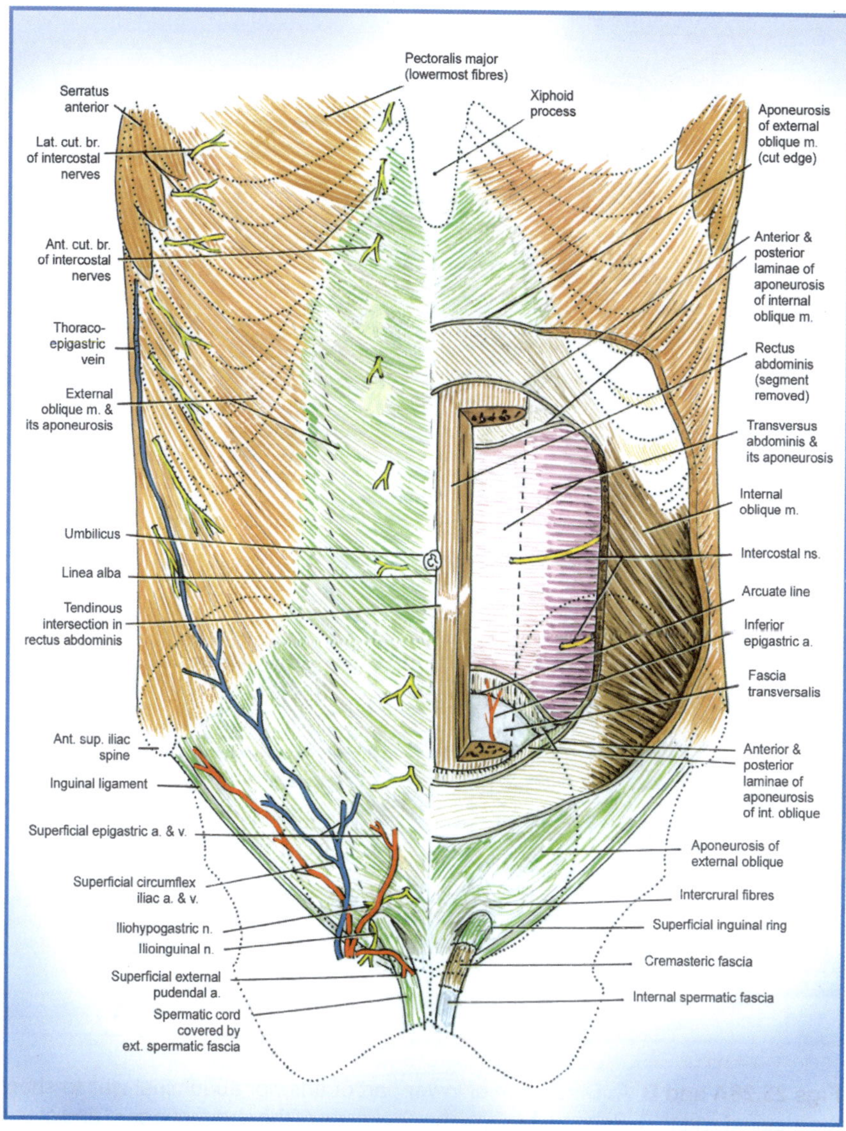

Fig. 25.27 Anterior abdominal wall. In the left half of the figure skin and fasciae have been removed to expose the external oblique muscle and its aponeurosis. In the right half of the figure windows have been cut to display successive layers of the wall. Identify the internal oblique muscle, the transversus abdominis and the rectus femoris. The spermatic cord is seen entering the inguinal canal at the superficial inguinal ring.

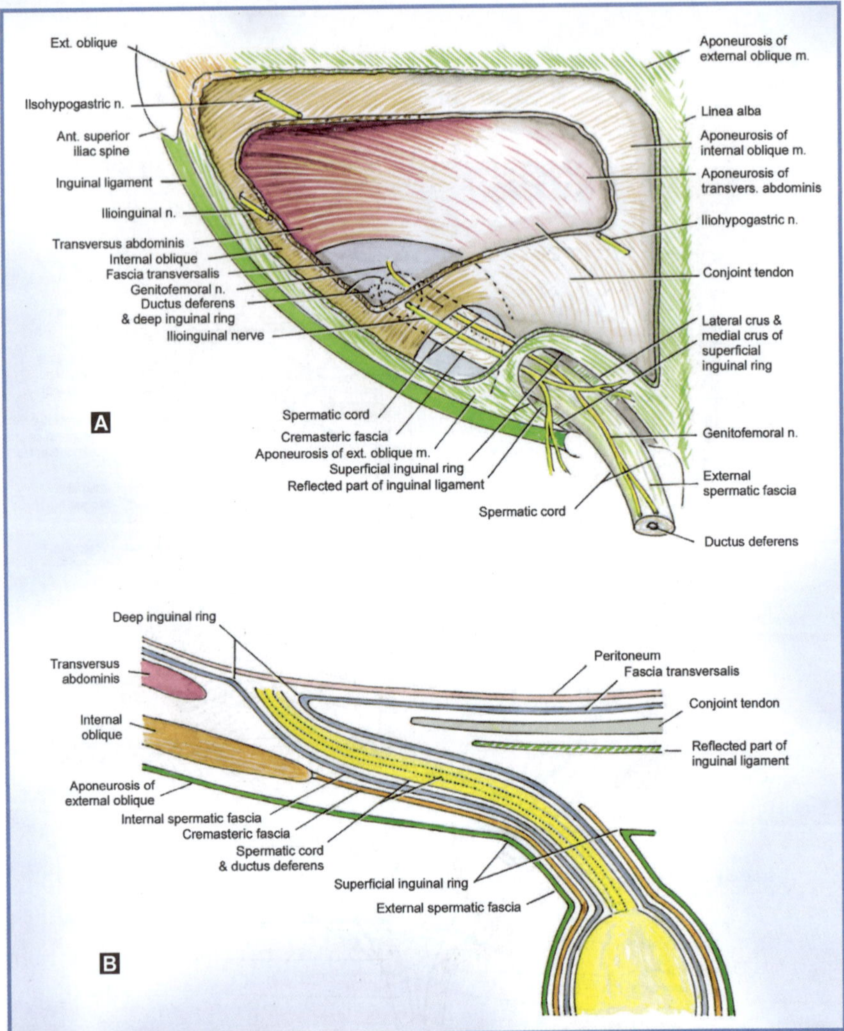

Figs 25.28A and B A. Dissection of lower part of anterior abdominal wall to show the inguinal canal; B. Scheme to show the coverings of the spermatic cord and of the testis. The anatomy of this region is of great importance in relation to inguinal hernia.

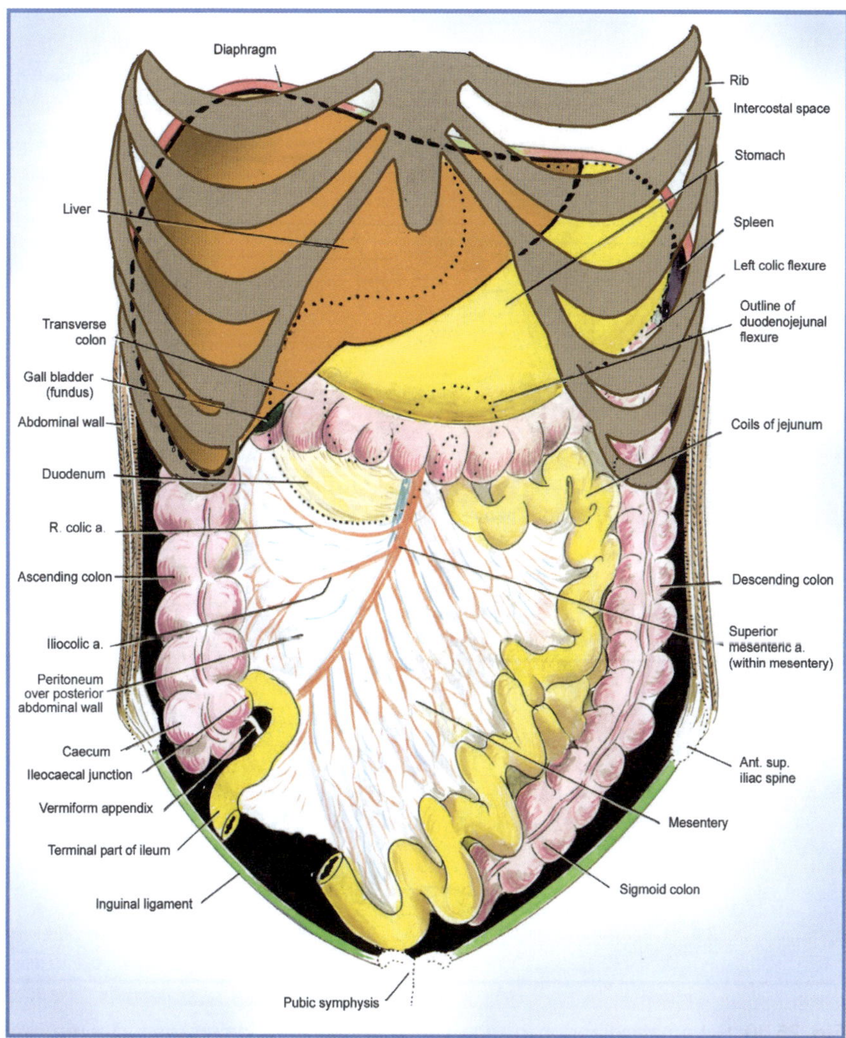

Fig. 25.29 Schematic diagram to show some superficial contents seen within the abdomen after removal of the anterior abdominal wall. The greater omentum and some coils of small intestine have been removed. Observe the position of the liver, part of the stomach, the large intestine and the mesentery.

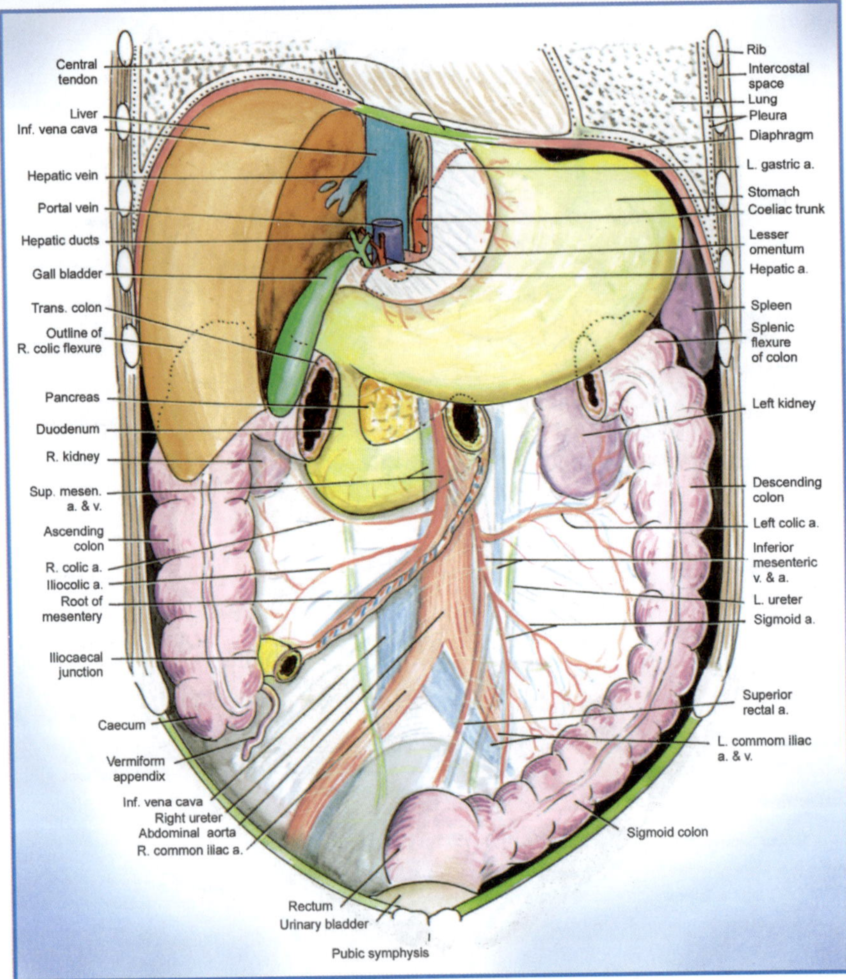

Fig. 25.30 Schematic diagram to show structures in the abdomen seen after removal of the jejunum and ileum, and most of the mesentery. Removal of part of the liver brings the entire stomach and duodenum into view. Note the position of the gall bladder (behind the liver). Identify the inferior vena cava and the spleen. The aorta is seen through overlying peritoneum.

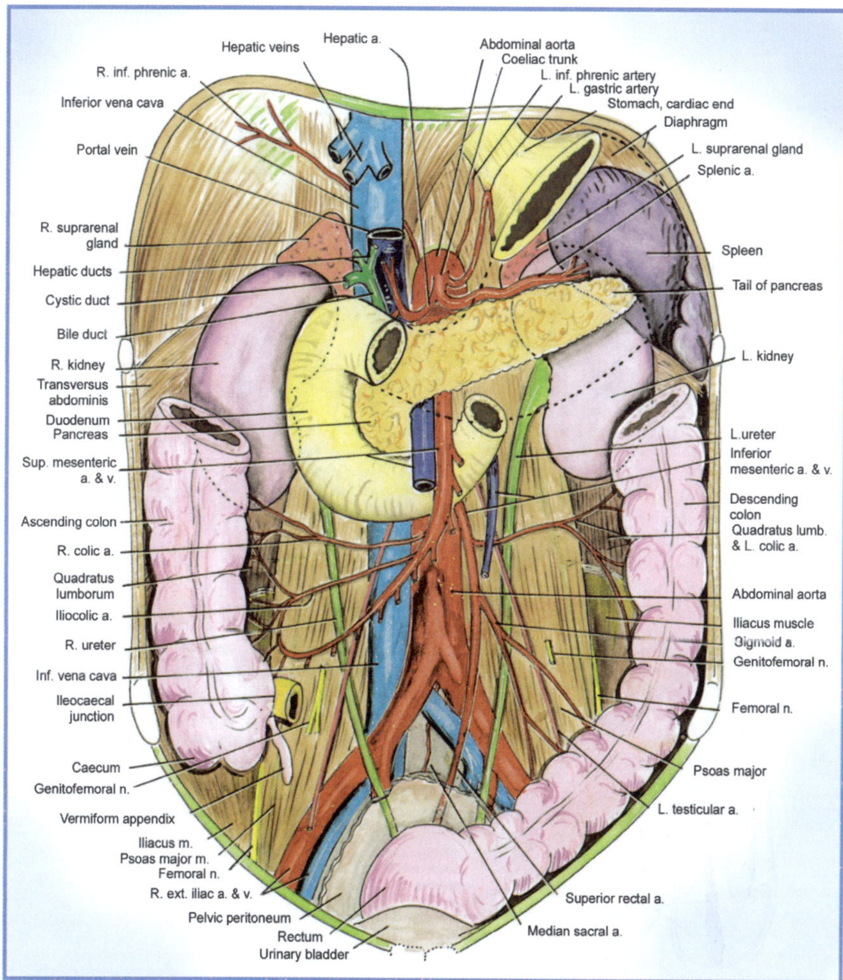

Fig. 25.31 Diagram showing the posterior abdominal wall and viscera related to it, after removal of overlying peritoneum. Observe the 'C'-shaped duodenum, the pancreas, the kidneys, the spleen, the abdominal aorta. the common iliac and external iliac arteries, and the inferior vena cava. Also identify the suprarenal glands and the ureters.

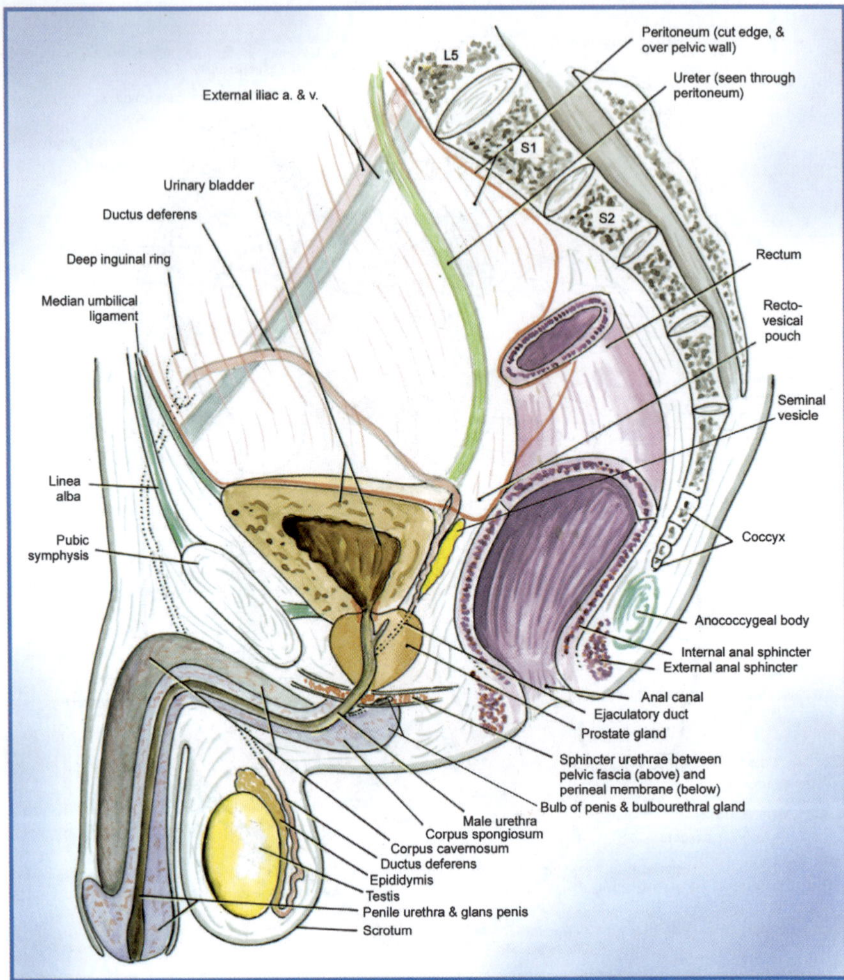

Fig. 25.32 Sagittal section through male pelvis showing viscera. First identify the rectum and anal canal. In front of the rectum there is the urinary bladder. Just below the bladder we see the prostate gland. Trace the urethra from the urinary bladder through the prostate and the penis. In the scrotum identify the testis, the epididymis and the ductus deferens.

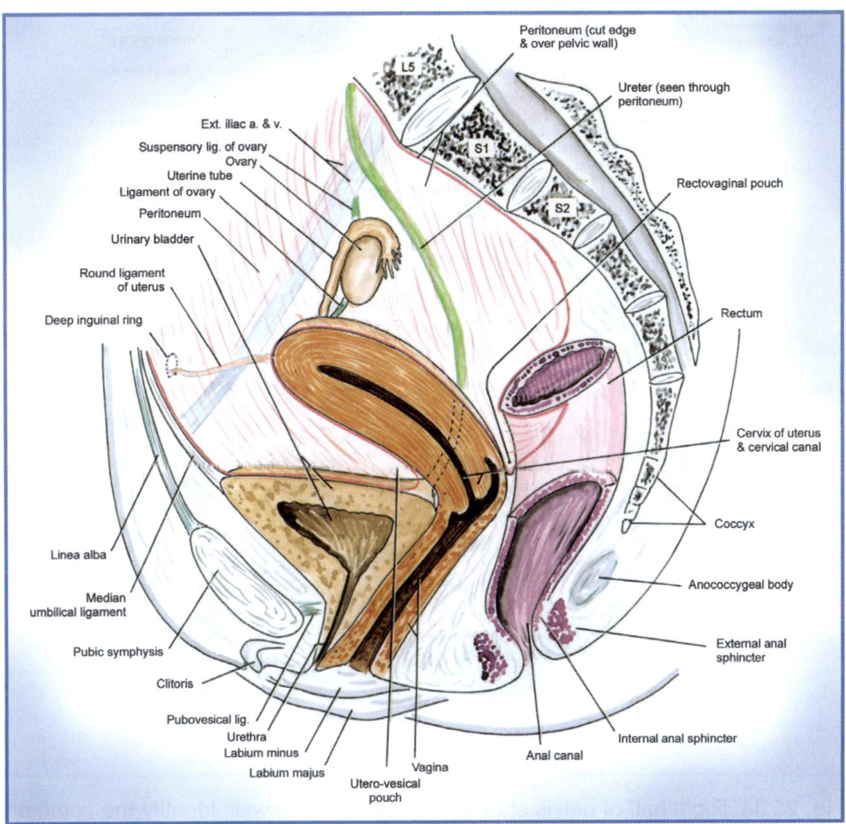

Fig. 25.33 Sagittal section through the female pelvis showing viscera. Begin by identifying the rectum and anal canal. Anterior to these identify the uterus (above) and the vagina (below). In front of the vagina there is the urinary bladder and the female urethra. The urinary bladder lies just behind the symphysis pubis.

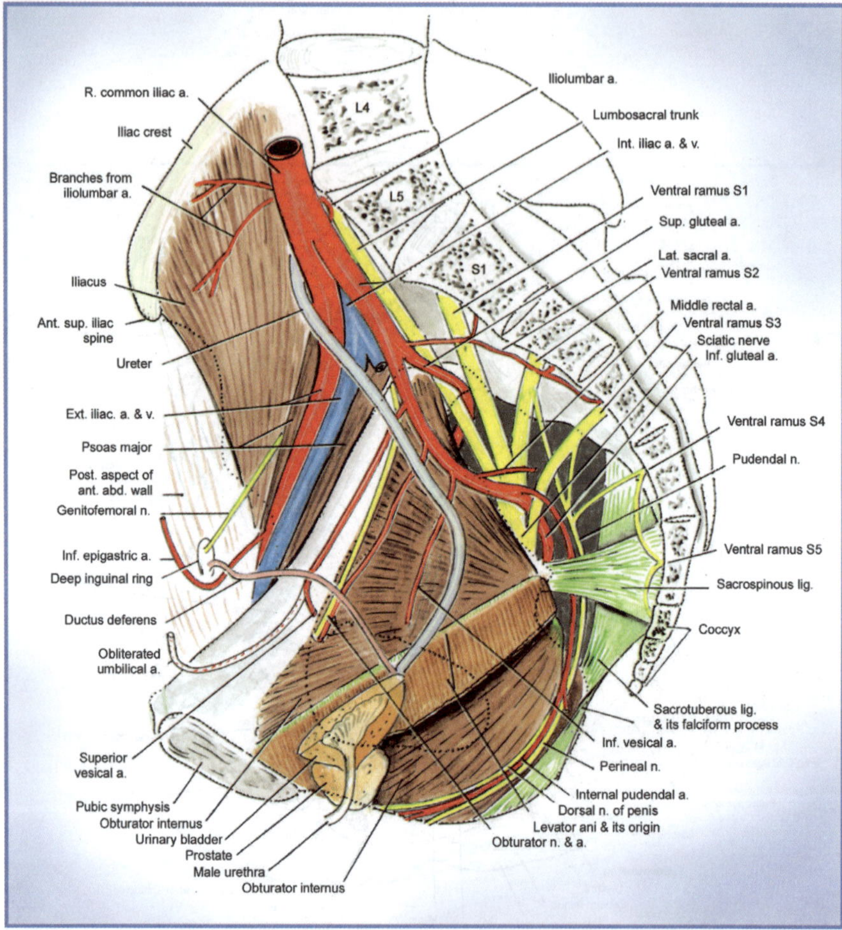

Fig. 25.34 Right half of pelvis showing structures in its wall. Identify the common iliac, external iliac and internal iliac arteries. See how the ureter descends through the pelvis to reach the urinary bladder. Note the various muscles shown. Finally note the position of the ductus deferens.

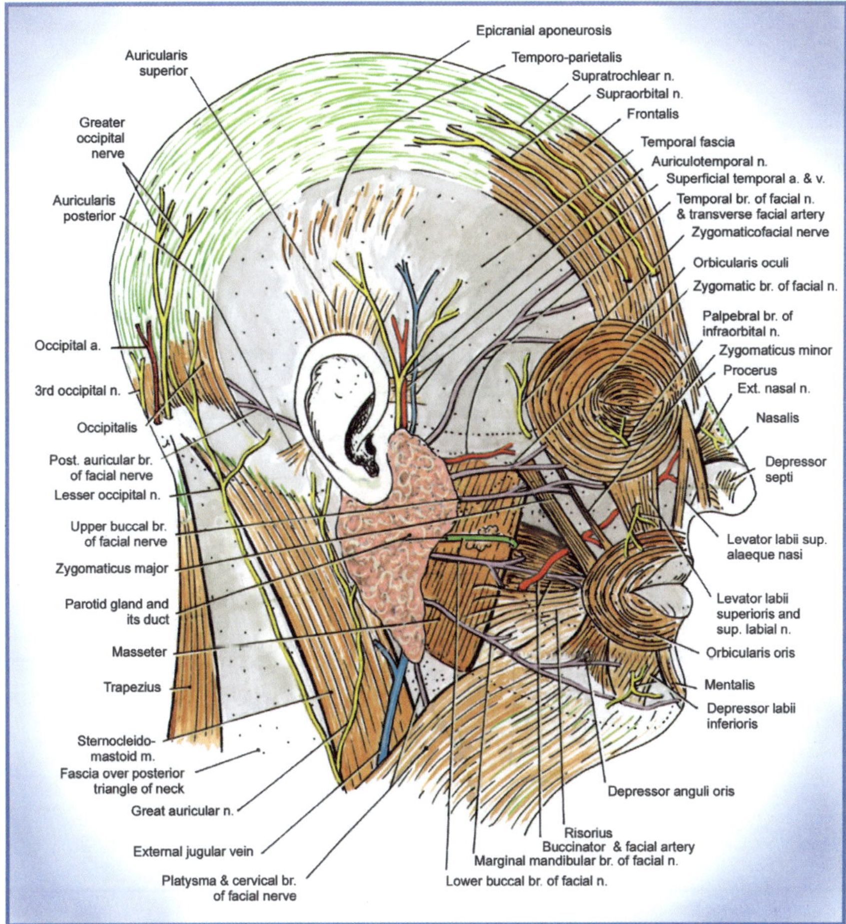

Fig. 25.35 Superficial dissection of the face, scalp, parotid region and temporal region. Branches of the facial nerve are shown in violet. Other nerves are yellow. Identify the parotid gland and its duct, the auricle of the ear, the epicranial aponeurosis in the scalp, the orbicularis oculi, the orbicularis oris, the masseter, the buccinator, and sternocleidomastoid muscles.

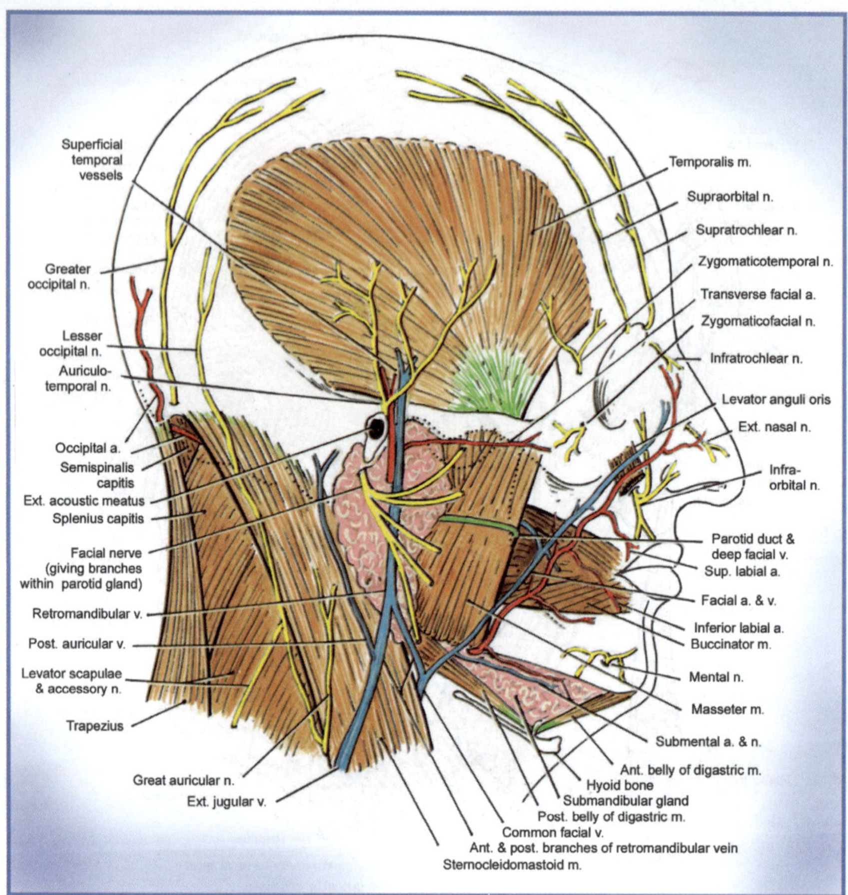

Fig. 25.36 Deep dissection of the face, and parotid region. A superficial view of the submandibular region is also seen. On the side of the head identify the large temporalis muscle. Just in front of the parotid gland identify the masseter. These two muscles help in chewing of food. In front of the masseter we see the buccinator muscle which forms the substance of the cheek. The facial artery and vein run over it. Behind the parotid we see part of the sternocleidomastoid muscle. Below the mandible you see the submandibular salivary gland.

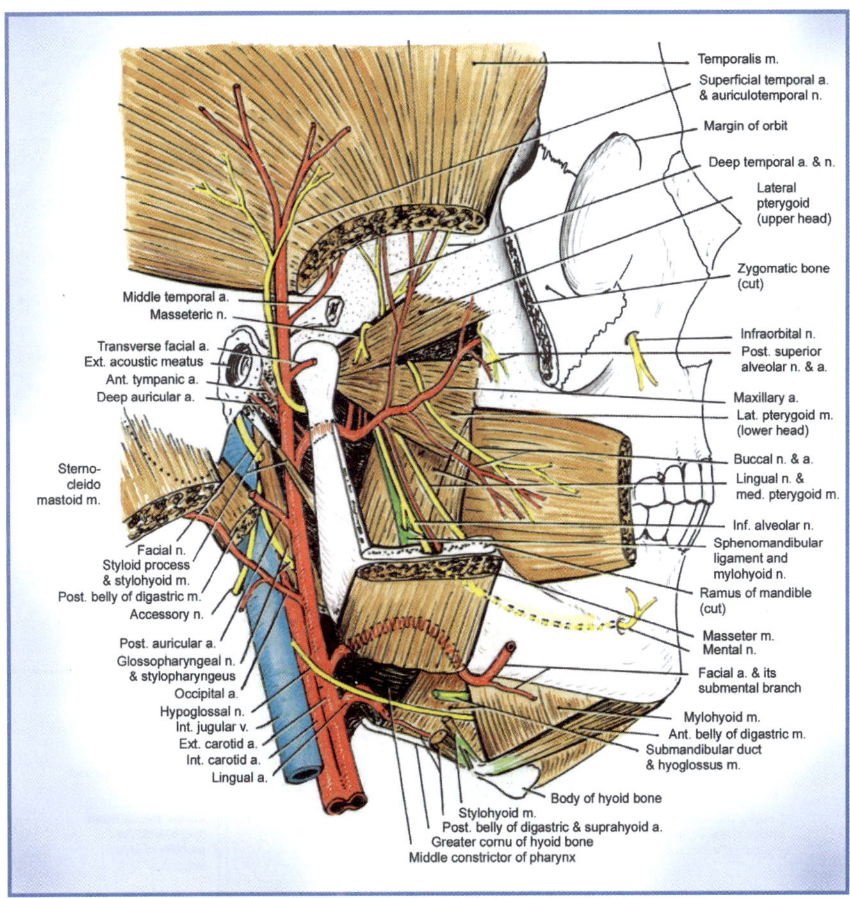

Fig. 25.37 Dissection of the side of the head. The infratemporal, temporal and submandibular regions are seen. Removal of the sternocleidomastoid brings the internal and external carotid arteries, and the internal jugular vein into view. Note the various branches of the external carotid artery. Deep to the ramus of the mandible we see the lateral and medial pterygoid muscles. Along with the temporalis and the masseter they are called muscles of mastication as they help in chewing of food.

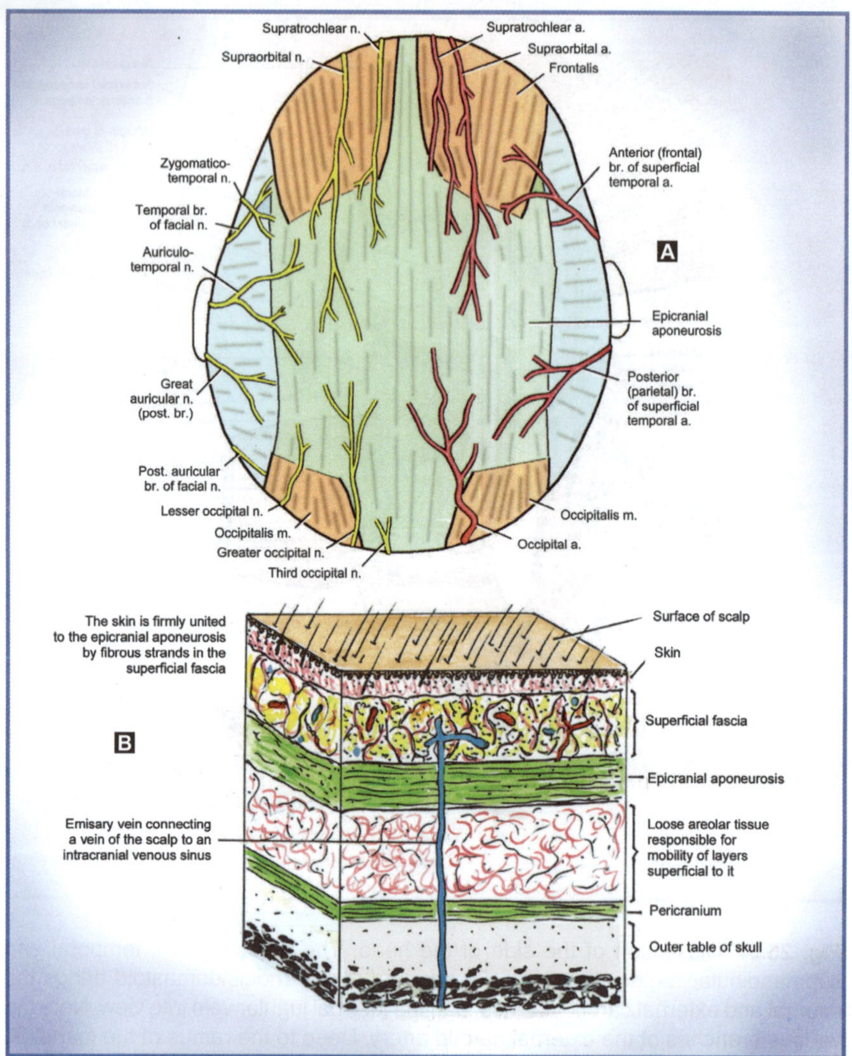

Figs 25.38A and B A. Nerves and arteries of scalp seen from above; B. Scheme to show the layers of the scalp.

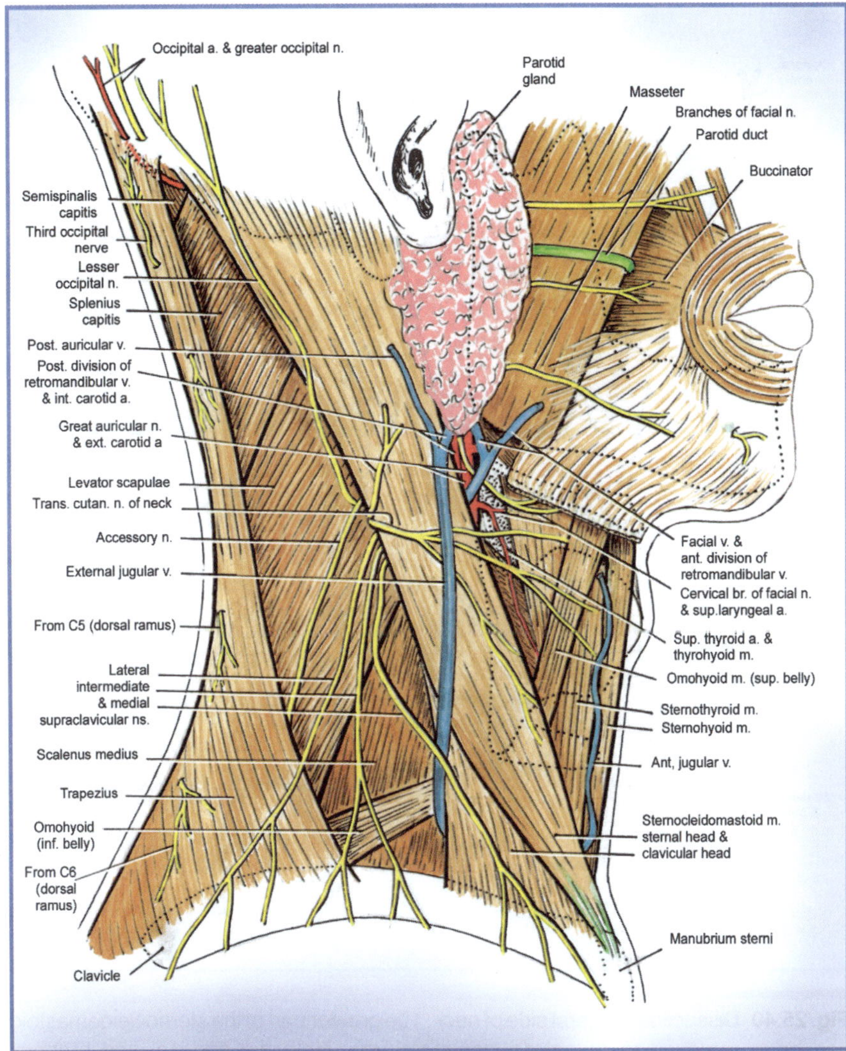

Fig. 25.39 Lateral side of the neck. Note the sternocleidomastoid muscle dividing the side of the neck into anterior and posterior triangles, and the various muscles present in these triangles. Identify the external jugular vein running down across the sternocleidomastoid. The anterior jugular vein can be seen some distance in front of the sternocleidomastoid. Observe the supraclavicular nerves emerging at the posterior border of the sternocleidomastoid muscle. They run downwards, cross the clavicle and enter the pectoral region.

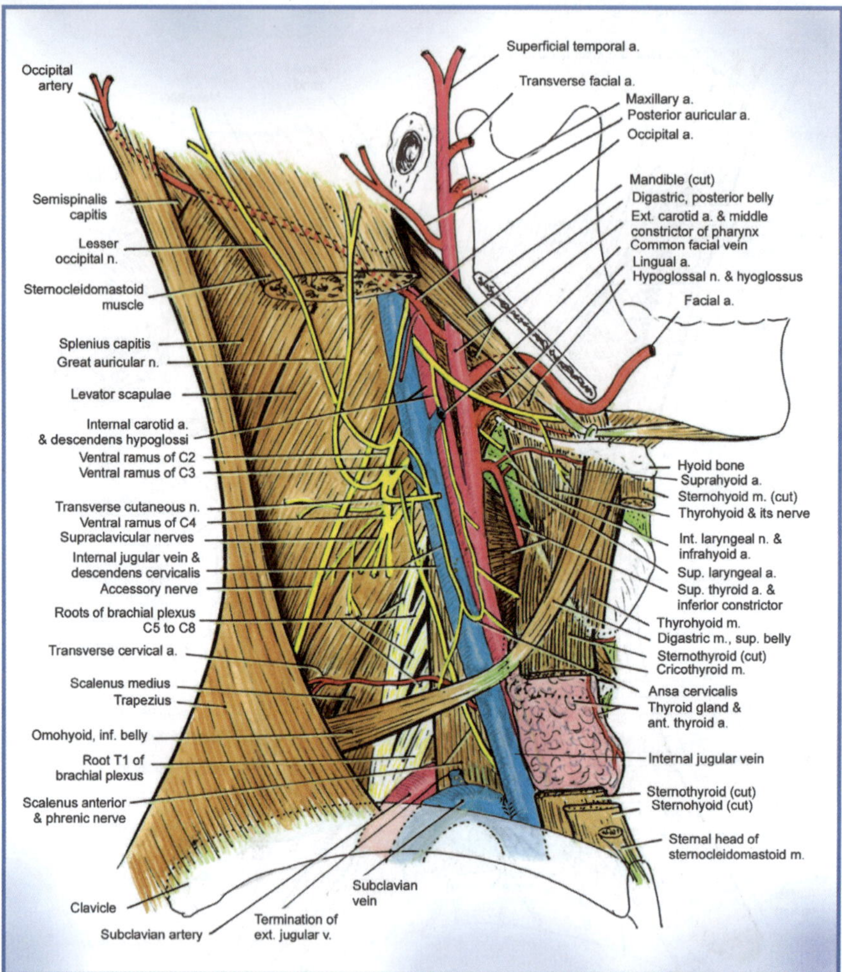

Fig. 25.40 Dissection of lateral side of neck. The greater part of the sternocleidomastoid has been removed to reveal deeper structures. Note the cervical and brachial plexuses, the accessory nerve,♥ the carotid arteries, the internal jugular vein and the subclavian vessels. Part of the thyroid gland is also seen.

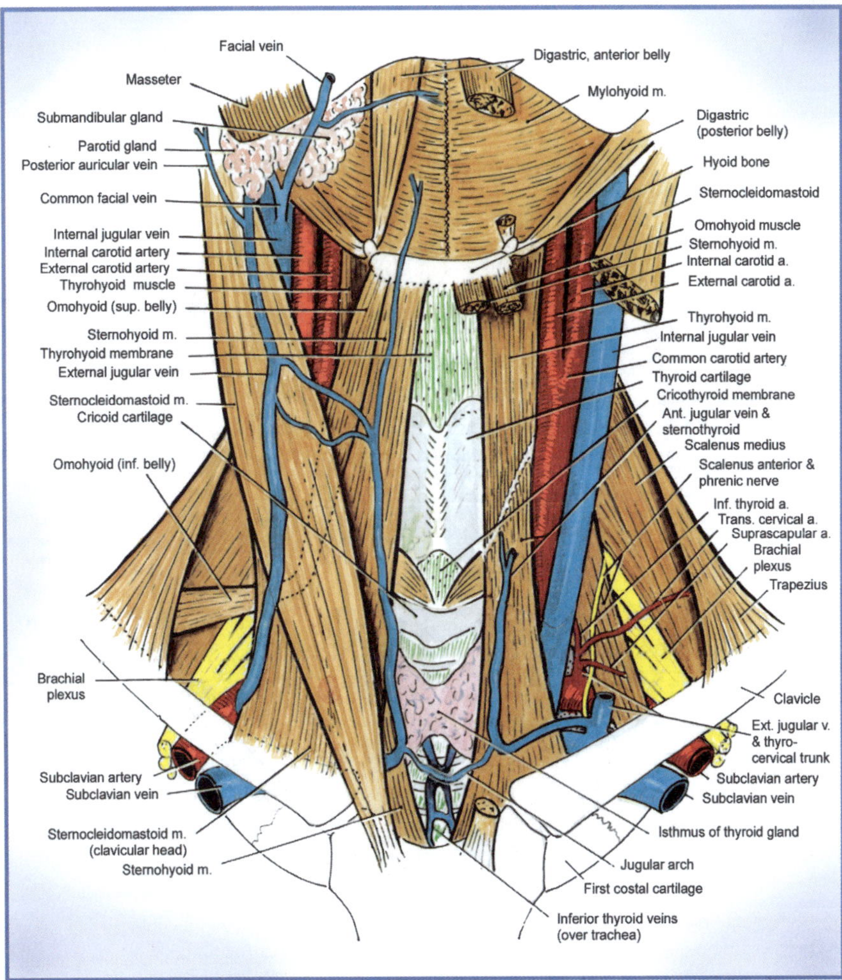

Fig. 25.41 Neck and submandibular region seen from the front. The left half of the drawing shows a superficial view, while in the right half the sternocleidomastoid muscle and some other muscles have been removed. Identify the various nerves and vessels shown.

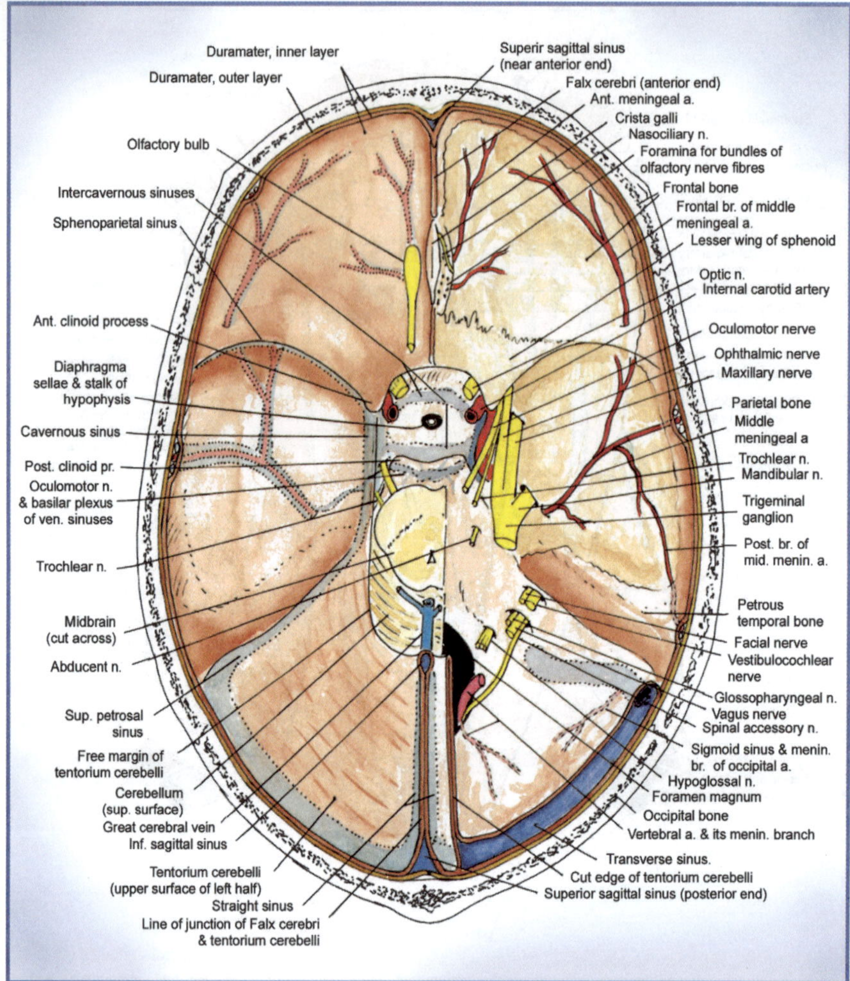

Fig. 25.42 Dissection to show the cranial fossae. The vault of the skull and the cerebral hemispheres have been removed. In the right half of the drawing the tentorium cerebelli and the cerebellum have also been removed. A number of cranial nerves and venous sinuses are shown. Identify each of them.

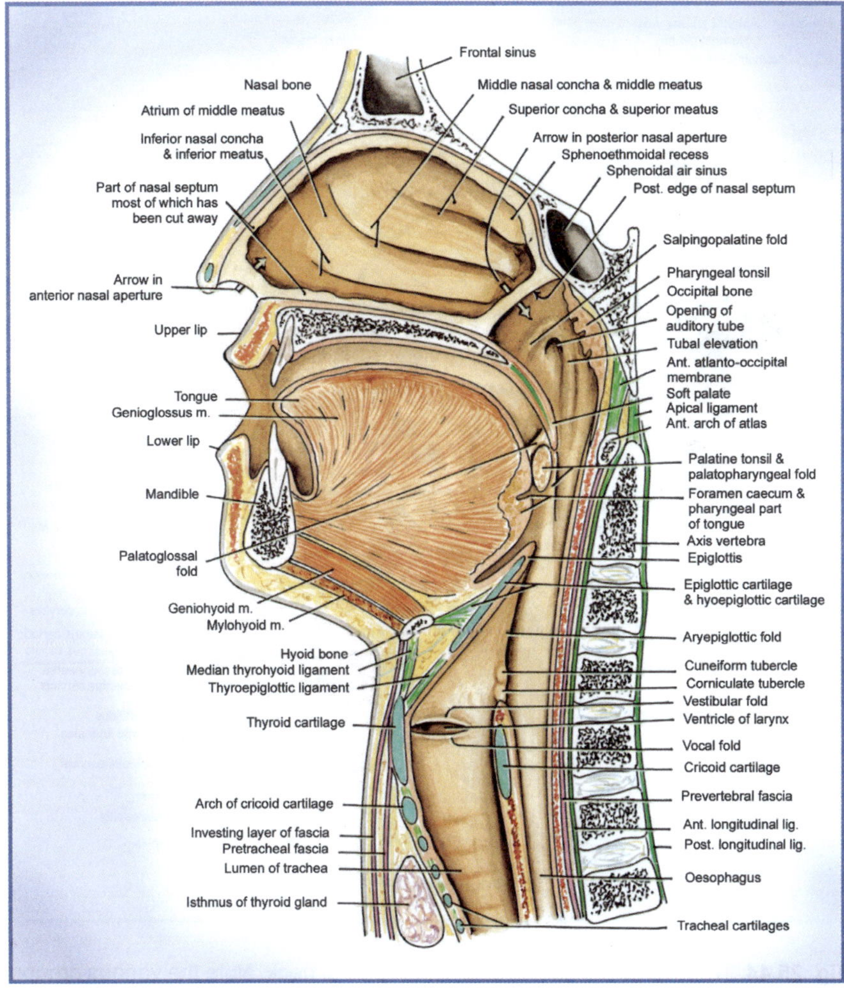

Fig. 25.43 Median section through the neck and anterior part of the head to show the interior of the nose, the mouth, the pharynx and the larynx.

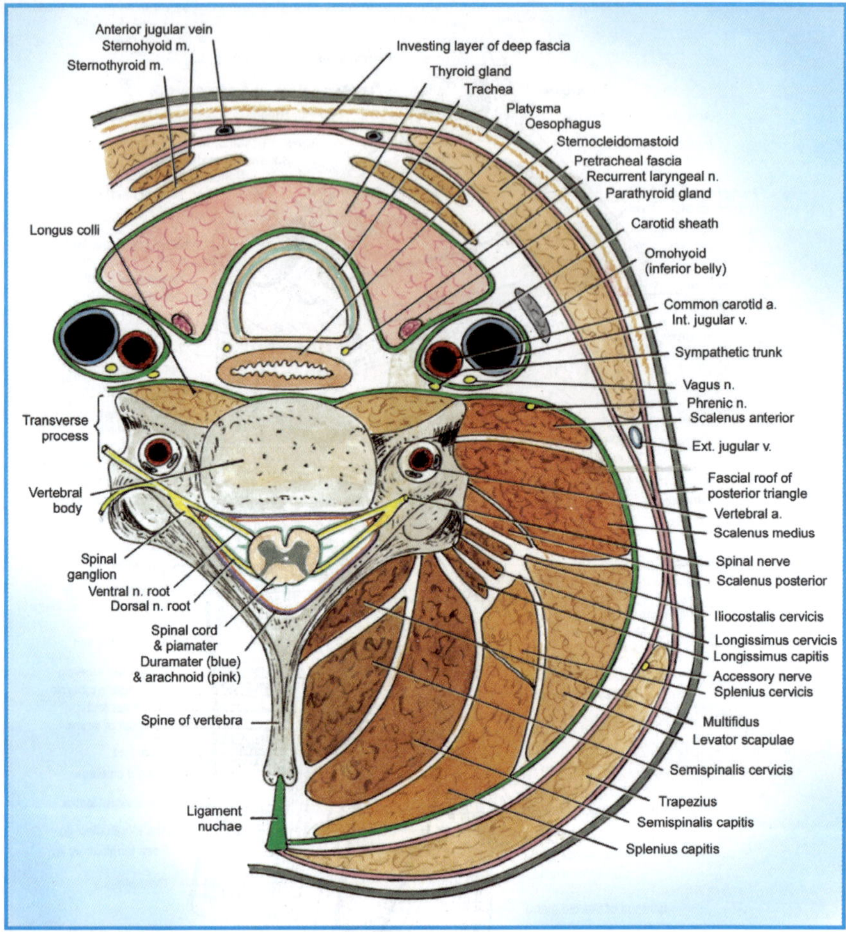

Fig. 25.44 Transverse section through lower part of neck. Note the various groups of muscles, the trachea and oesophagus, the thyroid gland, the carotid sheath, and the layers of cervical fascia.

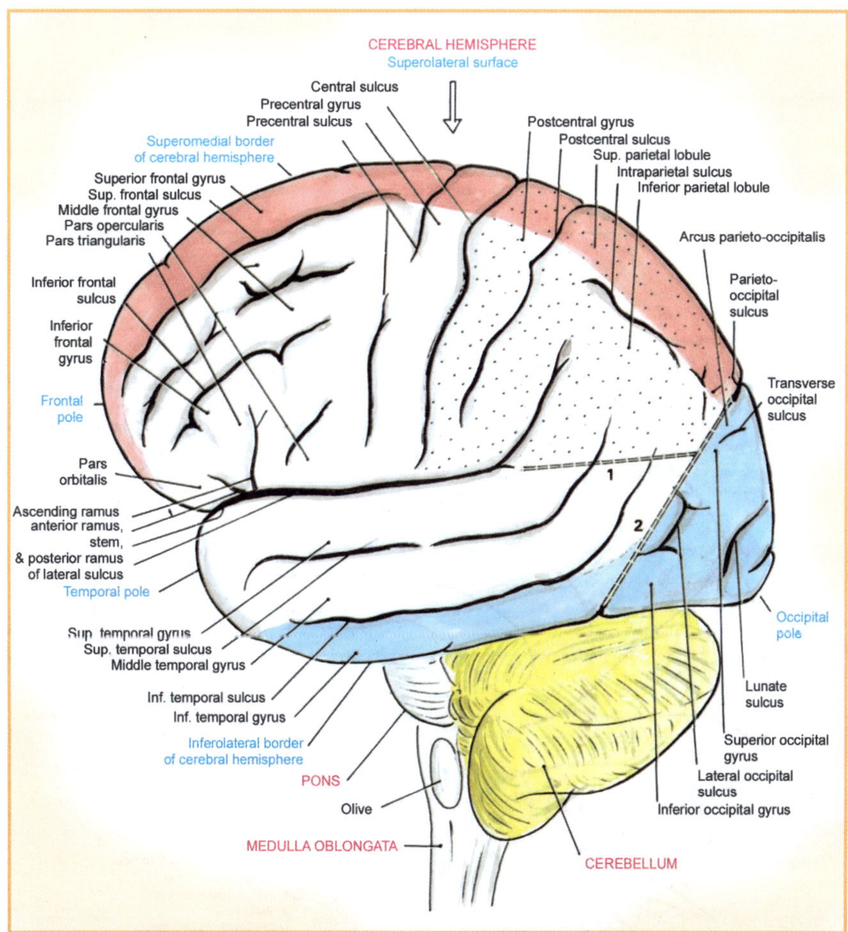

Fig. 25.45 Brain viewed from the lateral side (simplified). The interrupted double lines are imaginary: they are used to demarcate lobes. The area shaded in dots is the parietal lobe. The areas in front of it (above the posterior ramus of the lateral sulcus) is the frontal lobe. The temporal lobe is the area below the posterior ramus of the lateral sulcus and the imaginary line (1) that continues backwards in the line of the main part of the sulcus. The occipital lobe lies behind the parietal and temporal lobes being separated from them by the obliquely drawn imaginary line (2). The area of the cerebral cortex shaded pink is supplied by the anterior cerebral artery, and that shaded blue is supplied by the posterior cerebral artery. The uncoloured area is supplied by the middle cerebral artery.

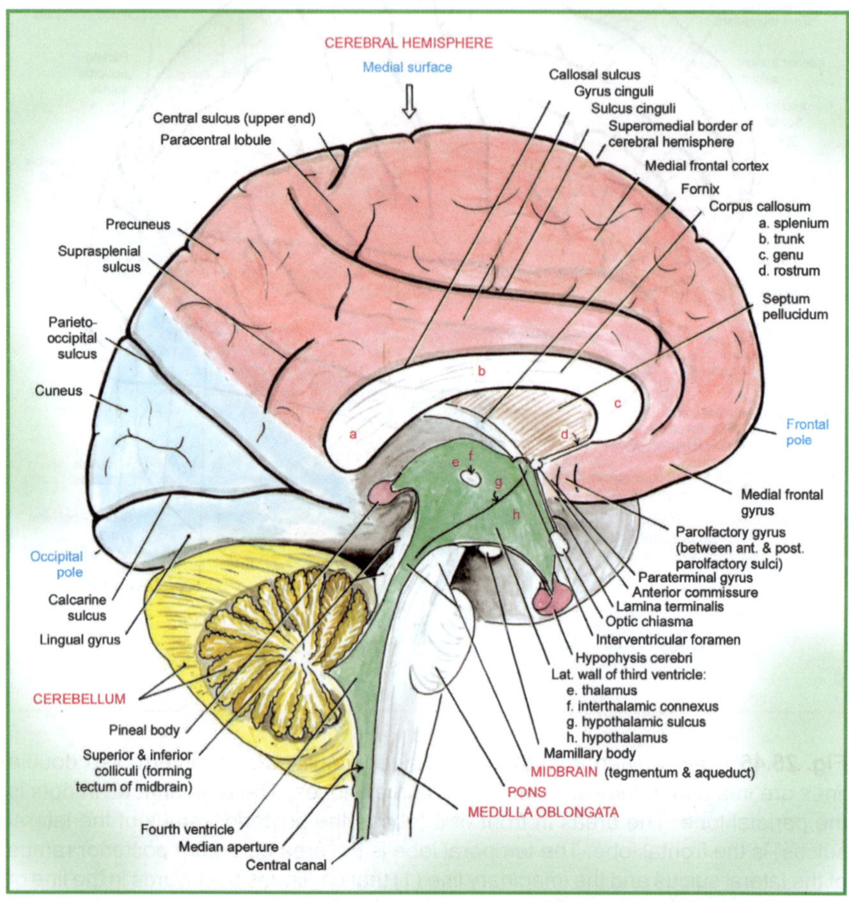

Fig. 25.46 Brain viewed from the medial side, after cutting it through the middle line (simplified). The area shaded in pink is supplied by the anterior cerebral artery, and that shaded blue is supplied by the posterior cerebral artery.

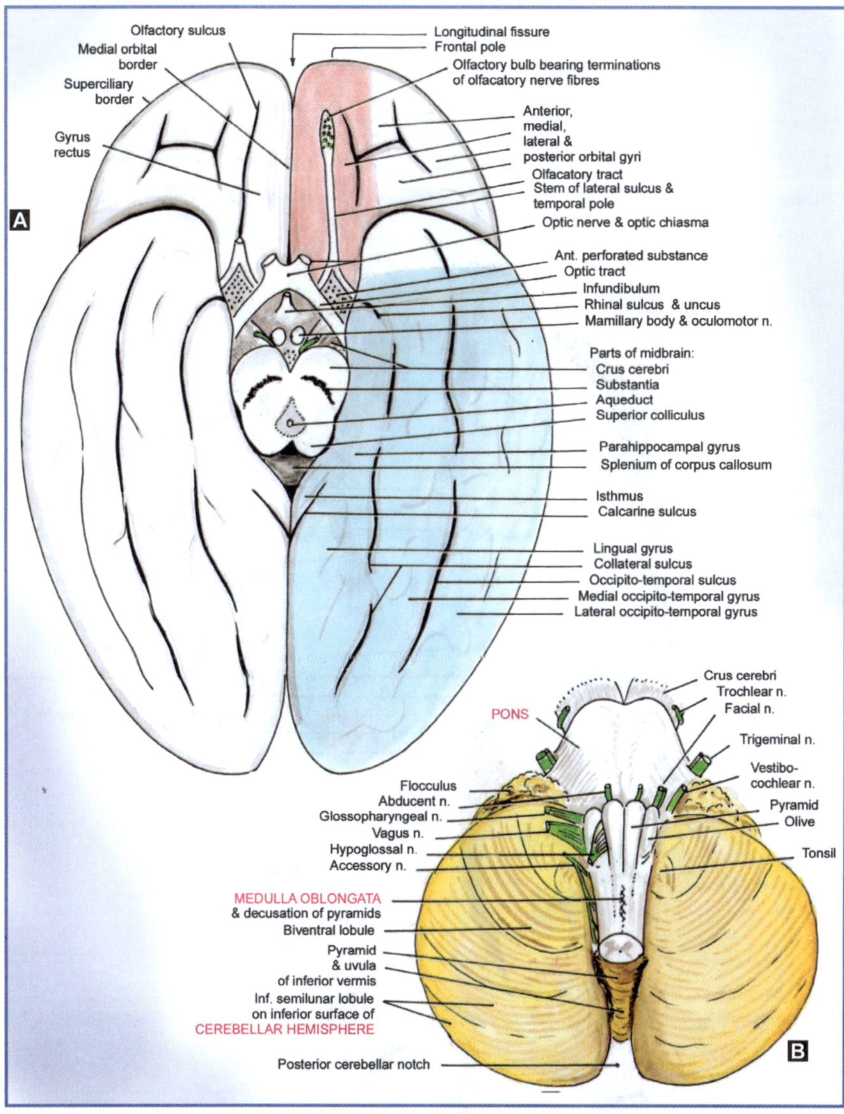

Figs 25.47A and B A. Cerebrum seen from below. The area shaded in pink is supplied by the anterior cerebral artery, and that shaded blue is supplied by the posterior cerebral artery; B. Cerebellum and brainstem seen from below and in front.

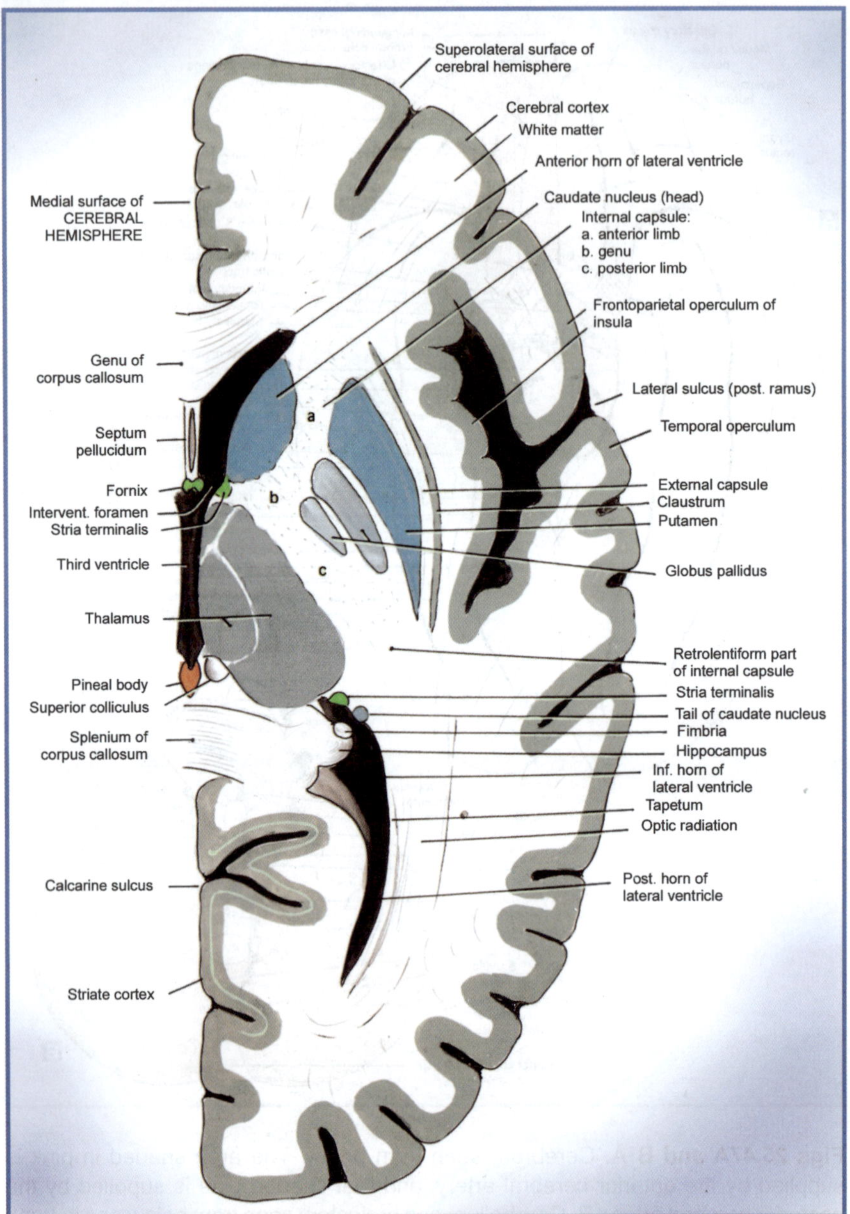

Fig. 25.48 Horizontal section through cerebral hemisphere to show the main features within it.

CHAPTER
26

Some Important Bones

THE CLAVICLE

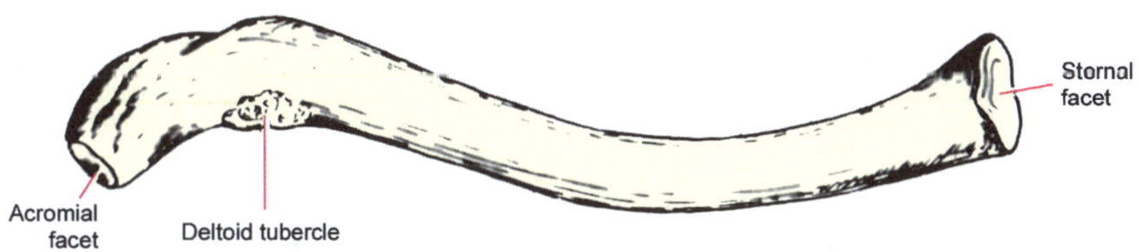

Fig. 26.1 Right clavicle, seen from above. Note the medial (or sternal) and the lateral (or acromial) ends. The shaft has an S-shaped curve.

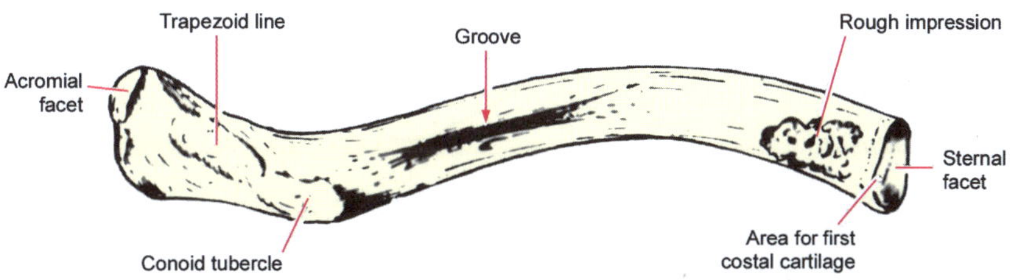

Fig. 26.2 Right clavicle, seen from below.

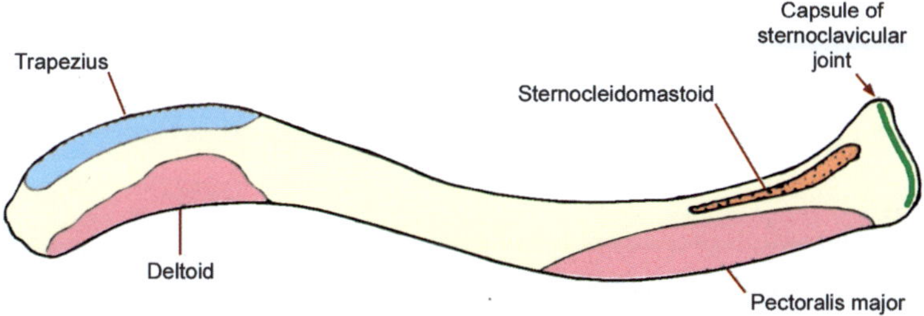

Fig. 26.3 Attachments on the right clavicle seen from above. The muscles attached include the pectoralis major, the deltoid, the trapezius and the sternocleidomastoid.

THE SCAPULA

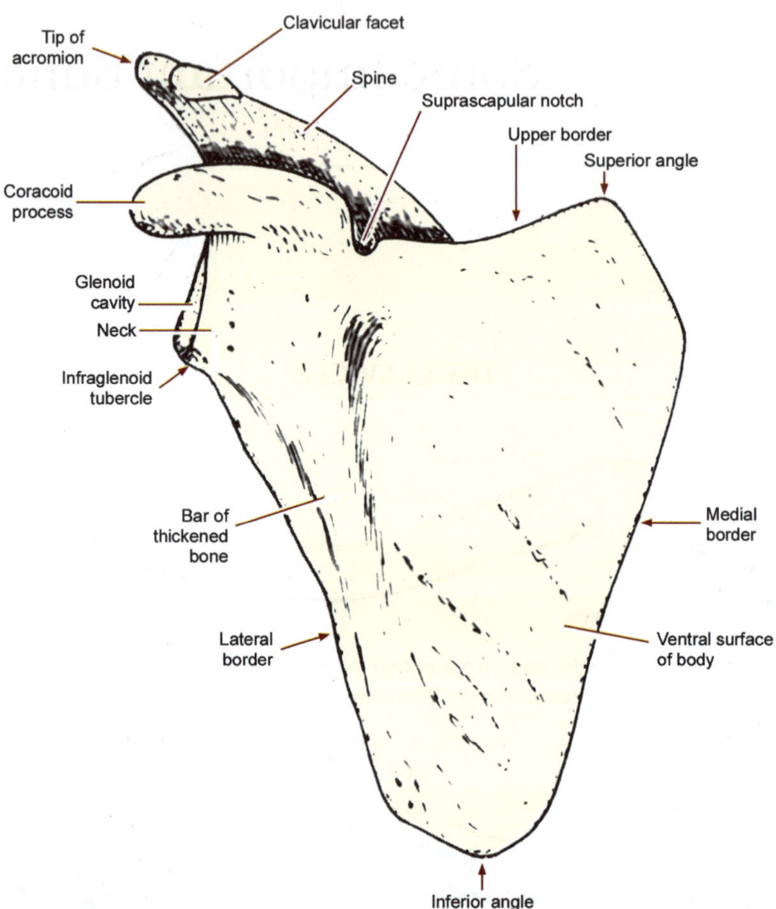

Fig. 26.4 Right scapula seen from the front.

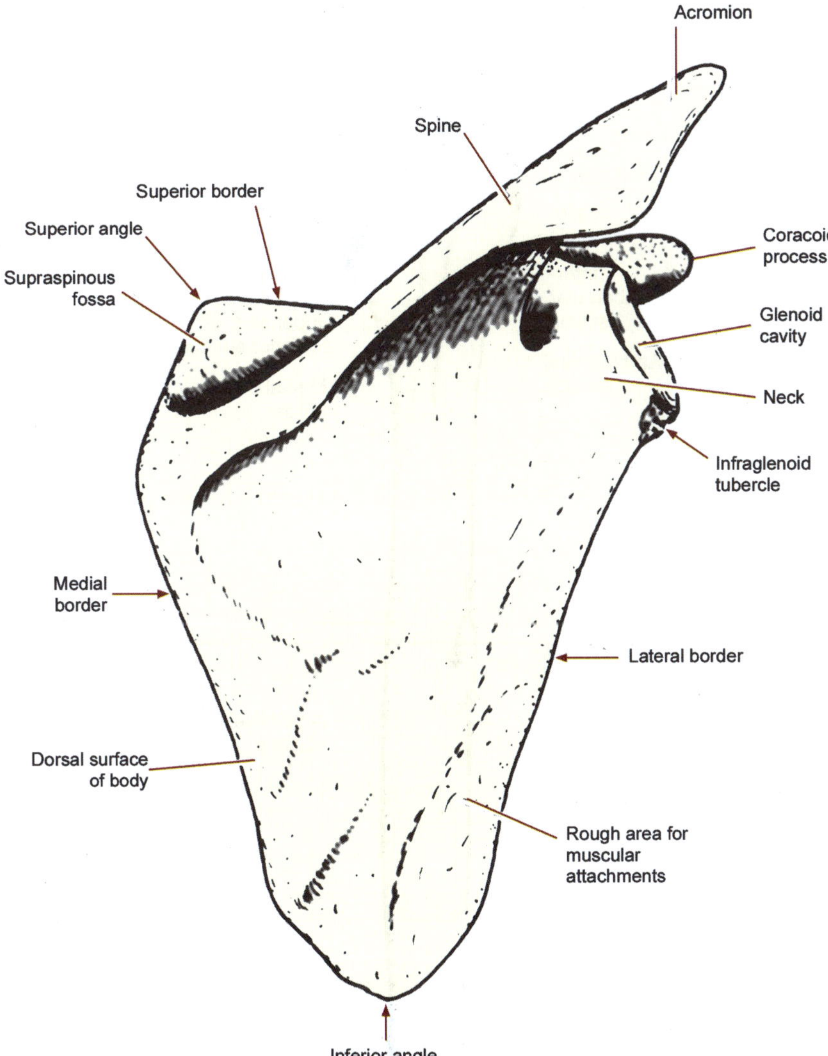

Fig. 26.5 Right scapula seen from behind. In Fig. 26.4 and 26.5♥ observe the triangular flat plate which forms the body of the scapula. The spine is a projection attached to the posterior aspect of the body. At the lateral angle of the body there is the glenoid cavity that takes part in forming the shoulder joint. Also identify the acromion, and the coracoid process.

THE HUMERUS

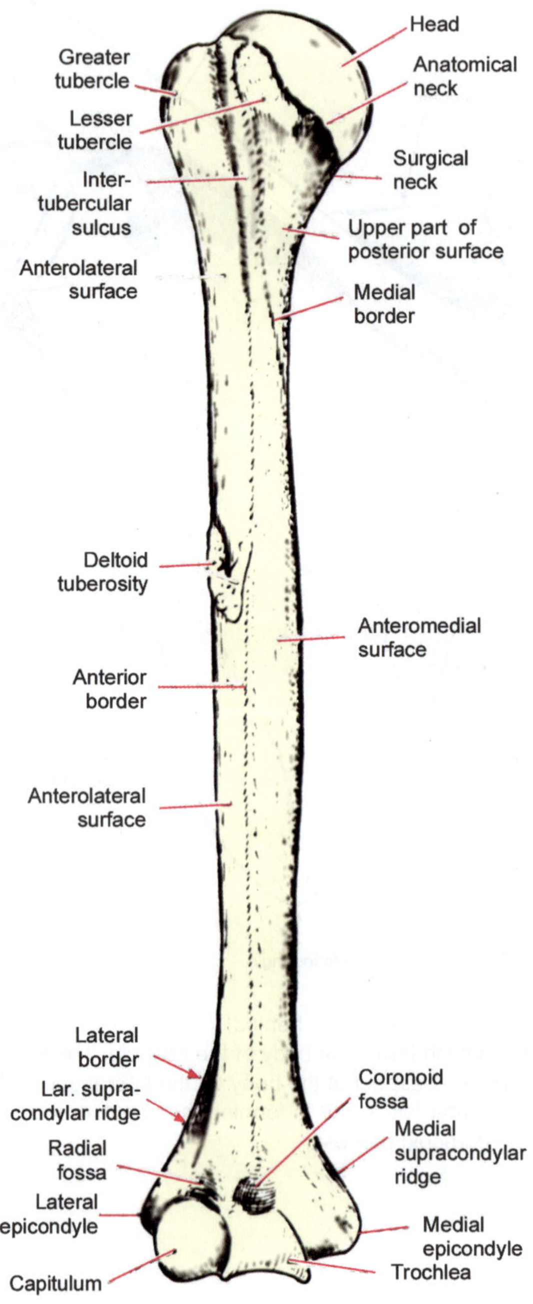

Fig. 26.6 Right humerus seen from the front.

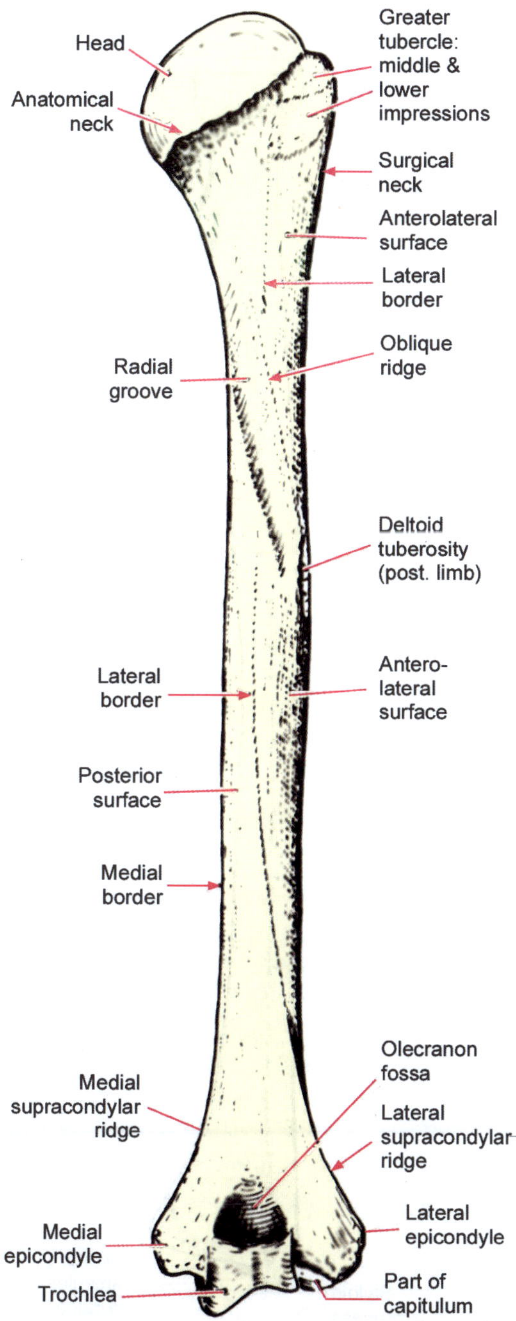

Fig. 26.7 Right humerus seen from behind.

THE RADIUS

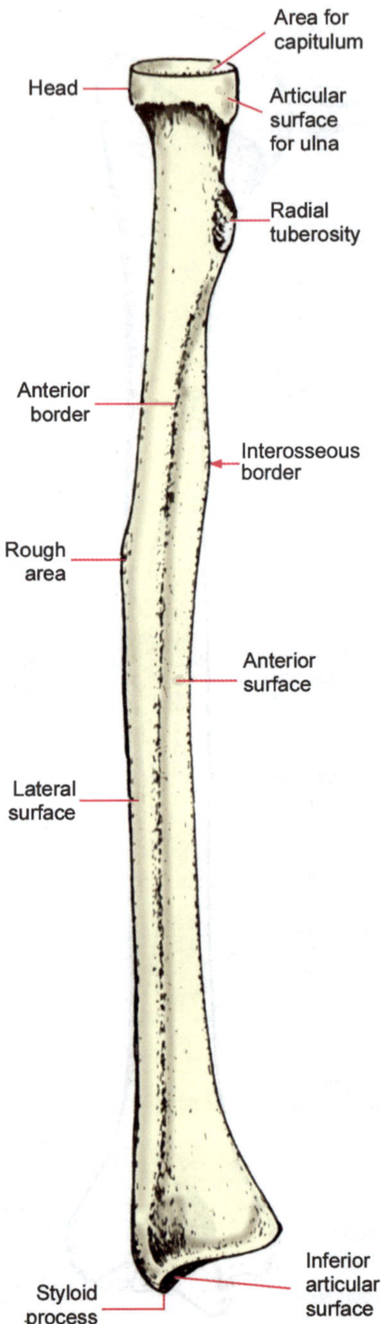

Fig. 26.8 Right radius seen from the front.

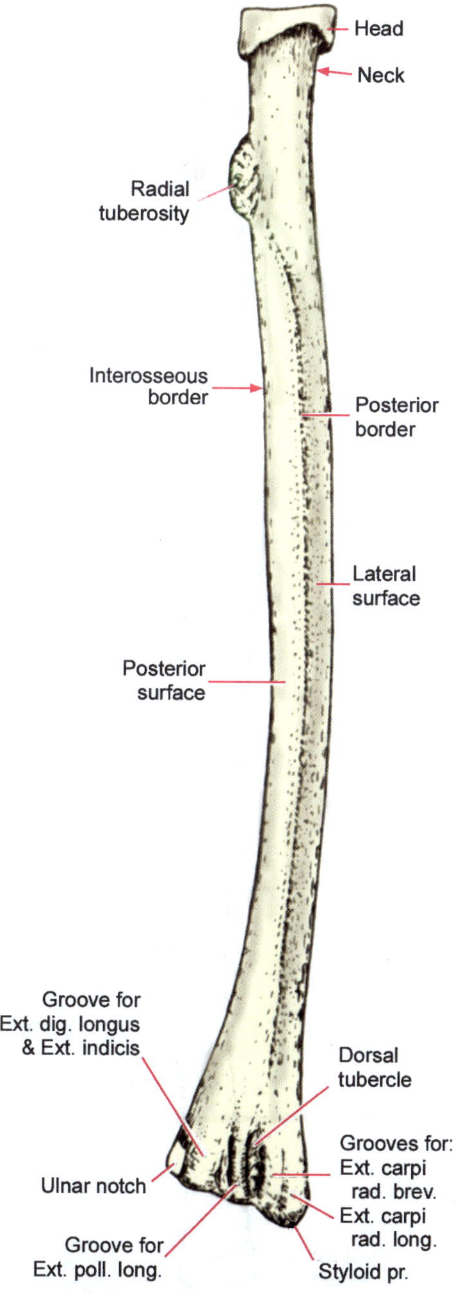

Fig. 26.9 Right radius seen from behind.

THE ULAN

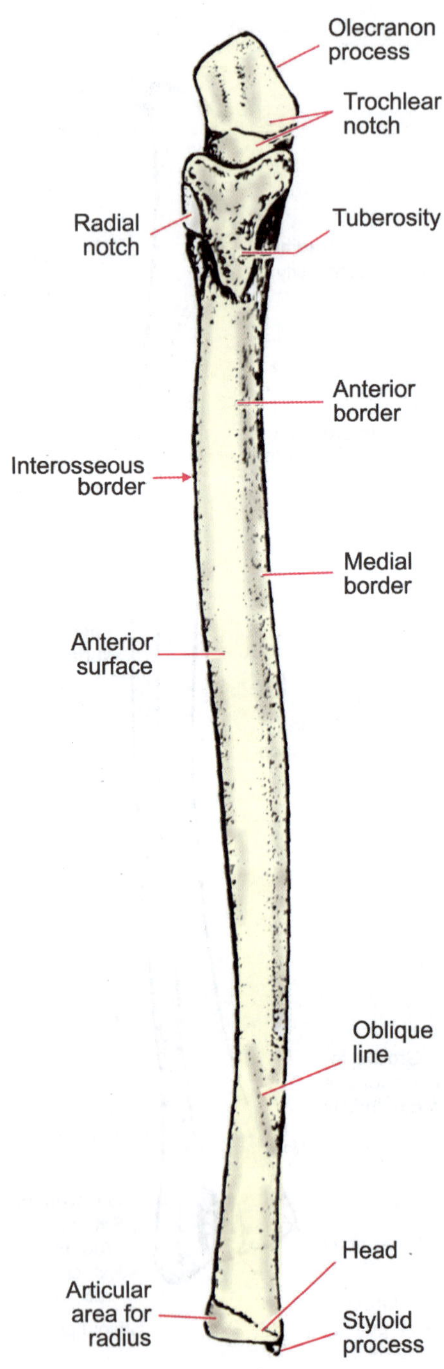

Fig. 26.10 Right ulna seen from the front.

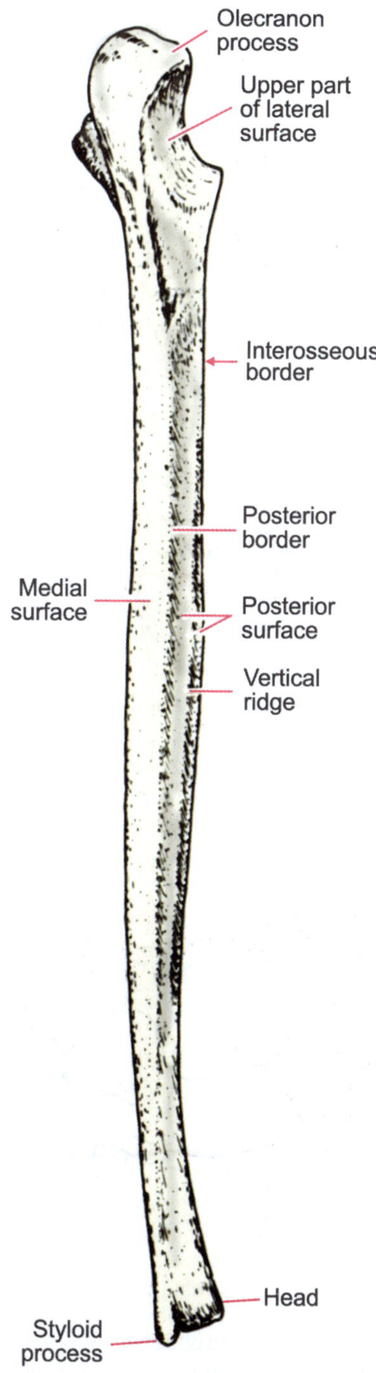

Fig. 26.11 Right ulna seen from behind

BONES OF THE WRIST AND HAND

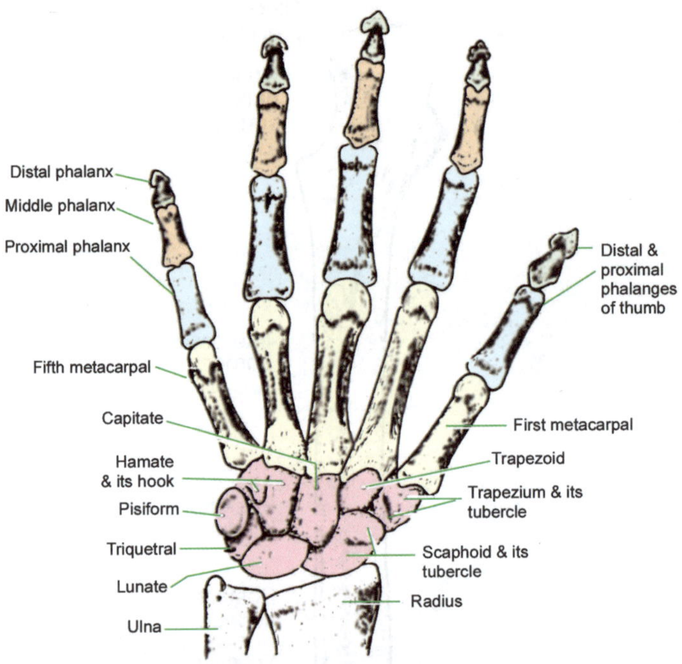

Fig. 26.12 Skeleton of the hand seen from the front (palmar aspect).

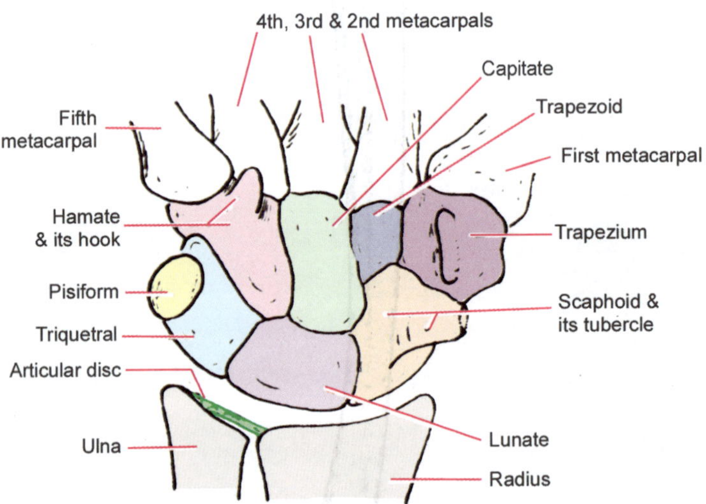

Fig. 26.13 Bones of the wrist (carpus) seen from the front.

In these figures identify the bones and observe the order in which they lie. Note that the carpal bones are arranged in two rows. The bones of the proximal row articulate with the lower end of the radius and ulna to form the wrist joint. The bones of the distal row articulate with metacarpal bones.

THE HIP BONE-1

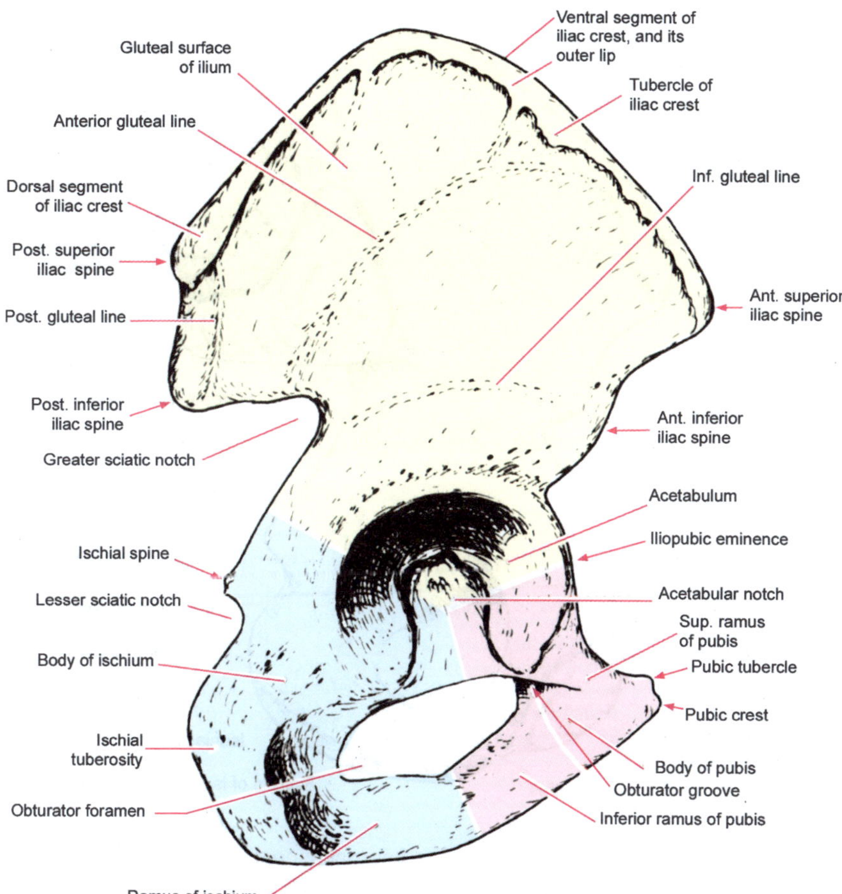

Fig. 26.14 The hip bone has one surface facing outwards, and an inner pelvic surface. In this figure we see the right hip bone from the external aspect. The part shaded yellow is the ilium. The part shaded blue is the ischium. The part shaded pink is the pubis. Note the large circular depression, the acetabulum. The head of the femur fits into it to form the hip joint.

THE HIP BONE–2

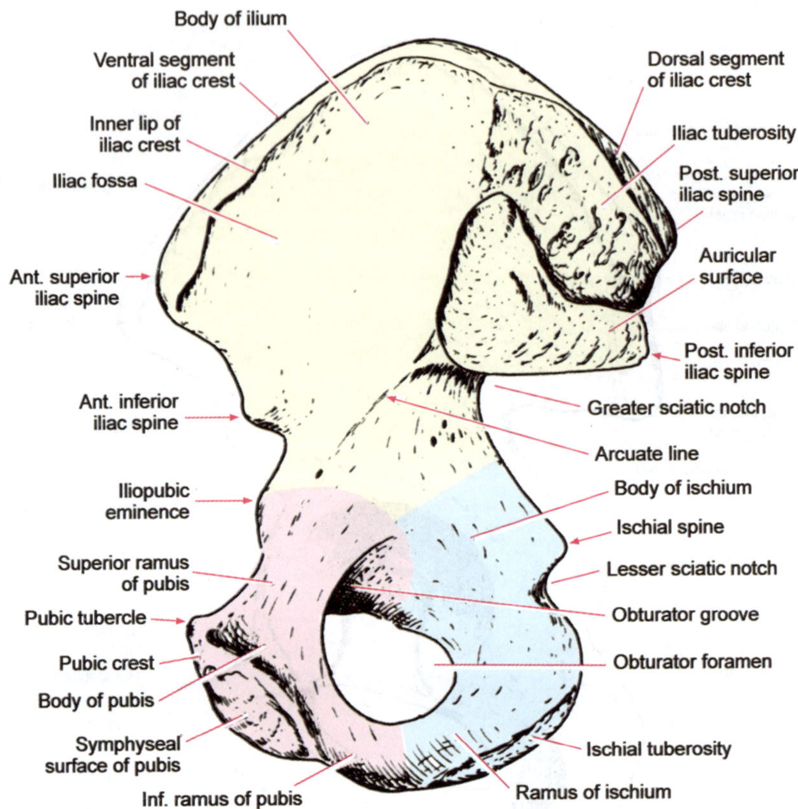

Fig. 26.15 Right hip bone seen from the internal aspect. The ilium, ischium and pubis are shaded as in Fig. 26.14.

THE PELVIS

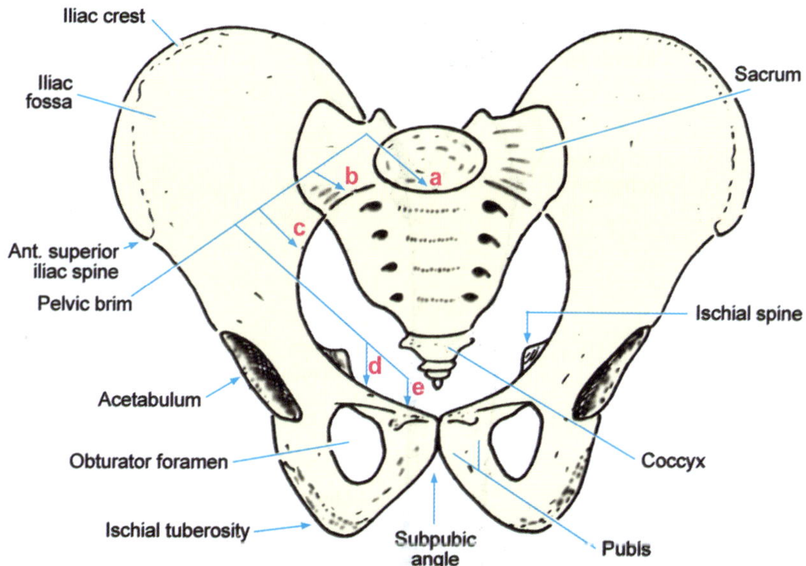

Fig. 26.16 Bony pelvis seen from the front. It is formed by right and left hip bones that join each other anteriorly (at the pubic symphysis). Posteriorly, the hip bones are separated by a gap into which the sacrum fits. The coccyx is attached to the lower end of the sacrum.

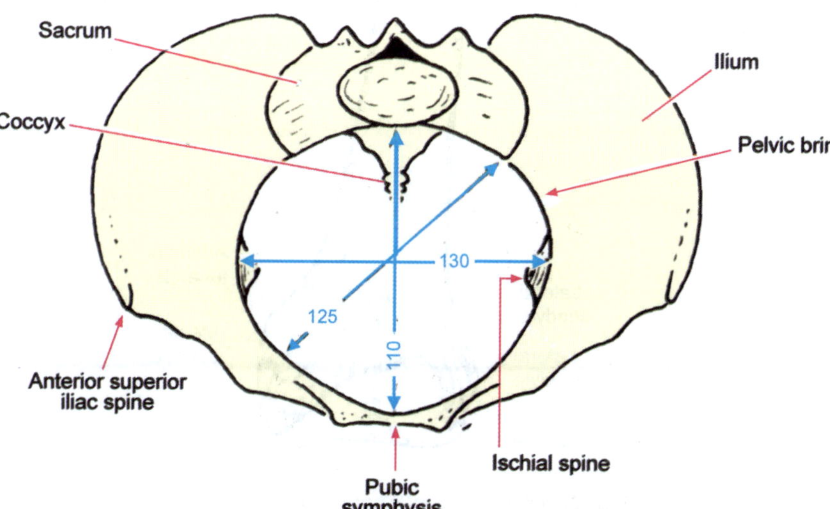

Fig. 26.17 Pelvis seen from above and in front. The round aperture seen is the pelvic inlet. During child birth the head of the child passes through it. The dimensions of the inlet are, therefore, very important.

THE FEMUR

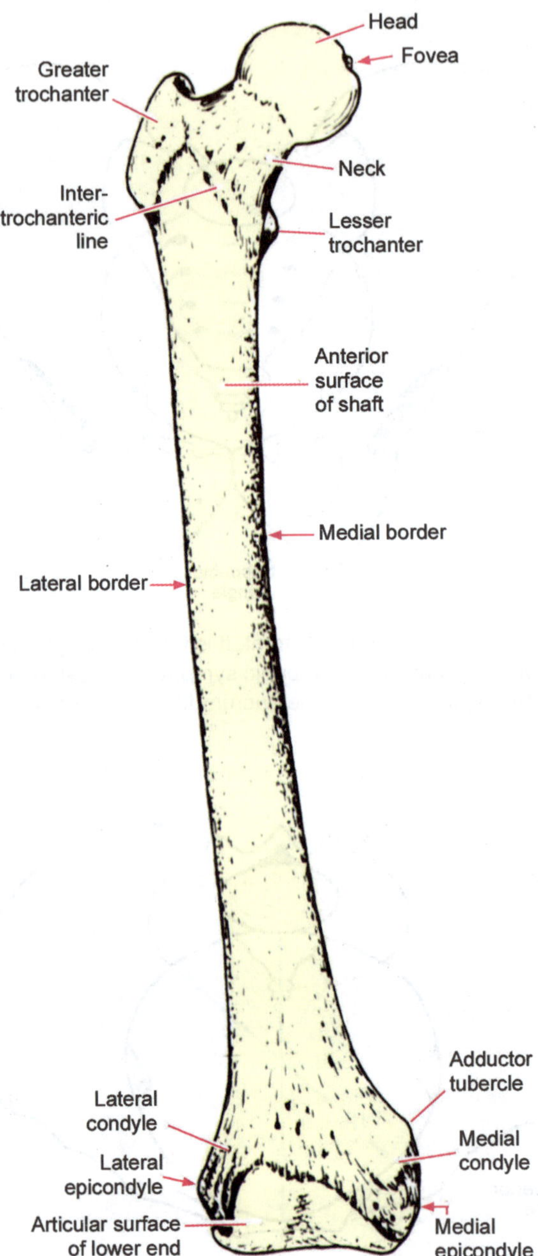

Fig. 26.18 Right femur seen from the front.

Note the large spherical head that fits into the acetabulum to form the hip joint. The enlarged lower end is made up of medial and lateral condyles that take part in forming the knee joint.

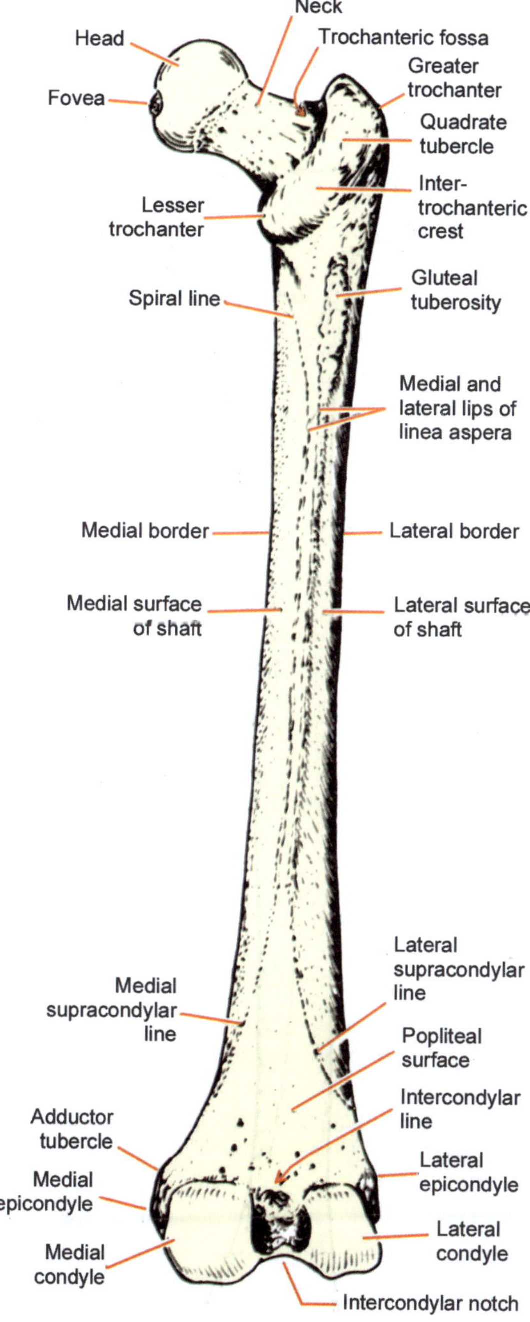

Fig. 26.19 Right femur seen from behind.

Note the large spherical head that fits into the acetabulum to form the hip joint. The enlarged lower end is made up of medial and lateral condyles that take part in forming the knee joint.

THE TIBIA

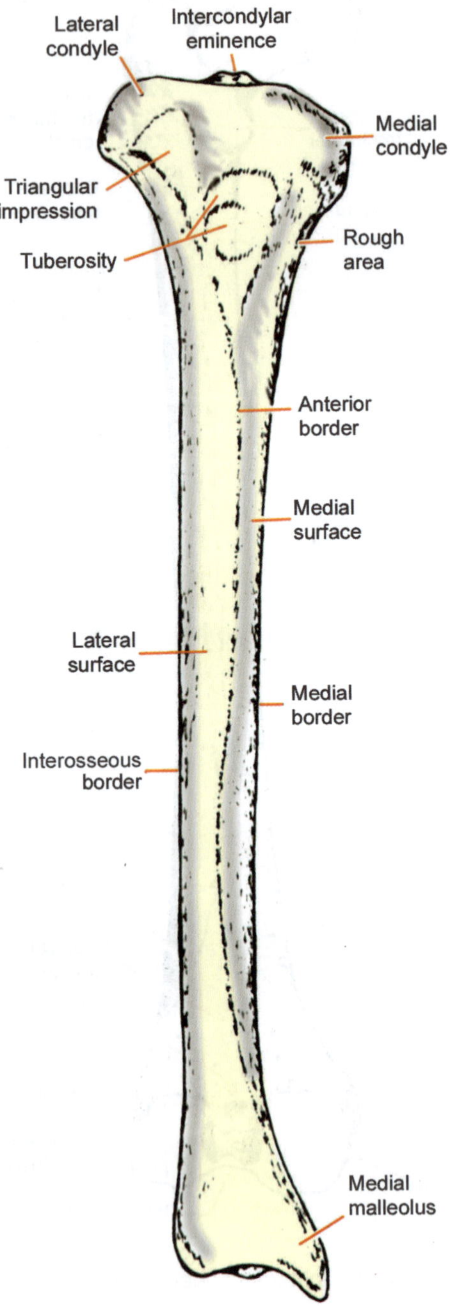

Fig. 26.20 Right tibia seen from the front. The upper end joins the femur to form the knee joint. The lower end takes part in forming the ankle joint.

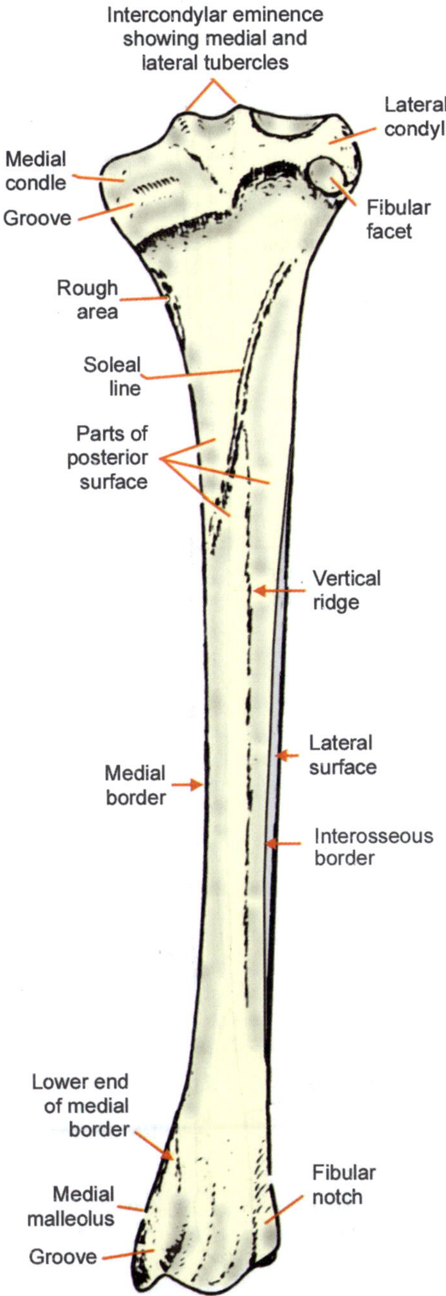

Fig. 26.21 Right tibia seen from behind. At the lower end, note the projection called the medial malleolus. You can feel it easily in your own body.

THE FIBULA

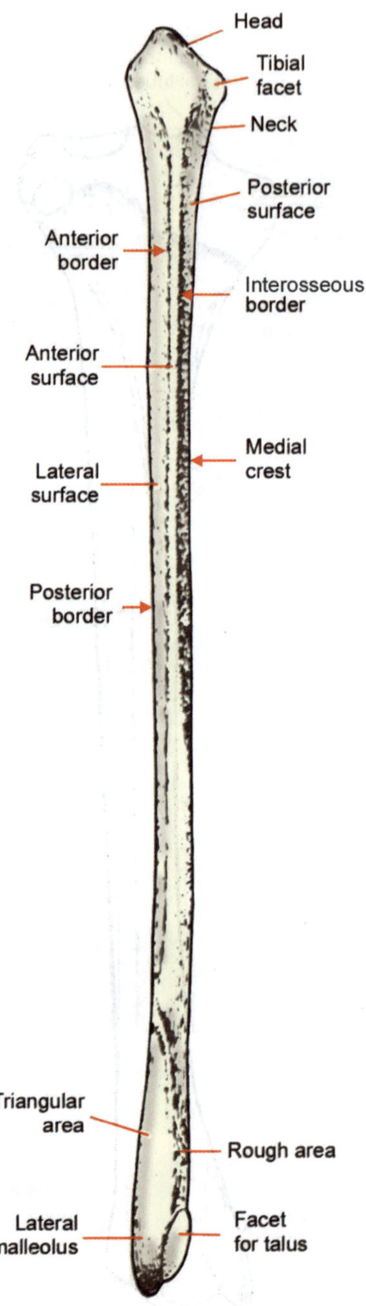

Fig. 26.22 Right fibula seen from the front. The fibula is much thinner than the tibia. Its lower end forms the lateral malleolus, that can felt in your own body.

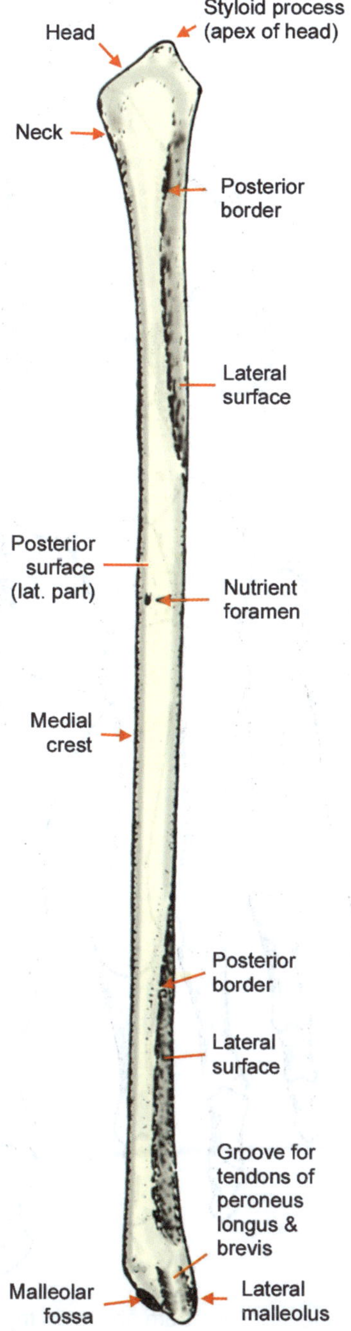

Fig. 26.23 Right fibula seen from behind.

BONES OF THE FOOT

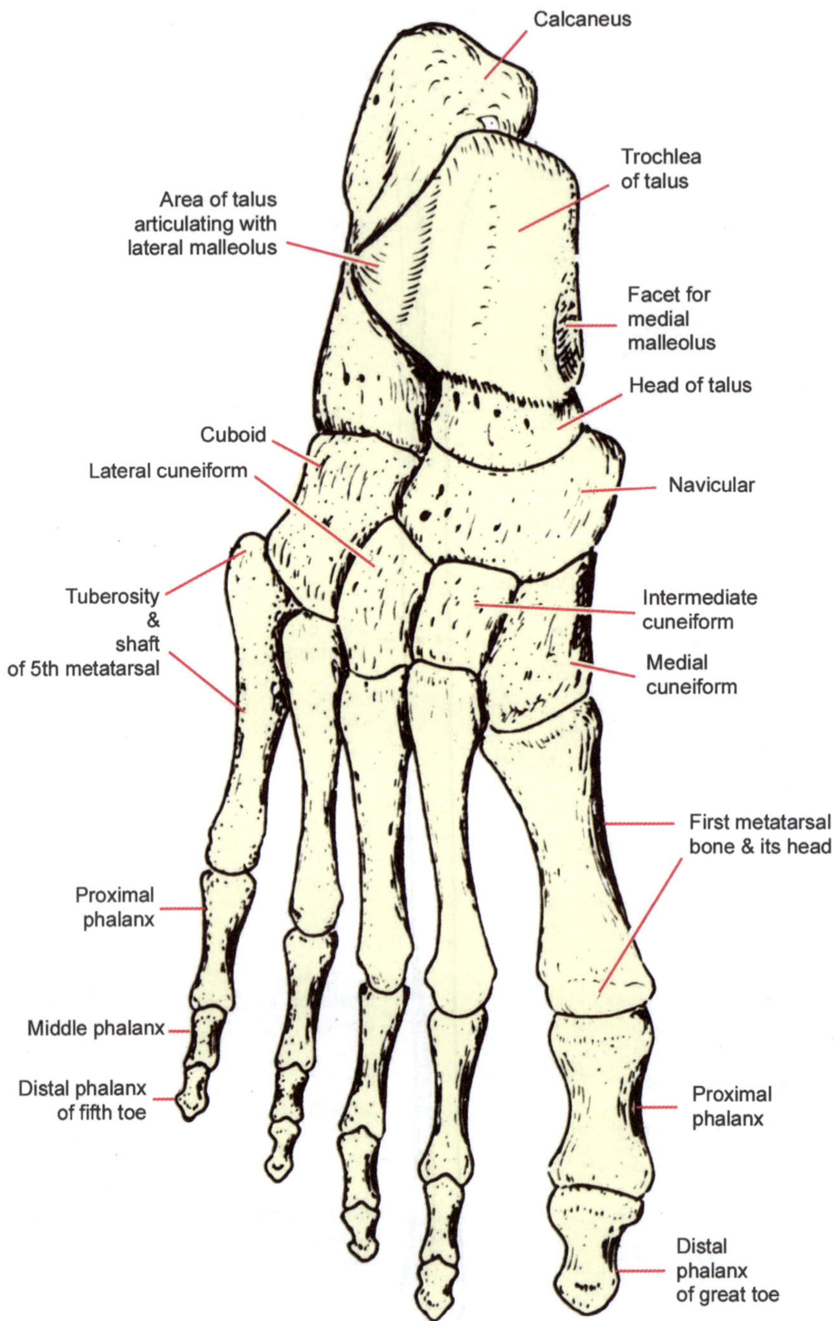

Fig. 26.24 Skeleton of the foot seen from above. In the upper part of the figure we see the tarsal bones. The largest of these are the calcaneus (which forms the heel), and the talus which articulates with the lower ends of the tibia and fibula to form the ankle joint. Identify the metatarsal bones and the phalanges.

TYPICAL THORACIC VERTEBRAE

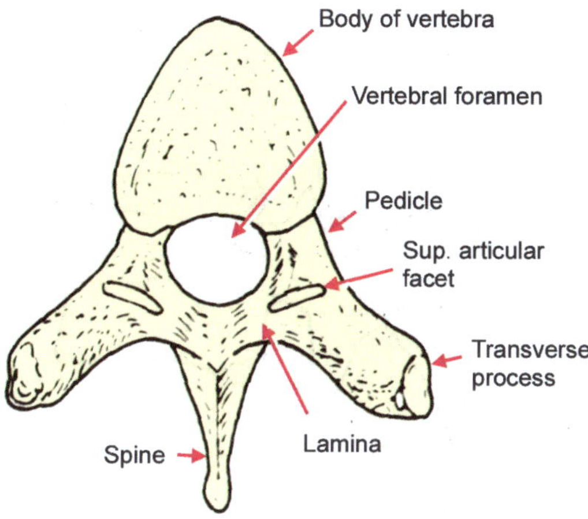

Fig. 26.25 Typical thoracic vertebra seen from above. Note the body, transverse processes and spine. The spinal cord passed through the vertebral foramen.

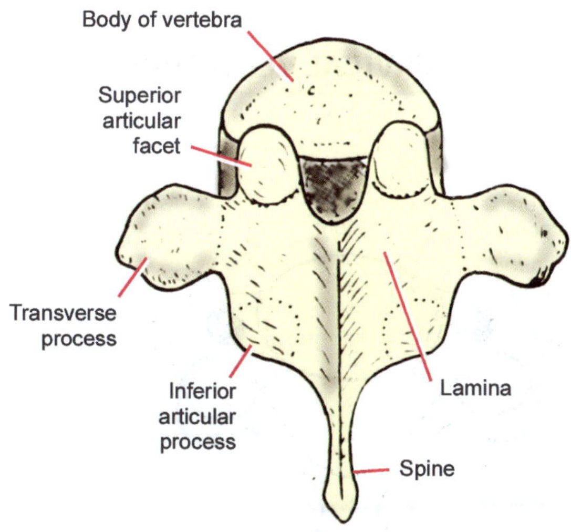

Fig. 26.26 Typical thoracic vertebra seen from behind.

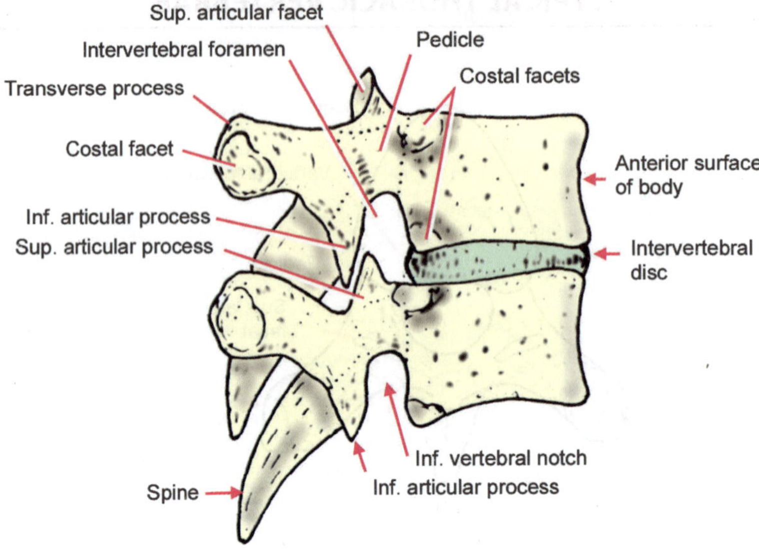

Fig. 26.27 Typical thoracic vertebrae seen from the lateral side. Note the intervertebral disc uniting the bodies of adjacent vertebrae. Spinal nerves pass out of the vertebral canal through intervertebral foraminae.

CERVICAL VERTEBRAL

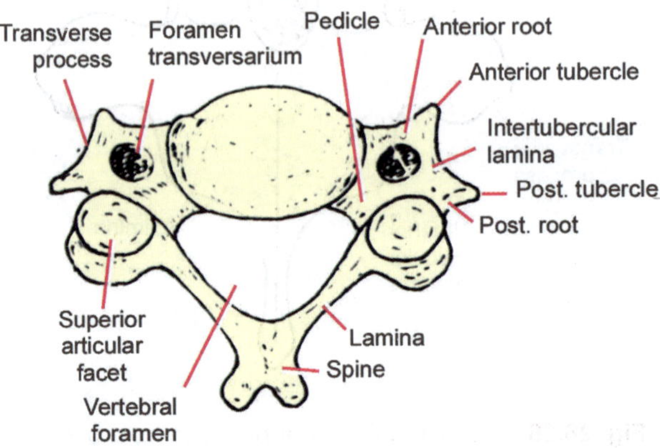

Fig. 26.28 Typical cervical vertebra seen from above. Note the foramen in the transverse process. The vertebral artery passes through it.

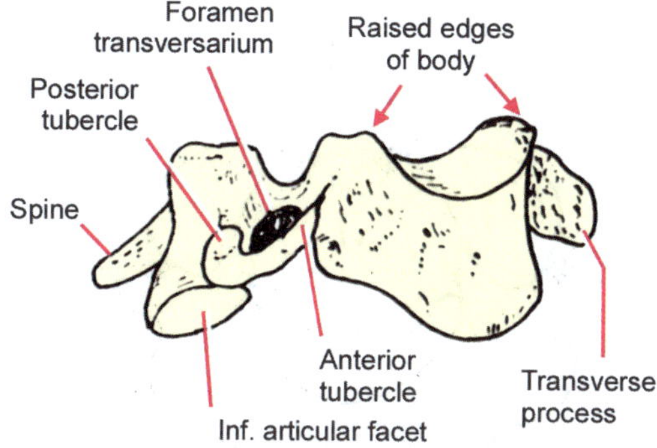

Fig. 26.29 Typical cervical vertebra seen from the anterolateral side.

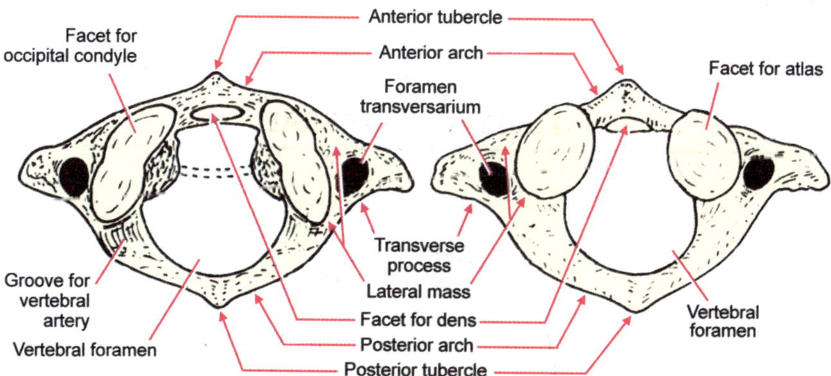

Fig. 26.30 The first cervical vertebra (atlas) seen from above (left) and from below (right). The upper surface articulates with the skull at the atlanto-occipital joint. The lower surface articulates with the second cervical vertebra at the atlanto-axial joint.

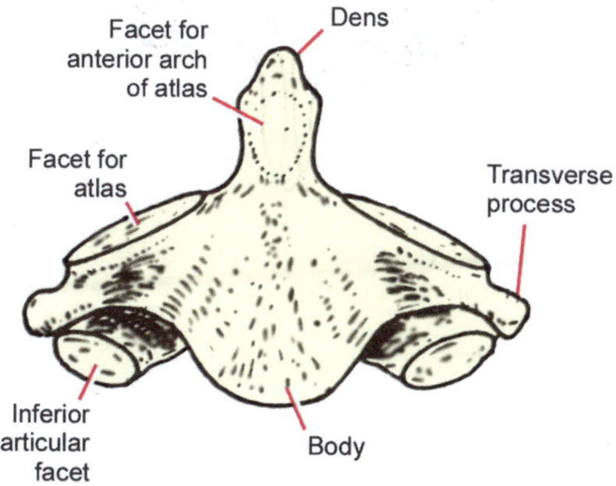

Fig. 26.31 The second cervical vertebra (axis) seen from the front. Note the rod like process called the dens.

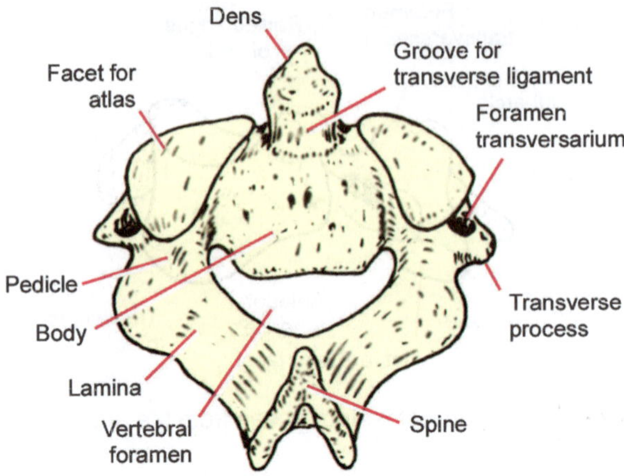

Fig. 26.32 The second cervical vertebra (axis) seen from the posterosuperior aspect.

LUMBAR VERTEBRAE

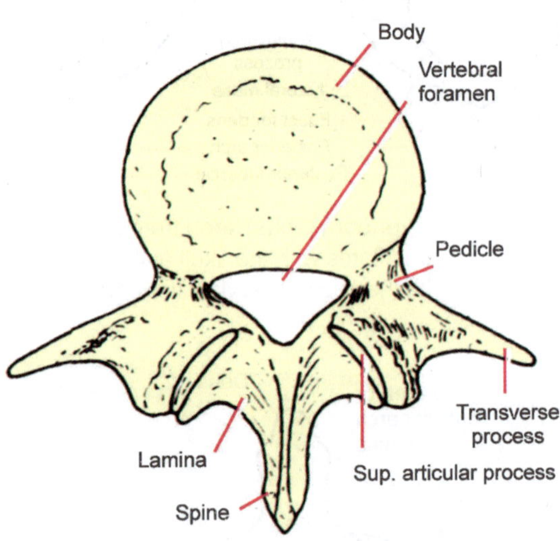

Fig. 26.33 Typical lumbar vertebra seen from above. The body is large. The transverse processes are small.

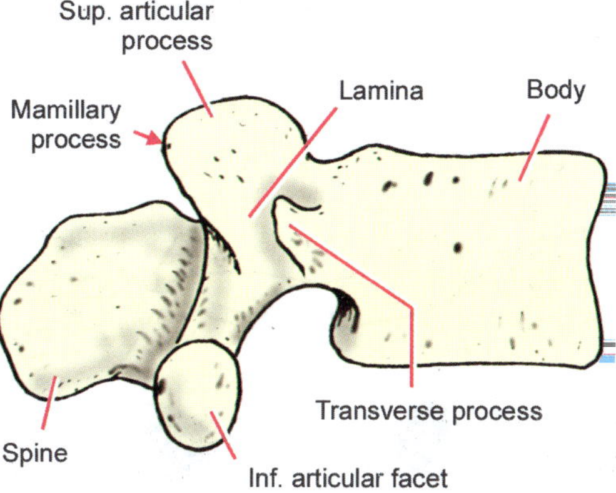

Fig. 26.34 Typical lumbar vertebra seen from the lateral side.

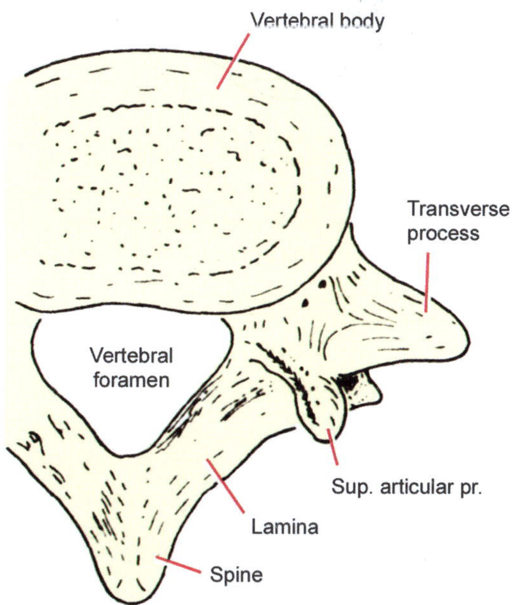

Fig. 26.35 Fifth lumbar vertebra seen from above. This vertebra articulates with the sacrum (lumbosacral joint). The body is very large.

THE SACRUM

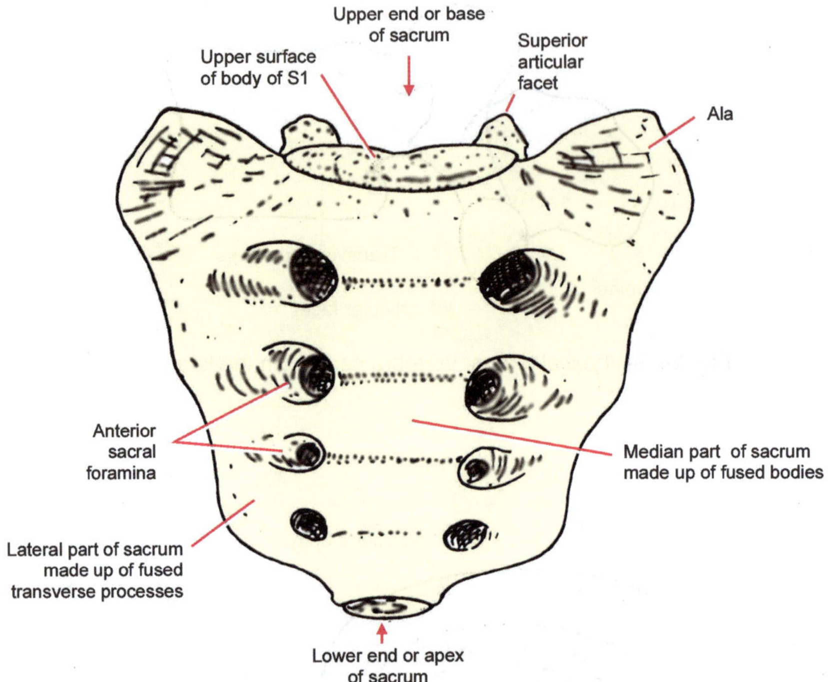

Fig. 26.36 Sacrum seen from the front. It is made up of five sacral vertebrae that have fused together. Nerve roots emerge through the sacral foramina.

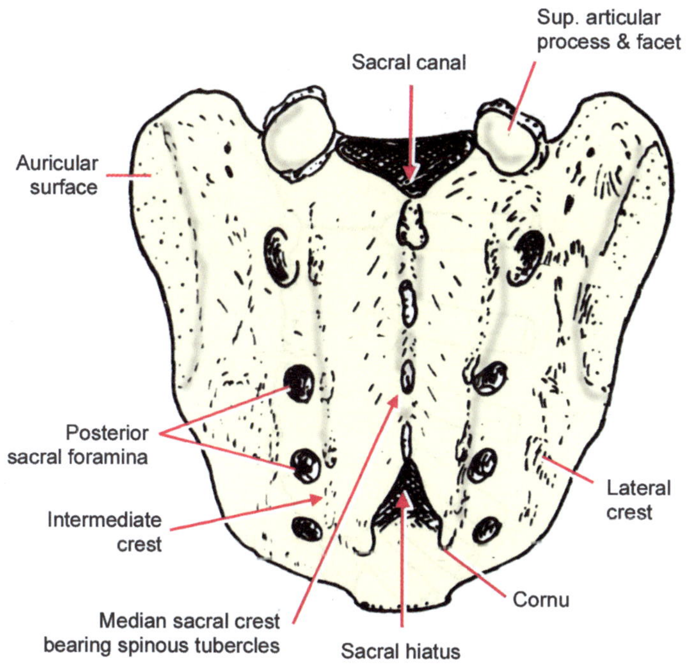

Fig. 26.37 Sacrum seen from behind. The rough posterior surface gives attachment to muscles and ligaments.

THE STERNUM AND RIBS

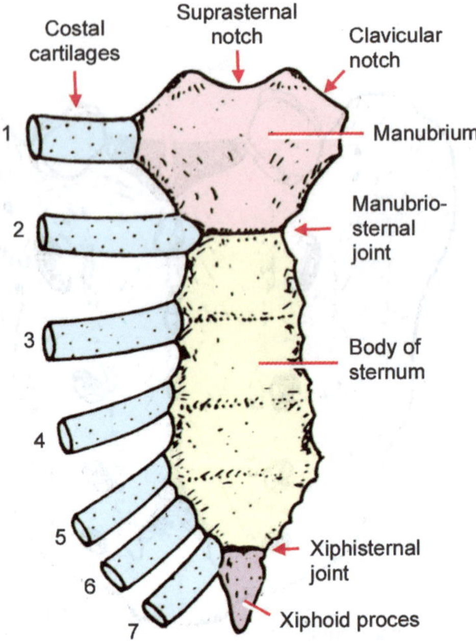

Fig. 26.38 Sternum and costal cartilages seen from the front. The sternum consists of three parts. The manubrium sterni is shaded pink. The body of the sternum is shaded yellow. The xiphoid process is shaded violet. It is cartilaginous in young persons. The first costal cartilage is attached to the manubrium sterni. The second cartilage is attached at the junction of manubrium and body. The seventh cartilage is attached at the junction of body with the xiphoid process. The clavicular notch of the manubrium sterni articulates with the medial end of the clavicle.

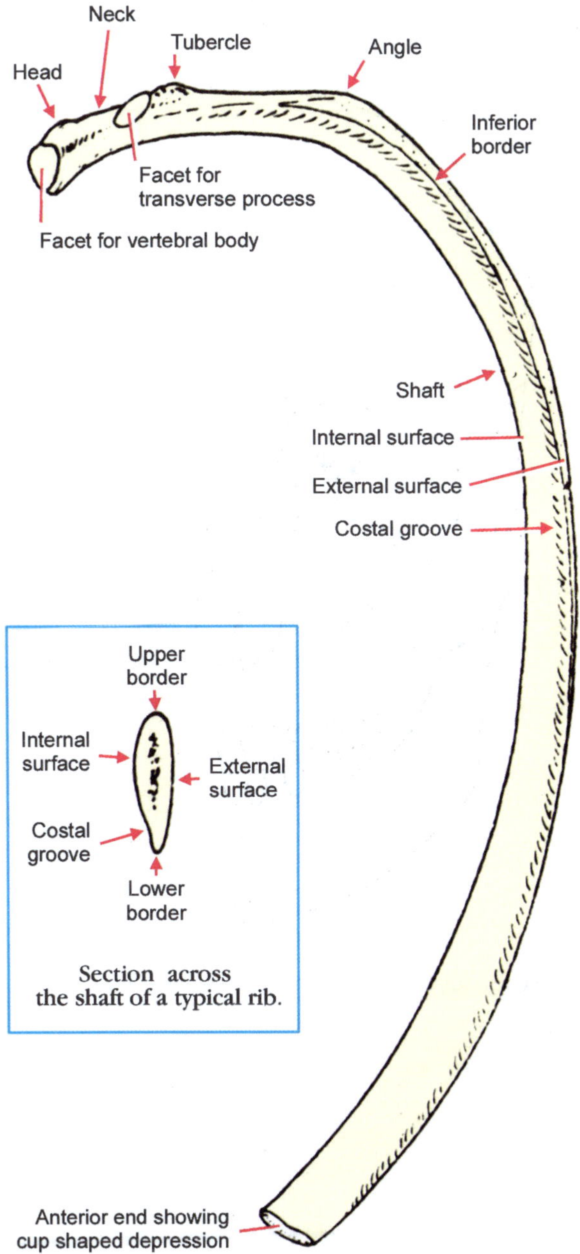

Fig. 26.39 A typical rib seen from below. Its posterior end is attached to the vertebral column. The anterior end is attached to a costal cartilage.

THE SKULL

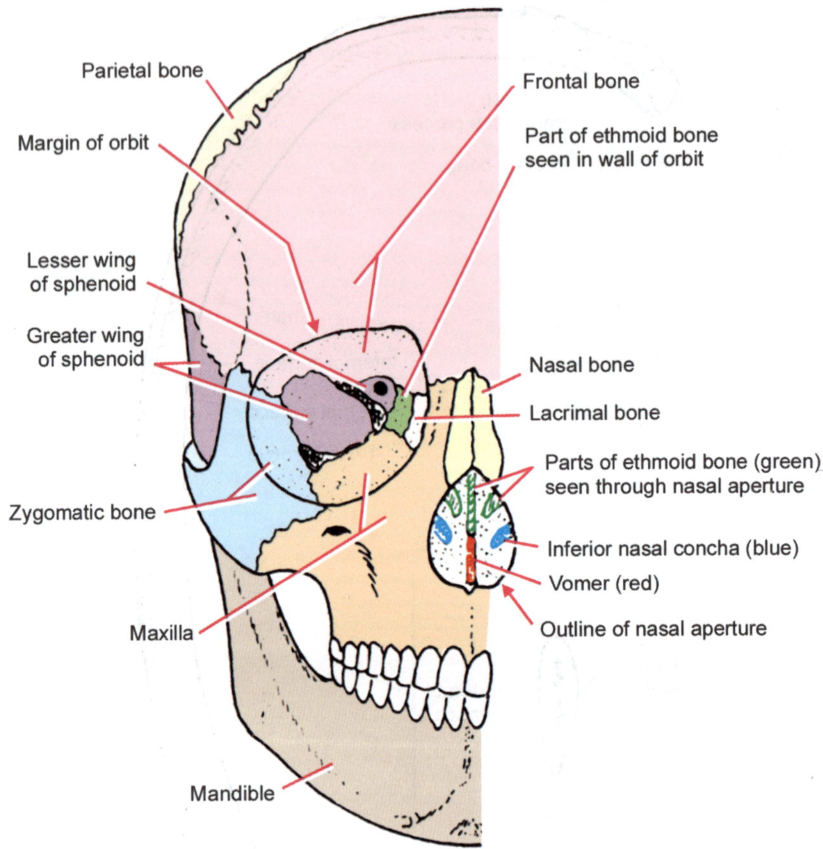

Fig. 26.40 Bones of the skull that can be seen from the front.

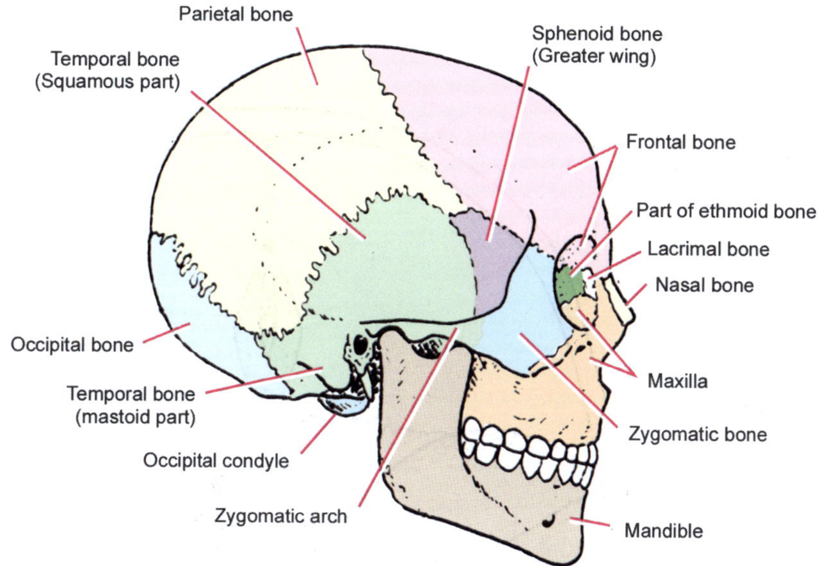

Fig. 26.41 Bones of the skull that are seen from the lateral side.

CRANIAL FOSSAE

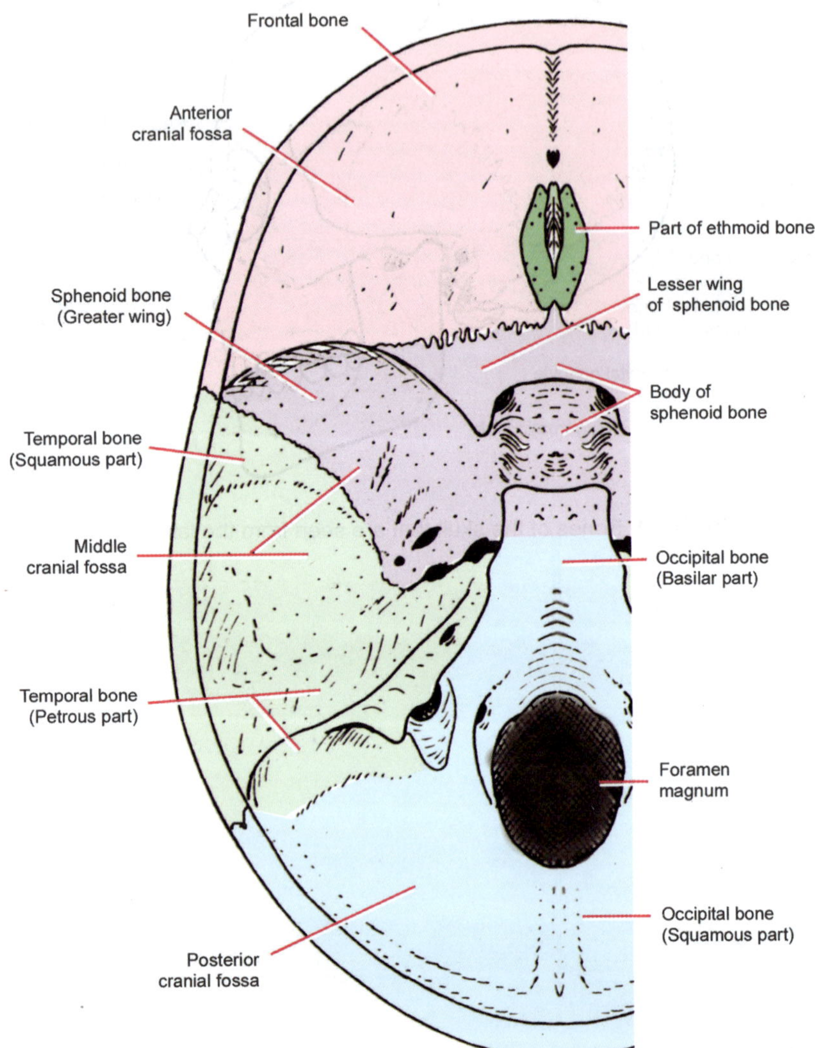

Fig. 26.42 Floor of the cranial cavity seen from above, after removing the roof (or vault). The floor of the cranial cavity is made up of three depressions called the anterior, middle and posterior cranial fossae. The frontal lobe of the brain rests on the anterior cranial fossa. The middle cranial fossa is occupied by the temporal lobe. The posterior cranial fossa contains the cerebellum and the brainstem.

THE MANDIBLE

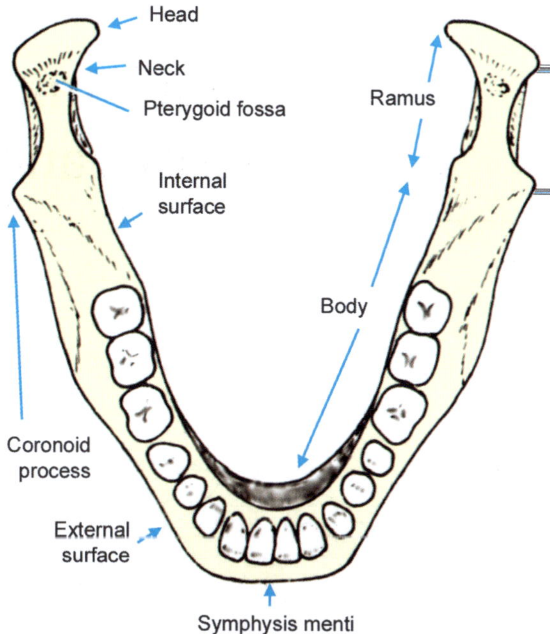

Fig. 26.43 The mandible seen from above. This bone forms the lower jaw, and gives attachment to the lower teeth. Note its subdivisions.

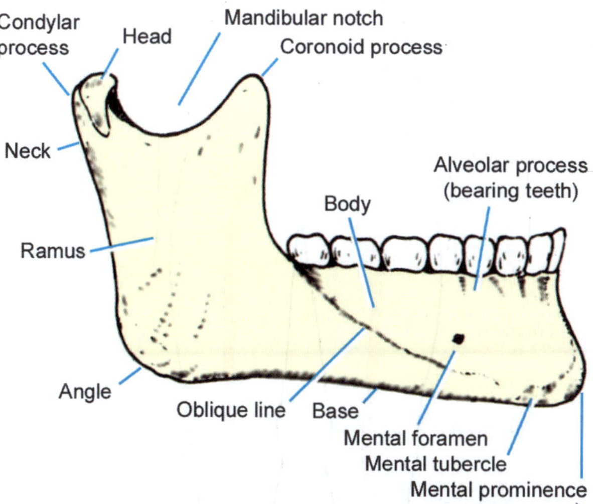

Fig. 26.44 Right half of the mandible seen from the lateral side. Note that the bone is L-shaped. The vertical part, placed posteriorly, is called the ramus. The anterior part is the body. At the upper end of the ramus there is the head that articulates with the temporal bone at the temporomandibular joint.

CHAPTER

27

Some Important Arteries and Veins

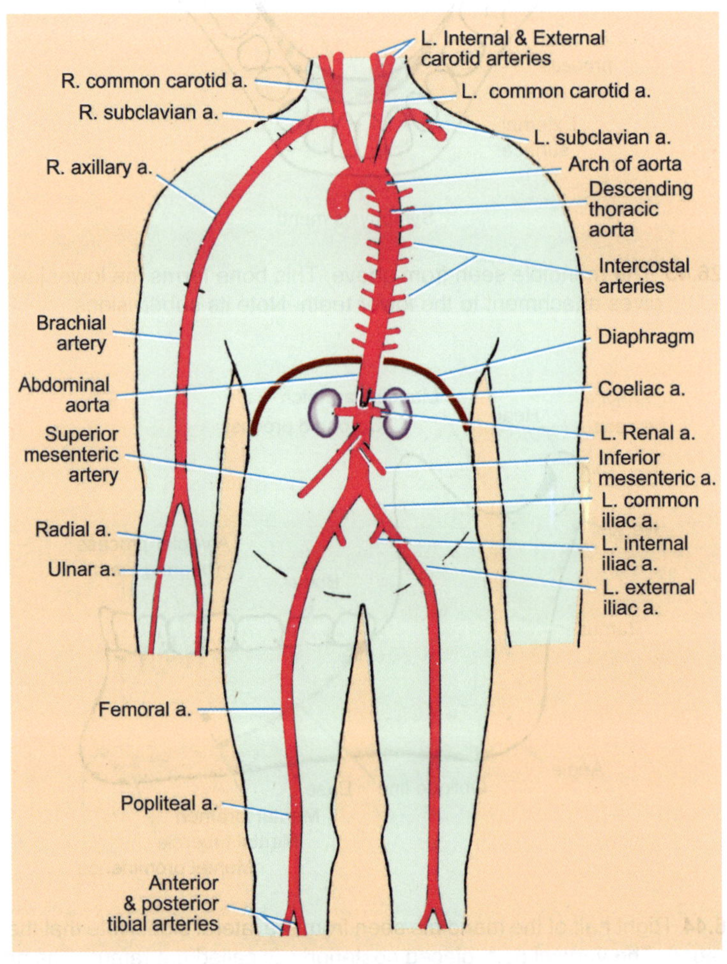

Fig. 27.1 Main arteries of the body

MAIN ARTERIES OF THE BODY

We have seen that oxygenated blood leaves the left ventricle through the aorta. After leaving the heart the aorta forms an arch convex upwards: this is the ***arch of the aorta*** (Fig. 27.1). The aorta then runs downwards in relation to the lower thoracic vertebrae as the ***descending thoracic aorta***. At the lower end of the twelfth thoracic vertebra the aorta pierces the diaphragm and passes into the abdomen where it is called the ***abdominal aorta***.

Three large branches arise from the arch of the aorta. The first branch is the ***brachiocephalic artery***. It ends by dividing into the ***right common carotid artery*** (which supplies the right half of the head and neck) and the ***right subclavian artery*** (which carries blood to the right upper limb). The second branch of the arch of the aorta is the ***left common carotid artery*** (for the left half of the head and neck); and the third branch is the ***left subclavian artery*** (for the left upper limb).

On each side the common carotid artery ascends into the neck and ends by dividing into the ***internal carotid artery*** and the ***external carotid artery***. The internal carotid arteries supply the brain and other structures within the cranial cavity. Each external carotid artery gives off numerous branches to tissues of the head and neck.

The right subclavian artery lies in the lower part of the neck. The left subclavian artery first runs upwards through the upper part of the thorax and then lies in the lower part of the neck. Here it gives off some branches the most important of which is the ***vertebral artery***. This artery takes part in supplying the brain and spinal cord.

Each subclavian artery is the first part of a long arterial trunk that supplies the upper limb. From the lower part of the neck this trunk enters the axilla (arm pit) and is now called the ***axillary artery***. From the axilla the artery enters the arm and is then called the ***brachial artery***. In front of the elbow the brachial artery ends by dividing into the ***radial artery*** and the ***ulnar artery*** both of which descend into the forearm. The tissues of the upper limb are supplied by branches of the axillary, brachial, radial and ulnar arteries. A few branches arising directly from the subclavian artery also enter the upper limb.

The descending thoracic aorta gives off many branches the most conspicuous of which are the ***intercostal arteries***. There are eleven pairs of intercostal arteries, one for each intercostal space (i.e., the space between two adjoining ribs). Another branch, the ***subcostal artery***, is similar to the intercostal arteries, but runs along the lower border of the twelfth rib. The abdominal aorta gives off several branches. On either side it gives off a ***renal artery*** to the corresponding kidney. From the front of the aorta three unpaired arteries arise to supply structures belonging to the digestive system. These are ***coeliac trunk***, the ***superior mesenteric*** and the ***inferior mesenteric*** arteries.

The coeliac trunk is responsible for supplying the liver, the spleen, the stomach, and parts of the duodenum and pancreas. The superior mesenteric artery supplies almost the whole of the small intestine. It also supplies the caecum, the ascending colon and part of the transverse colon. The inferior mesenteric artery supplies the rest of the large intestine.

Apart from the large branches named above the abdominal aorta gives off a number of smaller branches to other structures.

At it lower end the abdominal aorta ends by dividing into the right and left ***common iliac arteries***. Each common iliac artery divides into an ***external iliac artery*** and an ***internal iliac artery***. The internal iliac artery gives off branches to structures in the pelvis,

The external iliac artery is the uppermost part of a long arterial trunk that supplies the lower limb. It lies in the pelvis. Its continuation into the front of the thigh is called the ***femoral artery***. The femoral artery winds round the medial side of the femur to reach the back of the knee. The part of the arterial trunk that lies behind the knee is called the ***popliteal artery***. The popliteal artery ends by dividing into the ***anterior tibial artery*** and the ***posterior tibial artery***. These two arteries descend into the leg and foot.

MAIN VEINS OF THE BODY

Blood from the upper limb is drained through a number of small veins that join to form the ***axillary vein*** (lying alongside the axillary artery). The axillary

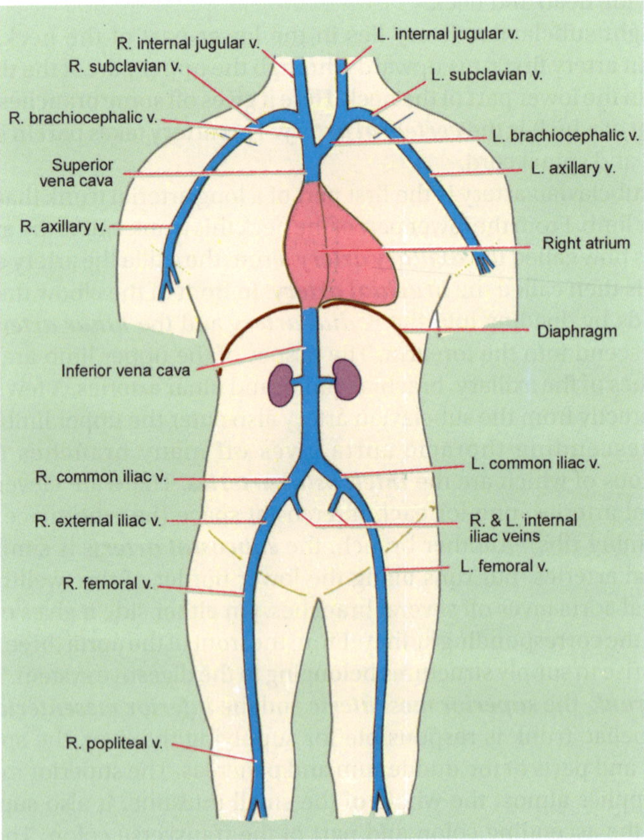

Fig. 27.2 Main veins of the body.

vein continues into the neck as the ***subclavian vein***. The main veins from the head and neck are the right and left ***internal jugular veins***. Each internal jugular vein joins the corresponding subclavian vein to form the right or left ***brachiocephalic vein***. The two brachiocephalic veins join to form the ***superior vena cava*** which opens into the right atrium of the heart. From the above it follows that all blood from the head and neck and from both upper limbs enters the heart through the superior vena cava.

The lower limbs are drained through small veins that join to form the ***popliteal vein*** at the back of the knee joint. The popliteal vein ascends into the thigh where it becomes the ***femoral vein***. The popliteal and femoral veins lie alongside the corresponding arteries. At the upper end of the thigh each femoral vein enters the abdomen and is now called the ***external iliac vein***.

Structures in the pelvis are drained by the ***internal iliac veins***. The external and internal iliac veins of each side join to form the corresponding ***common iliac vein***. The right and left common iliac veins join to form the ***inferior vena cava***. The inferior vena cava ascends alongside the abdominal aorta. At the upper end of the abdomen it pierces the diaphragm to end in the right atrium of the heart.

Some additional features of arteries and veins are given in the illustrations that follow.

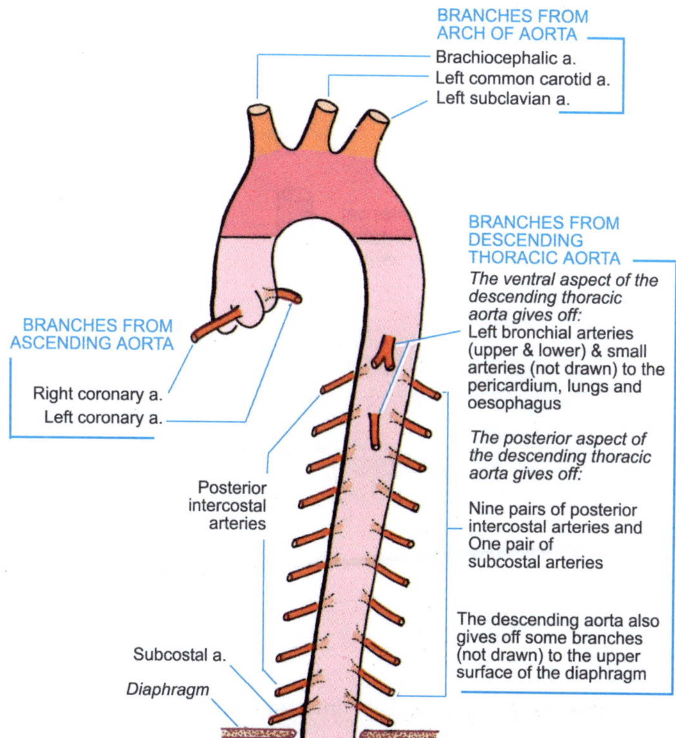

Fig. 27.3 Branches of the thoracic aorta.

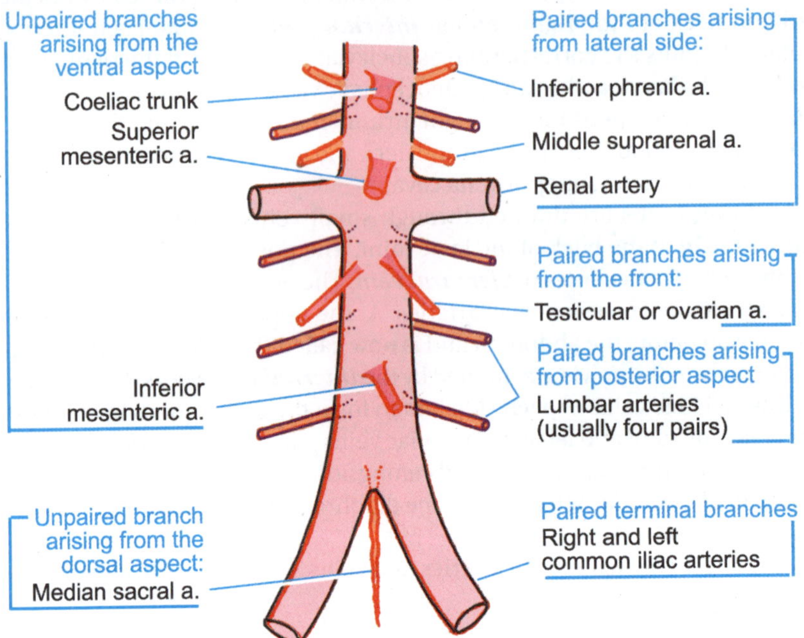

Fig. 27.4 Branches of the abdominal aorta.

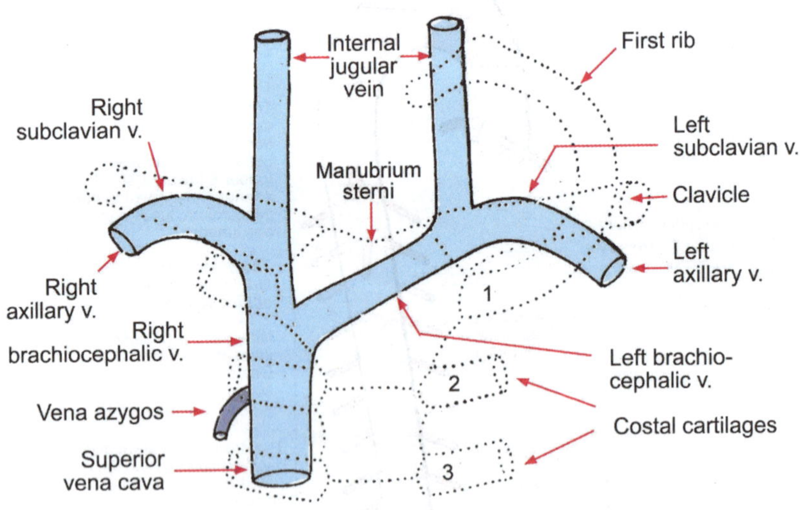

Fig. 27.5 Superior vena cava and its connections.

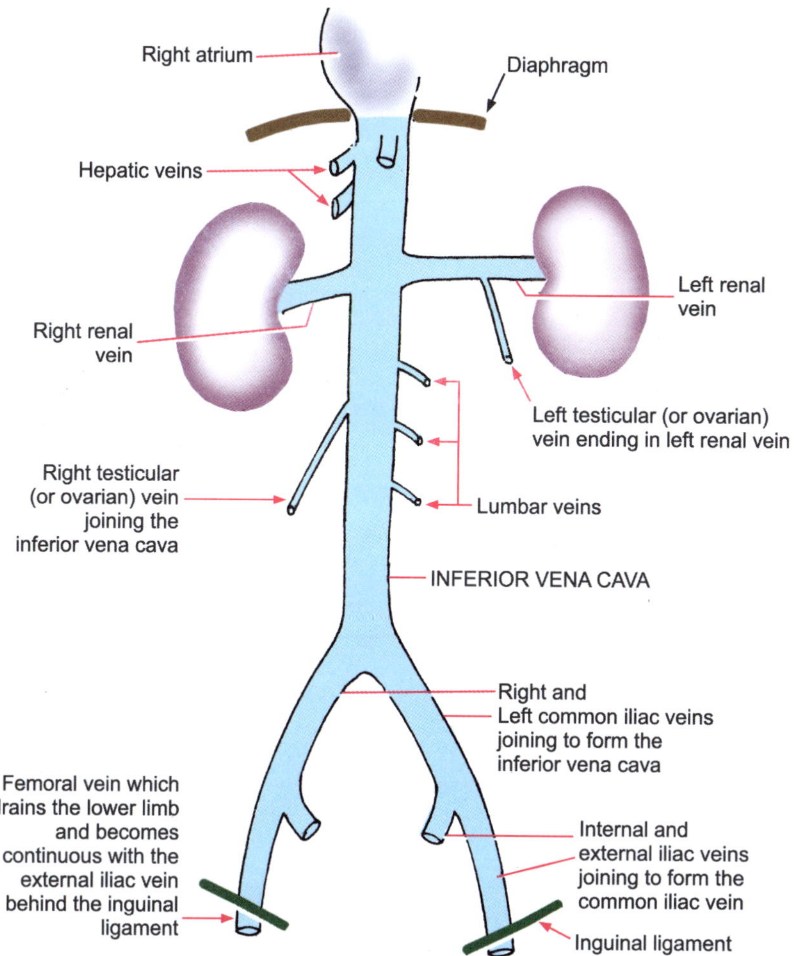

Fig. 27.6 Inferior vena cava and its tributaries.

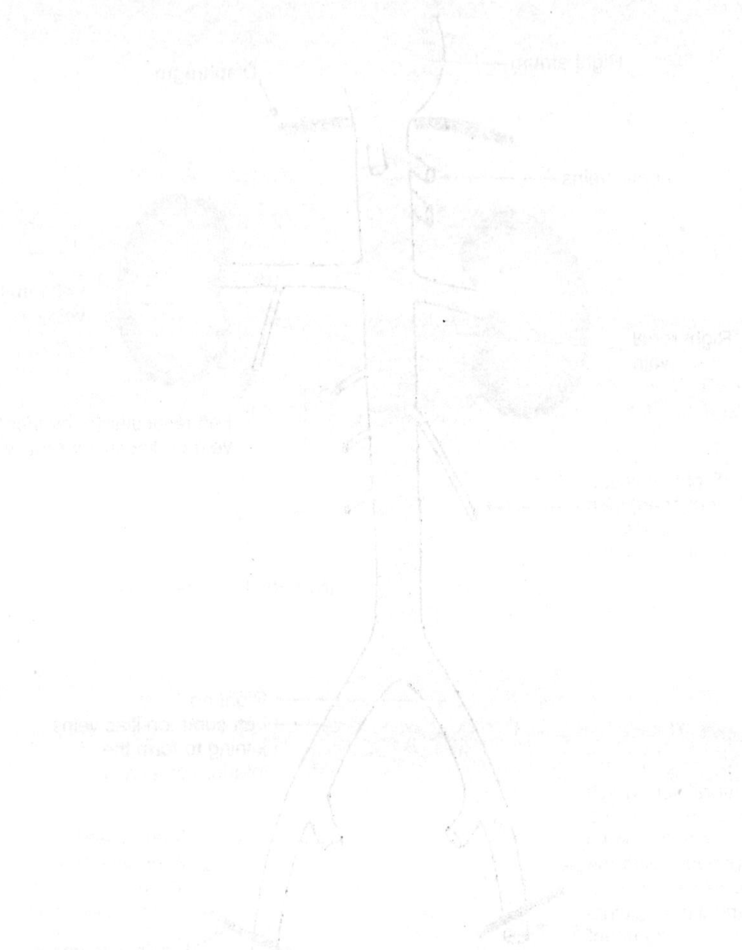

Index

Page numbers followed by *f* refer to figure.

B

C

J

K

L

N

O

P

T

U

V

W

Z